Let us hope that before the last sands have run out from beneath the feet of the years of the nineteenth century it will have become a model of its kind, and that upon the centennial of its anniversary it will be a hospital which shall still compare favorably, not only in structure and arrangement, but also in results achieved, with any other institution of like character in existence.

John Shaw Billings,
address at the opening of
The Johns Hopkins Hospital,
May 1889

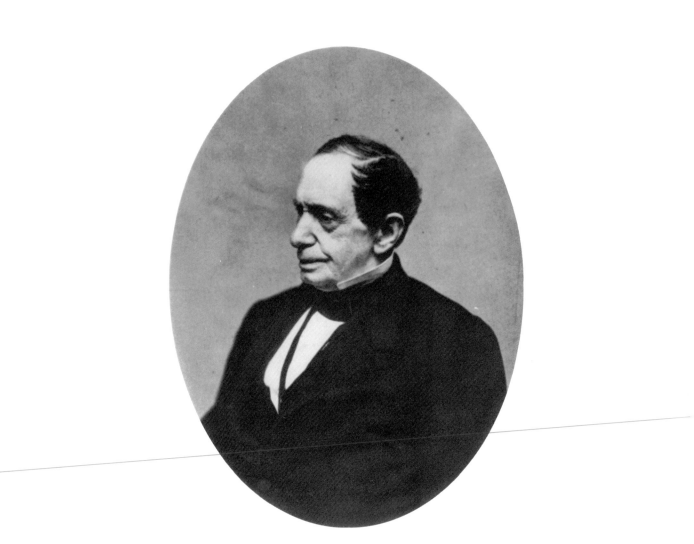

Johns Hopkins

A Model of Its Kind

Volume I
A CENTENNIAL HISTORY OF MEDICINE AT JOHNS HOPKINS

A. McGehee Harvey, Gert H. Brieger, Susan L. Abrams, and Victor A. McKusick

The Johns Hopkins University Press
Baltimore and London

©1989 The Johns Hopkins University Press
All rights reserved
Printed in the United States of America
The Johns Hopkins University Press
701 West 40th Street
Baltimore, MD 21211
The Johns Hopkins Press Ltd., London

The paper used in this publication meets the minimum requirements of
American National Standard for Information Sciences—Permanence of
Paper for Printed Library Materials, ANSI Z39.48-1984.

Library of Congress Cataloging-in-Publication Data

A Model of its kind.

Includes index.
Contents: v. 1. A centennial history of medicine at Johns Hopkins—
v. 2. A pictorial history of medicine at Johns Hopkins.
1. Johns Hopkins Medical School–History. I. Harvey,
A. McGehee (Abner McGehee), 1911–
R747.J62M63   1989   610'.7'117526   88-46064
ISBN 0-8018-3794-4 (v. 1 : alk. paper)
ISBN 0-8018-3816-9 (v. 2 : alk paper)

*To all the members
of the Johns Hopkins medical community
who have contributed to its success over the past century*

CONTENTS

ACKNOWLEDGMENTS

We would like to express our deep appreciation to Nancy McCall and the staff of the Alan Mason Chesney Medical Archives, who provided help, resources, and advice.

We also wish to thank those whose generous gifts of time and expertise contributed greatly to this book: S. William Appelbaum, J. Thomas August, Theodore M. Bayless, David A. Blake, David Bodian, John L. Cameron, Louise A. Cavagnaro, Carleton B. Chapman, J. Michael Criley, Daniel B. Drachman, Susan T. Edmunds, Joel Elkes, Elizabeth Fee, Nicholas J. Fortuin, Irwin M. Freedberg, Harriet G. Guild, Harold E. Harrison, Robert H. Heptinstall, Robert M. Heyssel, Kimishige Ishizaka, Teruko Ishizaka, Carol J. Johns, M. Daniel Lane, Terry Langbaum, Dale R. Levitz, Lawrence M. Lichtenstein, Guy M. McKhann, Linda Mishkin, Vernon B. Mountcastle, Gilbert H. Mudge, Gene Nakajima, Daniel Nathans, Philip A. Norman, Arnall Patz, Thomas D. Pollard, Donald L. Price, Julia Ridgely, Richard S. Ross, Murray B. Sachs, Solomon H. Snyder, Kim Solez, Edith B. Stern, Paul Talalay, Caroline Bedell Thomas, Thomas B. Turner, Mackenzie Walser, Henry N. Wagner, Jr., Nancy Wagner, Patrick C. Walsh, Myron L. Weisfeldt, George D. Zuidema.

Our thanks also to Harold A. Williams for permission to reprint photographs from his book, *Baltimore Afire,* and to W. Bruce Fye for permission to quote from his unpublished manuscript, "Daniel Gilman, John Shaw Billings and the Foundation of Johns Hopkins."

Finally, we thank our superb copyeditor, Miriam Kleiger.

A Model of Its Kind

Volume I
A CENTENNIAL HISTORY OF MEDICINE
AT JOHNS HOPKINS

INTRODUCTION

"What a combination of good luck and wisdom attended the founding of the Johns Hopkins University and the Johns Hopkins medical school," wrote Abraham Flexner in 1943. "The first was Gilman's own work, the second was the work of the Hospital Trustees, Gilman, Billings, and Welch. Dr. Thayer used to say, 'Chance is God.' Certainly God in the form of chance had a finger in the pie when the Johns Hopkins University and the Johns Hopkins medical school were established."[1]

Flexner ended his letter with this homely metaphor, but without further explanation. In his enthusiasm he is not alone, however; many other judicious men and women have been similarly ebullient over the years. The opinion of one historian who recently identified the founding of the Johns Hopkins University as "perhaps the single most decisive event in the history of learning in the Western hemisphere" is judged by a colleague as "extravagant, but not unreasonable."[2] Another contemporary historian terms the establishment of the medical school "the most spectacular innovation in the history of American medical education."[3] Even when the hospital and the medical school opened—the Johns Hopkins Hospital on May 7, 1889, and the Johns Hopkins University School of Medicine on October 2, 1893—scientists, physicians, and educators heralded them as offering the best medical education available in America at the time.

As John Shaw Billings had hoped, these two institutions, the medical school and the hospital,

became models of their kind. Yet the model of Hopkins medicine was not a composite of entirely new concepts and methods but a cohesive, effective union of ideas, several of which had already been tried elsewhere. In the stimulating environment created by the early leaders of Hopkins, these ideas were merged in a novel way.

The pillar of the model was the stipulation that the hospital form part of the medical school of the university, a connection specified by Johns Hopkins himself and one that has been vital to the institutions' development through the years. This astute and highly original idea ensured the fullest possible cooperation between the hospital and the medical school, and thus between the practice and the learning of medicine. It was a unique link that enabled the medical school and the hospital to adopt many of the ideals of the Johns Hopkins University. Like the university, the hospital and the medical school offered an exciting scientific atmosphere and emphasized the goal of advancing rather than merely transmitting knowledge.

The character of the parent university has been as important to medicine at Johns Hopkins as the link between the hospital and the university. When it was founded in 1876, the Johns Hopkins University was the first institution of higher learning in the United States to emphasize graduate education. Under the leadership of President Daniel C. Gilman, it attracted an excellent faculty and promising students and gave them the time, the facilities, and the money to conduct research.

Like the university, the medical school became a home for scientific investigators. Most other medical schools chose their faculty from among the local practitioners, but Hopkins' faculty members were selected from around the world on the basis of their research accomplishments. First in the preclinical sciences and then in the clinical fields, professors became "full-time" faculty, relinquishing private practice to devote their primary effort to the work of the medical school.

In addition, entering students were held to high educational standards: the medical school was the first to make a baccalaureate degree or its equivalent a prerequisite for admission, and a sound preliminary education in the sciences was also required. Bridging the gap between faculty and students were the graduate students: fellows (in the preclinical sciences) and residents (in the clinical sciences). The result was a community of scholars, students and faculty alike, engaged in generating new knowledge and transmitting it to the medical profession at large.

This community was housed in the most advanced facilities of the day. For the care of patients, John Shaw Billings designed the Johns Hopkins Hospital to enhance recovery and prevent the spread of disease. As the clinical laboratory of the medical school, the hospital contained laboratories and classrooms in close proximity to the wards.

It was thus a teaching hospital, and the embodiment of Johns Hopkins' wish. For each discipline, a single individual was placed in charge of both the medical school department and the corresponding clinical department in the hospital. One person therefore controlled the teaching facilities, the structuring of the curriculum, the care of patients, and the organization of the research program—a new arrangement for the time. Through this administrative arrangement, medical students easily became an integral part of the hospital staff, and residency programs flourished.

The early leaders of the hospital and the medical school had the satisfaction of recognizing the attainments of the institution they had shaped. By 1914, the twenty-fifth anniversary of the hospital's opening, all the features of the model were in place, and the Hopkins approach to medical education was spreading throughout the United States. The addresses of William Osler, William Henry Welch, and others at this event offer their perceptions of the reasons for Hopkins' success.

Welch credited the advances made by Hopkins' predecessors, advances that Hopkins wanted to surpass:

> The state of medical education when the Johns Hopkins School was started was most favorable for the development of such a school as we had in mind. As early as 1880 there had been efforts to improve the character of the medical schools of this country. . . . By 1880, Harvard Medical School, the school at Ann Arbor and a few other medical schools had already taken steps to improve the standard. There was consequently an eagerness on the part of the medical profession to see the establishment of a school of a higher order than any which existed at the time. We felt that to add one more similar medical school to the list of those already existing would be of little service to the community or to the country, or to the cause of medicine.[4]

"It was not the men," Osler wrote, "though success could not have come without them, so much as the method, the organization, and a collective new outlook on old problems." He continued:

> That part of the university which, with the hospital, forms the medical school has only had twenty-five years of existence, not a generation, a mere fraction of time in the long history of the growth of science, so that it seems presumptuous to claim any powerful influence on the profession at large. The feeling, however, is strong, too strong to be passed over, that the year 1889 did mean something in the history of medicine in this country. One thing certainly it meant, as originally designed by that great leader Daniel C. Gilman, that the ideals of the men on this side of Jones Falls [the medical school] were to be the same as those of the men in the laboratories of North Howard Street [the University], that a type of medical school was to be created new to this country, in which teacher and student alike should be in the fighting line. That is lesson number one of our first quarter-century, judged by which we stand or

fall. And lesson number two was the demonstration that the student of medicine has his place in the hospital as part of its machinery just as much as he has in the anatomical laboratory, and that to combine successfully in his education practice with science, the academic freedom of the university must be transplanted to the hospital.[5]

Beyond the specifics, there was what Osler called "the spirit of the place" that bound together everyone connected with the hospital and the medical school. It was a "sweet influence," Osler wrote, "whence we knew not, but teacher and taught alike felt the presence and subtle domination. Comradeship, sympathy one with another, devotion to work, were its fruits, and its guidance drove from each heart hatred and malice and all uncharitableness."[6] Welch echoed Osler's thoughts as he looked to the future: "All who are here today from those early years feel that there was an environment, an atmosphere and ideals which will always be cherished and will continue to be an abiding influence."[7]

This book discusses the innovations that made Johns Hopkins "a model of its kind." Part 1 identifies the features that distinguished the hospital and the medical school, and places them in chronological context. These features were substantially altered by federal support for training and research after World War II, and Part 1 includes a discussion of the influence of the federal government as a prelude to the story of the last forty-five years. Readers familiar with the early history of Hopkins will find old friends in Part 1, which introduces the characters and sketches the events as a prelude to the thematic section of the book. Part 1 thus sets the stage for Part 2, which traces the development of each innovation from the past century to the present.

So much has been written about medicine at Johns Hopkins that, despite the excuse of a centennial celebration, still another book on the subject hardly seems justified. Yet our intent is not to add new facts but to take a fresh look at what is known. The success of the model is largely appreciated and needs no further substantiation; instead, we are interested in the innovations that

made up the model, some of which deserve new emphasis. This is not a book of "firsts": although some of the components of the model were brand new, others were adapted from other hospitals and medical schools. It is the combination of parts that is important in the story of Johns Hopkins, not the uniqueness of each one.

We do not attempt to tell yet again the entire story of the founding and early years of the Johns Hopkins Medical Institutions—a story thoroughly documented by Alan M. Chesney and Thomas B. Turner and amplified by the many useful biographies and autobiographies of Hopkins' faculty members.

Nor is the book an exhaustive chronicle of events in the recent past. The "inner history" of the medical institutions will also not be found here. The thematic approach necessarily diminishes the emphasis on features not unique to Hopkins, and many subjects thus cannot be covered in sufficient detail to do them justice. For example, we have often omitted information about the departure of individual faculty members and about their subsequent careers. On a larger scale, there is a chapter concerning women in the medical school but relatively little about the admission of blacks.

The chapter on research discusses some of the scientific work done at Hopkins. Particularly in this chapter, examples must suffice to tell the story, as it is not possible to mention all the important discoveries that members of Hopkins' faculty have made over a century of productive investigation. Omissions in this chapter are not intended as historical judgments. Space constraints also prohibit us from considering the accomplishments that emanated from Hopkins in the context of contemporary achievements in other research-oriented medical schools. The chapter on the export of Hopkins-trained physicians, however, documents the idea that much of the research done elsewhere, particularly in the first half of the century, was generated by scientists trained in Baltimore.

Finally, although the hospital and the medical school are only part of what has become the Johns Hopkins Medical Institutions, the histories of the School of Nursing and the School of Hygiene and Public Health—the two remaining components—have been told in separate volumes.[8] We do not, therefore, discuss these schools except as they relate to our themes.

Instead, this book considers some of the representative discoveries, decisions, and activities that shaped the Johns Hopkins University School of Medicine and the Johns Hopkins Hospital in their first century. It is inevitably the story of people—members of the Hopkins medical community through whom Flexner's combination of "good luck and wisdom" has extended to the present day.

Part I

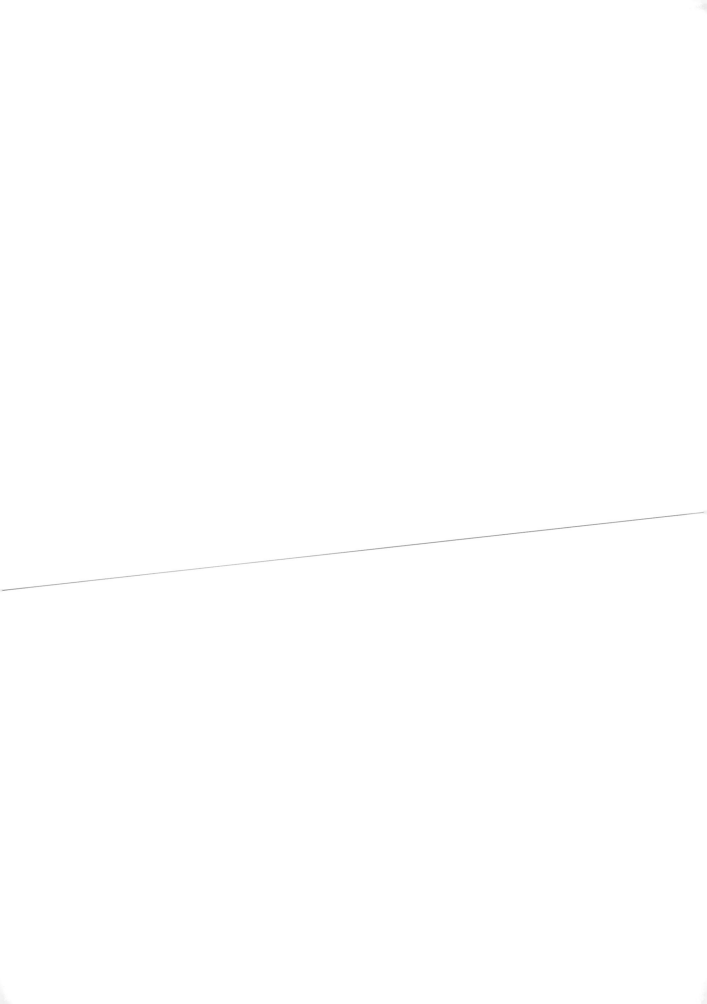

CHAPTER 1

THE OPENING OF THE HOSPITAL
AND MEDICAL SCHOOL

*The opening of The Johns Hopkins Hospital in 1889 marked a new de-
parture in medical education in the United States. It was not the hospital
itself, as there were many larger and just as good; it was not the men
appointed, as there were others quite as well qualified; it was the organization. For the first time in an English-speaking country a hospital was
organized in units, each one in charge of a head or chief. The day after
my appointment I had a telegram from Dr. Gilman, President of the
university, who had been asked to open the hospital, to meet him at the
Fifth Avenue Hotel, New York. He said to Dr. Welch and me: "I have
asked you to come here as the manager is an old friend of mine, and we
will spend a couple of days; there is no difference really between a hospital and a hotel." We saw everything arranged in departments, with responsible heads, and over all a director. "This," he said, "is really the
hospital and we shall model ours upon it. The clinical unit of a hospital is
the exact counterpart of one of the sub-divisions of any great hotel or
department-store."*

—William Osler

The Vision of Johns Hopkins

"*In all your arrangements in relation to this Hospital,*" stated Johns Hopkins in a letter to the hospital trustees, "*you will bear constantly in mind that it
is my wish and purpose that the institution shall ultimately form a part of the Medical School of that university for which I have made ample provision by my
will*" (italics added).[1]

The man who articulated this far-reaching
"wish and purpose" was neither a scholar nor a
physician but a successful Baltimore merchant
and banker, a Quaker who saw his fortune as a
trust and believed that it should be turned to the
benefit of his fellow citizens. Of English descent,

Johns Hopkins was born in Anne Arundel
County, Maryland, in 1795. His first name was
the family name of a great-grandmother on his father's side. The family plantation, "White Hall,"
was part of an original grant of land from the king
of England to a member of the Hopkins family;
but when in 1807 Johns' father freed his slaves, in
accordance with the beliefs of the Society of
Friends, the plantation could no longer support
the Hopkins family. Young Johns showed some
aptitude for business, and at the age of seventeen
he was sent to Baltimore to live with his uncle, a
wholesale grocer.[2]

When his uncle denied him permission to
marry his daughter (the Society of Friends did not

permit marriages between first cousins), Johns Hopkins moved out of the house and established his own grocery business. Its success allowed him to accumulate enough capital to lend money, and he abandoned the grocery business to become a banker. He prospered in this endeavor, too, and became Baltimore's leading financier.

A bachelor all his life, Johns Hopkins was able to use the whole of his wealth for philanthropic purposes. He decided to divide his $7-million fortune into two equal parts, for the founding of a hospital and a university. In 1867, he selected twelve Baltimoreans to form a corporation known as "the Johns Hopkins University," whose purpose was "the promotion of education in the state of Maryland." A similar process led to the incorporation of "the Johns Hopkins Hospital," all but two of whose twelve trustees were also trustees of the university. The naming of two interlocking boards was concrete evidence that Hopkins wanted the corporations to work closely together.

These projects probably ripened in Johns Hopkins' mind over many years. He was no doubt influenced by the example of other philanthropists, such as George Peabody of Baltimore, but he also obtained the views of friends and acquaintances about both general and specific aspects of the projects. In planning to link the hospital and the university through a school of medicine, Johns Hopkins may have considered the views of Dr. Patrick Macaulay, a fellow director of the Baltimore and Ohio Railroad. Macaulay's 1832 address "Medical Improvement" specified five essentials for the betterment of medical education in the United States, including the lengthening of the course of instruction leading to the medical degree, the broadening of its scope, and the application of science at the bedside. The address was reprinted in a book found among Johns Hopkins' possessions at his death.[3]

Johns Hopkins chose the site for the hospital and bought the land, giving it to the hospital's trustees along with a letter of instruction. Written less than a year before his death in 1873 at the age of seventy-eight, this letter set forth his wishes explicitly (italics have been added):

I have given you, in your capacity of Trustees, thirteen acres of land, situated in the city of Baltimore, and bounded by Wolfe, Monument, Broadway and Jefferson streets, upon which I desire you to erect a Hospital.

It will be necessary to devote the present year to the grading of the surface, to its proper drainage, to the laying out of the grounds, and to the most careful and deliberate choice of a plan for the erection and arrangement of the buildings.

It is my wish that the plan thus chosen shall be one which will permit symmetrical additions to the buildings which will be first constructed, in order that you may ultimately be able to receive four hundred patients; and that it shall provide for a Hospital, which shall, in construction and arrangement, compare favorably with any other institution of like character in this country or in Europe.

It will, therefore, be your duty to obtain the advice and assistance of those, at home or abroad, who have achieved the greatest success in the construction and management of Hospitals.

I cannot press this injunction too strongly upon you, because the usefulness of this charity will greatly depend upon the plan which you may adopt for the construction and arrangement of the buildings.

It is my desire that you should complete this portion of your labor during the current year, and be in readiness to commence the building of the Hospital in the spring of 1874.

It will be your duty, hereafter, to provide for the erection upon other ground, of suitable buildings for the reception, maintenance and education of orphan colored children.

I direct you to provide accommodation for three or four hundred children of this class; and you are also authorized to receive into this asylum, at your discretion, as belonging to such class, colored children who have lost one parent only, and, in exceptional cases, to receive colored children who are not orphans, but who may be in such circumstances as to require the aid of the charity.

I desire that you shall apply the yearly sum of twenty thousand dollars, or so much thereof as may be necessary, of the revenue of the property which you will hereafter receive to the maintenance of the Orphans' Home intended for such children.

In order to enable you to carry my wishes into full effect, I will now, and in each succeeding year during my life, until the hospital buildings are fully completed, and in readiness to receive patients, place at your disposal the sum of one hundred thousand dollars.

In addition to the gift, already made to you, of the thirteen acres of land in the city of Baltimore, upon which the hospital will be built, I have dedicated to its support and to the payment of the annual sum provided to be paid for the support of the Orphan's Home, property which you may safely estimate as worth, today, two millions of dollars, and from which your corporation will certainly receive a yearly revenue of one hundred and twenty thousand dollars; and which time and your diligent care will make more largely productive.

If the Hospital and Orphans' Home are not built at my death, it will be your duty to apply the income arising from the property so dedicated to their completion. When they are built the income from that property will suffice for their maintenance.

The indigent sick of this city and its environs, without regard to sex, age, or color, who may require surgical or medical treatment, and who can be received into the Hospital without peril to the other inmates, and the poor of this city and State, of all races, who are stricken down by any casualty, shall be received into the Hospital without charge, for such periods of time and under such regulations as you may prescribe. It will be your duty to make such division of the sexes and patients among the several wards of the Hospital as will best promote the actual usefulness of the charity.

You will also provide for the reception of a limited number of patients who are able to make compensation for the room and attention they may require. The money received from such persons will enable you to appropriate a larger sum for the relief of the sufferings of that class which I direct you to admit free of charge; and you will thus be enabled to afford to strangers, and to those of our own people who have no friends or relations to care for them in sickness, and who are not objects of charity, the advantages of careful and skilful treatment.

It will be your especial duty to secure for the service of the Hospital, surgeons and physicians of the highest character and greatest skill.

I desire you to establish, in connection with the Hospital, a training school for female nurses. This provision will secure the services of women competent to care for the sick in the Hospital wards, and will enable you to benefit the whole community by supplying it with a class of trained and experienced nurses.

I wish the large grounds surrounding the Hospital buildings to be properly enclosed by iron railings,

and to be so laid out and planted with trees and flowers as to afford solace to the sick, and to be an ornament to the section of the city in which the grounds are located.

I desire that you should, in due season, provide for a site and buildings, of such description and at such distance from the city as your judgment shall approve, for the reception of convalescent patients.

You will be able in this way to hasten the recovery of the sick, and to have always room in the main Hospital buildings for other sick persons requiring immediate medical or surgical treatment.

It is my especial request that the influences of religion should be felt in and impressed upon the whole management of the Hospital; but I desire, nevertheless, that the administration of the charity shall be undisturbed by sectarian influence, discipline, or control.

In all your arrangements in relation to this Hospital, you will bear constantly in mind that it is my wish and purpose that the institution shall ultimately form a part of the Medical School of that university for which I have made ample provision by my will.

I have felt it to be my duty to bring these subjects to your particular attention, knowing that you will conform to the wishes which I thus definitely express.

In other particulars I leave your Board to the exercise of its discretion, believing that your good judgment and experience in life will enable you to make this charity a substantial benefit to the community.[4]

No other documents signed by Johns Hopkins, including his will, mention any relationship between the Johns Hopkins Hospital and the Johns Hopkins University. The idea was nevertheless the key element in the success of both the medical and the educational enterprises, with far-reaching effects on American education. More than any other specification it was this connection that determined the future of the two institutions.

It may seem surprising that a man with so little formal education could set forth visionary ideas about relatively unfamiliar fields. The businessman is evident in this letter of instruction, in the stipulations concerning the allotment of funds. So, too, is the social reformer, in the specification that no black child should be denied assistance because he or she did not fall into the defined category of "orphan." Most of all, the letter reveals a reflective and highly intelligent man. Although Johns Hopkins never attended college, he had grown up in a family that revered books, he had received an excellent primary and secondary-school education, and as an adult, he had read extensively.[5]

Although Johns Hopkins sought advice from many, he ultimately made his own decision. He felt that he owed a duty to the community in which his business life had been spent, and he selected, from among his friends and business acquaintances, the men who he thought were best able to initiate the new enterprises.

The Trustees of the Hospital and the University

Johns Hopkins' death left the responsibility for executing his plans entirely on the trustees' shoulders. Six of the fourteen hospital and university trustees were businessmen, two were judges, another three were lawyers, and only one was a physician. Three were related to Johns Hopkins either by blood or by marriage. At least ten had received some college or university education.[6]

The most influential of the group appears to have been Francis T. King, long-time confidant of Johns Hopkins, president of the hospital board and head of its building committee. King was said to have been privy to Hopkins' plans long before they were made public, and he is among those credited with influencing Hopkins to choose a hospital and a university as beneficiaries.[7]

Charles Morris Gwinn was a prominent Maryland lawyer, later to become the state's attorney general. He drew up Johns Hopkins' will and is believed to have drafted the letter of instruction to the hospital trustees. Another distinguished jurist among the trustees was George Washington Dobbin, dean of the law faculty at the University of Maryland and a judge of the Supreme Bench of Baltimore City. His interest in natural science was probably of considerable importance to the new university, as Dobbin maintained a laboratory at his summer home and kept

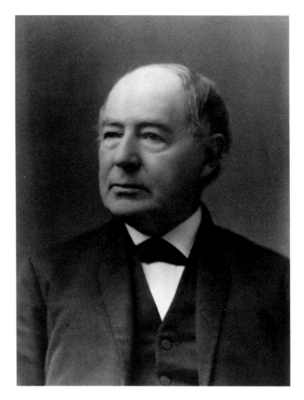

Francis T. King. (*Source:* The Ferdinand Hamburger, Jr., Archives, The Johns Hopkins University.)

up with the scientific literature. Reverdy Johnson, Jr., was the only member of the board who had studied abroad. A graduate of St. Mary's College and of Heidelberg University, Johnson was the son of an attorney general of the United States who had also served as minister to Great Britain. Other trustees included Galloway Cheston (head of the university board), George W. Brown, Francis White, William Hopkins and Lewis N. Hopkins, John Fonerden (who died before the opening of the university and was replaced on the board by James Carey Thomas), Thomas M. Smith, and John W. Garrett.[8]

Two months after Johns Hopkins died, the university trustees met to adopt bylaws and appoint committees. The executive committee—Johnson, Dobbin, Brown, Gwinn, and Thomas—then set out to consult with experts in education and medicine. They toured Harvard, Yale, Cornell, the University of Michigan, and the University of Virginia, and met in Baltimore with presidents Eliot of Harvard, White of Cornell, and

Angell of Michigan. Their desire for advice also led them to acquire a collection of books about current controversies in medical education.

One of the trustees' first tasks was to select a president for the university. Eliot, White, and Angell stated, independently, that the best choice was Daniel Coit Gilman of California.[9]

The First President of the Johns Hopkins University: Daniel Coit Gilman

Daniel C. Gilman came to Baltimore in 1875 from the University of California, where he had spent almost four years as president after leaving a faculty position at Yale. Gilman's ideas about medical education had crystallized by the time he arrived in Baltimore.[10] His inaugural address at the opening of the Johns Hopkins University on February 22, 1876, criticized the educational standards of existing medical schools but ended hopefully:

> We need not fear that the day is distant . . . which will see endowments for medical science as munifi-

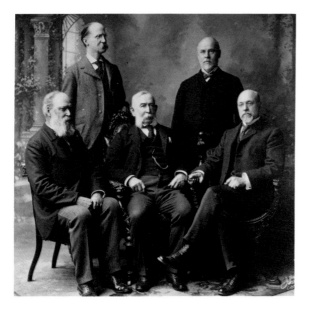

Daniel Coit Gilman with some members of the original faculty: *sitting, left to right,* Basil Gildersleeve, Daniel C. Gilman, Ira Remsen; *standing, left to right,* Henry A. Rowland, William H. Welch. (*Source:* The Ferdinand Hamburger, Jr., Archives, The Johns Hopkins University)

cent as those now provided for any branch of learning, in schools as good as those now provided in any other land.

> It will doubtless be long after the opening of the university, before the opening of the hospital; and this interval may be spent in forming plans for the department of medicine. But in the meantime we have an excellent opportunity to provide instruction antecedent to the professional study of medicine.[11]

A graduate of Yale University, Gilman became professor of physical and political geography at Yale's Sheffield Scientific School in 1853, and a short time later, secretary of the school's executive committee. From this vantage point, he developed a philosophy of education that he disseminated through articles in national magazines. It was during his tenure that the Sheffield School developed its pioneering biology course for prospective medical students.[12]

Gilman had also spent a winter at the University of Berlin in the mid-1850s, and he intended to incorporate its policies toward faculty into his new university: seeking out professors with proven abilities as investigators, ensuring that their teaching responsibilities would not be burdensome so that they could pursue their research, and encouraging them to publish their results. Gilman believed in the independence of the university's faculty. As he wrote to the Board of Trustees after his appointment:

> As the spirit of the University should be that of intellectual freedom in the pursuit of truth and of the broadest charity toward those from whom we differ in opinion it is certain that sectarian and partisan preferences should have no control in the selection of teachers, and should not be apparent in their official work. . . .

> We should hope that the Faculty soon to be chosen will be so catholic in spirit; so learned as to what has been discovered and so keen to explore new fields of research; so skillful as teachers; so cooperative as builders; and so comprehensive in the specialties to which they are devoted,—that pupils will flock to their instruction, first from Maryland and the states near to it,—but soon also from the remotest parts of the land. In seeking this result, the Board may rely on my most zealous cooperation.[13]

Five of the university's first six key faculty members were what would now be called "university" or research professors: Basil L. Gildersleeve in classics, James J. Sylvester in mathematics, Ira Remsen in chemistry, Henry A. Rowland in physics, and Henry Newell Martin in biology. All were promised freedom in research and the company of a few exceptional students.[14]

A spirit of unity prevailed under Gilman's leadership, not only among the faculty but between faculty and students. Gilman referred to them as "masters and pupils, not two bodies but one body, a union for the purpose of acquiring and advancing knowledge."[15] It was the fellows, as participants in the university's system of postgraduate education, who bridged the traditional gap between faculty and students. The fellowship system was the key to the new university's success as an institution dedicated to the advancement of knowledge.[16]

Hopkins' fellowship system was unique. Few American colleges offered fellowships, and those available were given only to the schools' own graduates. Hopkins lacked alumni, and Gilman intended to draw fellows from all parts of the country. The Kirkland and Parker fellowships at Harvard encouraged study abroad, but nowhere else in America in 1876 was there any program offering stipends so consistently large or numerous as at Johns Hopkins—and nowhere else in the country was there as good an opportunity for free graduate education.[17]

The success of the Johns Hopkins University in setting a new educational standard derived from a fortunate combination of circumstances. First, there were the financial resources, a single bequest, divided equally between the university and the hospital, as large as the endowment of any other American college. There was also the university's freedom from religious and governmental control, through its status as a private, nonsectarian institution. The Johns Hopkins University was also unfettered by the limitations of tradition, free from the handicap of antiquated ideas. Its benefactor had attached few conditions to his bequest, and the university had no entrenched faculty to be replaced.[18]

Johns Hopkins had selected the university's trustees wisely, and Gilman himself was a perspicacious choice. He saw the potential for establishing a true university in Baltimore. Although three eminent university presidents—Eliot of Harvard, Angell of Michigan, and White of Cornell—recommended that the new institution offer nothing above the level of college and technologic education, Gilman believed that advanced training and research were immediately feasible.[19]

Finally, there was the temper of the times. In 1876, the nation was ready for the establishment of a new kind of school. The third quarter of the nineteenth century was a time of technologic innovation in the United States. Americans had begun to appreciate the importance of research for applied science and the need for science in an industrial society, and improvements in public education were giving students the background that would enable them to undertake a university education.[20]

If Gilman had had the same funds available to obtain the very same faculty fifty years earlier, said one historian, the Johns Hopkins University would not have flowered.[21] By the last quarter of the nineteenth century, the opportunity to pioneer was available to several institutions, but it was the Johns Hopkins University, under Gilman's leadership, that seized the chance to innovate.

To Gilman, the medical school and the hospital were parts of the university. "It is impossible to have a hospital without its becoming a place for medical education," Gilman said.[22] When the medical school opened, the emphasis on research and on graduate studies characteristic of the Johns Hopkins University served as a model for its programs. The presence of postgraduate fellows in the laboratories of the medical school's faculty, the clinical residency system, the four-year graded medical course, and the methods of appointing faculty and of admitting students all reflected the influence of the parent institution.

The Design of the Hospital

Upon assuming the presidency in 1875, Gilman applied himself to the planning of the Johns Hopkins University. "[T]he glory of the University should rest upon the character of the teachers and scholars here brought together, and not upon their number, nor upon the buildings constructed for their use," he said.[23] The hospital trustees did not have the luxury of considering faculty and buildings in sequence, however, since the medical school could not offer a clinical program without the appropriate facilities. The construction of the hospital, therefore, became the hospital trustees' next important task.

In 1875, Francis T. King, the hospital board's president, invited five consultants to submit plans for buildings suited to the site Johns Hopkins had chosen. King asked them to address seven specific points: (1) the merits of the "pavilion" system (detached, permanent units, two or more stories tall—a system common in England) and of the "barrack" system (temporary, one-story structures that could be destroyed and replaced economically); (2) the best location for the training school for nurses (within the hospital buildings, or elsewhere); (3) accommodations for the medical classes, which would be held in the hospital; (4) the location of the buildings of the university's School of Medicine (near the hospital or near the rest of the university, or at a distant site); (5) provisions for accident cases and outpatients; (6) the best methods of heating and ventilating the hospital buildings; and (7) the management of the hospital.[24]

All five of the consultants were experts in hospital design. One of them, John Shaw Billings, was one of the outstanding men of his generation. In his forty-six-page essay, the most elaborate of the five responses, Billings clearly related the construction of the hospital to its philosophical underpinnings, fastening on the key point in Johns Hopkins' letter of instruction: the plan of the hospital must depend upon the extent and manner of its use as an instrument of medical education and upon the more or less intimate connection it is to have with the medical school.

In addressing the trustees' specific questions, Billings dealt with heating and ventilation in great detail, presenting sketches for the proposed pavilions and alternative plans for various buildings; but his report also ranged far afield from architectural details, pointing up the opportunity presented by Johns Hopkins' bequest to develop a new type of medical school. Many of Billings' ideas echoed Gilman's. Billings advocated small classes, high standards of admission, a four-year course, rigid examinations, and practical work in the various departments of the hospital. His plans included a first-class physiological laboratory, with ample facilities for chemical and microscopic work. Billings also stressed that the hospital must do more than care for the sick and educate medical personnel—it must also promote discoveries in science and medicine and make these discoveries known for the common good. "If we are ever to advance in accurate knowledge of the laws of health and disease," Billings wrote, "it will be by the application of instruments of precision and of graphic measurement to the secretions and motions of the body. . . ."[25] Too often, he lamented, American physicians and investigators who are qualified and eager to conduct original investigations lack the means or the time to do so. Like Gilman, he wanted to encourage the dissemination of scientific information by publishing an annual volume of reports about the more interesting cases seen in the hospital.

It was obvious to the hospital trustees that in Billings they would have more than an architect, and in June 1876, the building committee recommended that he be employed to supervise the hospital's construction.

John Shaw Billings

In the development of the new university's medical school, no single individual played a more important role than Billings. He advised the university's president, trustees, and faculty during the organization of the hospital and the medical school; he helped to select the first faculty of the School of Medicine; and his ideas about the im-

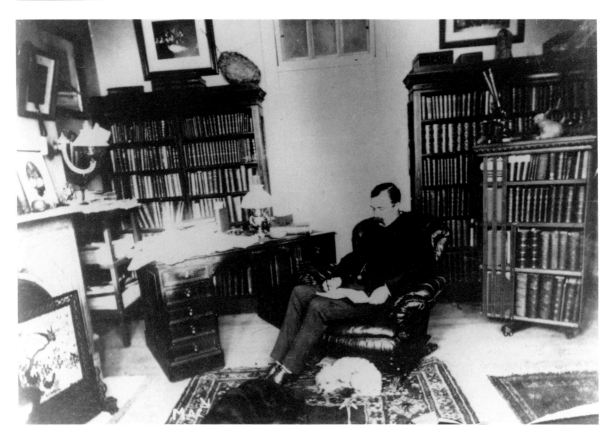

John Shaw Billings in his study in Georgetown. (*Source:* National Library of Medicine, Negative #66-264.)

portance of research were highly influential in the successful launching of these two institutions.

Billings' early career reflected his protean interests, foreshadowing not only his participation in the shaping of educational policy, his commitment to research, and his devotion to the training of investigators in both basic and clinical medical sciences, but also his contributions to hospital construction, medical bibliography, and public health. Billings' formal education was better than average for the time, but it was notably deficient in comparison with the education he was planning for the students at Johns Hopkins. A graduate of Miami University of Ohio in 1857, Billings entered the Medical College of Ohio the same year. His formal medical education consisted of two five-month lecture courses with essentially no patient-related instruction. Two years of clinical experience as a "house pupil" in two Cincinnati hospitals was followed by a year as a demonstrator of anatomy at the Medical College of Ohio.[26]

In 1861 Billings enlisted in the Union army as a medical officer. A six-month post at the Army General Hospital in Philadelphia, in 1862–63, introduced him to the new technique of microscopy, an interest that was to mature later in the decade. Billings' enthusiasm for the subject led him to laboratory investigation, and he published original observations on the morphology of fungi in diseases of cattle. In 1864, Billings was sent to the Surgeon General's office in Washington, D.C. —a turning point in his career. Although he had planned to join one of his former professors in the practice of surgery, at war's end he decided to remain in the army medical department.

Over the next decade, Billings immersed himself in the study of hospital design and management. A report he wrote in 1870 was distributed extensively, and his expertise became widely appreciated.[27] The connection that led to his appointment as advisor to the hospital trustees was made in 1871, when his colleague army surgeon

Alfred A. Woodhull introduced him to the president of the Board of Trustees, Francis T. King.[28]

Billings' official tenure began in July 1876, but he must have been gathering information about his new position during the preceding months, for on July 15, he presented the hospital trustees with his first report, which outlined his view of the role of the medical faculty and of the hospital. In this matter, too, his opinions echoed those of university president Gilman:

> The most difficult thing in forming this Hospital is not to plan the buildings . . . it is to find the proper and suitable persons to be the sole and motive power of the institution. . . .
>
> It is by no means certain that with increase of salary beyond a certain amount we can get correspondingly better medical service or scientific work. . . .
>
> We can much more certainly secure men who will minutely and patiently investigate individual cases . . . by showing them that they shall have space and apparatus to work with, that the resources of modern science and mechanical skill shall be at their command, and that any discoveries which they make shall be properly published, than by simply offering double pay.
>
> Again, to secure these skilled physicians; original investigators imbued with the true scientific spirit; gentlemen; a certain amount of experiment and probation will be necessary.[29]

Three months after his work at Hopkins formally began, Billings went to Europe to consult with luminaries in medical education and to visit hospital facilities and medical schools in such centers as London, Leipzig, Berlin, Vienna, and Paris. The focus of his trip was the integration of medical education and hospital construction. Billings found much to admire, but his admiration was not unreserved.[30] Of the laboratories at the University of Leipzig, for example, he wrote to Gilman:

> In some respects they surpass anything I have seen, yet there is plenty of room for improvement. . . . Upon the whole I am surprised that the Germans should have been able to effect so much as they have done for Medicine. It is by no means easy for a student to take advantage of the Materials and apparatus here. Two American Students went round with me at Leipzig, and they assured me that in a year

they had not been able to see so much as they did in the five hours they were with me.[31]

The English schools seemed best for the undergraduate medical student, Billings said. The German schools, in contrast, seemed to force, rather than fit, students to do original work. Students were encouraged to think that their highest aim should be to do some experiment that no one had done before. In pursuit of this goal, they would often emerge from a year in the laboratory with little of the knowledge they went there to obtain.[32] Billings' impressions were relatively superficial, gained from a whirlwind tour of the great laboratories of Europe. His somewhat negative view of the German system was counterbalanced at Hopkins by the more measured opinion of William H. Welch, the first professor of pathology, who had spent months at the bench in German laboratories. Welch recognized the value of the German system's emphasis on the scientific basis of medicine.

Billings returned from abroad having absorbed the best of the European approaches. He had left his mark on his hosts as well: the development of medicine at Johns Hopkins would be watched closely by the medical leaders of Europe.

To Billings can be attributed many of the enduring themes of the Johns Hopkins University School of Medicine. He was sometimes even more demanding than Gilman in considering the medical school's standards and curriculum. In 1878, Billings complained to Dr. John Warren in Boston: "With President Gilman the interests of medical science, and of the medical profession are, of course, held very secondary to what he believes to be the interests of the University, and it must be inferred that he does not think it specially necessary that a physician should possess the culture which is presumed to belong to an AB or BS in the Hopkins University."[33] Specifically, Billings disapproved of Gilman's intention at the time to award the degree of bachelor of medicine (particularly to persons who had studied no medicine but only declared their intention to do so), to remove anatomy and physiology from the medical curriculum, and, worst of all, to apply lower standards for matriculation in the medical school than prevailed in the rest of the university.[34]

Billings envisioned the Johns Hopkins Hospital and the Johns Hopkins University School of Medicine as the first American home of original medical research. No university, college, hospital, or asylum in the United States was conducting systematic, scientific investigation in the sciences basic to medicine. The new hospital and medical school would thus be the first to provide institutional and moral support for investigators.

Foreshadowing the advent of full-time professorships, Billings advocated allocating money and facilities to investigators so that they would not have to support their efforts by earning a living in other ways (usually by medical practice), and he expressed the hope that Hopkins would nurture a community of scientific investigators whose assistance, companionship, and sympathy would furnish the encouragement and stimulus necessary for most scientists.[35]

Prospective investigators would learn mainly from observation, experiment, and personal investigation—not from textbooks or lectures. Proper buildings would be crucial to this training: the new medical school would require many rooms and adequate instruments and apparatus, facilities that did not exist in any other medical school in the nation.[36]

The object of encouraging original research was not to retain these well-trained investigators at Hopkins, however. Billings intended Johns Hopkins to produce "men fitted to make research, and who will take the habit of, and taste for inquiry which they have acquired here—into, we will hope, wider and more extensive fields of usefulness."[37]

Delays in the Opening of the Hospital and the Medical School

The opening of the Johns Hopkins Hospital had originally been planned for October 1885, with the opening of the medical school soon to follow. In preparation, a joint committee of three hospital and three university trustees was formed to oversee all matters pertaining to the School of Med-

icine. In 1883, the committee appointed three members of the medical school's founding faculty—Henry Newell Martin, Ira Remsen, and John Shaw Billings—who met with Gilman several times during the next year to establish preliminary guidelines for the School of Medicine. Martin was professor of physiology, Ira Remsen was professor of chemistry, and John Shaw Billings was professor of hygiene. Remsen and Martin both had medical degrees.

Yet the trustees' plans languished as the hospital and university's financial fortunes waned. Only the annual income from Johns Hopkins' bequest could be used for construction costs, and the amount available was insufficient to permit the hospital's rapid completion. October 1885 passed, and the hospital was still not ready. The trustees came under great pressure to open the hospital before it was finished—even the mayor of Baltimore made a formal request that the hospital begin admitting patients.[38]

It was not a shortage of medical facilities that fueled the general impatience, as Baltimore had sixteen hospitals and seven dispensaries.[39] The great anticipation focused on the superior quality of care that the Johns Hopkins Hospital would provide. As Baltimore's *Medical Register* declared in 1885, "This institution will, when completed, be one of the finest in the matter of appointments in the world."[40]

Unfortunately, the following year saw a financial setback so serious that all pressure to open the hospital disappeared. The Baltimore and Ohio Railroad, whose stock represented almost one-half of Johns Hopkins' bequest, reduced its dividend in 1886, halved it again in 1887, and eliminated it entirely from 1888 to 1891.[41]

Preparations for the opening of the hospital and medical school continued nevertheless. On the hospital grounds, the Pathological Laboratory was completed in 1886; William Henry Welch, who had been appointed professor of pathology in 1884, returned to Baltimore after a year in Europe and took on fellows. Early in 1889, John Shaw Billings drew up a list of staff positions and responsibilities for the hospital, including, in addition to the medical staff, a director, a resident superintendent, resident physicians, a superintendent of nurses, a matron (or housekeeper), an apothecary, an engineer, and a steward (or storekeeper).

The Johns Hopkins Hospital opened in the spring of 1889, but the university's reduced income prevented the medical school from opening concurrently. Four more years elapsed before the medical school admitted its first class.

The Founding Faculty of Medicine

So far in advance were the members of the medical faculty appointed that none of the three actually served as professors at the medical school. Billings' background has already been discussed. Remsen, although he held the M.D. degree, had little influence on the School of Medicine. In contrast, Martin was a key figure in the school's development.

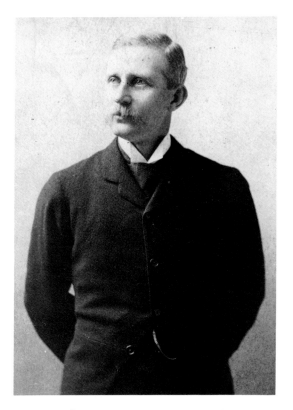

Henry Newell Martin. (*Source:* The Ferdinand Hamburger, Jr., Archives, The Johns Hopkins University.)

Henry Newell Martin had been invited to become professor of biology at the opening of the university in 1876, a post he accepted with the idea that he would eventually join the faculty of the School of Medicine.

Born in Ireland in 1848, Martin matriculated at the University of London before he was sixteen; after graduation, he became an apprentice to a London physician while studying medicine at University College Hospital. In 1870, Martin obtained a scholarship to Trinity College in Cambridge. There he received a doctor of science degree, becoming one of the first to take the degree in physiology. His first publication, on the structure of the olfactory membrane, appeared in the *Journal of Anatomy and Physiology* in 1873. The following year he helped to introduce Thomas Huxley's course in elementary biology at Cambridge; he subsequently acted as assistant to Huxley himself.

Martin was thus launched on a distinguished scientific career in Cambridge when Gilman invited him to Baltimore. Martin was only twenty-eight years old at the time, and like the other members of the founding faculty, he seemed to fit into Gilman's category of "young men who would be heard from."[42]

Gilman's appointment of a professor of biology (who would later occupy the chair of physiology) to the medical faculty reflected one of Billings' beliefs: the primacy of the biological sciences. Martin, whose major field of interest was experimental physiology, fit the trustees' description of an ideal faculty member, with his "devotion . . . to some particular line of study and the certainty of his eminence in that specialty; the power to pursue independent and original investigation and to inspire the youth with enthusiasm for study and research; a willingness to cooperate in building up a new institution and the freedom from tendencies toward ecclesiastical or sectional controversies."[43]

As head of the Department of Biology in the Faculty of Philosophy, Martin had established a well-organized premedical and graduate training course, the so-called Chemical-Biological Program.[44] The course was heavily influenced by the model that Gilman had helped to create at Yale. As Gilman said in his inaugural address at Johns Hopkins in 1876, "But who can doubt that a course may be maintained, like that already begun in the Sheffield School at New Haven, which shall train the eye, the hand, and the brain for the later study of medicine?"[45]

Premedical students at Johns Hopkins were advised to complete courses in physics and chemistry before proceeding to courses in biology. (Students were allowed to select a plan of study from one of several schedules listed in the university catalog.) Excellent facilities were provided for the study of a few key areas of biology and physiology in accordance with university policy, which sought to complement rather than rival other educational efforts; the areas chosen were those less commonly available in other schools. The university considered the teaching of physiology one of its particular strengths and prided itself on supplying the costly array of accurate instruments required for modern physiological research. Most universities could not afford to equip students with such instruments; accordingly, most students had only a rudimentary and secondhand knowledge of the important principles of physiology.[46]

An associate professor of biology, William K. Brooks, taught students about morphology and comparative anatomy, leaving Martin free to teach physiology and conduct his own research. Rounding out the department were the fellows; of the twelve fellowships offered by the university, three were allotted to biology.[47] Attesting to the success of Martin's program was the excellence of his students. Two were eventually appointed to the first faculty of the School of Medicine: William Henry Howell, professor of physiology, and John Jacob Abel, professor of pharmacology.

Martin's laboratory was controversial. Prominent naturalists condemned its emphasis on physiology, which they believed detracted from the study of morphology. They were joined by antivivisectionists, who objected to the laboratory for reasons of their own. Nevertheless, the enthusiasm of physiologists and scientifically oriented physicians attested to the growing belief in laboratory instruction as an important part of medical education.[48]

According to Martin, the mission of his department was "to advance our knowledge of the laws of life and death; to inquire into the phenomena and causes of disease; to train investigators in pathology, therapeutics and sanitary science; to fit men to undertake the study of the art of medicine. . . ." He continued, "these are the main objects of our laboratory. I do not know that they can be better summed up than in the words of Descartes, which I would like to see engraved over its portal: 'If there is any means of getting a medical theory based on infallible demonstrations, that is what I am now inquiring.' "[49]

Martin's research in Baltimore focused on the effects of drugs on the mammalian heart. For this purpose he developed a new method, which has been acclaimed as one of the most important contributions ever made in a laboratory of physiology in this country. Martin described the genesis of this technique:

The fact was impressed upon me that the mammalian heart is no such fragile organ as one is usually inclined to assume, but possesses a very considerable power of bearing manipulation. On the other hand, I knew of various unsuccessful attempts to isolate the mammalian heart and study its physiology apart from the influence of extrinsic nerve centres, in a manner more or less similar to the methods so frequently used for physiological investigations on the heart of a cold-blooded animal; the mammalian heart, however, always died before any observations could be made on it. Thinking over the apparent contradiction, it occurred to me that the essential difference probably lay in the coronary circulation; in the frog . . . there are no coronary arteries or veins, the thin auricles and spongy ventricles being nourished by the blood flowing through the cardiac chambers, but in the mammal the thick-walled heart has a special circulatory system of its own and needs a steady flow through its vessels, and cannot be nourished . . . by merely keeping up a stream through auricles and ventricles. The greater respiratory needs of the heart of the warm-blooded animal also needed consideration; the lungs ought either to be left connected with it or replaced by some other efficient aërating apparatus. . . .[50]

Daniel C. Gilman assessed Martin's stature:

> He came to Baltimore and established the first American biological laboratory. A score of successors followed. . . . To this study [of biology] Dr. Martin gave a noteworthy impulse, and the methods which he introduced were soon followed in other parts of the country. In the Johns Hopkins University it was soon determined that no one should be encouraged to enter upon the study of medicine without a careful previous training in a physiological laboratory. The improvements now common in medical schools are largely based upon the recognition of the principle that living creatures, in their normal and healthy aspects, should be studied before the phenomena and treatment of disease, and credit should always be given to Dr. Martin for the skill with which he introduced among Americans the best methods of study.[51]

As the eminent pathologist J. George Adami said, Henry Newell Martin's work in Baltimore was of basic importance in laying the foundation for medical science in America.[52]

In 1884, the three members of the medical faculty—Martin, Remsen, and Billings—met to consider the goals and requirements of the new medical school. They decided to accept as candidates for the degree of doctor of medicine only students with a general liberal education. As they defined it, a liberal education consisted of a knowledge of Latin, mathematics, English, physics, chemistry, general biology and physiology, and history; and enough French and German to enable the student to translate ordinary French and German prose. They also agreed to encourage research in the scientific branches of medicine, to open the research laboratories to all qualified persons wishing to become expert in these sciences—not just to medical students—and to admit for advanced study individuals with the M.D. degree. In addition, they decided that the medical school should adopt the university's fellowship system.[53]

It was not surprising that these men envisioned the new medical school as they did. As participants in a successful experiment in higher education—the original Faculty of Philosophy, directed by Gilman—they planned the next

school at the Johns Hopkins University along the same lines as the first.[54]

Failing health due to alcoholism forced Martin's resignation just before the medical school opened in 1893. He returned to England and died soon after, at the age of forty-five.[55] Remsen had decided to remain in the Department of Chemistry at the university; Billings was unable to accept the professorship of hygiene because of his connection with the United States Army. The first appointed professor who actually served on the faculty of the medical school was William Henry Welch, professor of pathology.

William Henry Welch

Gilman had gone to Europe in 1883 to gather information about the relationship of medical schools to hospitals and to hunt for a possible professor of pathology. The choice of a pathologist as the key member of the medical faculty reflected the preeminence of pathology in the 1880s. It was

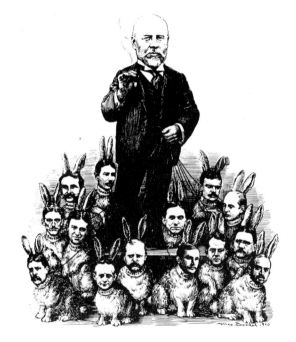

"Some Welch Rabbits," drawing by Max Broedel. (*Source:* Alan M. Chesney Medical Archives, The Johns Hopkins Medical Institutions.)

considered the basic science of medicine, and it was the specialty of most academic physicians of the time. When he was in Germany, Gilman tried to consult Julius Cohnheim, but they were not able to meet. The following year, however, Cohnheim wrote to Gilman recommending William H. Welch, a former student, for the professorship of pathology. Welch was then running a small pathological laboratory at the Bellevue Hospital Medical College. Billings had met Welch in Leipzig. Now he talked with Welch in New York, and Gilman then invited Welch to Baltimore for an interview. In the spring of 1884, William H. Welch was appointed to the faculty of the Hopkins medical school.[56]

Welch brought with him to Baltimore comprehensive experience in many facets of medicine. After graduating from the Columbia University College of Physicians and Surgeons in 1875, he had gone to Strasbourg, where he studied histology with Waldeyer, physiological chemistry with Hoppe-Seyler, and postmortem demonstrations with von Recklinghausen. After work in physiology with Ludwig and Kronecker in Leipzig, he studied pathology with Cohnheim in Breslau. Returning to New York, Welch accepted a professorship at the Bellevue Hospital Medical College, where he organized the first experimental laboratory in pathology in the country. He was well settled at an established medical school in New York, with promising students and good laboratory facilities, and his friends warned him that a move to Baltimore would be the ruination of his career. What lured Welch to Hopkins was the prospect of a full-time salaried position.[57]

Like the importation of Martin from England, Welch's invitation demonstrated Gilman's intention to nationalize the faculty. Had local physicians been antagonized by this policy, the new medical school could have been off to an inauspicious start; but Welch was immediately popular in Baltimore, partly because of his ability to charm and persuade—and partly because of his refusal to engage in practice or consultation of any kind.[58]

When Welch arrived in Baltimore in the fall of 1885, the Johns Hopkins University consisted of one school, the Faculty of Philosophy, with a flourishing university spirit and much optimism for putting medicine on a similarly high level.[59] Welch's Pathology Building at the hospital was not yet ready, so he moved into Martin's biology department for a brief period. Martin's laboratory, part of the main campus of the university, was then located on Howard Street near Center Street in downtown Baltimore, about two miles from the hospital.

Welch's association with the scientists on the university faculty reinforced his idea that the Johns Hopkins Hospital should be devoted not simply to the practice of medicine but also to the investigation of scientific issues. The original plans for the Pathology Building had reflected the assumption that the study of pathology could take place anywhere on the medical school grounds. The plans were changed, however, when Welch insisted that the activities of the Department of Pathology were so important to the work of the hospital that they should be conducted in close proximity to the wards. He also persuaded the trustees to include more laboratory space in the two-story structure and to add other facilities, such as an "autopsy theater" with an elaborate table.[60]

In this building, Welch began formal instruction in pathology in 1886 with his first assistants, William T. Councilman and Franklin P. Mall. Although most of Welch's first pupils were the younger members of the hospital staff, others came to Baltimore primarily to attend his courses in pathology and to participate in the research of his laboratory.[61] Welch had already done the last of his own important studies in the laboratory by the time the medical school opened (see chapter 11). His main interest was in training postgraduate students, or fellows—who found in his laboratory an investigative atmosphere verging on anarchy.

Welch deviated from the German practice of establishing a common theme for his laboratory's research by permitting his workers to go their own way unless they asked for advice. This laissez-faire attitude nevertheless produced important results: W. T. Councilman's discovery in

1887 of the crescent phase of the malarial parasites; Arthur G. Blachstein's finding in 1890 of the chronic carrier of typhoid bacilli in the biliary passages, and recognition of the relationship between typhoid infection of the gallbladder and the formation of gallstones; Councilman and LaFleur's contribution in 1891 to the understanding of the role of pathogenic amebae in producing amebic dysentery; Walter Reed's investigation in 1895 of the lymphoid nodules of the liver in typhoid fever; T. S. Cullen's demonstration in 1896 that adenomyoma of the uterus had its origin, in spite of the contrary opinion of von Recklinghausen, in the endometrium; T. C. Gilchrist's discovery in 1896 of the skin lesions caused by the *Blastomyces* fungi; W. G. MacCallum's demonstration in 1897 of the sexual conjugation of the malarial organism; Eugene L. Opie's proof in 1901 of a connection between the islets of Langerhans and diabetes in human beings; and MacCallum and Voegtlin's demonstration in 1908–9 that removal of the parathyroid glands leads to a calcium deficiency and that the accompanying postoperative spasms may be controlled by the administration of calcium—the first insight into the function of the parathyroids. Welch's laboratory has been characterized as "disjointed and lacking in direction," but its record is remarkable.[62]

Although Welch rarely suggested topics of study for his pupils, sometimes his recommendations launched careers. He urged Simon Flexner to study the spirochete of syphilis; it was Flexner's associate, Hideyo Noguchi, who later established the relationship of the spirochete to neurosyphilis.

Welch also called Walter Reed's attention to the demonstration by others that foot-and-mouth disease of cattle was caused by a filterable virus. Reed and his associate James Carroll then found that a filterable virus was also responsible for yellow fever—the first indication that a specific human disease was caused by this type of organism.[63] Welch was thus peripherally involved in the discovery that yellow fever is transmitted by mosquitos, credit for which belongs to the Yellow Fever Board. Walter Reed was the board's chief. Its members included James Carroll, Jesse Lazear,

and Aristides Agramonte—all, except for Agramonte, closely associated with Hopkins. Lazear, who was the first person to produce an undoubted case of experimental yellow fever with the mosquito, was an assistant resident physician and later an assistant in clinical microscopy. Carroll came to Welch's laboratory for two years of training in pathology and bacteriology, and Reed's study with Welch of the hog-cholera bacillus enabled him to recognize the resemblance between this bacterium and the microorganism erroneously claimed by Sanarelli to be the cause of yellow fever. Both Reed and Carroll maintained their ties with Welch's laboratory throughout their careers.[64]

Welch's Pathological Laboratory was a magnet for residents, fellows, and, later, other faculty members. In the process of following their own scientific interests, they linked the preclinical with the clinical departments of the medical school, and the medical school with the other science departments of the university. Welch's first assistant in pathology, William T. Councilman, was one of Henry Newell Martin's students, as were army surgeons George M. Sternberg and Walter Reed. William S. Halsted (the first professor of surgery at Johns Hopkins) and Franklin P. Mall (a fellow in pathology who later became the first professor of anatomy at Hopkins) worked together in Welch's laboratory to develop the distinctive suture that bears Halsted's name (see chapter 2).[65]

Welch also trained Thomas S. Cullen, the fifth resident of Howard A. Kelly, who was the original professor of gynecology at Hopkins. Cullen was also Kelly's successor as professor of gynecology. Cullen took with him from the Pathological Laboratory the conviction that no one should qualify in gynecologic surgery without first spending a year studying gynecologic pathology with Welch. Kelly agreed, and every successive resident in gynecology was thus exposed to Welch's teachings. William Osler's interest in malaria also led him to Welch's laboratory, where he learned of Councilman's discovery of malarial crescents. Even a member of the Department of Obstetrics, J. Whitridge Williams, began his career in Welch's laboratory, retaining a life-long interest in pathology as a result.[66]

It was Welch, more than anyone else, who created an invigorating atmosphere that focused attention on the revolutionary changes taking place in Baltimore. Through Welch's efforts, when the hospital opened, it quickly became recognized as an institution dedicated to the advancement of scientific medicine, and it became a powerful base for the immediate success of the School of Medicine.

The Recruitment of Halsted, Osler, and Kelly

As the hospital buildings inched toward completion, the trustees were eager to conclude the appointment of the hospital and medical school staffs. At the end of 1885, a subcommittee of hospital and university trustees was formed to select professors of medicine and surgery, whose appointments would be approved by the full boards of trustees of both the hospital and the university. In keeping with Johns Hopkins' intention to link the hospital and the medical school, Gilman and the trustees had devised a unique system of joint appointments. In other hospitals, several physicians alternated as chief of service, dividing the number of beds among them. In contrast, Gilman and the trustees envisioned one permanent chief of each service, who would also be professor of the respective department in the medical school. As a further link between the hospital and the medical school, each chief's salary would be paid by both.

Billings's first choice as surgeon-in-chief and professor of surgery was Sir William Macewen of Glasgow, the successor to Lord Lister. Macewen accepted the invitation, but negotiations fell through when he insisted on bringing his own nurses with him, intending to retain them entirely under his control. Welch was waiting with his own candidate, William S. Halsted, who with Welch and T. Mitchell Prudden had transported the German system of medical instruction to New York during the early 1880s. Despite his obvious surgical skills, Halsted's career had been marred by tragedy. Experimenting with cocaine as a local

anesthetic, Halsted had become addicted and underwent treatment for a year in a sanitarium. On his release in 1886, Welch invited Halsted to live with him in Baltimore and work in his laboratory. Welch persuaded the medical faculty to appoint Halsted as associate professor of surgery in 1889, and the following year he was made surgeon-in-chief of the hospital and professor of surgery in the medical school.[67]

Welch and Billings both supported the appointment of William Osler in 1888 as professor of medicine and physician-in-chief. Born and educated in Canada, Osler came to Hopkins from a professorship of medicine at the University of Pennsylvania. As physician to the Montreal General Hospital, Osler had founded a medical society, organized a student medical club, brought the medical school closer to the university, introduced the modern methods of teaching physiology and clinical skills, edited the first clinical and pathologic reports of a Canadian hospital, recorded nearly a thousand autopsies and preserved the most important specimens, written countless articles, and worked at biology and pathology as well as practicing medicine at the bedside. Osler had studied abroad, but not for long. He had never formed any close ties with the scientific community in Germany; instead, he represented the best of the English hospital schools as they had been transplanted to Canada. As Osler was the consummate clinician and teacher, his appointment strengthened the influence of the English tradition of clinical medicine at Hopkins.[68]

The final member of the "Big Four" at Hopkins, Howard A. Kelly, was not invited to Johns Hopkins until after the hospital had opened, Gilman had initially made no provision for a gynecologist, but late in 1889, the trustees empowered Osler to lead the search for one. Kelly was American in his training and outlook. A graduate of the University of Pennsylvania School of Medicine in the Class of 1882, Kelly had served as prosector to the paleontologist Joseph Leidy. Kelly then became the gynecologist at the Kensington Hospital in Philadelphia; his skill as a surgeon was renowned, and Osler recruited him to the University of Pennsylvania faculty. At Hopkins, Osler

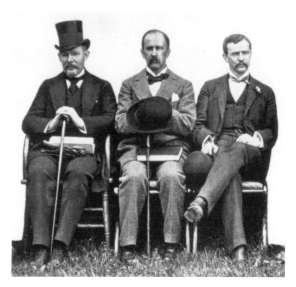

William S. Halsted, William Osler, Howard A. Kelly. The photograph was taken by James Mitchell, a member of the Class of 1897, the medical school's first class. (*Source:* Alan M. Chesney Medical Archives, The Johns Hopkins Medical Institutions.)

backed Kelly for the chair of gynecology and obstetrics just as Welch had backed Halsted for the chair of surgery. Neither Welch nor Billings knew Kelly, but they were willing to rely on Osler's high opinion of his skills in asking him to join the faculty.[69]

The Appointment of Gilman as Hospital Director

After twelve years of construction, the hospital was approaching completion in 1888, but the trustees were uncertain about the best method of putting the institution into active operation. Billings was the natural choice for director, but he declined to take on the full responsibility of running the hospital. (He did agree to serve as "consulting director.") In the winter of 1888–89, Francis T. King, the president of the hospital's Board of Trustees, himself now in failing health, came up with another candidate: Daniel C. Gilman, the president of the Johns Hopkins University.[70]

Gilman agreed to accept the dual responsi-

bility, and he began to divide his day between the university and the hospital. He plunged into an exhaustive study of hospital organization, familiarizing himself with the literature on the subject and corresponding with experts at home and abroad. He visited hospitals and large hotels in other cities to see their methods and details of management, to study their kitchens, laundries, and linen rooms.[71]

Gilman recommended establishing a Medical Board, which would consist of the chiefs of medicine, surgery, and pathology along with Alan P. Smith of the hospital trustees and James Carey Thomas of the university trustees, both of whom were physicians. Each department would pass along its nominations for subordinate officers to the Medical Board, which would in turn send them along to the Board of Trustees. In this way, the Medical Board would retain control over the hospital's staffing, nominating its physicians and appointing its interns.

The Opening of the Hospital

The Johns Hopkins Hospital was formally opened on May 7, 1889. "Magnificent in her beauty and her glory stood The Johns Hopkins Hospital yesterday," began the lead article in the next day's *Baltimore American*. The Baltimore *Sun* described the different multicolored tickets that admitted male Baltimoreans, out-of-town guests, women, important personages, physicians, and members of the press. A marble bust of Johns Hopkins stood in a corner of the hospital's rotunda, "twined with smilax"; smilax hung from the chandeliers; and the octagonal faces of the first gallery were hung with floral baskets and "festooned with evergreens." Luminaries crowded the rotunda, the hallways, and the galleries at the opening ceremonies, which consisted mainly of addresses interspersed with music. Francis T. King's talk was a brief account of Johns Hopkins' provision for the building of the hospital. The principal addresses, by John Shaw Billings and President Gilman, were philosophical and even prophetic, discussing the opportunities that the hospital would offer not only for the care of the sick but also for the education of physicians and the investigation of disease.[72]

Henri LaFleur, Osler's first resident physician, described Osler's satisfaction at the opening of the hospital:

It was a brilliant day, and notabilities, medical and otherwise, from Baltimore and the principal medical schools of America were grouped under the vast dome of the administration building to witness the inauguration of what was confidently believed to be the last word in hospital construction and management for the scientific study and treatment of disease. There was a feeling of elation—one might even say of exaltation—that the structure which had taken twenty years to evolve, absorbing the energies and thought of so many able minds, had at last become a *fait accompli*. And to none more than to Dr. Osler was this a red-letter day. To blaze a perfectly new road, untrammelled by tradition, vested interests, or medical "deadwood"—best of all, backed by a board of management imbued with a fundamental and abiding respect for scientific opinion and commanding an ample budget—what more could the heart of man desire?[73]

A "small-potatoes" impression of the event, as she called it, was given by John Shaw Billings' daughter Margaret:

It was a beautiful early spring day, sunny and mild. My father had announced, somewhat pontifically, a few days before, that he was taking the entire family over to Baltimore for the day. This was a great excitement for me, age 16, because I was the youngest, and Baltimore seemed a very long way from our home in Georgetown, D.C. The others took it in stride—my oldest sister Claire being an exalted 25, the twins—Dot and Daisy—were 22, and my brother John was a freshman at college.

We girls had our new Easter dresses, little summer prints of "India silk" (now called foularde), made at home by our family dressmaker. I did not think my mother had good taste—she dressed me like a barrel. But I felt gay and excited with my beautiful new straw hat covered with flowers that looked fresh enough to pick.

Speaking of flowers, we girls were eternally fed up with wearing the many blooms from mother's otherwise excellent garden. We wanted hot-house cor-

sages, but on this day we had nothing, not even a jonquil.

We all took the street-car from Georgetown to the B & O railroad station, a family of seven. Father, on a Major's pay, could not afford the luxury of owning or hiring a carriage. We travelled, oh wonder of wonders, in a Pullman car, to minimize, I suppose, the ravages of coal smoke, dust, and perspiration, for the day was warm. Ladies' rest rooms . . . so necessary for "repairs" after a journey, were few and far between and distinctly unprepossessing. To make matters worse, Father never allowed any of us to use cosmetics—no lipstick, rouge, not even powder. Ladies using such "artificial" aids to beauty in our set were apt to be considered "fast." Our speed must have been barely above a crawl.

On arriving at the Johns Hopkins Hospital I felt almost overcome with emotion. Father had been working on the plans in our study at home all through my childhood years. Discussion and conferences on it filled his—and our—days. He would often come home late in the evening from a meeting with the trustees and architects in Baltimore, mother would bring him a bowl of crackers and milk and he would tell her of progress.

The dream went slowly. The dour and conservative old Quakers who were raising the money would not let anything be built until the full amount of cash was on hand. So the hospital grew slowly, almost like a cathedral. I literally "grew up" with it.

But to return to the dedication. It was held in the large rotunda with many chairs facing a raised platform on which notable men of medicine, the Trustees and other distinguished guests were seated. We had "family seats" just to the right of the platform so close that I could plainly see the faces—many of them quite familiar to me—of the speakers. Several had visited our house many times and Father had taken me to their homes. I remember Dr. Osler, Dr. Welch, Dr. Kelly, Dr. Halsted.

Opening off of the rotunda were a series of corridors, like the spokes of a wheel, leading to the various wards, operating rooms, etc.—a most impressive sight. And standing at the partially opened door of every ward or room down these vistas was a starchly uniformed trained nurse. . . .

Speeches followed one another in endless succession and I don't remember a single immortal word of any of them—not even of my father's. They were far above my head. There were no funny stories—at least not to me—it was all too awe-inspiring. I remember Mr. Francis King spoke, also President Gilman of Johns Hopkins University, whose speech I thought was dry as dust for a person so distinguished. (Such are the critical faculties of age 16.)

After these formal festivities we enjoyed a gala buffet lunch, typical menu for Maryland in Spring —chicken salad, cold ham, ices and fresh strawberries with cream. I stuffed myself shamelessly.

Then we went on a tour of the new hospital. There were no patients, they began to arrive the next day. We saw—had pointed out to us—many of father's ideas and theories, based on his practical experience with sanitation, ventilation, lighting, and other problems in war hospitals.

Father had won a competition against 5 or 6 others for the best design for a hospital, and then had been retained as a consultant during its construction. Every ward had outside windows, sunlight and fresh air—no dark rooms. Corners of walls and floors had been rounded so as not to provide cracks for bugs and dirt. It was a dream that had evolved slowly—thoroughly—completely—a dream to have everything as perfect as possible, built to last, and planned as far ahead as it was then possible to see.[74]

The hospital was open to the public for several days after the dedication ceremonies, and elaborate arrangements were made to ensure that everyone who wished could tour the new institution. Many evidently did: contemporary accounts agree that the new hospital aroused great interest in the community. Seven days after the inauguration ceremonies, the Johns Hopkins Hospital admitted its second patient.

The first patient had been treated some ten years earlier, in the summer of 1879. John K. Bruff, a foreman of the bricklayers, was climbing a ladder on the Kitchen Building when he fell thirty feet into the cellar, breaking his right leg below the knee. He was moved to the basement of the Octagon Ward, and Dr. Alan P. Smith was summoned to set the fractured limb. Bruff convalesced for the next two months in the basement of the male private ward, later called Lower C, where temporary floors were laid and a room furnished to accommodate him. Samuel H. Kerr was employed to care for him, thus becoming the hospital's first "nurse." The hospital's additional expenditures for this unexpected patient included eighty cents for pills; fifty cents for ice, fruit, and sugar; ten cents for "liquor"; and seventy-five cents for brandy.[75]

The enduring attraction of the Johns Hopkins Hospital for out-of-state patients began early in its history: among its first patients was a Nebraska librarian with tuberculous peritonitis. During the first fractional fiscal year of seven and a half months (May 15 to December 31, 1889), nearly eight hundred patients were under treatment in the several available wards.[76]

The First Superintendent of the Hospital: Henry Mills Hurd

The hospital's superintendent, who would be in charge of its day-to-day activities, was not appointed until shortly after the hospital officially opened. Gilman himself undertook the task of finding this essential staff member. He chose Henry M. Hurd, the head of the Eastern Michigan Asylum in Pontiac. Then forty-six years of age, the oldest of the medical faculty, Hurd was a promi-

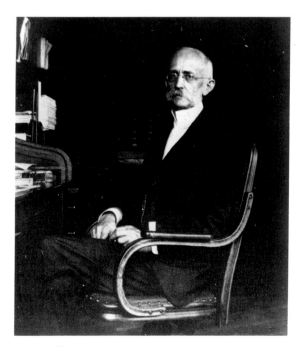

Henry Mills Hurd. (*Source:* Alan M. Chesney Medical Archives, The Johns Hopkins Medical Institutions.)

nent figure in American psychiatric circles. After attending Knox College in Illinois, Hurd finished his undergraduate education at the University of Michigan. He then began the study of medicine with his stepfather and graduated from the University of Michigan School of Medicine in 1866. The year after graduation, Hurd studied and performed hospital work in New York; he next moved to Chicago, where he spent two years as a general practitioner. Hurd was then appointed assistant physician to the Michigan Asylum for the Insane at Kalamazoo and rose to the position of assistant superintendent. Eight years at Kalamazoo were followed by eleven years as the first superintendent of the Eastern Michigan Asylum.[77]

The best of the asylums of that era were excellent training grounds in hospital administration. Hurd brought to Johns Hopkins not only great skill as an administrator but also literary attainments of a high order, a thorough medical training, and a keen knowledge of men—all of which enabled him to run the Johns Hopkins Hospital and maintain its relationship with the School of Medicine smoothly and efficiently. During his tenure at Hopkins, Hurd enthusiastically embraced the many new ideas taking hold in psychiatry, including abolition of the use of restraints on patients, employment of the mentally ill, and introduction of home comforts into institutional life. His most important literary effort was a four-volume history of hospitals for the insane in the United States and Canada, and he was the author of many papers published in the *American Journal of Insanity*.[78] Hurd's annual reports as superintendent of the Eastern Michigan Asylum were written in a masterly and polished style, revealing the skills he later displayed as editor of *The Johns Hopkins Hospital Bulletin*. As professor of psychiatry in the School of Medicine, he remained a contributor to the psychiatric literature during his superintendency.

Publications and Societies

Henry Hurd's editorial skills were particularly valuable at Hopkins when new publications and societies were founded to disseminate the results of research. Following the policy he had established in the Faculty of Philosophy, Gilman had promised to give investigators in the School of Medicine the means to disseminate their findings. In charge of manufacturing and distributing Hopkins' various publications was the university's so-called Publication Agency. In 1890, its name was changed to the Johns Hopkins Press, and it thus became the first university press so named in the United States.[79] In the medical realm, the trustees authorized the publication of two journals when the hospital opened in 1889: the *Johns Hopkins Hospital Bulletin,* which was expected to transmit news of the hospital, and the *Johns Hopkins Hospital Reports,* which would contain the results of the staff's scientific investigations. Although the *Bulletin* was intended for clinical studies, investigators in Welch's Pathological Laboratory used it to get their work into print. A new journal was begun in 1896, the *Journal of Experimental Medicine*. Edited by Welch, it was the nation's first journal devoted exclusively to medical research.

Investigators at Hopkins also spread their results through the Johns Hopkins Medical Society and through a journal club, both formed when the hospital opened. The journal club met weekly for years until it was fragmented into departmental endeavors.[80]

The Opening of the School of Nursing

Gilman appointed a superintendent of nurses, Isabel Adams Hampton, to run the Nurses Training School connected with the Johns Hopkins Hospital. This school was not one of the nation's first, but it had a formidable influence on the pattern of nursing education in the United States. Hampton had solid experience in her field: a graduate of the Bellevue Hospital Training School for Nurses, she had been head nurse at the Women's Hospital of New York City and had worked in Rome for two years at St. Paul's House for trained nurses. She came to Hopkins from a position as superintendent of the Illinois Training

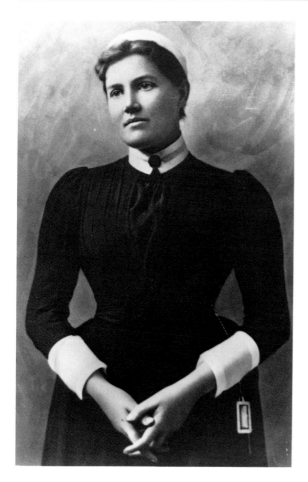

Isabel A. Hampton. (*Source:* Alan M. Chesney Medical Archives, The Johns Hopkins Medical Institutions.)

person in charge of corresponding hospital and medical school departments by naming Hampton the superintendent of nursing at the hospital as well as the head of the nursing school. He thus ensured that the nurses' training program would combine academic and service functions.

The Opening of the Medical School: The Women's Fund Committee Closes the Financial Gap

Although the hospital opened in 1889, sufficient funds were not available to get the medical school under way. It was unclear when—or whether—the school would open at all. Into the breach stepped a group of women, four of whom were trustees' daughters: Martha Carey Thomas, Mary Gwinn, Mary Elizabeth Garrett, and Elizabeth King. Led by M. Carey Thomas, they formed a Women's Fund Committee in 1890 to raise the rest of the money needed to open the medical school (see chapter 6). Gilman and the trustees doubted that they could raise the necessary funds,

School for Nurses in Chicago. Hampton joined the staff of the Johns Hopkins Hospital in time for the opening of the nursing school in October 1889, and remained until 1894, when she resigned to marry the first resident in gynecology, Hunter Robb, and moved to Cleveland. The nurses' home built in 1926 was named "Hampton House" in her honor.[81]

Under the administration of Hampton and her successor, Mary A. Nutting, the school set a new educational standard for the training of nurses nationwide. They lengthened the program from two to three years, included laboratory courses, introduced special programs in dietetics and psychiatry, and treated the trainees as students rather than employees. Gilman extended the innovative arrangement that placed a single

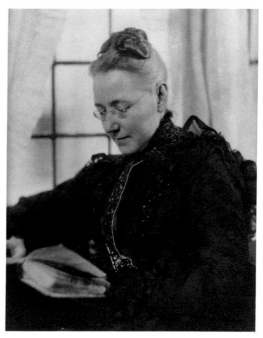

Mary E. Garrett. (*Source:* Alan M. Chesney Medical Archives, The Johns Hopkins Medical Institutions.)

but women across the country sent contributions. Prominent subscribers included members of the Adams, Bonaparte, Biddle, Drexel, and Widener families; Mrs. Louis Agassiz, the founder of Radcliffe College; Mrs. S. Weir Mitchell and Mrs. Samuel W. Gross (later Lady Osler); first lady Mrs. Benjamin Harrison; celebrated women physicians such as Emily Blackwell and Mary Putnam Jacobi; and women in the arts including Alice Longfellow, Julia Ward Howe, and Sarah Orne Jewett. Mary E. Garrett contributed $50,000, and in the fall of 1890 the women's committee was able to offer the trustees $100,000, with one stipulation: women must be admitted as students on equal terms with men. Gilman was privately opposed to accepting the gift, and Welch made his opposition public, but Halsted, Osler, and Kelly advised the trustees to accede to the terms of the Women's Fund Committee, and finally Welch went along.[82]

The women's contribution was accepted with the provision that the school would not open until a total of $500,000 had been obtained. By December 1892, less than $200,000 had been raised. The delay in the opening of the medical school had encouraged other schools to try to entice away members of the Hopkins faculty, and in mid-December, an anonymous benefactor pledged $1 million to McGill University if Osler would leave Johns Hopkins for Montreal. It was with immense relief, therefore, that the Hopkins trustees received Mary Garrett's letter late in December, in which she offered to make up the difference between the money raised and the total required to open the medical school.[83] From the Garrett fortune (which, ironically, derived from the earlier success of the Baltimore and Ohio Railroad), she contributed about $300,000.

Her additional gift came with its own stipulations, however. Persuaded by M. Carey Thomas, Garrett insisted that entering medical students have a bachelor's degree from a first-class college and a reading knowledge of French and German. These requirements echoed the terms of admission advocated by the founding preclinical faculty in 1884; but whereas eight years earlier they had merely been discussed, now they were formally accepted. The Johns Hopkins

medical school became the first in America with such stringent admission requirements; their unprecedented character led Osler to remark to Welch that they had been lucky to get in as professors, because neither of them could have been admitted as students.[84]

In establishing these entrance requirements, Johns Hopkins became the first medical school in the United States to demand a college degree for admission. As of 1900, only 15 or 20 percent of medical schools required even a high-school diploma of their entrants. Accordingly, many medical school courses were taught on an elementary level. At Johns Hopkins, in contrast, students would be expected to have mastered the basic elements of biology, chemistry, and physics, so that they could pursue their studies on a graduate level.

With Garrett's gift, funds were available to obtain professors of pharmacology, anatomy, and physiology, a task delegated to Welch. For this second round of appointments, Welch could turn to the first generation of students at the Johns Hopkins University. His candidate in anatomy was one of his own fellows, who had collaborated with Halsted; and his choices for pharmacology and physiology were students of Henry Newell Martin.

The First Professor of Anatomy: Franklin Paine Mall

Franklin P. Mall was never known to the public as a brilliant investigator, but his colleagues believed that he was the best of them all. He gave the field of anatomy a sound scientific basis, and he had a profound influence on medical education, training fellows who became the leaders of anatomy departments across the country (see chapter 9).[85]

Mall graduated from the University of Michigan School of Medicine in 1885. He then went to Germany, where he was educated by Wilhelm His and Carl Ludwig in anatomy, physiology, and embryology. Mall came to Johns Hopkins in 1886, and during the next three years he was first a fellow and then an assistant in pathology in Welch's laboratory. His studies of the stomach were done at this time, as well as his physiological investigations of the different types of contractions of the intestines and their effect on the local circulation of the blood.

Mall left Hopkins after his fellowship, becoming adjunct professor at Clark University. In 1892, he moved to the University of Chicago, and less than a year later, at the age of thirty-one, he accepted the professorship of anatomy at Johns Hopkins.

Mall thus spent his mature years at Hopkins. His research spanned three areas: embryology, the structural adaptation of adult organs to their function, and anthropology. He is best known for his work on the spleen, liver, and heart (see chapter 11), and he brought to its fullest development the idea that for each organ there is a structural unit that is a unit of function.[86] He also helped to found several anatomical journals, led scientific societies, and established a research institute for embryology.

The First Professor of Physiology: William Henry Howell

Of the first heads of the four preclinical laboratories at Johns Hopkins, William Henry Howell was the only one who had not studied abroad. He was nevertheless a prolific and accomplished investigator, publishing some fifty-five articles during his years at Johns Hopkins and five articles during his tenure at Ann Arbor and Harvard.

Howell was born and educated in Baltimore. Intending to practice medicine, he became a student in the new Johns Hopkins University's Chemical-Biological Program preparatory to the study of medicine, but lack of funds prevented him from pursuing the medical degree after graduation. Instead, he received from the university a scholarship that enabled him to undertake graduate studies. His thesis concerned the origin of fibrin formed in the coagulation of blood, a subject that was to interest him throughout his career (see chapter 11).[87]

Howell left Baltimore to become head of the Physiology Department at the University of Michigan in 1889; three years later, he accepted an appointment at Harvard as associate professor of physiology. He remained in Boston for only a year, as not long after his arrival, Gilman recruited him for the new School of Medicine.

Howell's career at Hopkins spanned thirty-eight years, twenty-five of them in the School of Medicine and thirteen in the School of Hygiene and Public Health. After a dozen years as dean of the medical school, Howell became assistant director and then director of the School of Hygiene and Public Health, where he remained from 1918 until his retirement in 1931.

Howell was best known to two generations of medical students for his *Textbook of Physiology,* which first appeared in 1905 and went through fourteen editions. His own research accomplishments were many. He is honored eponymously by the Howell-Jolly bodies, particles in red corpuscles that take nuclear stains. Howell was also among the first investigators to suggest that the two lobes of the pituitary gland are functionally different and to provide evidence for the chemical nature of the nervous influences that control the heart rate. After 1909, his research was devoted almost exclusively to the study of blood coagulation (see chapter 11).

America's First Full-Time Pharmacologist: John Jacob Abel

John J. Abel was above all an investigator, whose great enthusiasm and passionate devotion to research dominated his life. At the University of Michigan, he studied physiological chemistry with Victor Vaughan and physiology with Henry Sewall, a former student of Henry Newell Martin. Abel himself studied under Martin after receiving the doctoral degree from Michigan, moving to Baltimore in 1884 to work for a year in the Department of Biology at Johns Hopkins. Abel then went to Germany for seven years to study with the most distinguished scientists of the time. He returned to Michigan as professor of materia medica (as pharmacology was then known) but stayed only a year, joining the faculty at Johns Hopkins in 1893 as head of the Department of Pharmacology.[88]

Abel's research resulted in important and varied pharmacologic contributions. Four of his findings were particularly important to clinical medicine: his isolation of epinephrine, a benzoyl derivative of the active principle of the adrenal medulla; his method of renal dialysis, which he called "vividiffusion"; his experiments with phthalein derivatives; and his crystallization of insulin.[89]

Abel's courses, like those of his colleague Franklin P. Mall, departed from traditional methods of teaching. Neither relied on textbooks. Instead, using the original literature, Abel replaced lecture-room demonstrations with laboratory sessions that required the students' participation. Many of Abel's colleagues adopted his methods of instruction, including his assistant Walter Jones, who became head of the Department of Physiological Chemistry.

Abel also participated in the founding of some of the nation's first scientific journals, including the *Journal of Experimental Medicine* (with Welch), the *Journal of Biological Chemistry,* and the *Journal of Pharmacology and Experimental Therapeutics.* His eminence in his field led his colleagues to elect him the first president of the American Society for Pharmacology and Experimental Therapeutics.

The First Class

The opening of the medical school in October 1893 was announced at the university's Commemoration Day exercises the preceding February. Word spread beyond Hopkins in the in-

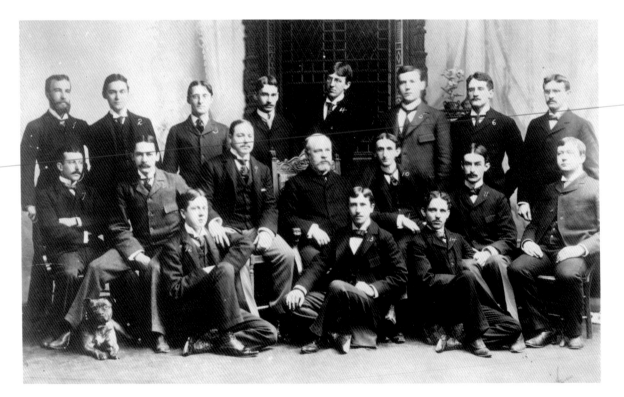

Class of 1897, School of Medicine (*not shown,* Mary S. Packard). *Second row, center,* William H. Welch; *indicated by numbers,* graduating members of class: (1) G. L. Hunner, (2) E. L. Opie, (3) C. R. Bardeen, (4) T. R. Brown, (5) O. B. Pancoast, (6) C. A. Penrose, (7) J. L. Nichols, (8) J. F. Mitchell, (9) R. P. Strong, (10) L. P. Hamburger, (11) I. P. Lyon, (12) W. G. MacCallum, (13) C. N. McBryde, (14) W. S. Davis. *Top row, unnumbered,* L. W. Day and W. W. McCulloh, who did not graduate. (*Source:* Alan M. Chesney Medical Archives, The Johns Hopkins Medical Institutions.)

tervening eight months: of the first sixteen applicants, only five were graduates of the Johns Hopkins University. On October 2, these sixteen brought their credentials to the university's Biological Laboratory for Welch's perusal. Welch must have been relieved to see so many applicants, for the Hopkins faculty had no idea how many students would be interested in enrolling in the new institution, and they were afraid that their stringent admission requirements would discourage or exclude prospective students. All sixteen applicants were admitted (some provisionally), and two more students were enrolled a few days later. The first class of the Johns Hopkins University School of Medicine therefore comprised eighteen students, three of whom were women.[90]

The Most Advanced Medical Institution of the Day

The essential element in the success of the hospital and medical school was the idea that the hospital should form a part of the medical school and thus a part of the university. Although Johns Hopkins had referred to this broad concept, the policies that created a medical school with a teaching hospital under its control were devised by Gilman, Billings, and Welch. As an instrument of medical education, the hospital was linked to the medical school in a unique way: a single individual headed both the hospital department and the corresponding department in the medical school. Instead of the responsibility for control of hospital beds being dispersed among a host of local practitioners, each hospital (and medical school) department would have a single chief.

This unity would be cemented by the actions of the Boards of Trustees of the hospital and the university. Although they operated independently, these boards had overlapping memberships, and they established several joint committees. Both boards were required to approve a chief's appointment and share the payment of his salary equally. Chiefs of service would themselves become members of two other unique organiza-

tional entities, the Advisory Board of the medical school and the Medical Board of the hospital. Comprising department heads and administrative chiefs of the medical school and hospital, respectively, these groups advised the trustees of appointments to the staff and other matters relating to patient care, education, and research.

The founder's desire to attract a staff of "the highest character and skill" led the trustees to turn their backs on the provincialism that marked most hospital and medical school appointments. Instead of merely selecting faculty and staff from Baltimore, or even from the well-known medical school in Boston, they searched worldwide for the most qualified individuals. Osler was a Canadian who had migrated from Philadelphia; Welch and Halsted came from New York; Hurd was imported from Michigan.

These men had a qualification new to American medicine: their proven ability as investigators. Most had studied in Germany, a center of research in the 1880s, and they brought back one of the most profound influences of German medicine upon America: the university ideal. It was in Baltimore that the trustees of the new university medical school created the conditions that allowed that ideal to flourish, and eventually to become the model for all medical schools.

The Hopkins faculty were capable not only of teaching what was known but also developing new knowledge and training others to do so as well. At Johns Hopkins, they were given both tangible and intangible encouragement. Well-equipped laboratories—facilities rare in other medical schools—were provided in the preclinical sciences, including pathology. Also provided were publications for the dissemination of the laboratories' findings. The journals created at Johns Hopkins for this purpose were among the first such publications in the United States.

The preclinical faculty was relieved of the necessity of earning a living from the practice of medicine—another unusual feature of the new hospital and medical school. To enable these faculty members to concentrate on research, the medical school and university paid their salaries, placing them on the so-called full-time basis. The decision to maintain a full-time policy was first tested in 1884, when negotiations were held with Matthew Hay, a candidate for the professorship of pharmacology. Hay wanted to continue treating private patients, but the trustees responded, "Medical Education in the United States now suffers from the fact that the [preclinical science] chairs are almost always filled by practitioners and consequently the scientific work of the Schools of Medicine has been less efficient than it should be. It is thought best here to initiate our Medical School by appointing several teachers who shall not engage in practice."[91] (Clinical professors also received a salary but were permitted to have some private patients.)

The students were seen not primarily as a source of revenue, as at proprietary medical schools, but as the recipients of existing knowledge and the faculty's partners in developing new knowledge. Women were accepted at the medical school on equal terms with men, by stated policy.

The hospital and medical school also included two advanced groups previously unknown in American medicine: the residents in clinical medicine and the research fellows in the preclinical sciences.

By 1893, most of the innovations that characterized the Johns Hopkins Hospital and the School of Medicine were in place, including the residency training program (see chapter 2). Like pieces of a jigsaw puzzle, these novel features fitted together to form a model for American medical education and medical care. These elements made the new Johns Hopkins University School of Medicine and the Johns Hopkins Hospital the most advanced institutions of the day.

CHAPTER 2

THE EARLY DAYS, 1893–1905

It was not the men, though success could not have come without them, so much as the method, the organization, and a collective new outlook on old problems. They were gathered here from all parts to do one thing, to show that the primary function of a university was to contribute to the general sum of human knowledge.

—William Osler

The Medical School Prospers

Billings, Gilman, and Welch had chosen well. With a talented faculty, a hand-picked student body, and William H. Welch as its first dean, the Johns Hopkins University School of Medicine was successful from the start.

As the school's first year ended, its financial picture was bright. In May 1894, Gilman reported to the Advisory Board that the school's income of $27,000 had exceeded its expenditures by $2,400, and the second entering class was nearly double the first in size.[1] The entering Class of 1898 comprised thirty students, and two more joined later in the year. Fifteen different colleges were represented. Seven students were graduates of Johns Hopkins; six were natives of Baltimore; and eight were women.

Two students who had completed the first year of medical school elsewhere joined the Class of 1897 in its second year. Eugene L. Opie and William G. MacCallum were admitted with advanced standing, after some hesitation by the Advisory Board. Opie's application had first been rejected but was reconsidered when a similar application from MacCallum was received a week later. Both men went on to distinguished careers in medical science, Opie at the Rockefeller Institute for Medical Research and Washington University, and MacCallum as Welch's successor as chief of pathology.

New Faculty in the Early Years

The medical school's early success attracted new faculty, many of whom later achieved international fame. Here, as elsewhere, representative examples must suffice. J. Whitridge Williams was appointed associate in obstetrics in 1893. A graduate of the Johns Hopkins University and of the University of Maryland medical school, Williams was appointed head of the new outpatient obstetrical service in 1895. He thus became the hospital's first obstetrician-in-chief and the medical school's first professor of obstetrics.[2]

Walter Jones, a brilliant lecturer and a pioneer in research on nucleic acids, was appointed assistant in physiological chemistry in 1896. When this section became an independent department, he was appointed to be its head. Ross G. Harrison, who became one of the outstanding

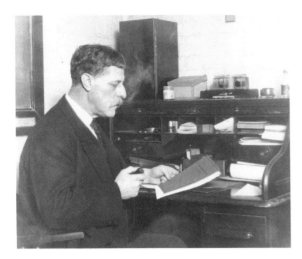

J. Whitridge Williams. (*Source:* Alan M. Chesney Medical Archives, The Johns Hopkins Medical Institutions.)

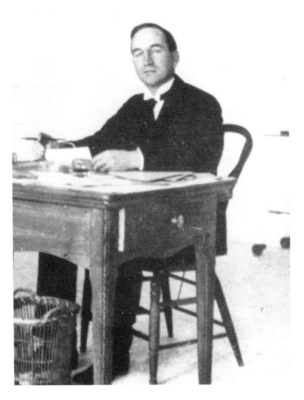

Hugh H. Young. (*Source:* Alan M. Chesney Medical Archives, The Johns Hopkins Medical Institutions.)

figures in American biology, was appointed instructor in anatomy in 1896. Harrison had obtained his doctorate from the Johns Hopkins University two years earlier, under Henry Newell Martin; he remained a member of the medical faculty until 1907.[3]

Others who became stalwarts of the clinical faculty first came to Baltimore as hospital residents. Hugh H. Young arrived in 1896 as an assistant resident surgeon. His first interest was general surgery, but Halsted nevertheless identified him as the man to develop the specialty of urology. Young recounted the conversation that changed his career, when in 1897, Halsted asked him to take charge of genitourinary surgery: "I thanked him and said: 'This is a great surprise. I know nothing about genitourinary surgery.' Whereupon Dr. Halsted replied, 'Welch and I said you didn't know anything about it, but we believe you could learn.'"[4]

The practice of giving young men with potential the responsibility for developing an unfamiliar field was characteristic of Halsted. Similarly, he chose Harvey W. Cushing to develop the field of neurosurgery. Cushing had originally sought a position on Osler's service but, receiving no reply, he applied and was accepted for training in surgery. Cushing arrived in 1896, and his next sixteen years at Hopkins laid the basis for his dis-

tinguished career. He introduced x-ray apparatus to the hospital, taking all the x rays at Johns Hopkins until he became resident surgeon in 1897; and he was renowned for his later work on the pituitary gland. Although Cushing specialized in neurosurgery, his wide-ranging interests gave

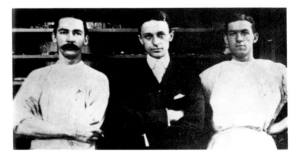

J. F. Mitchell, Harvey W. Cushing, and M. B. Clopton, members of the resident staff, 1899. (*Source:* Alan M. Chesney Medical Archives, The Johns Hopkins Medical Institutions.)

him—and Hopkins—an international reputation.[5]

Cushing also established and oversaw the Hunterian Laboratory, the laboratory for experimental surgery at Hopkins (see chapter 7). Instead of teaching students surgical technique on a cadaver, Cushing had them practice on living, anesthetized dogs. He likened the exercise to the actual performance of surgery on a human patient; his students wrote up the history, kept an ether chart as well as operative and postoperative notes, and performed a complete postmortem examination.[6]

Cushing remained in Baltimore until 1912, when he became professor of surgery at the newly opened Peter Bent Brigham Hospital in Boston. His career exemplifies one of Hopkins' most important accomplishments: the training of clinicians and investigators who assumed key posts in other university centers.

Thomas McCrae arrived at Johns Hopkins from Ontario about a month after Cushing. He had completed the medical course at the University of Toronto and came to Baltimore as one of Osler's assistant resident physicians. McCrae remained in Baltimore until 1912, when he accepted the chair of medicine at Jefferson Medical College in Philadelphia. His prime contribution at Hopkins was administrative, as he brought about the orderly arrangement of the histories of patients admitted to the medical service. Until 1897, old histories remained unsorted, and current histories were carried away by anyone who wanted them. From 1898 to 1902, McCrae labored to set the Department of Medicine's histories in order. Hundreds of missing ones turned up in the house of one faculty member (not Osler); many were found in other hospital departments. In 1907, McCrae was given a secretary to help with the work, and the preparation of a disease index was begun. After about eight years of work, the histories were arranged, indexed, and bound. McCrae also assisted Osler with the eighth and ninth editions of his textbook *The Principles and Practice of Medicine*; for the next three editions, which were published after Osler's death, McCrae was the sole author.[7]

New Buildings in the Medical School

The number of qualified students interested in the new venture in medical education surpassed expectations, and the trustees were hard pressed to provide them with laboratories and classrooms. As a temporary measure, third and fourth floors were added to the Pathological Building before the medical school opened in 1893 to accommodate instruction in anatomy and physiological chemistry for the first-year students.

Two new buildings were constructed on the medical school lot in the next few years. The first was the Women's Fund Memorial Building, known as the anatomy building, which was completed in time for the start of the school year in 1894. Mary E. Garrett had set aside "no more than $50,000" of her original gift for a building that would memorialize the contributions of the women's committee—and that was exactly how much the trustees allowed.[8] The second was the Physiology Building, which took its place beside the Women's Fund Memorial Building in 1899. The first six medical school classes had been forced to travel downtown to the university for their courses in physiology, and they complained of the time wasted in transit. With the completion of the Physiology Building, all instruction in the medical school was at last united on the East Baltimore campus.[9]

On the hospital grounds, Osler finally obtained a permanent clinical laboratory when two floors were added to the building connecting the Amphitheater and the Dispensary. In the original construction of the hospital, no provision had been made for clinical laboratories, and a temporary laboratory had been set up in the hospital basement; but the addition of a permanent laboratory at last rectified the initial oversight.[10] It was Osler who thought the laboratory should be near the hospital wards—an innovation considered to be one of his most important accomplishments. The laboratory was a key facility not only for the care of patients but also for instruction in clinical microscopy, a course that had just been added to the curriculum for third-year students.[11]

The Curriculum in the Preclinical Years

Before the students reached the clinical years, they were immersed in rigorous, if informal, courses taught by the professors of anatomy, physiology, pathology, and physiological chemistry. "The original heads of departments were relatively young and in their prime," recalled G. Canby Robinson, a student in the entering class of 1899, "and the spirit of youth was in the air."[12] So knowledgeable in their fields were these professors that they used the standard textbooks only as a point of departure. In the classroom, students in the first two years of medical school thus found themselves listening to investigators who were conducting pathbreaking research; and in the laboratories, students enjoyed a close professional relationship with these faculty members. Robinson described the exciting atmosphere in physiological chemistry, as taught by Walter Jones:

> Jones was a spirited and, on occasions, a dramatic talker. He gave us an idea of the vehemence a scientific controversy could arouse, as he was at that time in the midst of a polemic with a professor in a German university and his arguments bubbled over in his lectures, giving them life and interest. One of our classmates, Arthur Loevenhart, was an advanced student of biochemistry. . . . When the subject of his previous research fitted into the course, Jones asked him to lecture to the class—an example of the comradeship that existed among students and teachers in the medical school.[13]

First-year students took courses in anatomy, physiology, and physiological chemistry; pathology was saved for the second year, when students actually worked with bacteria in the laboratory. Even students in the early years of medical school were thus able to participate in "learning by doing." Under Welch's direction, students attended postmortem examinations in the hospital and studied specimens and microscopic sections in the laboratory.[14] Eugene L. Opie's notes from his second year of medical school illustrate Welch's solicitousness:

> In Bact. from Oct. 1894 to Jan. '95 Dr. Welch gave all of the lectures, that is 24. These were systematic lec-

tures including a consideration of the history of bacteriology, morphology and physiology of bacteria, immunity (4 lectures) and bacteria on the exposed surfaces of the body. . . . Dr. Welch discussed in the laboratory with each student his cultures and preparations made from them. It was my impression at the time that he liked this form of demonstration and was quite unhurried in his progress from student to student. . . . Of the lectures in Pathology . . . what Dr. Welch said could be readily followed and gave an insight into the subject that I could not obtain from any text book.[15]

The Curriculum in the Clinical Years

Although other schools relied on lectures as the primary method of instruction in the final two years, at Hopkins, courses in the final two years continued to emphasize student participation. Third- and fourth-year students were the beneficiaries of a varied program. The highlight of the third year was probably Osler's medical clinic. As one former student described the class:

> In our third year, we had two classroom exercises with him at 12. noon on Tuesdays and Thursdays, and an amphitheatre clinic on Saturday at 12.00 noon. On these occasions he acted as a fellow student with us, guiding us in our examinations of the patient, causing us to see what we had not previously noted and making us realize that the Hippocratic dictum "to see, to touch and to hear," was not all in making a diagnosis, for Laennec introduced the words "to auscult" and so revealed further facts. But he showed us that all of this went for naught if we did not follow what Louis, the great French clinician, had taught us "to record." He made us make careful notes of our findings.[16]

Fourth-year students were divided into four groups, each spending two months in medicine, surgery, obstetrics, and gynecology. George J. Heuer, a member of the Class of 1907, described his rotation in surgery with Dr. Halsted:

> The teaching of surgery to medical students was also a departure from the common practice in medical schools of this country. Instead of only reading assigned textbooks, attending lectures and "dry" clinics at which the professor demonstrated surgical

diseases, or viewing operations which were performed with dexterity and rapidity and often with an eye on the clock, the undergraduate student through a "clinical clerkship," was assigned to the surgical wards and came into direct contact with patients. It was his responsibility to take complete histories and to make careful and thorough physical examinations and such other tests as blood counts and urine analyses. All this became part of the permanent hospital record and the need for careful work was stressed and the work itself checked by interns and residents. It was expected that the student would "read up" on his cases so as to become familiar with the surgical diseases they represented; and it came about that an interested student could, through discussions with his fellow students, become familiar with all the patients in the wards. On ward rounds by the professor or his resident it was the student who presented the history and physical examination and he usually knew all the details of the cases. This very practical clinical work was supplemented by ward rounds, by an operative clinic held by Dr. Finney on Friday morning and by a "dry" clinic held by Dr. Halsted Friday at noon, by work in the surgical outpatient dispensary, and by a course in operative surgery on animals given in the Hunterian Laboratory.[17]

Work in the Department of Medicine also involved students heavily in the daily routines of the hospital.[18] This was Osler's "natural method of teaching," as he called it, in which "the student began with the patient, continued with the patient, ended his studies with the patient, using books and lectures as tools, as means to an end."[19] For the clinical years, Osler made the hospital the laboratory of the medical school, and the students lived and worked in the hospital. By taking careful histories of their patients' illnesses, performing thorough physical examinations, conducting the routine laboratory tests, following the moment-by-moment course of their patients' conditions, and making suggestions regarding management, they obtained personal experience, rather than mere textbook familiarity, with disease and therapy. Students were not expected to learn all the facts about medical diseases but were expected to master the "principles of practice," a phrase so important to Osler that he adapted it for

the title of his textbook, first published in 1892.[20]

Osler's teaching devices reflected the English system of medical education, although he changed the European ideas to fit Hopkins' egalitarian American setting. At eminent teaching hospitals in England, clerks were a student aristocracy; the majority of students had to be content with merely walking the wards. Similarly, in France, although residency in the hospital had become established as the desirable way to learn surgery and medicine, the hospital residency was reserved for an elite selected by competitive examination. In Germany, medical students were not permitted to work in the laboratory, as opportunities for research were given only to advanced students.[21]

The unique idea in American medicine, in contrast, was that the ideal medical education should be available to every medical student, not to just a few. Osler believed that a solid foundation was necessary for all medical students who wanted to become competent practitioners, not just for those who would become teachers and investigators. Similarly, in the basic sciences, Mall argued that every student should acquire good habits in working, observing, and thinking through proper laboratory instruction, regardless of the student's future career. Thus, at Johns Hopkins, elitism marked the admissions process, not the subsequent years of education.

Students could have been overwhelmed by this abundance of intellectual riches. Instead, "they all seemed animated by a desire to master all that was known about man and his ailments," in the words of Rufus I. Cole, a graduate of the Class of 1899:

> The professors made little or no effort to urge them to work. The example of the perfectionists who founded and organized the school and of those who were then directing its activities, seemed to be a sufficient stimulus. . . . It was surprising how happy they all seemed in the unremitting and arduous toil of preparation. The explanation is that they had all been converted to perfectionism. Moreover, a fellowship developed among these disciples like that which is present among the followers of a religion. There was little or no envy or spirit of rivalry, nor

was there evident any undue ambition for future personal success. For the present, the work was all absorbing.

A large group of the students then lived in the houses facing Jackson Place [a one-block square between Fairmount Avenue and Fayette Street]. After working all day in the hospital and laboratories, they had dinner in the near-by boarding houses, and then, especially on pleasant evenings, they were accustomed to congregate about the fountain which stood in the middle of the Square. There they engaged for a short time in gossip and banter, and in conversation, some of it high, some of it not so high. But there existed among them an indescribable spirit of high endeavor. There was an atmosphere of otherworldliness like that which must have been present in the monasteries of old. One was conscious of the other world across town, with its pleasures and distractions, but for the time being that other world seemed distant and unreal. There were then no movies to attend, no automobiles to carry one quickly into the midst of bright lights and gaiety. These interludes did not last long. Soon, one by one, the men would depart. Like horses, eager for the race, they hastened to get back to their studies, and lights would appear here and there in the windows overlooking the Square, and one knew that behind each one was a student eagerly trying to acquire the knowledge that had been accumulated by the workers of the past.[22]

The first students to undergo this peculiarly American form of education—the members of the first graduating class of the Johns Hopkins University School of Medicine—received their degrees on June 15, 1897. President Gilman presided at the ceremony, which took place not at the medical school but in the Academy of Music, one of Baltimore's largest theaters, located near the university on Howard Street.

The Residency System

From the fifteen members of the first graduating class, the Advisory Board chose eleven men and one woman as the hospital's first interns. The Advisory Board decided that interns (known as house medical officers) would spend four months each on the medical, surgical, and gynecological services (and one month of the gynecology rotation would be spent on the obstetrical service). Above them would be a resident physician, surgeon, and gynecologist, who would be supported by assistant residents.[23] After 1900, the interns spent the entire year on a single service.

Of the remaining three graduates, Charles R. Bardeen and Joseph L. Nichols had already accepted faculty appointments in anatomy and pathology, respectively. The third, Richard P. Strong, was appointed in October to fill the place of Charles N. McBryde, who resigned from his internship because of illness. All the places available were thus taken by Hopkins graduates; not until 1914 did graduates of other medical schools begin to fill a substantial proportion of the internships at Johns Hopkins.[24]

It was Osler who introduced residency training at Hopkins, adapting the German system that permitted a physician to spend an indefinite number of years living in the hospital to complete his specialized training. Hopkins medical residents remained for so long that during his sixteen years at Johns Hopkins, Osler trained only five resident physicians (the last of whom, Rufus I. Cole, remained for only a year). The first, appointed at the hospital's opening, was Henri A. LaFleur. His successor, William S. Thayer, was resident physician for the next seven years. During that time, he was in charge of the medical service in the hospital when Osler was absent. Thayer's tenure revealed the wisdom of the residency plan: he acquired the experience and skill to take over much of the teaching of third- and fourth-year students and was well-prepared to care for patients when he left to enter private practice.

The first resident surgeon was Frederick J. Brockway, who had been an intern at the Roosevelt Hospital in New York. The head surgeon, Charles McBurney, had recommended Brockway in response to an inquiry from Halsted. Brockway remained in Baltimore for only a year and a half, leaving to take a post in anatomy at the College of Physicians and Surgeons of Columbia University.[25]

Hunter Robb, the first resident gynecologist, had served as a resident under Kelly in Philadelphia from 1884 to 1886. Robb spent five years

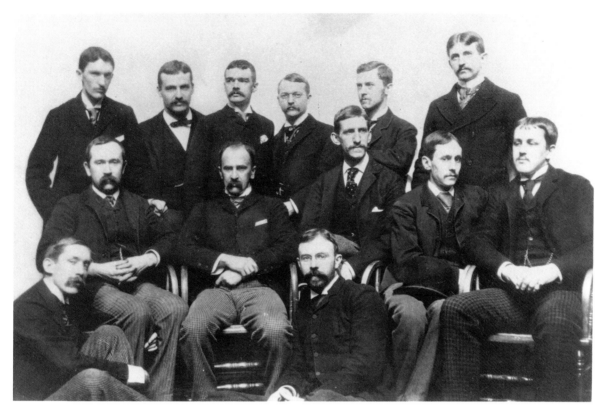

William Osler (*center*) with the first resident staff, 1889–90. *Back row, left to right,* Albert A. Ghriskey, J. M. T. Finney, Alexander Abbott, Hunter Robb, George E. Clark, William Baltzell. *Middle row, left to right,* Frederick J. Brockway, William Osler, Meredith Reese, Henri A. LaFleur, William W. Farr. *Bottom row, left to right,* J. Allison Scott, Harry Toulmin. (*Source:* Alan M. Chesney Medical Archives, The Johns Hopkins Medical Institutions.)

at Johns Hopkins, the first three as resident and the remainder as a member of the hospital staff. He departed for the professorship of gynecology at Western Reserve University in 1894.[26]

Changes at the Turn of the Century

The turn of the century was marked by several "firsts" at the medical school and hospital. The first gift for medical research, $750 a year for five years, was awarded in 1898 for the study of tuberculosis, to be carried out in the outpatient department by C. D. Parfitt. Osler had obtained this grant from an anonymous donor. Two years later, the first endowed professorship in the university was created as the result of a bequest of $24,000 given by Henry Willis Baxley, a well-known physician in Baltimore, on his death in 1876. The in-

terest had been allowed to accumulate, so that by the time the Baxley Professorship in Pathology was established, the fund contained more than $50,000.[27]

The Herter Lectures were inaugurated in the 1903–4 academic year, becoming the first of many endowed lectureships at Johns Hopkins. This series has remained Hopkins' best-endowed and most prestigious lectureship. Its principal purpose is to disseminate the research of foreign investigators in medical science, and lecturers are selected by a standing committee representing the Departments of Pathology, Medicine, and Physiological Chemistry. The first Herter Lecture was delivered by the renowned German scientist Paul Ehrlich, who was in the process of discovering his remedy for syphilis, "Salvarsan," and had already developed his method for staining blood corpuscles, his "side chain theory" of immunity to diseases caused by bacteria, and his concept of specific chemotherapy for infectious diseases. Ehrlich delivered his lecture, "The Mutual Relations between Toxin and Antitoxin," in German, a detail that illustrates the linguistic proficiency expected of Hopkins physicians at the time.[28]

In the hospital, in 1897, staff surgeon J. M. T. Finney was allowed to admit his private patients for treatment—the first time a staff member other than one of the chiefs of service was given this permission. Finney was considering an offer from the University of Maryland, and this privilege, along with an increase in his salary, persuaded him to stay at Johns Hopkins. For years afterward, hospital policy continued to prevent most members of the visiting staff from using the hospital in this way, and Kelly even established his own hospital to accommodate his numerous private patients.[29]

For the first time, beginning in 1898, patients on the private medical wards were charged a fixed amount each week; the Medical Board hoped that this revenue would balance the hospital's deficit for the previous year. The hospital trustees also decided to charge outpatients and "house cases" for medical attention. (House cases were patients who could pay for their care but came directly to the hospital rather than to a private physician; they were assigned to medicine, surgery, or gynecology and were cared for by the chief of the service and his associates.) As more and more private patients came to the hospital, the admitting office began to refer house cases to staff members with so-called private ward privileges—the chiefs of service and Finney. Consequently, the hospital's income from this source diminished as the staff's income increased.

New specialties emerged, as obstetrics and orthopedics were recognized as independent fields of study. A separate Department of Obstetrics was established in the hospital in 1899, the fulfillment of Kelly's long-time wish; and a clinic devoted to orthopedic surgery was created when William S. Baer joined the Dispensary staff in 1900. Surgical pathology had become the first, albeit unofficial, specialty division of the Department of Surgery in 1895, when Halsted appointed

his fourth resident, Joseph C. Bloodgood, to develop this field. Bloodgood knew little about surgery when he arrived for a surgical internship in 1892, having completed a year as resident physician at the Children's Hospital of Philadelphia. Sent to visit the surgical clinics of Europe, he returned with a microtome for cutting frozen sections of tissue and first-hand knowledge of how to stain them. A tireless worker, Bloodgood spent every hour he could spare from private practice working in his laboratory, teaching undergraduate and graduate students, and analyzing cancers of the breast, bone tumors, and other pathological conditions.[30]

At the turn of the century, the medical school and the hospital were starting to reach outside their walls. Postgraduate courses, which had begun before the opening of the medical school, were organized more systematically—with a corresponding increase in enrollment by local physicians. The university also sponsored a commission that studied tropical diseases in the Philippines. In 1899, two members of the faculty—Simon Flexner and Lewellys F. Barker—and two medical students—Joseph Marshall Flint

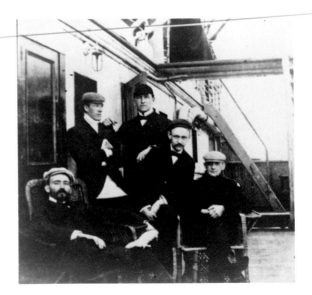

Left to right, John Garrett, Lewellys F. Barker, Joseph M. Flint, Frederick P. Gay, Simon Flexner. (*Source:* The Ferdinand Hamburger, Jr., Archives, The Johns Hopkins University.)

and Frederick P. Gay—traveled with John W. Garrett (who was interested in the political situation in the Philippines) to Manila. There they were met by Richard Strong, a graduate of the medical school's first class who was in charge of the laboratory at the First Army Reserve Hospital in Manila. The commission's work resulted in the isolation by Flexner of the bacillus found in cases of acute dysentery, the organism that now bears his name.[31]

By 1900, the first group of interns at the Johns Hopkins Hospital were moving into faculty positions. This progression from student to faculty member at Hopkins was a natural outcome of the restriction of internships to Hopkins medical school graduates. Few other physicians would qualify as teachers, given the new standards that Hopkins had set. Bardeen and Nichols, members of the first class, had joined the faculty immediately after graduation. After residency, MacCallum and Opie, also members of the first class, were appointed to the staff of the Department of Pathology; Thomas Brown and Louis P. Hamburger joined the faculty in the Department of Medicine; and Percy Dawson received an appointment in the Department of Physiology. One of the most outstanding graduates to join the medical school faculty in this era was Joseph Erlanger, a member of the Class of 1899, who later shared the Nobel Prize in Physiology or Medicine with another Hopkins graduate, Herbert S. Gasser (see chapters 9 and 11).

New special fields of surgery and new procedures developed at Hopkins drew attention to the hospital's surgical services, and patients referred by other physicians swelled the department's inpatient population. The original hospital buildings soon became confining. The Department of Surgery was particularly cramped; in 1901, 1697 patients were treated for surgical disorders. Surgery in the hospital was performed in the Amphitheater, a one-story building with seating space for two hundred persons. The science of surgery had changed since the Amphitheater was constructed, however, and aseptic conditions could not be attained without a separate operating room. As a result, additional facilities were built:

an operating room measuring eighteen by twenty feet, well lighted from the south and east; an "etherizing" room; a recovery room; a surgeons' room; a small three-bed ward; and an "accident reception room," which contained two beds.[32]

The Department of Surgery still needed its own amphitheater, however, where students could observe operations. The improvised arrangements became increasingly unsatisfactory, and Halsted requested a separate building. The high cost led the trustees to demur, but they relented under pressure from the Medical Board. By 1904, Halsted's new building was ready, at a cost of $159,573.53. None of this amount was contributed by the university—the hospital assumed the entire expense.

The senior members of the surgical staff held their own dedication, in the new main operating room on the building's fourth floor. The "ceremony" was a resection of the femur performed by Halsted. James Mitchell, J. M. T. Finney, Harvey Cushing, Joseph Bloodgood, Hugh Young, Richard H. Follis, and F. H. Baetjer replaced the residents as assistants. Cushing referred to this operation as the "All-Star Performance."[33]

Construction of the Henry Phipps Tuberculosis Dispensary was completed a year after the surgical building was ready. A two-story building on Monument Street, it was connected to the Dispensary Building by a corridor. The Phipps Building replaced one of the original hospital structures—the stable.

The Great Baltimore Fire

The progress of the hospital and the medical school came to a sudden halt on February 7, 1904, when a fire swept the city, demolishing much of Baltimore's business district. The fire began in the office building of one of the hospital's trustees, John E. Hurst, who had died just the month before. Fire companies came from as far away as New York. Before the fire was extinguished, two days after it began, more than seventy city blocks in downtown Baltimore were destroyed. The damage to property was estimated to

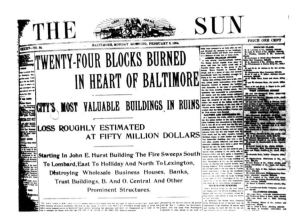

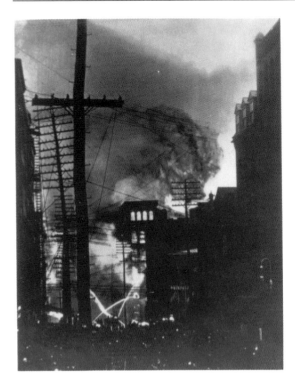

The headline in the Baltimore *Sun*, February 8, 1904. The edition was printed in Washington, D.C., and rushed back to Baltimore by train. (*Source:* Harold A. Williams, *Baltimore Afire* [Baltimore: Schneidereith, 1954; repr. 1979].)

Baltimore afire. Photograph taken seventeen minutes after the first alarm shows the Hurst Building already a blazing ruin. The fire began in this building owned by John E. Hurst, one of the hospital trustees. (*Source:* Harold A. Williams, *Baltimore Afire* [Baltimore: Schneidereith, 1954; repr. 1979].)

be between $125 and $150 million; although the fire did not reach the hospital buildings, to the east of the city, it consumed more than sixty buildings given in Johns Hopkins' will.[34]

The resulting financial strain was considerable. The hospital trustees' immediate response was to ask the staff to economize as much as possible, and to increase the hospital's income by temporarily allowing Drs. Bloodgood, Cushing, and Young to admit private patients. The staff volunteered to work without pay so that the hospital could continue to function, but help arrived from another quarter.

A few years earlier, Osler had received an unsolicited letter from Frederick T. Gates, the financial advisor to John D. Rockefeller, telling him how important his textbook of medicine had been in the founding of the Rockefeller Institute for Medical Research. At the time of the fire, William

Welch was head of the institute's Board of Scientific Advisors, and after the fire, he wrote to Gates soliciting help on behalf of the hospital. Rockefeller dispatched a representative to Baltimore to assess the situation, but before he had reached a decision, articles began appearing in the Baltimore newspapers announcing Rockefeller's intention to give Hopkins a substantial sum. Although these articles caused Welch much embarrassment, they did not deter Rockefeller, who donated $500,000. At the same time, the Maryland legislature authorized a $40,000 grant to the hospital, but Rockefeller graciously declined to reduce the size of his gift.[35]

The End of an Era

One year after the Great Baltimore Fire, Osler accepted the Regius Professorship of Medicine at Oxford University and departed for England. Welch had resigned as dean of the medical faculty in 1898, and Osler had been prevailed upon to succeed him. Osler spent only one year in the deanship before stepping down, weary with the responsibility of running both the entire School of Medicine and the Department of Medicine in the hospital. (He was succeeded by William H. Howell, who served as dean until 1910.)

The deanship had worn down Welch as well:

during his five years as dean, he had organized the school and opened it for classes—all practically unaided. His official correspondence was in longhand, and in fact no carbon or original of a typed letter written by Welch during his deanship has ever been located. Welch's filing system reflected his many responsibilities. As the surgeon Hugh Young described it:

One day I called on Dr. Welch and was admitted to his library. There was no place to sit down. Every one of the eight chairs was piled high with mail, most of it unopened, and so was the desk. Dr. Welch apologized for the appearance of the room. He explained that while I might think his study was in a state of disorder, he really had an excellent system. "On that armchair there I have the letters that have come during the past week; I hope to read these in the near future. On that chair I have the letters that have come within the past month. On the other chairs are letters and magazines anywhere from six months to a year old which I hope to get to sometime." As to the desk, he said that when it got too cluttered up he would open a newspaper, and spread it over the letters and manuscripts, and start afresh. I counted four such layers. There was one little corner of his desk pad which was vacant—just room enough to place a small sheet of note paper on which he wrote in his cramped handwriting.[36]

Welch thus appreciated Osler's decision:

[I]t had become apparent that he could not carry on the whole work which had fallen upon his shoulders. He never neglected the hospital, but gradually there grew up a very large consulting practice, no small part of which consisted of consultations in cases of physicians themselves who came to him from all over the country, so that together with the conduct of the clinic, the care of patients in the hospital, the teaching of the students, and on the other hand a burdensome practice, the weight became too heavy. Physically, in justice to himself, he could not continue. In a sense, then, his acceptance of the call to Oxford was a kind of retirement from this very active clinical work.[37]

Osler left with warm and laudatory feelings for Hopkins. In his valedictory address, he said, "The character of the work of the past sixteen years is the best guarantee of its permanence.

. . . Personally I feel deeply grateful to have been permitted to join in this noble work and to have been united in it with men of such high and noble ideals."[38]

Osler was the first of the original department heads to go. Although his departure removed the most influential member of the clinical group, by 1905 the course of the hospital and the medical school had been set, and he was leaving behind a strong, flexible institution. Since its opening, the hospital had admitted almost 50,000 patients to its wards, and more than 900,000 had been seen in its Dispensary. The resident staff had grown from 10 at its opening to 27; the Dispensary staff from 12 to 62; and more than 350 nurses had been graduated from the Nurses Training School. Similarly, the medical school, which had opened with 9 professors and 6 associates, now had 10 professors, 7 clinical professors, 15 associate professors, 4 lecturers, 13 associates, 12 instructors, and 21 assistants—82 individuals in all. The school had graduated 9 classes totalling 371 doctors of medicine, and classes now contained between 47 and 57 members each.

The Directorship of Lewellys F. Barker: The Department of Medicine Accepts Responsibility for Clinical Science

Osler was a master clinician and diagnostician in the great nineteenth-century British tradition, and he believed that experimental work should be confined to the preclinical science departments. At the same time, he was a proponent of the new medicine, sympathetic to the opinion that experimental studies should supplement work on the wards. As an old-style naturalist-observer, he neither undertook nor vigorously promoted studies of the fundamental nature of disease.[39] His deliberate disregard of the investigation of underlying disease processes may be partly attributed to the lack of adequate facilities for the study of disease, but along with most of his contemporaries in the United States, he did not fully appreciate the rapid progress taking place in physiology and chemistry or the potential of these developments as the basis for important advances in clinical medicine. Investigators in the preclinical sciences likewise believed that medical research could be carried out only in their departments, as clinicians had neither the time nor the training for such activity.

Osler's successor as director of medicine and physician-in-chief was a new type of clinician. Lewellys F. Barker was trained in the basic sciences, coming to Johns Hopkins from a professorship of anatomy. He was instrumental in bringing laboratory investigation into clinical medicine, first at Hopkins, later, by extension, throughout American medicine.

The appointment of a relatively inexperienced clinician to follow in the steps of a master was the outcome of several months of speculation and maneuvering. The manner in which Osler's successor was chosen illustrates the rather informal way in which many of the administrative tasks of the medical school and hospital were handled at the time.[40]

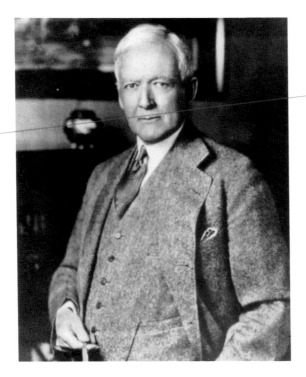

Lewellys F. Barker. (*Source:* Alan M. Chesney Medical Archives, The Johns Hopkins Medical Institutions.)

After Osler had declared his intention to leave Hopkins, Welch bypassed the Advisory Board to write unofficially to Barker. A rumor had reached him, Welch wrote, that Barker was being considered for a position by another university, and Welch hoped that Barker would let him know before accepting any other offer. "I should not write this if I did not consider it fairly probable that an offer would come to you from our medical school, but at the same time," Welch wrote, "I have no assurance of this."

Meanwhile, Welch himself was proposed as the new director, in a memorandum sent to the trustees by William T. Howard, Jr., a graduate of the Hopkins medical school who was then professor of pathology at Western Reserve. The matter soon got into the local newspapers, and the public took it for granted that Welch would be the new department head. Howard's efforts looked as though they might succeed, but Welch finally refused to be recruited.

By the end of 1904, the path was finally clear for Barker, and in December, Mall wrote him an encouraging letter. When the Advisory Board met in January, however, and again two weeks later, no decision was forthcoming. A special meeting of the board was called for March 2, 1905, and Ira Remsen, who had become the university's president, asked for nominations in writing from its members. Mall suggested Barker as "the man who is most likely to raise our department of medicine to a higher level"—a comment that reflects the unhappiness of some members of the preclinical faculty with the conduct of the Department of Medicine under Osler.

William H. Howell, the professor of physiology, recalled that although a majority favored Barker, a minority group inclined toward George Dock, professor of medicine at the University of Michigan. Prolonged informal discussion ensued; no vote was taken. The minority group felt that it had enjoyed the fullest opportunity to express its views, and to make its appreciation manifest, it fell in with the majority to make the vote for Barker unanimous.

Barker's appointment was approved at the

meeting on March 2, and Mall telegraphed him, "Welch will write you the good news." Welch invited Barker to confer with some members of the Advisory Board. The meeting took place in Washington instead of Baltimore, as the Hopkins authorities wished to keep the matter completely secret until they had obtained Barker's acceptance.

Later that month, at its regularly scheduled monthly meeting, the Advisory Board took formal action, making the appropriate recommendation to the university's Board of Trustees. Ten days later, the Medical Board of the hospital recommended to the hospital trustees that Barker be appointed physician-in-chief. Both appointments were promptly approved.

Osler's choice was neither Dock nor Barker, but his former resident William S. Thayer, associate professor of medicine at Hopkins. Thayer was under serious consideration for the post, but the Advisory Board may not have wanted to set the precedent of giving a directorship to the next person in line. When the Advisory Board voted to recommend Barker, it also recommended the appointment of Thayer as professor of "clinical" medicine. Neither the official records of the Advisory Board nor those of the university trustees indicate that Barker and Thayer would share the chair of medicine. That was nevertheless the impression given to the public by the announcement that appeared in the morning edition of the Baltimore *Sun* on April 4, 1905—an announcement that pleased Osler with its inclusion of Thayer as an equal. There was no division of the chair of medicine in 1905, however, when Barker took the helm. Barker was chief of medicine and physician-in-chief, first in the chain of command and under no obligation to consult Thayer in the conduct of the affairs of the department relating to either the hospital or the medical school.

A graduate of the University of Toronto, Barker had interned for one year in Canada and had come to Baltimore in 1891 to work in the Johns Hopkins Hospital. A year in Osler's clinic was followed by a fellowship in pathology under Welch. After the opening of the School of Medicine in 1893, Barker had joined Mall in the anatomical

laboratory, and for the first time he appreciated the excitement of laboratory work, demonstrating the presence of iron in eosinophil cells. Barker was soon promoted to assistant resident pathologist, associate in anatomy, and in 1899, to resident pathologist.

After eight years of close association with Osler, Mall, and Welch, Barker traveled to Germany to study under Von Frey. In Leipzig he carried out a detailed study of the localization of the sensory points in the skin of the arm. This was the beginning of his interest in the nervous system. A pioneer in this field, he soon became an authority. Before he became chief of medicine at Johns Hopkins, Barker's career included membership in Flexner's Commission to the Philippine Islands, a professorship of anatomy at the University of Chicago, and another sojourn in Germany.

Barker and his close colleague Franklin P. Mall were outspoken advocates of the full-time system in clinical departments (see chapter 8). Barker had hoped for a full-time professorship, but the university's endowment was insufficient. He therefore assumed the directorship under the same conditions as his predecessor.

The choice of Lewellys F. Barker as director of the Department of Medicine represented a move from one era to the next. Osler had reported new syndromes, but he had not applied the new scientific knowledge of biochemistry and physiology to the study of disease. Mall in particular knew what the new era should bring, and he wanted Osler replaced—not for any personal reason, but because he believed that Osler would not carry medicine forward. As one of the few who understood what had to be done to advance the science of medicine, Barker had no real competitors for the position. In retrospect, though, he seems poorly qualified for the directorship, having had little experience in caring for patients. It is said that he learned about clinical medicine on the job, from his resident physician Rufus I. Cole. Moreover, he had not demonstrated an outstanding talent for research. Yet Barker was able to seize control of the department, and by selecting outstanding faculty and impressing on them his vision of scientific progress, he made it a model for American medicine.

Barker's Laboratories for Clinical Research

Barker organized three full-time research divisions within the Department of Medicine to provide his staff with opportunities for investigation. Barker's laboratories were unique because they were established for this specific purpose. They were the start of a movement that changed the character of university clinics in the United States and helped to create the scientific base of modern medical practice.

In justifying the need for his three research divisions, Barker spoke of the relation between pure science and practical result, harkening to the technologic progress under way in metallurgy, brewing, and electrical engineering. "Technology has demonstrated how necessary it is for the promotion of the individual arts to secure investigators trained in the so-called sciences of physics, chemistry, and biology," he said, "who will devote themselves to the application of the methods and principles of these sciences to the solution of the special problems by which those who wish to advance the industrial arts are concerned."[41]

The Physiological Division, the first of Barker's three facilities to become operational, opened in 1905. Its purpose was to study individual cases of disease from the standpoint of function. One of its small rooms was located in the Surgical Building, near patients, and employed the special machinery in use in physiological laboratories, particularly graphic methods such as electrocardiography. A second laboratory was situated in the Hunterian Building of the medical school. There, conditions seen in the medical wards could be reproduced in animals and studied physiologically.

Arthur D. Hirschfelder, a graduate of the Hopkins medical school in 1903, was placed in charge of the Physiological Division. After an internship at Hopkins, Hirschfelder had returned to his native San Francisco as assistant in medicine at Cooper Medical College, where his father was a member of the faculty. One year later,

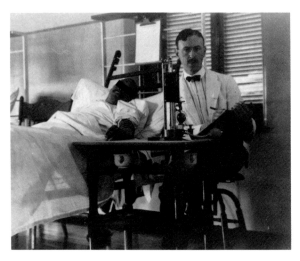

Arthur D. Hirschfelder. (*Source:* Alan M. Chesney Medical Archives, The Johns Hopkins Medical Institutions.)

Hirschfelder came back to Johns Hopkins as an assistant in the Department of Medicine.

As director of the physiological laboratories, Hirschfelder concentrated on disturbances of the heart and the circulation. His volume *Diseases of the Heart and Aorta,* published in 1910, was one of the earliest monographs in cardiology. Hirschfelder left Hopkins in 1913 to join the University of Minnesota as professor of pharmacology.[42]

The Biological Division opened in 1906, under the direction of Rufus I. Cole. Cole had been resident physician at Hopkins since 1904. After completing his second year as resident, he devoted his full time to the new Biological Laboratory, which applied bacteriologic and immunologic methods to the study of patients. During Cole's tenure, the facility occupied three rooms in the southeastern corner of the Surgical Building's second floor. Cole remained at Hopkins until 1910, when he became the first medical director of the Hospital of the Rockefeller Institute.[43]

The Chemical Division also opened in 1906. It was supervised by Carl Voegtlin, a native of Switzerland, whom Barker had recruited from the University of Wisconsin. Osler had a hand in the funding of this third laboratory, asking the university trustees to contribute the $1000 he had donated to Hopkins during a campaign for funds. The trustees responded by adding $1000 of their

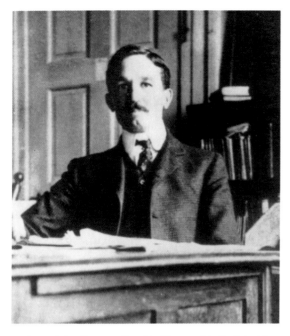

Rufus I. Cole. (*Source:* Alan M. Chesney Medical Archives, The Johns Hopkins Medical Institutions.)

own. The Chemical Laboratory was a neighbor of the Biological Laboratory, occupying a large room on the second floor of the Surgical Building. Voegtlin headed the laboratory for four years; as the culmination of his career, he later became the first director of the National Cancer Institute.

As one of his first efforts in the Chemical Laboratory, Voegtlin demonstrated the value of a high-calorie diet in the treatment of typhoid fever, a debilitating disease also under study in the Biological Laboratory. It was rampant in cities along the Atlantic seaboard, including Baltimore, and Voegtlin's discovery was the first definitive approach to its management. Voegtlin's most important work at Hopkins, done in 1908–1909, provided the first insight into the workings of the parathyroid glands. With William G. MacCallum, he demonstrated that removal of these glands leads to calcium deficiency and that the accompanying postoperative spasms can be controlled by administering calcium.[44]

All three divisions operated on stringent budgets. The Chemical Laboratory, for example, had no stenographer and no assistant. Voegtlin wrote all his manuscripts in longhand and washed the glassware himself. The laboratories were nevertheless the site of pathbreaking investigations. They diversified Hopkins' approach to the study of disease and provided facilities for the training of young physicians interested in clinical methods and scientific investigation.

As the Johns Hopkins Hospital and the Johns Hopkins University School of Medicine entered the twentieth century, they offered the best of American medicine at the time. The innovations that seemed excellent in the early 1900s have retained their luster to the present day, and so embedded have Hopkins' contributions become in the traditions of medical education, practice, and research that today we accept them as ordinary.

Osler's "natural method of teaching" was one of these contributions. The idea that students should begin, continue, and end their studies with the patient, using books and lectures only as tools, seems contemporary and fresh even today. Osler himself identified the innovation in teaching as the best idea to emerge from Johns Hopkins:

> By far the greatest work of the Johns Hopkins Hospital has been the demonstration to the profession of the United States and to the public of this country of how medical students should be instructed in their art. I place it first because it was the most needed lesson, I place it first because it has done the most good as a stimulating example, and I place it first because never before in the history of this country have medical students lived and worked in a hospital as part of its machinery, as an essential part of the work of the wards.[45]

Similarly, other medical schools adopted Osler and Mall's belief in the other facet of "learning by doing," the idea that students should acquire good habits in working, observing, and thinking through first-hand laboratory experience.

Self-education under guidance was the goal of this new brand of medical education, and the faculty at Johns Hopkins believed that it should be available to every student. This was the American achievement in medical education: the application of democratic principles to the training of physicians.[46]

Medical educators have also singled out as particularly effective the graded residencies put in place by Osler, Halsted, and Kelly. This system melded the needs of patients with the needs of medical education. What patients lost in privacy they gained in the quality of care, as they were observed by a hierarchy of physicians rather than by a single physician. The pyramidal Hopkins system required many of the residents to finish their training elsewhere, spreading Hopkins' ideas of medical practice to other hospitals. More than any other factor, the advanced clinical training developed at Johns Hopkins has been identified as the reason for the preeminence of American medicine.[47]

Placing the preclinical departments on a full-time basis was another important innovation. The chairs of anatomy, physiology, pharmacology, and pathology were full-time positions, requiring the physician who filled them to give up his outside income for a lower salary. Welch had correctly predicted that the best scientists would be attracted by the school's laboratory facilities and the prospect of having the time to use them. The success of the full-time system improved medical education, professionalized the preclinical sciences, and thus paved the way for the growth of the research-oriented university school of medicine.

Barker's organization of full-time research laboratories in a clinical department, another innovation at the medical school, laid the foundation for the emergence of clinical science. He created a new academic breed, the clinical scientist, who bridged the gap between the preclinical investigator and the practicing physician. Barker's divisions were adapted by his protégé, Rufus Cole, at the Hospital of the Rockefeller Institute, and Cole's program of research and clinical care, in turn, served as a model for the training of a new generation of clinical chiefs.

At the hospital, Kelly and his associates and successors—Hunter Robb, Thomas S. Cullen, and Guy L. Hunner—revolutionized gynecological surgery in the United States and developed a pathologic laboratory in his department that became a model of its kind. Halsted advanced the practice of surgery with his careful handling of tissues and his original techniques and equipment. In a final break with the age-old tradition that surgery was simply an empirical skill, he related surgery to physiologic research.

Few additional innovations were applied to the organization and operation of the Johns Hopkins hospital and medical school until 1914, when full-time professorships were inaugurated in the clinical departments. The Johns Hopkins hospital and medical school had been started on a good course by wise leaders, whose contributions would endure even after their departure.

CHAPTER 3

CONSOLIDATION AND GROWTH, 1905–1942

That part of the university which, with the hospital, forms the medical school has only had twenty-five years of existence, not a generation, a mere fraction of time in the long history of the growth of science, so that it seems presumptuous to claim any powerful influence on the profession at large. The feeling, however, is strong, too strong to be passed over, that the year 1889 did mean something in the history of medicine in this country.

—William Osler, at the twenty-fifth anniversary of the opening
of the Johns Hopkins Hospital, 1914

Despite the evident sense of progress at Johns Hopkins, the year of Osler's departure for England, 1905, saw American medical education slowly stirring from its slumbers. Osler himself had spoken publicly about its deficits. For the past four decades, individuals and organizations had been considering the standards and training of physicians in this country, with pockets of improvement across the country.

The changes that Osler had hoped for began to occur on a larger scale not long after his departure. Joining forces in the effort to improve medical education in the United States were professional organizations and philanthropic foundations. Both would turn to Johns Hopkins as a model of the best in medical education.

Two organizations, the Association of American Medical Colleges (AAMC) and the American Medical Association (AMA), were attempting to raise the quality of medical education in this country. The AAMC, founded in 1876 with twenty-two schools as members, had tried to en-

courage higher educational standards but, unable to achieve a consensus, it disbanded for seven years. It was revived in 1890, when it was asked to send delegates to a conference on the improvement of medical education, sponsored by five medical schools in Baltimore and the staff of the Johns Hopkins Hospital. Four years later, the AMA conducted a survey that attracted national attention, prompting a series of articles that exposed fraudulent medical institutions and emphasized the poor quality of clinical training generally available for interns and medical students.[1]

During the next decade, the preeminence of German medicine and the example of the Johns Hopkins University School of Medicine contributed to a general rise in standards. By 1900, the AAMC required its member colleges to offer a graded curriculum at least three years in length and to admit only students with a high-school diploma or those who could pass a thorough examination. By 1905, the AMA had devised an "ideal standard" for medical education. Like the

AAMC's, its prerequisites for admission to medical school included a high-school education and a year's training in several of the basic sciences. For medical training itself, the AMA recommended four years of medical school and a year's internship.

Based on these standards, the AMA grouped the nation's medical schools into four classes, A to D, published the results, and distributed them to all medical schools. It drafted a model bill that states could use to license medical practitioners and tried to persuade states not to approve graduates of schools in the lowest category. Finally, the AMA arranged for an independent survey of American medical education, and the Carnegie Foundation for the Advancement of Teaching selected Abraham Flexner to carry it out. The result was the Flexner Report of 1910.[2]

The Flexner Report of 1910

Abraham Flexner was a Kentucky schoolmaster, a writer throughout his ninety-two years, a reformer but not a revolutionary. When he began his famous survey of American medical education, he was forty-two years old, with two decades of varied professional experience behind him. He thus brought to his task considerable experience and a broad perspective. Born in 1866, Flexner graduated from the Johns Hopkins University with a bachelor's degree at the age of nineteen. (His older brother, Simon, also studied at Hopkins, in Welch's Pathological Laboratory). Abraham Flexner then taught high school in his native Louisville, founded and ran a private school, and spent one year in graduate study at Harvard and two more years in Germany. Returning to the United States, Flexner published his first book, a critical study of the American college. His report for the Carnegie Foundation fueled the movement for change already underway by 1910.[3]

"Medicine is part and parcel of modern science," Flexner wrote.[4] His point of departure was the observation that medicine had entered the scientific era. Physics, chemistry, and biology provide the intellectual basis of modern medicine,

Flexner said, but the scientific method—that is, the well-planned experiment—applies to medical practice as well as research. He believed that, for medical students, the best introduction to the scientific method and the most direct route to the acquisition of scientific knowledge was "learning by doing" (see chapter 7).

Flexner's greatest effect on medical education in the United States derived from his advocacy of a particular type of medical school—one with good laboratory facilities for each subject in the preclinical years, and with control of a hospital that would offer students in the clinical years first-hand experience with patients. Flexner envisioned a school that would admit only academically qualified students, who would be exposed to professors who were full-time teachers and investigators. It was therefore important that the medical school be part of a university. Although some criticized his specifications as elitist, they were quite the opposite: Flexner was emphasizing the education of all physicians, not just the brightest. His model system of medical education would provide the best available training to every physician—to bridge the great gap between what was known to medical science and what was known to the average practitioner.[5]

Flexner's report is notable for its scathing indictment of American medical education. Of the 150 medical schools then in existence, he had lukewarm praise for only 5. Of Johns Hopkins, however, he said: "This institution, fortunate in its freedom from all entanglements, in its possession of an excellent endowed hospital, and, above all, in wise and devoted leadership, set a new and stimulating example precisely when a demonstration of the right type was most urgently needed."[6]

Flexner's specifications were formed in the course of long conversations with many individuals in medical education, including members of Hopkins' faculty. Advising Flexner, and thus acting as consultant to the Carnegie Foundation, was William Henry Welch. The reputation of Johns Hopkins made Welch a powerful figure in foundation circles, and Welch was also an adviser to the General Education Board.

The General Education Board and the Rockefeller Foundation

The creation of the great foundations in the first quarter of the twentieth century had important implications for the Johns Hopkins Hospital and the School of Medicine. Through the donations of Johns Hopkins, Mary Garrett, and other individual Baltimoreans, buildings had been constructed and the two facilities had opened. The growing reputation of Johns Hopkins coincided with the creation of large philanthropic funds in the United States. By the early 1900s, the hospital and the medical school had become so well known that they could attract these donors nationwide. The General Education Board provided the support for the major innovation at Johns Hopkins that followed the Flexner Report: the inauguration of full-time professorships in the clinical departments in 1913.

The General Education Board was the second of the several independent philanthropic organizations created by John D. Rockefeller and his advisor, Frederick T. Gates. The first was the Rockefeller Institute for Medical Research, chartered in 1901. The following year, the General Education Board was organized for "the promotion of education within the United States of America, without distinction of race, sex, or creed." The Rockefeller Foundation was incorporated in 1913; in 1928, when several of the Rockefeller family charities were consolidated, the Rockefeller Foundation absorbed the General Education Board.

Flexner came to the attention of Rockefeller and Gates after the publication of his Report of 1910, known as the Carnegie Foundation's "Bulletin Number Four." Gates invited Flexner to lunch, and as Flexner recalled, the conversation at the luncheon was simple and brief:

> Mr. Gates wasted no time on preliminaries. He said:
> "I have read your 'Bulletin Number Four' from beginning to end. It is not only a criticism but a program."
> I replied, "It was intended, Mr. Gates, to be both, for you will remember that it contains two maps: one showing the location and number of medical schools in America today; the other showing what,

in my judgment, would suffice if medical schools were properly endowed and conducted by a well-trained personnel."

> "What would you do," asked Mr. Gates, "if you had a million dollars with which to make a start in the work of reorganizing medical education?"
> Without a moment's hesitation, I replied, "I should give it to Dr. Welch."
> "Why?"
> "With an endowment of four hundred thousand dollars," I answered, "Dr. Welch has created, in so far as it goes, the one ideal medical school in America. Think what he might do if he had a million more. Already the work Dr. Welch and his associates have done in Baltimore is having its effect in reorganizing the personnel of medical schools elsewhere, and we must not forget that but for the Johns Hopkins Medical School there would probably be no Rockefeller Institute for Medical Research in New York today."
> "Would Pritchett [head of the Carnegie Foundation] release you long enough to go to Baltimore to make a detailed study of the situation and report to me?"
> "I think he would," I replied.[7]

Flexner's ensuing visit resulted in the introduction of full-time clinical professorships at Johns Hopkins.

Full-Time Clinical Professorships

As the Johns Hopkins Medical Institutions prospered, the number of faculty members increased; and as the preclinical fields grew more complex, the need to integrate their new knowledge into the clinical fields grew more pressing. Nevertheless, investigators in the preclinical sciences believed that medical research could be carried out only in their departments and that clinicians had neither the time nor the training for such activity. Welch, Mall, and Barker promulgated the idea of salaried clinical professors as a way of repairing the widening breach between clinicians and laboratory investigators.

In the twenty years preceding Flexner's investigation, instruction in the preclinical sciences in medical schools had changed dramatically.

Formerly the province of physicians whose primary occupation was the practice of medicine, by 1910 all the preclinical sciences in the acceptable schools were taught by full-time professors. The clinical departments, in contrast, were still staffed by part-time faculty. These departments, therefore, entered the post-Flexnerian era at a disadvantage compared to their preclinical counterparts.

The idea that experimental methods could be applied to research in clinical disciplines was nevertheless gaining wide currency. Young clinical scientists shared the same academic values as their colleagues in the preclinical departments: increasing numbers aspired to careers in teaching and research, rather than in private practice. The full development of clinical science awaited the recognition that, like anatomy, biochemistry, and physiology, the clinical disciplines were valid university subjects.

Welch and his colleagues attributed the problem to the isolation of the clinical staff, whose private practices kept them from participating fully in the hospital's teaching and research. Welch's solution was to appoint clinicians with investigative experience as chiefs of the clinical services. Clinical chairs would thus resemble the other professorships, and clinical services would be fully absorbed into the university programs.

Yet the concept of full-time clinical professors generated widespread opposition. Many felt that the clinician who accepted a full-time salary would be poorer and sadder—as would the school that had to pay his salary. Abandoning a private practice would also cut the clinician off from valuable experience and deprive patients of his superior services. Osler was a particularly eloquent critic of the proposed full-time plan for the clinical departments. The large fortunes made by members of the clinical staff were "largely illusory" anyway, he wrote to Ira Remsen, then president of the university:

> The truth is, there is much misunderstanding in the minds, and not a little nonsense on the tongues, of the people about the large fortunes made by members of the clinical staff. At any rate, let the Univer-

sity and Hospital always remember with gratitude the work of one "prosperous" surgeon, whose department is so irritatingly misunderstood by Mr. Flexner. I do not believe the history of medicine presents a parallel to the munificence of our colleague Kelly to his clinic. Equal in bulk, in quality, and in far-reaching practical value to the work from any department of the University, small wonder that his clinic became the Mecca for surgeons from all parts of the world, and that his laboratory methods, perfected by Drs. Cullen and Hurdon, have become general models, while through the inspiration of Mr. Max Brödel a new school of artistic illustration in medical works has developed in the United States. And, shades of Marion Sims, Goodell and Gaillard Thomas! this is the department which the "Angel of Bethesda," in the fullness of his ignorance, suggests should be, if not wiped out, at any rate merged with that of Obstetrics![8]

Welch persevered: In 1910, when the Hospital of the Rockefeller Institute opened with a staff of full-time clinicians, Welch began negotiations with the Rockefeller officials and the Hopkins faculty. Flexner arrived the next year as an emissary of the General Education Board. It took three years for Welch to win the faculty's support, however, and not until 1913 did he have sufficient backing at home to ask the General Education Board for aid. Then, assisted by a $1.5 million grant from the General Education Board, Hopkins placed its Departments of Medicine, Surgery, and Pediatrics on a full-time basis. This was another turning point in American medicine (see chapter 8).

The plan went into effect immediately in the surgical department, and Howland in pediatrics also accepted the new arrangement. Theodore C. Janeway became the first full-time professor of medicine in 1914. As funds became available, additional clinical chairs were made full-time: obstetrics in 1919, psychiatry in 1923, and ophthalmology in 1925.[9]

Full-time status did not cut clinicians off from their private patients entirely. They were permitted to serve as consultants, but all fees were paid to the university and held for the benefit of the medical school. This avoided some criticisms but engendered others, as the plan placed medical school faculty in competition with private physicians.

It is important to emphasize that the full-time system in the clinical departments applied only to a few members of the staff with professorial rank. The rest of the clinical faculty remained on a part-time basis. This diversity was beneficial to the medical school and hospital inasmuch as the very existence of the plan pressured all clinical professors to value research, and the presence of part-time associates maintained private practice as an important influence. With the completion of the Marburg Building in 1913, more beds became available for private patients, and the part-time faculty flourished.[10]

The system of full-time clinical professorships at Johns Hopkins led to rapid change nationwide, as the General Education Board used Hopkins as a model to introduce similar arrangements at other medical schools. By the 1920s, the caliber of medical education in the United States had greatly improved, thanks in part to financial assistance from foundations such as the General Education Board. Many clinical professors, like professors in the preclinical departments, had become full-time teachers and investigators. The critical mass of Hopkins-trained faculty in certain American medical schools was sufficiently great to cast them in the Hopkins image, and the movement of Hopkins faculty and students undoubtedly accelerated the rate at which the full-time system became entrenched in American medical education. Although national acceptance of the full-time system was not easily won (the American Medical Association and its Council on Medical Education opposed it as "extreme") and some schools delayed for many years, most medical schools eventually adopted some version of it (for a fuller description, see chapter 8).[11]

For Hopkins, the program represented a final step in integrating the medical school with the university. After the controversy had subsided, Welch told Flexner that even if the full-time scheme were utterly abandoned, clinical teaching in America could never retreat. Like the preclini-

cal departments, the clinical departments had become a home for research.[12]

The First Full-Time Department of Medicine

Barker had asked Welch for a full-time appointment when he was offered the directorship of the Department of Medicine in 1905, but at the time the money for his salary was not available. When funds for this purpose were finally in hand in 1913, Barker was unwilling to give up his large private practice, and he declined the full-time chair in medicine. This was a surprising reversal, since it was Barker's 1902 speech that had roused so many to support the full-time system. Barker made it clear, however, that personal reasons, not a change in attitude toward the full-time system, had dictated his decision (see chapter 8).[13]

Barker, therefore, stepped down as director of medicine. Succeeding him as head of the department was Theodore Caldwell Janeway. The son of Edward G. Janeway, one of the foremost

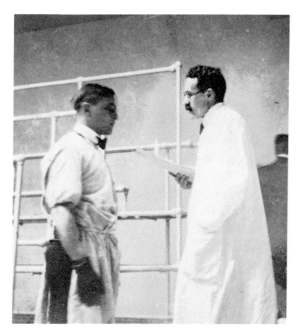

Right, Theodore Caldwell Janeway, the first full-time professor of medicine; *left,* Milton Winternitz, a protégé of Welch, who became professor of pathology and dean of the Yale Medical School. (*Source:* William Thomas, M.D.)

physicians of his day, Theodore Janeway had attended Yale University, where he came under the influence of the great biochemist Russell H. Chittenden. Three years after graduating, in 1895, Janeway received the medical degree from the Columbia University College of Physicians and Surgeons. In 1909, he became Bard Professor of Medicine at Columbia, and two years later, he succeeded Christian A. Herter as the representative of internal medicine on the board of scientific directors of the Rockefeller Institute.

As a clinician, Janeway was one of the first modern internists to think in terms of the natural history of a disease and its dynamics, and the first to measure blood pressure routinely in his office. Janeway defined treatment as "a therapeutic experiment based on a theory. This theory we call a diagnosis." Moreover, his belief that the experimental approach was "the only sure basis for the successful practice of the art of medicine" was unique for the time.[14]

Janeway's greatest contribution to clinical science was his work on blood pressure: he was among the first in America to study hypertension and its relation to the heart and kidneys clinically and experimentally. His treatise on hypertension, published in 1904, is a classic.[15] He was also one of the first to advocate the long-term use of digitalis for minor grades of cardiac insufficiency, and in 1914, at least five years before anyone else mentioned the subject, he prescribed digitalis for patients who had normal cardiac rhythm but cardiac insufficiency secondary to prolonged high blood pressure.

As a teacher, Janeway emphasized the rational interpretation of symptoms and the importance of pathological physiology. He was among the first in the United States to teach the concept of disease as a deviation from the physiological normal, an idea well known decades earlier in Germany.[16] In style, Janeway's instructional approach was an improvement over the customary memorization- and recitation-based educational method to which medical students were usually subjected.

The bare bones of Janeway's accomplishments do not convey the qualities of intelligence,

leadership, and energy that explain his success in the several aspects of medicine. At Columbia, he became the leader of a younger group of "physiological clinicians" who helped to transform American medicine.

Hopkins had obviously acquired an outstanding physician of the day as one of its first full-time department heads. For his part, Janeway considered the professorship of medicine at Hopkins particularly appealing because his post at Columbia afforded him little time for experimental work. Arriving in 1914, Janeway found a medical clinic organized largely in accord with his ideals for patient care, laboratory work, teaching, and investigation, a clinic existing alongside others similarly organized and associated with strong departments in the preclinical sciences. Janeway maintained Barker's three research divisions, adding Herman O. Mosenthal as associate professor in charge of the Chemical Laboratory. He also retained nearly all of the staff already in the department and quickly made the readjustments necessary to put the department on a "full-time" basis.

Janeway nevertheless became disillusioned

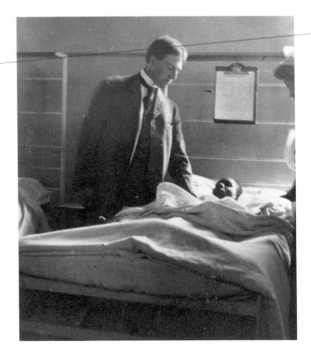

William S. Thayer. (*Source:* Alan M. Chesney Medical Archives, The Johns Hopkins Medical Institutions.)

with the full-time plan. Despite improved facilities for research, he suffered financial hardship because of the restrictions on his income. In 1917 he resigned his professorship at Hopkins with the idea of returning to New York. He died suddenly, from pneumonia, before leaving Baltimore, and Mosenthal assumed the temporary directorship of the department.[17]

William S. Thayer, clinical professor of medicine, was appointed director in early 1918, but he was studying typhus in Europe and could not assume the post until the following year. Louis Hamman replaced Mosenthal as department head until Thayer's return in 1919 (see chapter 8).

Thayer's training had been predominantly clinical. After receiving the medical degree from Harvard in 1889, he served as a house officer at the Massachusetts General Hospital. He then spent time studying in Germany, coming to Johns Hopkins as an assistant resident physician in 1890. He was appointed chief resident in 1891 and remained in that post for seven years.

In Germany, Thayer had acquired expertise in using Ehrlich's new technique of staining blood cells, and he became one of the first clinicians to employ blood cultures in the study of patients with fever and heart murmurs. Thayer thus attracted many physicians to the clinical laboratory to study with him. He was primarily interested in malaria, a disease rampant in Baltimore in the 1890s. The discovery of the malarial parasite by Alphonse Laveran had been confirmed in America by William T. Councilman and William Osler. Thayer's investigations with John Hewetson, another member of the Department of Medicine, enlarged the knowledge of the subject, and his lectures on malarial fever, published in 1897, carried the new knowledge through the English-speaking world.[18]

Thayer's career spanned the transition between the old school and the modern school of "physiological medicine," and his ideas about research and departmental organization reflected his familiarity with both perspectives. Although a sound basis in the fundamental sciences was desirable for the trained and scholarly physician, it was not a shortcut to the practical experience es-sential to making a good diagnostician, a good doctor, and a good clinical teacher. This type of experience, Thayer said, must be gained by prolonged and systematic training in ward and outpatient departments, and through studies in pathological anatomy and in physical diagnosis. Thayer thus brought the perspective of a clinician to the directorship of the department.

The First Full-Time Department of Pediatrics

Not until 1912 was a separate facility established at Hopkins for the care of children. When the hospital opened, the Department of Pediatrics was a part of the Department of Medicine. The number of sick infants and children with diarrhea and nutritional deficiencies soon exceeded the available hospital beds, although an outpatient clinic tried to fill the gap by performing diagnostic studies and prescribing treatment for parents to carry out at home.

Construction of a separate facility near Hopkins, to be named the Harriet Lane Home for Invalid Children, was specified by the will of Mrs. Harriet Lane Johnston, a resident of Baltimore whose two sons had died in their youth. The home was first planned as a permanent residence for crippled and chronically ill children, but by 1905, the idea of a hospital had evolved. If an adequate site was to be purchased, buildings erected, and a sum set aside for a permanent endowment, however, Mrs. Johnston's bequest would provide a hospital able to care for only about twenty-five children at a time. An alliance with the Johns Hopkins Hospital therefore seemed mutually advantageous, and a formal agreement was proposed and accepted. Hopkins would supply a site for the buildings and provide for the medical care of the patients. The Harriet Lane Home, for its part, would contribute a modern, 100-bed hospital building, adapted for the treatment of children's diseases.

Barker wanted to obtain a director for the new Department of Pediatrics immediately, to supervise the building and the organization of its facilities. At Barker's suggestion, the university established a professorship of pediatrics and appointed Clemens von Pirquet, a thirty-four-year-old native of Vienna, to fill the post. Von Pirquet had already made significant contributions in infection and immunity, extending his investigation of serum disease (begun with Bela Schick) to a study of the results of reinoculation with smallpox virus. To his discovery of the phenomenon of acquired hypersensitivity he gave the name "allergy," and he developed the cutaneous test for tuberculosis that bears his name.[19]

Von Pirquet came to Baltimore in 1909; the next year he was offered the professorship of pediatrics at the University of Breslau and took a leave of absence to consider the post. He had agreed to let Hopkins know his decision by the end of the year, but made his return contingent upon a raise in salary from $7,500 to $10,000 per year, which the trustees were unwilling to provide. In the midst of negotiations, von Pirquet was offered a professorship of pediatrics in Vienna—which he accepted.[20]

The Hopkins trustees had anticipated von Pirquet's defection, and the Medical Board immediately authorized Welch to offer the position to John Howland, professor of pediatrics at Washington University in Saint Louis. In 1912, Howland replaced Samuel Amberg, the acting chief, as director of the Harriet Lane Home and professor of pediatrics. A grant from the General Education Board established the position on a full-time basis in 1913.

Under Howland's direction, research in pediatrics at Hopkins flourished. It was Howland's teacher, L. Emmett Holt, who had laid the foundation of biochemical investigation in pediatrics in the first decade of the twentieth century. Holt had been a member of the original Board of Scientific Advisors of the Rockefeller Institute for Medical Research, and the Institute supported Holt's well-equipped laboratories at the Babies Hospital in New York. Howland had studied in these laboratories after graduating from Yale University and the New York University School of Medicine. An internship and two years of residency training at Presbyterian Hospital in New York were followed by another year's internship at the New York Foundling Hospital, where Howland encountered

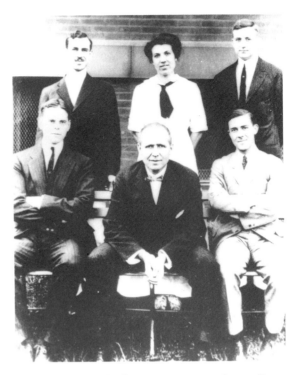

John Howland and the first Harriet Lane resident staff. *Standing, left to right,* Arthur L. Walters, Eleanor B. Wolf, and William B. McClure (interns); *seated, left to right,* Edwards A. Park, director of outpatient services; John Howland, professor of pediatrics; and Kenneth D. Blackfan, resident pediatrician. (*Source:* Alan M. Chesney Medical Archives, The Johns Hopkins Medical Institutions.)

Holt. Further study in Berlin and Vienna inspired Howland to become an investigator rather than a practitioner, and upon his return to the United States in 1902, he was appointed Holt's assistant.[21]

Howland was given the professorship of pediatrics at Washington University in 1910. To prepare for this appointment, he returned to Europe to study under the most distinguished pediatrician of the time, Adalbert Czerny. Here he developed his interest in the nutritional disorders of children and began to appreciate the use of chemistry as a research tool. He returned to Saint Louis in 1911, leaving six months later for Baltimore.

Howland's full-time status at Johns Hopkins allowed him to establish the nation's preeminent research laboratory in pediatrics. For the first time, the techniques of biochemistry were applied systematically to the study of diseases in childhood. With no preexisting pediatric staff, Howland was able to select his own group—Edwards A. Park, Kenneth Blackfan, Grover Powers, and W. McKim Marriott—every one of whom later headed his own department of pediatrics.[22]

The Medical Institutions in World War I

Work in laboratories and clinics was interrupted as about 700 Johns Hopkins medical graduates served in the armed services during World War I. The Johns Hopkins medical community contributed to the war effort on several fronts. Hopkins faculty members were active in policy-making in Washington—Welch as president of the National Academy of Sciences, Hospital Superintendent Winford Smith as chief of the hospital division of the Surgeon General's Office, and Theodore C. Janeway as medical consultant in the Surgeon General's Office. Many faculty members were stationed overseas and in camps throughout the United States. In 1918, one third of all faculty members were on active duty; of the full time, younger faculty members, more than half served in this country or abroad. When the Armed Forces reached France, several Hopkins men received important assignments. Finney was made chief consultant in surgery to the American Expeditionary Forces (AEF). Boggs was placed in charge of the medical service of the Aviation Corps. Hugh Young, designated director of the AEF's division of urology, accompanied General Pershing to Europe.

The Second Faculty

As World War I ended, age and attrition began to erode the original medical faculty. Kelly became emeritus in 1919; Mall died in 1917, Halsted in 1922. Of the original senior faculty, the only members still active in the 1920s were Abel and Jones from the preclinical departments; Williams from the full-time clinical faculty; and Finney, Barker, Cullen, and Thayer of the part-time faculty.

Shifts in leadership had placed Hopkins stalwarts in new positions within the medical institutions. Hurd had retired as hospital superintendent in 1911, after a tenure of twenty-two years. His successor was his deputy, Winford Smith, who remained until after World War II. (Midway through his tenure, the title of superintendent was abolished, and the head of the hospital became known as its director.) Welch had left the School of Medicine for the School of Hygiene and Public Health. So had Howell, who was replaced by J. Whitridge Williams as dean of the medical school in 1911.

The need to replace many senior faculty members, coupled with the abundant financial resources available from the General Education Board and a bequest in 1919 from Joseph R. De Lamar, led to a time of rapid change at the medical school and the hospital. Between 1916 and 1927, new department heads were appointed for anatomy, medicine, gynecology, pathology, pediatrics, physiological chemistry, physiology, and surgery—and the faculty grew as these new department heads brought in junior associates. The creation of two new departments—the Wilmer Ophthalmological Institute in 1925 and the Institute of the History of Medicine in 1929—further increased the number of faculty members.

In selecting the new department heads, the Advisory Board usually carried on the informal tradition at Johns Hopkins of obtaining "the best man wherever he could be found." They chose faculty from outside the institution, not simply promoting to the chair the next most senior faculty member in line. Senior part-time staff members naturally favored appointing local physicians with superior clinical ability, but the preclinical faculty has traditionally preferred a candidate with a strong background in research as well, and the full-time clinical staff tended to side with the preclinical faculty. Investigative accomplishment has thus been a prime requisite for department heads at Johns Hopkins.

The best candidate was often a Hopkins graduate who had been exported to another medical school. When the General Education Board helped schools such as Washington University in

Saint Louis and Yale University to reorganize their clinical departments on a full-time basis, Hopkins provided much of the staff (see chapter 9). Hopkins' relatively long experience with the full-time system had allowed it to educate a substantial number of faculty members, and the choice of Hopkins-trained individuals by other medical schools reflected the preponderance of Hopkins physicians in the pool.

The early house officers, fellows, and junior faculty members at Hopkins set the pattern that persists to this day: most departed from Baltimore to advance in other medical schools. The Hopkins graduates who returned were only a small fraction of those who left to fulfill John Shaw Billings' hope that Hopkins-educated physicians would "spread the influence of such training far and wide." Hopkins' informal tradition of obtaining its own graduates as department heads gave rise to the generally accepted notion that for a Hopkins man to become a department head at his own school, he had to win his spurs elsewhere.

The new department heads and their associates were known as the "second faculty" because they replaced the original group of department leaders. According to some assessments, this second group was second-best, their abilities and achievements eclipsed by those of their predecessors. Others have disagreed, including the eminent neurologist Stanley Cobb:

> Many physicians speak of an earlier time as the "Golden Age of Medicine" when Osler, Welch and Halsted developed a great center of American medicine. In 1915, we still had Halsted, Howell and Abel, with Barker, Howland, Thayer, Janeway, Meyer and McCollum [sic]. They were the teachers who drew us to Baltimore and inspired us. But it was the *young men* who made that time so exciting. Blackfan, Park, Gamble, Mariott [sic] and Powers at the Harriet Lane; Bloomfield, Austrian, Levy, Thomas, Pincoffs and King in Medicine; Heuer, Reid and Dandy in Surgery; Moore, Watson, Richter, Lewis, Greenacre with me at the Phipps; and across the street in the Medical School laboratories: Drinker, Lamson, Binger, Bayne-Jones, Rivers, Richardson, Wilson, Weed, and Clark. These are only a few of those who made this time great.[23]

The first two decades of the twentieth century are often characterized as years of relative decline for Johns Hopkins, years when the pace of innovation and the pursuit of excellence slackened. More accurately, these were the years when other schools rose to its level.

As a group, the second faculty was relatively young—but not as young as the first faculty had been. As investigators, they and the junior faculty members they attracted continued, and even exceeded, the investigative accomplishments of their predecessors; in the new, more technologically advanced era of medical research, they were on the cutting edge.

Lewis H. Weed had been at the top of his medical school class at Johns Hopkins. He accompanied Harvey Cushing to Boston in 1912, returning to Hopkins two years later; and in 1917, Weed replaced Mall as head of the Department of Anatomy.[24]

Welch's successor as head of the Department of Pathology was William G. MacCallum, a member of the first class to graduate from the Hopkins medical school; MacCallum completed a rotating internship at Hopkins, joined Welch's staff, and then left to become head of the Department of Pathology at the Columbia University College of Physicians and Surgeons.[25]

E. Kennerly Marshall, Jr., received both a doctorate in chemistry and a medical degree from Johns Hopkins; he returned to Hopkins from Washington University in Saint Louis to succeed William H. Howell as head of the Department of Physiology. Marshall was one of the first Hopkins faculty members with both M.D. and Ph.D. degrees.[26]

William M. Clark followed Walter Jones as head of the Department of Physiological Chemistry in 1927; Clark was not a physician, but he had received his doctorate in chemistry from Hopkins and was at the time of his appointment professor of chemistry at what later became the National Institutes of Health.[27]

In the Department of Medicine, Thayer was replaced first in 1921 by G. Canby Robinson (who took the position on a temporary basis) and then

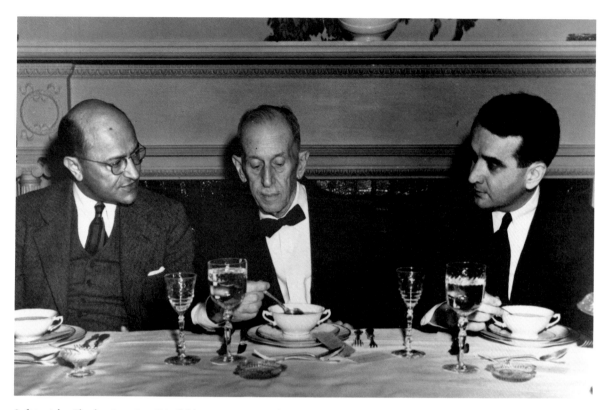

Left to right, Charles Austrian, Warfield T. Longcope, and A. McGehee Harvey (1946).

finally the next year by Warfield T. Longcope, who was forty-four years old when he assumed the directorship.[28]

After receiving the A.B. and M.D. degrees from Hopkins, Longcope had joined the staff of the Ayer Laboratory at the Pennsylvania Hospital. Under the direction of Simon Flexner, Longcope began investigations in immunology. His work included training in pathology, biochemistry, bacteriology, and serology. He also visited the wards frequently, giving advice about diagnosis and treatment. In 1911, Longcope moved from an assistant professorship at the University of Pennsylvania to an associate professorship at Columbia University College of Physicians and Surgeons, where he succeeded Theodore Janeway as Bard Professor when Janeway departed for Baltimore.

Thayer had brought a clinician's point of view to the directorship and Robinson, an educator's. As their successor, Longcope was a uniquely

trained academician who set a new standard of learning in several scientific disciplines, all of which merged in a broader approach to the problems of disease and a comprehensive etiologic and pathophysiologic understanding of its nature. His training and decisions reflected the outlook of the clinical investigator—a renaissance man with the ability to perform skillfully in both the laboratory and the clinic. By stimulating research activity in clinical fields, Longcope was a bridge between the old-time clinician and the modern clinical investigator. He identified the investigation of the fundamental processes that form the basis of disease in human beings as the most fertile field of work for physician investigators.[29] (For more information about Thayer and Longcope, see chapter 8.)

Edwards A. Park, who succeeded John Howland as head of pediatrics in 1927, met Howland when Park was a resident at the New York Foundling Hospital. In 1911, Park joined Howland in

Baltimore as associate and then associate professor; he became professor at Yale in 1921, returning to Hopkins six years later.

The department changed considerably under Park's direction, mainly because of his decision to establish a number of subdivisions, including cardiology, endocrinology, neurology, and psychiatry (see chapter 9). Park realized that medicine was becoming increasingly specialized, and he moved to bring his department into the forefront of progress. The department's early success seemed to bolster his predecessor's decision not to segregate patients in clinics by type of illness. Some of the physicians on the staff of the Harriet Lane Home therefore thought that specialty clinics would weaken the pediatric dispensary, but Park relied on the resulting improvement in patient care to bring more children to the hospital. As he expected, word of the new divisions traveled rapidly, and a growing number of children with severe and unusual conditions came to the clinics.[30]

In the Department of Surgery, J. M. T. Finney was made acting head of the department when Halsted died in 1922, and Robert T. Miller, Jr., was appointed associate professor on a full-time basis. A poll of the department unanimously recom-mended Finney as permanent department head, but he declined to be considered because of his age (he was almost sixty years old). As a compromise, he agreed to serve as chief for an additional two years.[31] Dean DeWitt Lewis, the next permanent chief of surgery, had no prior connection with Hopkins, having come to Baltimore from Chicago, where he was professor of surgery at the University of Illinois and surgeon-in-chief at the new university hospital.[32]

The heads of the Departments of Gynecology and Obstetrics were links between the first and second faculties. J. Whitridge Williams directed the Department of Obstetrics from 1899 until his death in 1931.[33] Kelly's successor as head of the Department of Gynecology in 1919 was Thomas S. Cullen, who had come to Johns Hopkins in 1891, just two years after the hospital opened; he remained a member of the faculty until his death in 1953.[34]

New Departments and Programs

The new institutes, departments, and programs added between 1905 and 1930 contributed to the final fundamental shape the Johns Hopkins Med-

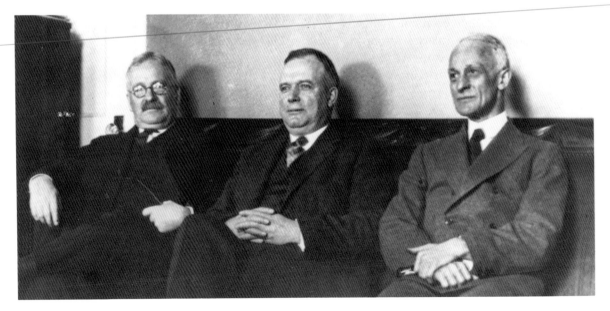

Members of the Department of Surgery. *Left to right,* J. M. T. Finney, Dean DeWitt Lewis, and Harvey W. Cushing. (*Source:* Alan M. Chesney Medical Archives, The Johns Hopkins Medical Institutions.)

ical Institutions would assume until the surge of specialization that followed World War II. They included the Johns Hopkins School of Hygiene and Public Health; the medical school's Departments of Psychiatry, Ophthalmology, and the History of Medicine; the Program in Art as Applied to Medicine; and, in the hospital, the Social Service Department.

The Social Service Department

Although Johns Hopkins was not the first hospital to have an organized social service department, the degree of the department's integration into a large general hospital was unique for the time. The Social Service Department was founded in 1907 under the direction of Helen B. Pendleton. She remained for only a year, as did her successor, Helen S. Wilmer. The third head of the department, Margaret S. Brogden, served until her retirement in 1931. Under her leadership, the department expanded to include dozens of paid staff members and volunteers.

Margaret Brogden's retirement coincided with the Great Depression, Lacking permanent leadership and an adequate budget, the department fell into decline, just at a time when its services were particularly needed by patients affected by the difficult economic climate. The amount budgeted for salaries dropped from $41,700 in 1931 to $10,000 in 1934. The work load increased while the staff was curtailed, and as a result, most social service was offered in the outpatient clinics rather than on the wards.

The Social Service Department was revived in the late 1930s through the efforts of G. Canby Robinson, then a member of the Department of Medicine. He obtained additional funds for staff, and a new full-time director, Amy Greene, arrived in 1939. Brogden's training as a nurse had reflected the orientation of the social services before the 1930s. In contrast, the sociological training of Greene and her staff marked them as a new generation of medical social workers. Greene centralized the social service activities within the hospital (the Phipps and Harriet Lane social services were maintained separately), standardized

the varied sources of salaries so that all social workers were paid by the hospital, and worked toward acquiring a formally trained staff.[35]

Art as Applied to Medicine

The program in Art as Applied to Medicine was funded in 1910 by Henry Walters, a Baltimore businessman with a deep interest in art. Thomas S. Cullen, a faculty member in the Department of Gynecology, had persuaded Walters to donate $15,000 to create a permanent home for Max Broedel, a gifted medical artist. Broedel had come to Hopkins in 1894, but sixteen years later he was considering an offer from a large private clinic. Cullen hoped that by obtaining funds from Walters, he could convince Broedel to remain as head of his own program.

Max Broedel had entered his profession by accident. A student at art schools in Leipzig, he had been called upon by Carl Ludwig in the summer of 1888 when Ludwig's regular artist became ill. At Ludwig's physiological laboratory, Broedel met and worked for Welch and Mall. A few years later, Broedel decided to come to the United States to continue this association.

When Broedel arrived in Baltimore, he found Mall too busy to use the services of an illustrator, and he was passed along to Howard Kelly, head of gynecology. There were no other artists at Johns Hopkins at the time, and Broedel was often "loaned" to other members of the faculty. Broedel believed that the training of other artists was as important as his own artwork. Beginning in 1905, he conducted a class in general technical sketching for histology, gross anatomy, and pathology, and he devoted several hours each week to teaching throughout the medical school.

Broedel's work for Kelly was finished in 1910, and he began to look for employment elsewhere. Cullen's offer, backed by Walters' support for a Department of Art as Applied to Medicine, enabled Broedel to train a new generation of medical artists, sparing these medical students and art students the years of trial and disappointment that their self-taught predecessors had endured.[36]

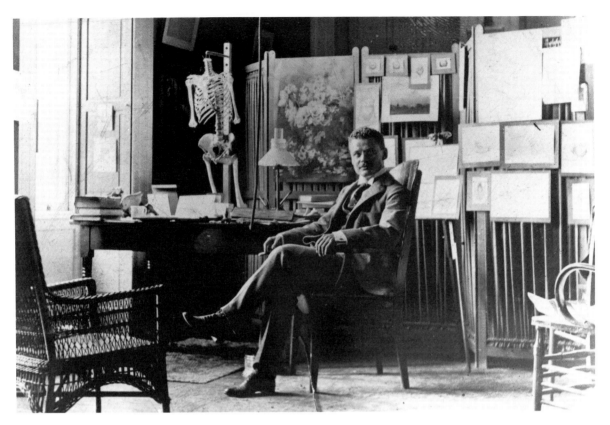

Max Broedel. (*Source:* Alan M. Chesney Medical Archives, The Johns Hopkins Medical Institutions.)

The First Department of Psychiatry

The funds for an institute of psychiatry at Johns Hopkins were donated by Henry Phipps, a Philadelphia trustee of the Johns Hopkins Hospital and a long-time contributor to the hospital's building program. Only two university psychiatric clinics existed in America before Johns Hopkins opened its facility, the first at the University of Michigan and the second in Boston.[37] Phipps' bequest enabled the hospital to build and maintain a psychiatric clinic and allowed the university to establish a post that combined the professorship of psychiatry with the directorship of the clinic.

The separation of the psychiatric patients in the new clinic reflected the nationwide effort by psychiatrists to distance their field from neurology. Before the construction of the psychiatric clinic, neurological and psychiatric cases had been treated and studied in the outpatient department by neurologist Henry M. Thomas and psy-

chiatrist Henry J. Berkley. Berkley was also head of the Bay View Insane Asylum, where medical students received instruction in the care of psychiatric inpatients. Although President G. Stanley Hall of Clark University, a Johns Hopkins University graduate, had been instrumental in introducing Freudian thought into the United States, it was the Phipps Psychiatric Clinic that transformed psychiatry from the almost exclusive concern of "asylum" superintendents into a university discipline.

This transformation was largely the work of the new head of psychiatry at Hopkins, Adolf Meyer. He assumed the post in 1909, in time to participate in the planning of the new clinic. Forty-one years old when he came to Hopkins, Meyer was a native of Zurich and had lived in the United States for fifteen years. He had served as pathologist to an asylum in Kankakee, Illinois, and as clinical director of the Worcester State Hospital in Massachusetts, where he taught stu-

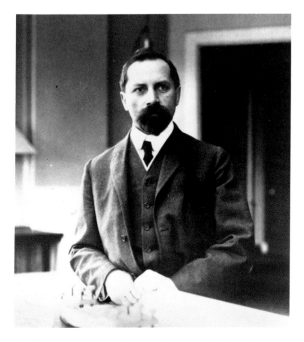

Adolf Meyer. (*Source:* Alan M. Chesney Medical Archives, The Johns Hopkins Medical Institutions.)

dents at neighboring Clark University. Meyer next moved to Ward's Island, in New York, where he was director of the Pathological Institute of the New York State Hospitals for the Insane. A concurrent appointment at Cornell Medical College kept him involved in academic life, and he published numerous articles in medical journals.

Meyer emphasized a biologic orientation, but he was one of the first to see the implications of the social sciences for medicine. His influence among professionals in these fields transcended his own institution, as his methods and ideals were adopted by many clinics throughout the nation.[38]

Meyer had been at Johns Hopkins for four years before the Phipps Clinic was completed. In that time, he was able to establish a comprehensive program of instruction for the medical students and design a useful plant that proved to be a model of psychiatric service. The Phipps Clinic provided facilities for the care of patients with all types of mental disorders (from the simplest psychopathological disturbances to the frank psychoses) as well as laboratories and other research facilities for the study of the somatic accompaniments of mental disorders, and for original investigations in neuropathology and psychopathology.

The Phipps Clinic was formally opened in 1913, but modern psychiatric concepts coexisted with superstition: the bronze plaque outside the building gave the year as 1912, because a year ending in thirteen was considered bad luck.

The clinic was located on the south side of the hospital lot and connected to the Harriet Lane Home by corridors at ground and basement levels. The clinic faced north, and its front part was devoted almost exclusively to administrative, laboratory, and staff quarters. Its outpatient department, for patients with milder disturbances, was located in the basement. The clinic proper, for inpatients, was situated in a five-story pavilion consisting of four superimposed wards extending to the south. Its basement contained facilities for hydrotherapy and mechanotherapy, and rooms for orderlies; the other floors contained wards, a recreation hall, and a roof garden. The clinic was a self-contained unit that served the Department of Psychiatry for almost seventy years, until the Meyer Building was finished in 1982.

The Johns Hopkins School of Hygiene and Public Health

Characterized by Frederick F. Russell as "the turning point in public health education, not only in the country, but throughout the world,"[39] the Johns Hopkins School of Hygiene and Public Health opened in October 1918. Existing schools of public health produced highly trained health officers, but the new school in Baltimore was intended to educate investigators and teachers as well as practitioners. It was the first formally organized program to span all the disciplines related to hygiene, including statistics, nutrition, public health administration, parasitology, and physiology—and to provide a faculty that was competent in all these fields. As a place where knowledge could be developed as well as transmitted, the school reflected Gilman's wishes for the Johns Hopkins Hospital and the School of Medicine.

As a research center, the school of hygiene was crucial to the professionalization of public health, helping to shape the field by generating organized research, developing new scientific knowledge, and training highly educated personnel to put this knowledge into practice. As a center for training international public health officers, it influenced the development of public health activities around the world. As the first of the series of national and international schools of public health funded by the Rockefeller Foundation, the Hopkins school, like its sister institution, was a model for those that followed.

When the school was founded, public health was institutionalized in city and state health departments, but few public health officers had any specialized training. Their paid, part-time positions were assigned largely by political patronage. Any knowledge of public health principles among these political appointees was fortuitous, the result of self-education and practical experience. Most public health officers had medical degrees, but some were engineers and others were lawyers, chemists, or biologists. Indeed, there was little agreement about what type of knowledge was necessary or desirable for public health practice.

The activities of the Johns Hopkins School of Hygiene and Public Health led to organized research and training that defined the content and practice of the field. Through Hopkins' effort, public health became both scientific and professional. Scientific training and new credentials increasingly allowed public health professionals to distance themselves from the volunteers and amateurs; they also were conducive to more secure positions, a reduction in political interference, and better pay. Finally, they brought public health from the field into the laboratory.

The man most responsible for the birth of this new school was William H. Welch. As a bacteriologist, Welch wanted to apply the new science of bacteriology to the public health, to guide and supplement general observation and environmental controls.[40] Since his arrival in Baltimore,

he had hoped to establish a division of public health at Hopkins in tandem with the medical school. When two of his chosen staff members, John Shaw Billings and Alexander C. Abbott, moved to the new School of Hygiene at the University of Pennsylvania, he was forced to wait. For thirty years, Welch bided his time, encouraging public health activities in Baltimore and serving as president of the Maryland State Board of Health.

Meanwhile, German scientists had begun to apply scientific principles to the study of public health. Young Americans who studied abroad were exposed to the brilliant work of Pasteur and Koch in their bacteriological laboratories, and the importance of the new science was soon impressed on the leaders of American medicine. Once the agents of particular diseases were visible under the microscope, the general American public also recognized the importance of scientific research.[41]

Welch was also an advisor to the Rockefeller Sanitary Commission. At a conference sponsored by the Rockefeller General Education Board in 1914 and attended by leaders in public health, Welch adroitly manipulated the proceedings. The meeting was convened to discuss the founding of a school of public health, and by the meeting's end, Welch and Wickliffe Rose, the sanitary commission's director, had been charged with working out a plan for the new school that would be sent to the other participants for their comments.

Not surprisingly, their proposed school resembled the School of Medicine at Johns Hopkins. Echoing Lewellys Barker's approach to clinical research, the new school would contain four "divisions": chemical, biological, engineering or physical, and statistical. The school's main purpose would be to cultivate and advance the science of hygiene and its various branches, not to meet the immediate needs of public health practice in the United States. Welch recommended that the school of hygiene be located close to a school of medicine, but that it not be part of a medical school. The "institute" for hygiene, as Welch referred to it, should also have access to a good general teaching hospital for study and training in preventive medicine. Its emphasis on research and on the training of graduate students in the experimental method echoed the principles that emerged from Martin's Department of Biology in the university and from the preclinical departments of the medical school.

Welch's emphasis on the teaching facilities of the medical school and hospital turned out to be the most important factor in the final decision about the school's location. Wickliffe Rose had asked Abraham Flexner to investigate possible sites for the new school; although Boston and New York were candidate cities, Baltimore was in an especially favorable position because of its administratively coordinated medical school and hospital. The need for medical schools to control hospital appointments was one of Flexner's most cherished principles, and the interlocking boards of trustees for hospital and medical school at Johns Hopkins reassured him that there would be no difficulty in using the hospital for research and training, or in opening up special hospital departments.

Early in 1916, the Rockefeller Foundation decided to award the new school of hygiene to Johns Hopkins. For his first faculty appointment, Welch turned to the medical school, selecting William H. Howell as head of the Department of Physiological Hygiene. Thus began a tradition of exchange and collaboration that persists to the present day.[42]

The Welch Medical Library and the Institute of the History of Medicine

A combined hospital and medical school library had been under consideration since 1919, but not until Welch's impending retirement from the School of Hygiene and Public Health in 1925 did plans for this building solidify. When a quiet movement began to induce Welch to lead a new Department of the History of Medicine, Hopkins asked the General Education Board for funds for both the library and the department. In 1926, the board gave $200,000 for a chair of the history of medicine, and Welch was appointed to fill it.

Next, the board appropriated $750,000 for the purchase of land, construction, and equipment for a central library, and it set aside another $250,000 for the library's endowment, provided the university could raise an additional half-million dollars. This sum was supplied by Edward S. Harkness, director of the Commonwealth Fund, in the same year.[43]

Welch went to Europe at the end of 1926 to study and to select books for the library. He intended to model the Institute of the History of Medicine after the one in Leipzig, which he considered "the only really important one anywhere." On his return in 1928, he appointed as lecturers in the history of medicine John R. Oliver, a psychiatrist and novelist, and Stephen d'Irsay, a young Hungarian medievalist who was working in the institute in Leipzig.

Fielding Garrison, the Welch Library's first librarian, was also appointed resident lecturer. Garrison's scholarship and deep interest in medical history emerged in his *Introduction to the History of Medicine,* the foremost American work of its kind.[44] When Garrison died in 1935, he was succeeded by Sanford V. Larkey, who had both a medical degree from the University of California at San Francisco and a master's degree from Oxford University. The library served the hospital, the medical school, and the school of hygiene, and the committee that managed it comprised representatives from these components of the medical institutions, along with the professor of the history of medicine and the medical librarian.[45]

Welch was succeeded as head of the institute in 1932 by Henry E. Sigerist, whom Welch had met in Europe and invited to lecture at Johns Hopkins. Sigerist's lectures to capacity audiences in Baltimore were brilliant; a few weeks later, while he was still in the United States, he was formally offered the professorship.[46] The growing political turmoil in Europe on his return led him to accept the post. He brought with him a young associate at the Leipzig Institute of the History of Medicine, Owsei Temkin, who later became director of the institute at Hopkins.

The Wilmer Ophthalmological Institute and the Department of Ophthalmology

The Wilmer Institute was the second of the quasi-independent medical institutes to be developed at Johns Hopkins, following the precedent set by the Harriet Lane Home. Three patients with eye ailments were responsible for the building and its endowment. The original idea came from Mrs. Ada deAcosta Root, a patient of William H. Wilmer, an ophthalmologist in Washington, D.C. She was instrumental in obtaining money from Wilmer's former patients to create the Wilmer Foundation, which was intended to erect and endow a "Wilmer Institute" in Washington. Consultation with Abraham Flexner steered Mrs. Root to Johns Hopkins, as Flexner had concluded that Wilmer should be professor of ophthalmology at either the Harvard or the Johns Hopkins medical school.

The second patient to become involved was Wallace Buttrick, head of the Rockefeller Foundation's General Education Board. Coming under the care of Alan C. Woods, an ophthalmologist and Hopkins faculty member, he proposed the creation of a large institute of ophthalmology at Johns Hopkins. Woods was enthusiastic.

The third patient, a former patient of Wilmer's admitted to Johns Hopkins, brought Woods and Wilmer together. The two ophthalmologists talked first about their mutual patient and then about the proposed institute. Wilmer wanted the facility located in Baltimore; Woods had no idea that Johns Hopkins was formally interested, but a conversation with the dean of the medical school, Lewis Weed, encouraged him to continue his discussions with Wilmer. In 1924, the Advisory Board recommended Wilmer as a full professor with membership on both governing boards. The General Education Board then gave Johns Hopkins $1,500,000 to match a like sum provided by the Wilmer Foundation to create the new clinic.[47]

Wilmer began to assemble a staff the following year. The Halsted type of residency prevailed: the senior resident was in charge of the ward service and was responsible only to the chief of the service. Woods was given offices in the institute and was paid $1,000 a year (an arrangement that would now be called geographical full-time). Leo J. Goldbach and Clyde A. Clapp, associates in clinical ophthalmology, were the other senior part-time staff members. Jonas Friedenwald was appointed instructor in pathological ophthalmology, and Earl L. Burky joined the staff as a researcher.

Wilmer also began to form a division of physiological optics, hiring Harold F. Pierce (as associate professor of research ophthalmology), Clarence E. Ferree (as director of the Laboratory of Physiological Optics), and Ferree's wife, Gertrude Rand (as associate professor of research ophthalmology). This group investigated perimetry, lighting, and visual acuity testing, and they were among the first to devise an instrument for checking and standardizing tonometers.

The Wilmer Institute Building was completed in 1928. It was created by enlarging and remodeling the original "female pay ward" at the south end of the front of the original hospital. Its five stories contained more than 68,000 square feet of floor space. In addition to ward, semiprivate, isolation, and nursery beds, the institute in-

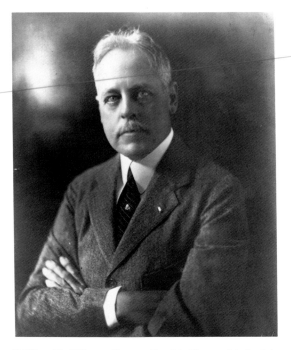

William H. Wilmer. (*Source:* Alan M. Chesney Medical Archives, The Johns Hopkins Medical Institutions.)

cluded an emergency operating room, a social service department, a machine shop, an outpatient department, patient examining rooms, administrative offices, rooms for instruction, a specialized library, research laboratories, and animal rooms.

A few clinical articles had been published by Wilmer, Bagley, MacLean, Goldbach, and Clapp before the institute opened. With additional space for research, the staff investigated such diverse topics as lens protein, the use of tuberculin in ocular tuberculosis, uveal pigment suspensions in sympathetic ophthalmia, periodic ophthalmia in horses, and syphilitic interstitial keratitis. A graduate of the Hopkins medical school, Jonas Friedenwald was a particularly distinguished investigator. His early contributions were descriptions of histopathologic abnormalities and clinical syndromes; later he worked on problems in optics; and during his last years, his primary interests were biochemistry and histochemistry. His studies of the dynamics of aqueous flow in the eye are classics and contributed greatly to the understanding of glaucoma. Joining the Wilmer Institute in the 1930s was Frank B. Walsh, who came to ophthalmology relatively late in his professional career, leaving general practice in Canada to train at Wilmer. Walsh was particularly interested in neuro-ophthalmology and worked closely with Johns Hopkins neurologist Frank R. Ford. Wilmer stepped down in 1934 at the mandatory retirement age of seventy and was succeeded by Alan C. Woods.

Like its parent institution, the Wilmer Institute was a model of its kind. Private donations enabled a recognized leader in ophthalmology to join the Hopkins family, and under Wilmer's leadership, the facility became an outstanding and integral part of the Johns Hopkins Medical Institutions.[48]

The Building Boom of the Twenties

The need for additional facilities at Johns Hopkins was so substantial after the World War I that Hopkins administrators considered reducing the size of entering medical school classes, which numbered about ninety students, until new hospital buildings could be provided. A $3 million grant from the General Education Board for physical expansion made this step unnecessary: Hopkins embarked on a building program, and in a single decade the medical institutions added buildings costing over $10 million and providing more than 800,000 square feet of new space. Other major philanthropies also contributed significantly to the building boom, which added twelve major facilities to the medical institutions in the years between the end of World War I and the onset of the Depression.[49]

The growing needs of medical education, the technological advances in support of patient care, and the surge in medical research on many fronts created a demand for renovation of existing space and new construction to keep the school and hospital in the forefront of medical progress. Like the Wilmer Institute and the Welch Medical Library, which were constructed during this building boom, each new building reflected a response to at least one of these needs.

The Woman's Clinic Building, completed in 1926, contained facilities for the Departments of Obstetrics and Gynecology. The problems connected with its design reflected the ambiguous relationship between the two departments. The General Education Board had offered an additional sum to the medical school if Hopkins would place the Department of Obstetrics on a full-time basis. Providentially, Lewellys F. Barker had interested a patient, Lucy Wortham James, in financing the construction of a clinic for the Department of Gynecology.

The resulting five-story building provided sixty obstetrical beds and sixty-six gynecological beds, each section divided equally between white and black patients. It also contained ten private rooms for obstetrical patients and seventeen cubicles for gynecological and obstetrical patients. Private gynecological patients were accommodated in the Marburg Building.

Plans had included a sixth floor for gynecological operating rooms, but chief of gynecology Cullen objected. Gynecology was a surgical specialty, he believed, and should not share quarters with obstetrics. Furthermore, he found the proposed operating-room facilities inadequate. Cullen preferred a new suite of operating rooms atop the new outpatient building, the Carnegie Dispensary.

It appears that Welch tipped the balance, by supporting the idea that the gynecology operating rooms should be located "in close proximity to the patients on this service and in the new Woman's Clinic." Several meetings and memoranda later, the final decision was made to construct the gynecological operating suite atop the Woman's Clinic Building.[50]

The cost of the Woman's Clinic (more than $500,000) exceeded the original estimate by $100,000, and the university made up the difference with a contribution from the principal of the De Lamar Fund.

The Pathology Building had long been outgrown, but its replacement became essential in 1920 when an apparatus for hydrogen ion determination built by Stanhope Bayne-Jones and Lloyd Felton exploded and the building burned down. An eight-story replacement was constructed on hospital property in 1922–23. Its cost was met by funds from both the university and the Rockefeller Foundation, and the annual maintenance costs were shared by university and hospital (three-fifths paid by the former and two-fifths by the latter).

A $2 million grant from the Carnegie Corporation enabled Hopkins to complete the Carnegie Dispensary in 1927. The building was originally planned as an outpatient department, primarily for the instruction of young physicians and surgeons, but under the terms of the Carnegie grant, its purpose was expanded and a diagnostic clinic for patients of modest means was organized (see chapter 10). The trustees also intended the dispensary and clinic to be closely related to the school of hygiene, emphasizing the prevention as well as the cure of disease.

The eight-story building had a usable open roof, a basement, and a sub-basement for major utility services. The basement contained the central record room of the hospital for many years, as well as locker rooms for nonprofessional staff, pharmacy stores, a shop for the manufacture of orthopedic appliances, and facilities for physical therapy. Admitting offices for the outpatient department were on the first floor, as were administrative offices, a pharmacy, and the orthopedic clinic. The next three floors were devoted to outpatient clinics; the fifth and sixth floors provided research and service laboratories for the full-time faculty. The main operating suites of the hospital were on the seventh floor, and at one end of the top floor were lounges and observation rooms for the surgical suites and two isolated animal rooms. The building featured a new and expensive automatic record-carrier system, which moved medical histories around the building by vacuum tube. Unique at the time, this system functioned for a few years but broke down as it was overwhelmed by the growing demands of the medical records system.

The cost of the building was $1.25 million, and the additional $150,000 above the Carnegie grant was provided by the medical school. Nine hundred thousand dollars of the Carnegie grant was earmarked as an endowment to defray operating costs.

Expansion of the medical school's teaching and clinical facilities required augmentation of the nursing staff, and new facilities for the nursing school were constructed in 1927, when the operating rooms were moved from the old Surgical Building to the Carnegie Dispensary. New housing for nurses was also completed in 1926, and an eight-story building, named for the first superintendent of nurses at Hopkins, Isabel Hampton Robb, provided single rooms for 235 nurses, with a few more spacious apartments for the officers of the nursing school. The $750,000 cost of construction was covered by a contribution from the General Education Board.

By 1921, the Department of Physiological Chemistry needed more research space than the original Physiology Building could provide. This building also accommodated the Departments of Physiology and Pharmacology, along with the medical school's administrative offices. Although a new physiology building was included in the

General Education Board's grant, a peculiarly long time elapsed between the planning, which began in 1921, the start of construction in 1927, and the building's completion in 1929. The reason for this remains unclear.

Never formally named, the new structure came to be known as "the new Physiology Building" until the original Physiology Building was demolished in 1959. Its six stories contained research laboratories, seminar rooms, offices, and animal rooms for the three departments. Meanwhile, the old building was renovated, and its teaching laboratories were expanded and reequipped.

About half of the General Education Board's $3-million gift had been spent by the late 1920s. The hospital trustees decided to use the remainder primarily for buildings to replace the medical and surgical wards. An additional endowment was needed to support activities in the new buildings. The trustees approached Edward S. Harkness of the Commonwealth Fund with a memorandum that stressed the importance of training more leaders in general medicine and surgery, extending Hopkins' research facilities, and adding enough free beds to care for indigent patients and provide a more comprehensive course of instruction for the School of Medicine. In early 1929, Harkness gave the Johns Hopkins Hospital $3 million in endowment for the new buildings. Estimates of construction costs again exceeded the funds available, and the General Education Board supplied the additional amount required—its last major contribution to Johns Hopkins. The resulting Osler and Halsted Buildings, dedicated in 1932, remain in service today.

The general plan called for a single edifice with two symmetrical wings, each seven stories high. On the ground floor, the main east-west corridor transected both wings, with the patient bed area situated along a north-south access south of the main corridor, and with elevators and laboratories north of the main corridor. As originally constructed, the Osler Clinic had a bed capacity of 150. It included sixteen-bed wards on each floor, with a few single-patient rooms and a few rooms for two or four patients. The first floor was

devoted to physical therapy and contained no beds; the fifth floor was set aside for clinical research and contained only one- and two-bed units; the seventh floor was designed as an isolation ward for patients with communicable diseases.

The Halsted Building contained two hundred beds, arranged mainly in two- and four-bed units. It had less research space than the Osler Building, and its first floor was devoted to bed patients (hence its higher total bed capacity). Later, the first floor was used for semiprivate medical and surgical patients. Postoperative recovery rooms were located on the seventh floor, near the main operating rooms in the Carnegie Building, which was connected at all floor levels with the Osler and Halsted Buildings.

Situated at ground level between the Osler and Halsted Buildings was the Henry M. Hurd Memorial Hall, a three-hundred-seat amphitheater that remains a facility of elegance and dignity. Funds for its construction were provided by George K. McGaw, a hospital trustee and friend of Hurd. McGaw originally intended that the building contain a library and a repository for hospital records, paintings, and photographs, along with an auditorium, but the Welch Library and the Carnegie Dispensary had assumed several of these functions. Upon its dedication in 1932, Hurd Hall was regarded as a most modern auditorium, one appropriate for both lectures and semipublic meetings. In that year, it was the site of Harvey Cushing's elucidation of the syndrome that bears his name.

Except for minor additions and renovations, no further major building projects or reconstructions were undertaken until the 1950s. The structures for teaching, research, and patient care erected during the 1920s thus formed the basic physical plant of the Johns Hopkins Medical Institutions for more than twenty-five years.

The Transmission of Medical Knowledge

With more buildings, faculty, and departments, communication within the Johns Hopkins Medical Institutions became more difficult. New ways of sharing medical knowledge were, therefore, developed and old ways strengthened.

Each of the major clinical departments customarily held weekly rounds for their staffs. The house officer in charge of the case would present from memory a detailed description of a patient who illustrated a particular feature or problem, and the professor or another faculty member with particular expertise would comment. Questions or remarks from the other staff members would follow. When the staff was small, into the 1930s, all would walk around the wards, stopping at the bedside of the patient selected for presentation.

Each department also had a journal club; at meetings, members summarized articles from specialized journals for the remainder of the staff.

Clinical-pathological conferences conducted by the Department of Pathology were initiated at Hopkins by Welch and continued by each of his successors. This discussion of all pre- and post-mortem information about a patient allowed the immediate validation of the clinician's conclusions. The clinicopathologic conference was developed at the Massachusetts General Hospital by Richard Cabot, following a suggestion by medical student Walter B. Cannon. It was a characteristically American exercise: no German *Geheimrat* would have risked correction by his colleagues in front of medical students and house staff.[51]

In the Hopkins version, the clinician who discussed the case was given only raw material—the patient's charts, x-rays, and so forth—and not a prepared summary of the case. After the clinician had made his diagnosis, the postmortem findings were discussed by a member of the Department of Pathology. For many years these conferences were conducted by William S. Thayer as clinician and William G. MacCallum as pathologist. After Thayer's death in 1933, Louis Hamman served as clinician and Arnold R. Rich as pathologist. When Hamman died in 1946, the conferences were taken over by A. McGehee Harvey, first in collaboration with Rich and then with Rich's successor, Ivan L. Bennett.

Endowed lectureships, too, were stimulating events for the faculty, covering all of medicine in topic and intent. The Herter series, inaugurated in 1903, was followed by the De Lamar, Dohme, Thayer, and Noguchi Lectures, all initiated before World War II. The De Lamar Lectures were established in 1918 under the auspices of the new School of Hygiene and Public Health; the Dohme Lectureship, funded by Ida S. Dohme in memory of her husband Charles, relates to chemistry in medicine; the William S. and Susan Read Thayer Lectureship is delivered by physicians distinguished in clinical medicine, pediatrics, neurology, or related branches of medicine; the Noguchi Lectures in the history of medicine, funded in 1929 by Emanuel Libman, honor Hideyo Noguchi, a scientist of the Rockefeller Institute for Medical Research. The Gould, Wilkins, Novey, Gilman, Bayne-Jones, Shelley, and Dale Lectureships were inaugurated after World War II.

Hospital and medical school publications were also important vehicles for the transmission of new knowledge. Welch founded the *American Journal of Hygiene* in 1920 to communicate the work and views of the faculty of the new School of Hygiene and Public Health. By this time, he had also been editor of the hospital *Reports* for twenty years, and under his editorship the character of that publication had changed (see chapter 1). Because he did not process submissions punctually, original contributions spilled over into the *Bulletin of The Johns Hopkins Hospital*, and the *Reports* became a place for lengthier articles. The Institute of the History of Medicine received its own publication in 1933, when the *Bulletin of the History of Medicine* began as a supplement to the hospital *Bulletin*. From 1935 to 1938, the institute was solely responsible for the new journal; since 1939, it has been jointly sponsored by the institute and the American Association for the History of Medicine.

Interdepartmental societies proliferated during the 1920s as well. The Johns Hopkins Medical Society was formed soon after the opening of the hospital and endured until after World War II. With Welch as its president, it offered a critical forum for the presentation of research results before they were subjected to scrutiny at national meetings. Welch was also elected as the first president of the Johns Hopkins Medical History Club (although Osler presided over its first meeting). The club was successful as long as Welch was alive and active, but with his death attendance declined. Interest in the club was revived by Henry Sigerist, and it will celebrate its centennial anniversary in 1990.

A Johns Hopkins Medical Alumni Association was created in 1910, but as a purely social undertaking, it did not survive after its first two meetings. The idea of an organization for alumni was revived in the 1920s, however, when director of surgery Dean D. Lewis organized the Johns Hopkins Surgical Society, and a few years later, the medical staff of the hospital formed the Johns Hopkins Medical Association. The two groups met together for the first time at a raucous dinner in 1930 and continued to meet biennially thereafter. All present and former members of the hospital's clinical staff and all medical school graduates were eligible to attend. At the second and successive meetings, the dinner followed the first of two days of scientific presentations. The two organizations merged in 1940, and the combined association has made sizeable donations to the School of Medicine's scholarship fund.

Student organizations provided eating facilities and housing for men and women. Some national fraternities—Nu Sigma Nu, Phi Chi, Alpha Kappa Alpha, and Phi Beta Phi (most established at Hopkins before the 1930s)—were once strong but have dwindled away. The oldest fraternity, the Pithotomy Club, still flourishes. This local social club was founded in 1897. Its escutcheon—a largely naked cherub astride a beer keg, in one hand a scepter around which a snake coils, and in the other a mug of beer from which the snake is lapping—was designed by Max Broedel. The club's annual show, which began in 1914 and continues to this day, has been more controversial. Always bawdy, sometimes clever, the show is merciless to dull or pompous faculty members.[52]

The first organization of Hopkins women medical students, Zeta Phi, was founded in 1906, part of a national group. Three years later, an association was established solely for Hopkins women medical students: the Women's Association of the Johns Hopkins Medical School. Members of both societies met to discuss the current medical literature, and memberships overlapped. The two groups merged in 1919 (see chapter 6), to become the Johns Hopkins Women's Medical Alumnae Association.

The students' social clubs shared the same few blocks of North Broadway with the rooming houses. Relations between the students and the community were basically good. The students saw many members of the community in the outpatient clinics and often helped to deliver their babies in their homes. Landladies in the hospital's environs were happy to have the students as tenants. A few became part of the Hopkins folklore, as depicted in Augusta Tucker's novel about a Hopkins boardinghouse, *Miss Susie Slagle's*.[53] Miss Jane Tydings, in particular, took countless medical students under her wing until her death in 1972 at the age of eighty-eight.

The Effect of the Depression on the Medical Institutions

At the start of the Great Depression, the Johns Hopkins Medical Institutions were stronger than ever before. The full-time system was in place in the clinical departments, and the School of Medicine had been broadened and deepened by new faculty, new departments, and a greatly improved physical plant. In the hospital, the original wards had been replaced with new facilities, and new buildings had been erected.

The strength of the clinical departments attested to the eminence and versatility of their part-time faculty, who compensated for the paucity of full-time staff. The Department of Surgery, for example, had only three full-time faculty members, excepting the senior members of the house staff, who held faculty appointments as instructors and assistants. The department's large part-time staff, however, included J. M. T. Finney, professor of clinical surgery, and Joseph C. Bloodgood, Richard H. Follis, and Robert T. Miller, Jr., associate professors. The excellence of these so-called "clinical" staff members was partly responsible for the informal blurring of official distinctions. By 1930, the medical school's catalog grouped full- and part-time faculty of like rank together. The next year, the catalog went one step further, removing the word "clinical" from academic titles.

In 1931, for the first time, a formal committee convened to examine the state of the hospital and the medical school.[54] The resulting survey affirmed that the innovations of earlier years were working well. The report advised these two institutions to remain dedicated to educating practitioners with a sound scientific background, while maintaining the liberal principles that had characterized the medical school since its inception. It stated that faculty should continue to experiment with educational procedure, and individual departments should retain the liberty to conduct their courses as they deemed fit.

With startling prescience, the committee sensed the advances to come in pharmacology, especially progress in chemotherapy. It visualized a laboratory devoted to the search for new therapeutic agents, a laboratory devoted primarily to testing them, and a biophysical division that would study physical agents with effects on humans or animals. As a harbinger of the specialization of the postwar years, it advocated new divisions in the Departments of Anatomy and Physiology. Foreshadowing the 1950s, when a single Department of Microbiology began to serve both the school of hygiene and the medical school, it recommended joint studies of microorganisms, as well as closer administrative and faculty contact between the two schools.

The committee also recommended a greater emphasis on preventive medicine; in 1939 a grant from the Rockefeller Foundation enabled Hopkins to establish a separate department in this area, under the direction of Perrin H. Long. When the grant ended ten years later, Long accepted the directorship of medicine at the Downstate Medical Center in New York, and the Department of Preventive Medicine at Hopkins was disbanded.[55]

Financial deficits incurred by the Johns Hopkins Hospital, the School of Medicine, and the School of Hygiene and Public Health through-

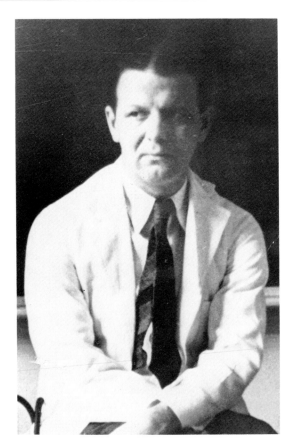

Perrin H. Long. (*Source:* Alan M. Chesney Medical Archives, The Johns Hopkins Medical Institutions.)

out the 1930s kept the medical institutions from putting most of the committee's recommendations into effect. Hospital expenditures had risen 50 percent during the 1920s, but the Depression caused soaring demands for hospital service without a concomitant increase in income. At the school of hygiene, research programs were sacrificed to balance the budget. Medical school expenditures rose 300 percent in the 1920s, a rise that was unmatched by additional endowments. The survey committee recommended additional bequests and endowments of $4 million in unrestricted funds and $20 to 25 million for improvements in all medical school departments, but these recommendations remained unrealized.[56]

During the Depression years, facilities were maintained but no new buildings were constructed, and the preclinical departments were allowed to remain small. For the first time, it was conceded that research must be generally funded from external sources. At the time, the sums that supported research were not large. Investigators required no more than modest gifts from grateful patients or small grants from pharmaceutical companies.

Expansion of clinical facilities was achieved not by expansion of the Johns Hopkins Hospital but by the development of affiliations with other institutions, such as the Sydenham Hospital for Infectious Diseases, Sinai Hospital, the Children's Hospital School, the Baltimore City Hospitals, and, for psychiatric rotations, Spring Grove State Hospital.

Keeping the School of Medicine on course during these trying years was Dean Alan M. Chesney, who had taken over the deanship from Lewis Weed on the eve of the Depression in 1929.[57] Weed had been dean for six years, succeeding J. Whitridge Williams in 1923. Chesney's prudent management of the medical school's finances in the 1930s included an insistence on maintaining a balance of funding among the departments. In 1935, the trustees decided to consolidate the separately invested endowment and other funds—a plan that would have penalized the medical school, whose invested funds had appreciated in value more than those of the other divisions. Chesney prevailed, and while the money was pooled, the medical school received shares in the consolidated account proportionate to the market value of its securities at the time of consolidation.

Despite budget and salary reductions, the faculty was not pressured to produce income for the School of Medicine during the 1930s. In fact, the survey committee discussed the need to relieve the Phipps staff—particularly Adolf Meyer —of the pressure to earn professional fees sufficient to balance the clinic's budget. Even under severe financial stress, the medical school maintained a nucleus of senior teachers who were free from the necessity of engaging in private practice to earn an income for themselves or for their institution.

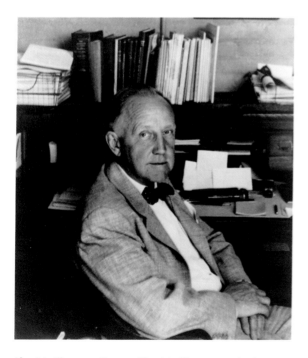

Alan M. Chesney. (*Source:* Alan M. Chesney Medical Archives, The Johns Hopkins Medical Institutions.)

The Retirement of William H. Welch

The deleterious effects of the Depression at Johns Hopkins were augmented by the final retirement of William H. Welch in 1930 at the age of eighty. His forty-five-year tenure at Hopkins had spanned all but the School of Nursing: he had been professor of pathology in the School of Medicine, pathologist-in-chief of the Johns Hopkins Hospital, dean of the School of Medicine and the School of Hygiene, and director of the medical school's Institute of the History of Medicine. It was largely through Welch's wisdom in shaping the Johns Hopkins Medical Institutions that they were able to survive his departure, but administrative problems beset every part of the medical institutions after his retirement.

The School of Hygiene and Public Health was locked into a three-year deanship, a policy that caused a lack of continuity in its leadership. Welch had relinquished the deanship of the school of hygiene in 1926; his successors were William H. Howell (1927–31), Wade H. Frost (1931–34), and Allen W. Freeman (1934–37).

The policy was changed in 1937, when Lowell J. Reed assumed the deanship for the next ten years.

At the medical school, Weed's successor as dean, Alan M. Chesney, never held the academic rank of professor throughout his professional career. As dean, he was extraordinarily dedicated and able, but he lacked formal academic or administrative tenure.

Although the medical school, the school of hygiene, and the hospital were dedicated to common goals, they increasingly went their own way after Welch's retirement. At certain vital points, they failed to act and react in concert or, perhaps more important, failed to look to the future by consulting a broad range of advisers.[58]

In the expansive four decades between 1905 and 1942, one innovation stands out: the advent of the full-time system in the clinical departments. This development solidified the scientific approach to clinical medicine and created the foundation for the future of the clinical departments, first at Johns Hopkins and later at medical schools around the country. The faculty at Johns Hopkins—the so-called second faculty—brought this scientific approach to fruition, particularly in the Department of Pediatrics, where Edwards A. Park developed strong specialty departments. New departments, institutes, and programs flourished, all supported by hospital, university, or private funds. These were the last years in which private funding would play such a large part in the expansion of the Johns Hopkins Medical Institutions—the last years in which Johns Hopkins would be entirely free to set its own course.

CHAPTER 4

THE WAR YEARS AND THE
POSTWAR EXPANSION, 1942–1968

We have limited funds available for research purposes. If you have investigators who need these funds, let us hear from you by return mail.

—Letter from National Institute of Health to deans of all
American medical schools, 1945

The War Years and Federal Support for American Medicine

Americans were enormously impressed by the practical, immediately useful contributions of research and concomitant technologic advances in World War II.[1] The death rate from wounds, for example, was half that in World War I, partly because of the availability of blood and plasma for the treatment of hemorrhage and shock, the use of sulfonamides and penicillin, the more rapid transportation of the wounded by motor ambulance and airplane to hospitals for surgical care, and the use of mobile surgical teams and well-staffed hospital ships in island-hopping operations. Once the development of the atomic bomb had demonstrated the potential of scientific research, it was only a short step to the belief that the nation's future would depend on the development of its intellectual capital.

These wartime advances were achieved despite a fragmented national policy. At the start of World War II, the several military services and the Public Health Service were unable to agree on a coordinated approach to medical problems. President Roosevelt's compromise was the creation of the Office of Scientific Research and Development

(OSRD) and two parallel committees, one concerned with national defense and the other with medical research. The Committee on Medical Research (CMR) undertook a comprehensive program to cope with the medical problems of the war. It was responsible for mobilizing the medical and scientific personnel of the nation; recommending contracts to be entered into with the universities, hospitals, and other agencies conducting medical research; and submitting recommendations concerning medical problems related to the national defense. Between 1941 and 1947, $25 million was spent through the six CMR divisions.[2]

The federal support during the postwar years could hardly have been predicted from wartime levels of support. Federal involvement in medical education and research during World War II was modest. The changes in medical education requested by the War Manpower Commission reflected the wartime need for more physicians. At Johns Hopkins, the Advisory Board condensed the process of medical education, eliminating the long summer vacation so that classes could graduate early without a reduction in class hours. Under the federal wartime program, the Advisory Board also temporarily contravened the provisions of Mary Garrett's gift to the medical school: for admission, students no longer needed a bachelor's degree, or competence in French and German. (The latter requirement was modified in 1952 for all applicants, who were now required to demonstrate competence in only one modern foreign language.)

During wartime, these new policies applied only to students who could participate in the training programs of the armed forces. Foreign nationals and those exempt from military service for physical reasons still had to meet the usual requirements. As in World War I, medical students enrolled in military training programs were subject to military discipline, and their medical work was supplemented by instruction in military matters. Tuition was paid directly by the federal government to the medical school, and the students received the same pay and allowances as enlisted personnel in the armed services.

By 1943, ninety-two faculty members had left to join the armed forces, most of them serving in the two original Johns Hopkins Hospital units. Many of the remaining senior faculty were dividing their time between Baltimore and Washington as members of civilian boards—notably Lewis Weed, who was appointed chairman of the National Research Council in 1939.[3]

The federal government also used the medical school for war-related research and teaching. For Navy physicians, Chalmers Gemmill taught a course in respiration and metabolism, related to problems of high-altitude flying and maintenance of efficiency in submarines. Dean Alan M. Chesney, with the approval of the Advisory Board, also offered the facilities of the medical school for research projects deemed important to the national defense.

The Rise of Federal Support for American Medicine

A second revolution in American medicine took place at the end of World War II, thirty-five years after the Flexner Report of 1910, the document that had affirmed and popularized the model in place in Baltimore. The genesis of this next radical change was an enormous infusion of federal dollars for medical research and training.[4] The Johns Hopkins University School of Medicine was the standard-bearer in the first revolution, but it was forced to assume a more passive role in the second. Rather than setting the course of American medicine, Johns Hopkins, like other medical schools, responded to the decisions of the federal government. These decisions evolved from the public perception at the end of the war that financing could speed up the conquest of disease and that support of scientific research could solve a variety of national problems.

The resulting conflicts and compromises were played out on a grand scale as the nation's population and wealth grew. Governmental support led to more of everything in American medicine: more students, interns, residents, and fellows; more faculty; more departments; more buildings; bigger budgets; and more committees to coordinate the ever-more-complicated administrative process.

At Johns Hopkins, many of the ensuing changes specifically affected the unique structure of the hospital and the medical school: their administrative equality and their place within the university. The administrative arrangement that Johns Hopkins had established proved to be strong enough to bend with the pressure, but no aspect of the two organizations was left untouched.

On the national level, control of federal funds quickly became the key question of the postwar years. The independence of American scientists was a principle stressed by Vannevar Bush, head of the OSRD, whom President Roosevelt had charged with planning government aid to science in the postwar period. Bush believed that federal money should be allocated for scholarships and research, but he insisted that science be kept free from the influence of pressure groups and from the necessity of producing immediate and practical results. He recommended the establishment of an independent national research foundation to coordinate all the nation's research needs and prevent government interference in the conduct of research in the private sector. Many of

Bush's ideas were realized by the creation of the National Science Foundation and by legislation, notably the Public Health Service Act of 1944, that gave the Public Health Service specific authority to award grants to individuals.[5]

Governmental agencies were, however, not ready to relinquish the power they had acquired during the war, especially in view of the intense public interest in the nation's health. Under the leadership of Rolla E. Dyer, assistant Surgeon General of the Public Health Service, programs in the medical sciences previously supported by the CMR were transferred to the Public Health Service's National Institute of Health (NIH), and those in the physical sciences were transferred to the Office of Naval Research. The Public Health Service thus acquired more personnel and a larger administrative budget. In 1946, Congress appropriated almost $8 million for the NIH—more than a tenfold increase over its annual funding at the start of the war and 30 percent of the total federal outlay for medical research. Between 1941 and 1951, the federal budget for medical research grew from about $3 million to $76 million. By then, the NIH was locked into place as the key peacetime mechanism for the support of medical research.[6]

The nation's relative affluence during these years encouraged the assumption that resources were almost infinite. Paul B. Beeson, a department head in those days, recalls thinking, "What *else* should I be asking for?"[7] From 1945 to 1964, the decision to fund any given scientific project turned entirely on the project's scientific merit.

International rivalries and tensions also fueled the federal support of science and technology, particularly after the Soviets' launching of Sputnik in 1957, which revealed the United States' scientific deficiencies. They were most evident in the physical sciences, and the sharp increase in funding for these branches of science reflected the nation's shame and consequent determination to match the expertise of the Soviet Union. Although biomedical science benefited from the nation's increased interest in science in general, the motivation for funding was less volatile, and the patterns of support differed accord-

ingly. Large annual budget increases for biomedical science began in fiscal year 1957, before the shock of Sputnik. Funding for biomedical science rose steadily during the Korean War, whereas funding for science in general dipped during those years. Moreover, biomedical research was perceived as the source of domestic social benefits; support for it was not a response to international tensions or a result of enthusiasm for technologic prowess.[8]

In funding for all sciences, the focus of federal attention was on research and development. In the biomedical sciences, "research" had an even narrower meaning, as an area separate from teaching and patient care. The federal government considered these other two areas the responsibility of the states or the private sector. Little federal money was allocated for teaching, largely because of the American Medical Association's opposition to governmental support of medical education.[9] A congressional committee warned the NIH in 1957 that funds for medical research were not to be spent for the general support of medical schools and medical education.[10]

The benefits of research grants spilled over into the schools' educational programs, but in return, much faculty time and floor space had to be given to the research effort. Clinical faculty did benefit from the influx of federal funds, as an increasing number of physicians were trained in specialty areas, but the federal emphasis on research caused a shift in the relation between clinical and basic-science departments. A generation earlier, surgeons had dominated medical schools in terms of financial resources. In contrast, in a typical research-oriented medical school of the 1960s, the budget for experimental work was five times the budget of the Department of Surgery.[11]

Moreover, the federal government was interested not only in research *per se,* but also in its products. Enthusiasm for the practical results of research—the concrete medical advances that emerged from World War II—was translated into the "categorical approach" of the 1950s. A peer-review system for evaluating grants kept scientists in control of the substance of research, but decentralized control of the federal funds left the support of scientific research open to influence by pressure groups of nonscientists, who were much more interested in cures for specific diseases than in basic research. A lay leader in the promotion of federal and private support for medical research was Mrs. Mary Lasker, whose efforts led to the drafting of legislation to create a National Heart Institute similar to the National Cancer Institute that had been founded in 1937.[12]

This "categorical" approach to funding was popular with legislators as well as with the public. Legislators realized that by giving their all-out support to medical research, they could show their concern for the advancement of medical science while avoiding controversial issues such as compulsory health insurance, governmental involvement in medical education, and the delivery of health services. Surgeon General Leonard Scheele was diplomatic in his view of the public's attitude, saying that it was hard to keep up with the enthusiasm of the lay members of the NIH's advisory councils.[13] Scientists leery of the categorical approach were labeled "over-cautious," and their "narrow views" were perceived as obstacles to progress. The preeminence of the categorical approach nevertheless fragmented the national research effort, as medical lobbyists went directly to Congress rather than to a unified science foundation.[14]

An emphasis on the conquest of specific diseases thus superseded the "undirected" approach to scientific investigation. Undirected research was not abandoned, however. For those basic research activities that did not fit neatly into specific disease categories, a Division of General Medical Sciences was formed in 1957. Renamed the National Institute of General Medical Sciences in 1962, it became the first noncategorical institute of the NIH.[15]

Some problems resulting from the funding policies of the federal government emerged immediately; others appeared only years later. It quickly became apparent that the three components of academic medicine—research, teaching, and patient care—could not easily be separated. The expansion of research programs required more scientists, who could be produced only through the expansion of graduate education. The federal response was the creation of research training programs and grants. These programs supported trainees with stipends, and departments were paid associated institutional costs. About half of such funds went to departments; although the programs were clearly limited to the training of scientists, they became an important source of operating funds for the departments involved.

Serious imbalances resulted from the policy makers' zeal for research coupled with their refusal to provide adequate support to the undergraduate teaching function of the institutions doing the research. Major departments were developed with federal funds, but the source of funds was precarious, requiring renewal usually every four to five years.[16] Medical schools often found it necessary to pay a significant part of the cost of doing the research, thereby reducing the funds available for educational activities. James A. Shannon, director of the NIH from 1955 to 1968, perceived a persistent ambivalence in Congress: Was research predominantly an academic function supported by public funds or a public function located in universities?[17] This ambivalence influenced the universities' own planning and development, their exercise of administrative responsibility, and their negotiations with philanthropic agencies.

Schools could pay their faculty only by bootlegging research dollars, by taking salary money from research and training grants—a "robbing-Peter-to-pay-Paul" practice that became one of the most destructive byproducts of NIH policy.[18] By 1970, half of the medical faculty in the United States were receiving at least part of their salaries from federal grants of this type.[19] Medical schools also turned to the care of patients to support faculty salaries, as corporations devoted to providing care for profit competed with academic institutions for the Medicare and Medicaid dollar.[20]

The government's decision to support the research of individual faculty members rather than their parent institutions fragmented medical schools as well. Rather than perceiving themselves as part of a university, faculty members in research-oriented medical schools were led to capture as much NIH funding as possible to enhance the research and training activities in their own departments. Universities were paid for overhead and for time-sharing of faculty salaries, but in dealing directly with individual investigators, the NIH deprived the universities of the chance to use federal funds to plan the broader programs that only an institutional perspective allows.[21]

The number of medical students in American medical schools grew by only 45 percent between 1960 and 1970, whereas the full-time clinical faculty increased by 167 percent.[22] Moreover, the faculty was enlarged not primarily to accommodate the needs of medical education but rather to respond to the demands of the research laboratory and its offshoots, graduate training and the specialty practice of medicine. Furthermore, as insurance took responsibility for the cost of hospitalization and not for outpatient care, individual patients spent less time in the hospital. This resulted in a more rapid turnover in the hospital census and required more house officers to carry out the increased number of admission work-ups. In 1957, hospitals were looking for more than 12,000 interns annually, but American medical schools were graduating fewer than 7,000 students a year.[23] By the 1960s, the perception of a "doctor shortage" led the federal government to institute a program of capitation grants, the first substantial direct federal aid to medical education.[24]

Uncontrolled expansion, as well as the imbalance of federal funding, led to unforeseen consequences in later years. Town-gown conflicts were intensified as medical schools, to attract faculty with a research base and good clinical facilities, began to expand their networks of affiliated hospitals. Local physicians were displaced as full-time faculty took over the posts of part-time clinical instructors and previous chiefs of staff at affiliated hospitals. Removal of local physicians was the cost of affiliation, as hospitals usually had to permit the medical schools to initiate or to approve staff appointments in order to acquire this link with a medical school. For their part, the medical schools believed they needed this authority to maintain the quality of their graduate education.[25]

In many of the research training programs, a majority of the trainees went into practice and were recruited by community hospitals to bring the latest medical knowledge to their institutions. It is ironic that the expansion of their postgraduate population thus caused university medical centers to relinquish their role as the sole repository of the latest in medical progress.

Although faculty and administrators were not unaware of the existing and potential problems associated with their increasing dependence on the federal government, several factors diminished the fear of government control.[26] In the health field, the government was not a monolithic structure. Its policies were diverse, its varied activities were subject to counsel from certain advisory groups (notably the Councils of the National Institutes of Health, which were composed of scientists, physicians, and lay representatives), and its administrative structure was decentralized. Even more reassuring was the leadership of NIH director James A. Shannon, who understood the type of relationship that would be effective in linking the government with private institutions.

More important, the relationship between the federal government and medical schools was basically harmonious. In the words of one participant, it was an "Augustan age."[27] No fundamental conflict arose between the two entities during the 1950s and 1960s. Each needed the other to reach their common objectives—the continuing improvement of health in America and the advance of medicine and biomedical science in general. The leaders of both groups realized that medical institutions constituted a national resource of great value to American society as a whole.[28]

For the scientists themselves, it was a time of excitement, determination, enthusiasm, and youth—all fueled by seemingly inexhaustible federal funds. Nurturing young scientists was the first priority in the allocation of research money. Young men and women were shielded from administrative responsibilities so that they could devote their energies to their research interests in the laboratory. As new technologic methods displaced the importance of clinical experience, the wisdom of older physicians was denigrated as "anecdotal" rather than "scientific." It became the nature of the experimental results rather than the researcher's age or position in the medical hierarchy that counted. Moreover, because new technologies could be learned more quickly than clinical expertise based on experience, younger physicians became knowledgeable more swiftly.[29] The Hopkins tradition of giving high academic posts to talented young men was now echoed nationwide as many of this new breed of young scientists went on to build new departments and divisions in leading medical schools.

The Response at Johns Hopkins

The greatest influence on the Johns Hopkins Hospital and the School of Medicine in the years after World War II was the overwhelming financial dominance of the federal government, which greatly affected the direction of medicine at Johns Hopkins—and indeed, at most academic medical centers in the United States. The numbers tell the story. At Johns Hopkins, the medical school's total grant receipts increased from $2,685,981 in 1947 to $7,003,536 a decade later, and they then increased fourfold between 1957 and 1968, to $27,959,878.[30] The hospital's receipts also grew, increasing threefold in the latter period, from $10,503,874 to $30,741,681. During Thomas B. Turner's deanship, the United States Public Health Service training and research grants received by the Department of Medicine alone increased from $620,102 in 1957 to $2,750,666 in 1967.[31]

The influx of federal dollars for medical research supported the hiring of additional faculty and fellows to carry it out. The number of full-time assistant, associate, and full professors at Johns Hopkins more than doubled between 1959 and 1968, from 131 to 304. The tide of federal money also permitted these faculty members to add postdoctoral students to their staffs; during these years, the number of fellows at Johns Hopkins grew from 393 to 616. At Johns Hopkins and its affiliated hospitals, the number of house officers increased from 235 in 1959 to 328 in 1968. Federal capitation grants to Johns Hopkins in the 1960s also increased the number of medical students per class, from 74 in 1957 to 95 a decade later.[32]

The increase in the number of interns, residents, and fellows in the clinical departments was initially viewed as only temporary and was attributed to an influx of men returning after the war to complete their training, but the number of house officers increased further in later years. There was a proliferation of training fellowships in medical specialties, particularly in medicine and pediatrics, as a response to the shortage of trained practitioners in these areas. Federal grants also made fellowships in pathology, pediatrics, preventive medicine, psychiatry, ophthalmology, and otology available to returning veterans.

Additional facilities were naturally needed to house the additional faculty, students, and fellows—along with the wave of house staff who had returned from the war to complete their training. New specialties were also created as faculty members carved out specific areas of expertise. Committees and other governing bodies consequently grew in size and number as these new departments and divisions demanded representation. Finally, administrative staff were added to assist in managing the expanded bureaucracy.

Although federal funding began to grow during the last years of Chesney's deanship and steadily increased during Philip Bard's four years as dean, Chesney and Bard were only on the cusp of change. It was the deanship of their successor, Thomas B. Turner, that coincided with Hopkins' receipt of more money from the federal government than ever before. From 1957 through 1968, Turner directed what he termed the "relentless expansion" of the hospital and medical school—a phrase encompassing the addition of more students, more fellows and house officers, more fac-

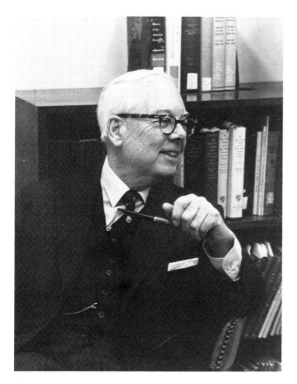

Thomas B. Turner. (*Source:* Alan M. Chesney Medical Archives, The Johns Hopkins Medical Institutions.)

ulty, more ancillary staff, more buildings, more complicated administrative arrangements, and bigger budgets than ever before.[33]

Turner envisioned some of the dangers of uncontrolled expansion and tried to put on the brakes:

> The dangers in excessive growth were obvious to me as dean, yet no ready formula by which to control or direct it was evident. Gradually, however, certain touchstones were developed to promote growth in an orderly pattern. Was the proposed new project consistent with the goals and scope of the Medical School's program, or was it opportunistic mainly because funds were available? What were the implications in terms of new senior faculty members to whom we would acquire a continuing obligation? Would the commitment of space, always in short supply, foreclose other developments which might be more productive? What impact would the new project have on the essential teaching functions of the Medical School? Having posed these questions, the answers were liable to be anything but obvious.[34]

Turner sought out private funding as one way of reducing Johns Hopkins' dependency on federal money. Income from foundations, individuals, associations concerned with special diseases, and pharmaceutical companies increased significantly. Through large and small gifts and bequests, and sound management, the value of the university's endowment funds set aside for the medical school increased from $45.0 million in 1957 to $83.7 million in 1968.[35] Turner also tried to lighten the pressure of government support on the school's policies by ensuring that the salaries of senior faculty members were paid primarily from nongovernmental funds.

Turner admits that he lost the last argument about containing growth, especially the growth of tenured positions. Yet Turner believed that Johns Hopkins had no choice but to accept the federal largesse:

> [I]t is probable that no one could have foreseen in the immediate post-war years the enormous infusion of Federal funds that was to come, or would have planned for it in a more adequate way. . . .
>
> Yet, the net result was an enormously enriched educational environment—enriched in terms of intellectual content, exciting new fields of endeavor, many fine faculty members, and doubtless, the easier recruitment of highly qualified young medical students. Not to have embraced the opportunity for such enrichment would have left Johns Hopkins in an educational backwash and pragmatically noncompetitive with the better medical schools in America. The choice was not consciously made, but rather arose from the collective intuition of the senior faculty. It was nevertheless a wise one and not to be regretted. That unbalances occurred is regrettable, that risks were entailed was inevitable, yet a contrary course would have been unthinkable.[36]

The deanship of the medical school emerged during this influx of federal support as the position of greatest authority and responsibility. The traditional spirit of cooperation between the medical school's administrative officers and its department directors allowed Chesney, Bard, and Turner to exercise their power sparingly and subtly. Turner described the Johns Hopkins University School of Medicine as "a loose affiliation of some 15 major departments, often going in different directions. The dean reigns but he does not rule."[37] As the budget officer of the School of Medicine, Turner was able to maintain the degree of fiscal control that gave the medical school the leadership it needed during his eventful tenure.

New Leadership in the Postwar Period

The new personalities who came to Hopkins in the years after World War II brought new ideas and new vigor at the same time that the changing national scene brought new problems. As the war ended and rapid demobilization began, members of the "second faculty" were replaced by younger men. The Hopkins model of scientific medicine that had been developed over the past fifty years had changed both the backgrounds of the candidates for faculty positions and the disciplines themselves. The legacy of Barker and Mall was a group of department heads with highly specialized training.

Most important to the medical school and hospital immediately after the war was the retirement of four of its leaders. Isaiah Bowman, the university's president, Winford Smith, director of the hospital, and Lowell Reed, director of the school of hygiene, stepped down between 1946 and 1948. Alan M. Chesney, dean of the medical school, retired only a few years later, in 1953. Their association with Hopkins, spanning parts of four decades, was marked by professional, scientific, administrative, and literary contributions to Johns Hopkins.[38]

Like Welch, who "retired" several times in the course of his career, Lowell J. Reed left the directorship of the school of hygiene to become vice-president of the university in 1946, vice-president of the hospital in 1949, and president of the university in 1953.

As director of the hospital since 1911, Winford H. Smith was the key liaison between the hospital's Medical Board and Board of Trustees. The hospital's physical plant was outmoded when he arrived, and his first priority was to improve

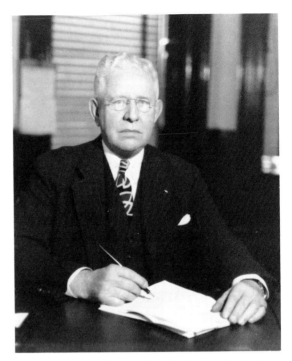

Winford H. Smith. (*Source:* Alan M. Chesney Medical Archives, The Johns Hopkins Medical Institutions.)

the housekeeping and administration of the existing facilities and to help plan for new ones. World War I took Smith to the Office of the Surgeon General. When he returned to Hopkins at the end of the war, he initiated the joint expansion program of the hospital and university (see chapter 3). Smith served on city and state agencies, helped to plan hospitals elsewhere, and worked to reduce the cost of medical care. Regarded by his peers as one of the nation's leading authorities in the field, he was elected president of the American Hospital Association. Nor were his interests confined to a narrow area of expertise, as his enthusiasm for all aspects of medicine involved him in issues of medical education and research.[39]

Smith's retirement in 1946 spared him the difficulties that beset his successors, Edwin L. Crosby and Russell A. Nelson. Like directors at other hospitals in the postwar years, Crosby and Nelson presided over an antiquated physical plant. Complaints about hospital service during this time were prevalent and well founded, as new department chiefs sought better facilities for patient care, instruction, and research.

Crosby knew the medical institutions well, having spent his entire career at Johns Hopkins. Before becoming the hospital's statistician in 1937, Crosby received a doctorate from the Johns Hopkins School of Hygiene and Public Health, and served on its faculty. In 1941, he became assistant director of the Johns Hopkins Hospital and was placed in charge of the outpatient department. Two years later, he was appointed Smith's principal deputy. Crosby was hospital director from 1946 to 1952, when he left to become head of the newly created Joint Commission for the Accreditation of Hospitals. He was succeeded by Russell A. Nelson, one of his early appointees.[40]

Like his predecessor, Nelson had been at Johns Hopkins since medical school. After graduating in 1937, he had taken an internship and residency in the Department of Medicine. Nelson was director of the hospital from 1952 until his retirement twenty years later. He presided over a period of great transition at Johns Hopkins, including expansion of the physical plant, sweeping financial adjustments, and expansion of outpa-

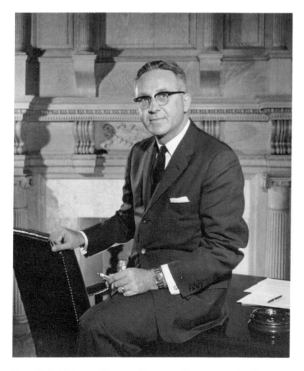

Russell A. Nelson. (*Source:* Alan M. Chesney Medical Archives, The Johns Hopkins Medical Institutions.)

tient services. During his tenure, the hospital plunged into comprehensive programs of health care in Columbia, Maryland, and East Baltimore (see chapter 10). Nelson was also a major figure in the field of hospital administration: he was chairman of the Executive Committee of the Association of American Medical Colleges, president of the American Hospital Association, advisor to state and federal governments and to major medical centers.

The choice of Henry Hurd's successors thus continued the Johns Hopkins tradition of selecting hospital directors with broad backgrounds. Smith, Crosby, and Nelson were knowledgeable about medical education and medical research, and appreciated the medical school and its primary teaching hospital as uniquely important components of the university.

The dean of the medical school from 1929 to 1953, Alan M. Chesney, enjoyed a career that spanned research and administration. He had graduated from the Johns Hopkins School of Medicine in 1908. He then had worked at the Rockefeller Institute for three years with Rufus I. Cole and Oswald T. Avery, producing a classic paper on the growth curve of the pneumococcus in broth culture. After serving in World War I, Chesney had headed the infectious disease service at Washington University in Saint Louis under George Dock. When Robinson moved to Hopkins in 1920, he recruited Chesney as associate professor of medicine and director of the newly created syphilis division. Chesney returned to the Rockefeller Institute for almost a year to prepare for this post, working under Wade Brown. During his first decade at Johns Hopkins, Chesney spent half his time caring for patients with syphilis and the other half investigating the basic mechanisms of immunity in that disease. In pioneering experiments, he was assisted by a succession of younger physicians, most of whom went on to make important contributions of their own. Chesney's other accomplishments include writing the standard history of the early years of the Johns Hopkins Hospital and School of Medicine and serving as president of the Association of American Medical Colleges.

Chesney's devotion to the medical institutions reached into his personal life as well. Described as a quiet academician, Chesney was said to have transformed himself into a practical ward politician and civic leader. He opposed a Baltimore City ordinance, supported by antivivisectionists, that would have crippled medical research in the city. When a supplier of laboratory animals was arrested on charges brought by the Society for the Prevention of Cruelty to Animals, Chesney and his wife pledged their home as bail security.

Chesney's good judgment and abiding sense of purpose kept the medical school on course from the Depression years to the beginning of the postwar expansion of government support for research. In keeping with the absence of bureaucratic complexity during these postwar years, Chesney lacked the title of full professor and served without assistant deans. He saw himself as the servant of the Advisory Board, and his deep devotion to the school and his sense of fairness were paramount.[41] Chesney's reluctant successor was Philip Bard, who from 1953 to 1957 sacrificed time in the physiology laboratory for the deanship.

Not only did four of Hopkins' most important staff members leave during the years immediately following the war, but the heads of the university and hospital Boards of Trustees also departed. Decisions to replace the directors of several departments had been deferred during the war, and now the preclinical Departments of Pathology, Pharmacology, Anatomy, and Physiological Chemistry acquired new directors, as did the clinical Departments of Medicine, Pediatrics, and Ophthalmology, and the Department of the History of Medicine.

The search for these new department heads placed new burdens on the search committees, which had to look beyond traditionally trained candidates for the directorship of basic science departments. The increasing emphasis on research expressed itself in increasing specialization, and the best candidates were now trained in specialized fields. In anatomy, for example, recent developments in histochemistry and other technical areas eliminated candidates trained solely in the traditional approaches to anatomy and histology.

Directors of clinical departments now had to develop complex progressive research programs, in addition to maintaining programs in teaching and patient care. The responsibilities seemed so great that the search committee selecting Longcope's successor even considered the idea of dividing the directorship of the Department of Medicine between two individuals: one to take charge of research and the other to oversee clinical practice and teaching. This approach would have had the advantage of diffusing the increasing administrative burden on the leader of a large clinical department, but it would also have fragmented the responsibility for the department's direction.

The Department of Medicine

After twenty years as head of medicine, Warfield Theobald Longcope was ready for retirement in 1942. He stayed on through the war years, however, as the turmoil of World War II prevented the medical institutions from appointing new faculty. Although Longcope was known as an outstanding clinician, his interest in research led him to publish meritorious articles on a variety of subjects, including glomerulonephritis, sarcoidosis, and atypical pneumonia. He was a member of the National Academy of Sciences, an honor given only sparingly to clinicians, and had received numerous honorary degrees and awards. His influence at Johns Hopkins was great: for a quarter of a century, scarcely any important decision was made at the medical institutions without his counsel.[42]

The committee in charge of finding his successor, chaired by Alfred Blalock, recommended to the Advisory Board the appointment of two co-directors of the department: Chester A. Keefer, a mature internist with an established reputation, and A. McGehee Harvey, a young man who was thought to have great promise. As mentioned earlier, the board decided to place the department under a single chief. That decision maintained two Hopkins traditions, as the Advisory Board rejected the idea of divided responsibility for the department and wagered on relative youth. The position was given to Harvey. He was thirty-four years old, compared to Keefer's forty-eight, and his appointment followed the precedent set by the appointments of Welch at the age of thirty-four, Kelly at thirty-one, Halsted at thirty-six, Osler at thirty-nine, Howell at thirty-three, Abel at thirty-five, and Mall at thirty-one.[43]

A. McGehee Harvey was a graduate of the Johns Hopkins University School of Medicine. He had served as a house officer on the Osler service, studied in England with Sir Henry Dale and at the University of Pennsylvania with Detlev W. Bronk, and returned to Hopkins in 1940 as chief resident in medicine. His residency was followed by a year at Vanderbilt University as an assistant professor. During World War II, he was on active duty with one of the Hopkins units.

Harvey led the Deparment of Medicine for twenty-seven years, from 1946 until his retirement in 1973. He brought into the department a number of young physicians who would later play important roles at Johns Hopkins. Philip A. Tumulty was his first resident on the Osler (ward) service, and William G. Speed, on the Marburg (private) service. Palmer H. Futcher, a graduate of the Johns Hopkins School of Medicine who had served on the medical house staff, took charge of the private outpatient service, which had been organized immediately after the war by James Bordley III.

Harvey also continued his research, begun during residency training, in the field of neuro-muscular problems. He and Joseph L. Lilienthal, Jr., were the first to advocate total thymectomy for the treatment of myasthenia gravis, and he and his group at Hopkins were the first to recognize the importance of the adrenocortical hormone in the management of patients with hypersensitivity diseases and to emphasize the clinical pattern of systemic lupus erythematosus.[44]

The Department of Pediatrics

When Edwards A. Park retired in 1946, he was succeeded as director of pediatrics by Francis F. Schwentker, a graduate of the Hopkins medical school who had served as chief resident pediatrician and then as director of the Sydenham Hospital, the City of Baltimore's hospital for communicable disease. He then became director of medical research for the Baltimore City Health Department and a member of the International Health Division of the Rockefeller Foundation.

Schwentker took over a department that bore Park's indelible stamp. Park had been chief of pediatrics since 1927. Contradicting the policy of his predecessor, John Howland, Park had established several specialty clinics in the pediatrics outpatient department, including cardiology, endocrinology, neurology, and child psychiatry (see chapter 9). Turner described Park as shy, hesitant, and retiring in appearance. He gave the impression of uncertainty, but a "vigilant thoroughness . . . characterized his approach to a sick child or a research problem."[45] He was the first of a group of academicians who took a particular interest in the problem of providing good medical care for all segments of the population.

Schwentker was chief of pediatrics for only eight years; he died in 1954, at the age of fifty. As department head, he made no indelible changes in the shape of the department, other than his transfer of Lawson Wilkins to full-time status. Wilkins, who was associate professor of pediatrics, consented to serve as acting chief of the department after Schwentker's death. He administered the department vigorously and sensitively, and convinced the medical school's Curriculum Committee that students would benefit from more time spent studying pediatrics.

In 1956, Robert E. Cooke took over the chair of pediatrics, allowing Wilkins to return to his research program. A graduate of the Yale University School of Medicine, Cooke came to Hopkins from an associate professorship of pediatrics at Yale. During his tenure at Hopkins, he designed and implemented novel programs that complemented the outstanding care furnished to sick children in the Children's Medical and Surgical Center (CMSC)—including a program that brought better medical care to inner-city mothers and their children. A major project was the construction of a new center for the habilitation of the handicapped, the Kennedy Institute for Handicapped Children, at the corner of Broadway and Monument streets.

Cooke developed an outstanding pediatric faculty and house staff. His perception of the important targets of pediatric research included an awareness of the increasing effect of the rapidly developing field of genetics, and he attracted a core of internationally known pediatric research scientists. Cooke's belief in the importance of surgical training for the pediatric house staff led him to initiate a novel program that integrated pediatric and surgical interns and residents. His drive to use the knowledge gained from medical research for the benefit of patients as soon as possible resulted in a screening program for the detection of Tay-Sachs disease and a program of lipid research. Cooke was particularly interested in the field of electrolyte metabolism, especially alkalosis. He left Johns Hopkins in 1973 for an administrative post at the University of Wisconsin medical center.[46]

Cooke's successor was John W. Littlefield, who moved to the directorship of the Department of Physiology twelve years later. The new director of pediatrics in 1985 was Frank A. Oski.

The Department of Ophthalmology

When Alan C. Woods retired in 1955 as head of ophthalmology, he was succeeded by Alfred Edward Maumenee, professor of surgery in ophthalmology at the Stanford University School of Medicine. A graduate of Cornell Medical College, Maumenee had studied with Woods as resident in ophthalmology at Johns Hopkins. He had progressed from instructor to associate professor at Hopkins before accepting a post at Stanford. Maumenee's research interests included problems related to corneal transplantation and the histopathology of ocular lesions produced by sulphur and nitrogen mustards.

Maumenee's twenty years as head of ophthalmology were an era of modernization, marked by the building of a research facility and by advances in ophthalmologic instrumentation. The devotion of his students is legendary, as ophthalmologists travel from around the world to attend the annual reunion of former Wilmer residents.[47]

Maumenee retired in 1979. He was succeeded by Arnall Patz (see chapter 11).

The Department of Pathology

When William G. MacCallum suffered a stroke in December 1941, the medical institutions were forced to consider a new head of pathology despite the war. First, Ernest W. Goodpasture declined the directorship, not wanting to move from Vanderbilt University at this late stage in his career. The search committee's second choice, Harry S. N. Greene, did not receive the unanimous support of either the committee or the Advisory Board. The hospital's Medical Board also hesitated before concurring with the recommendation—but Greene declined the post in any event, citing its uncongenial administrative requirements.

The Medical Board wanted to appoint Arnold R. Rich. As acting head, he was greatly admired by the medical faculty, which had presented the Advisory Board with a petition requesting that Rich be selected as director of pathology. Two members of the search committee favored Rich's nomination, while three wanted to defer a decision until the war was over. The Advisory Board agreed to delay its decision. The opposition to Rich probably stemmed from another Hopkins tradition, a reluctance to appoint to a faculty directorship the next man in line, particularly one whose entire career had been spent in Baltimore. Rich would also have become the first Jewish head of a department at Johns Hopkins, at a time when such an appointment was controversial in many American medical schools. As Turner commented, it was one of those rare instances in which the Medical Board of the hospital attempted to impose its will on the Advisory Board of the medical school in the selection of a department head. The Medical Board voted to reject the Advisory's Board's recommendation to wait, stating that further delay was not in the best

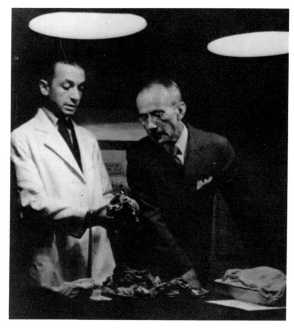

Arnold R. Rich and Louis Hamman. (*Source:* Alan M. Chesney Medical Archives, The Johns Hopkins Medical Institutions.)

interest of the medical institutions. Rich was promoted to the rank of full professor a few months later.[48]

Rich's promotion appeared to be a prelude to the directorship, as full professors other than department heads were rare at the time. But the university's president, Isaiah Bowman, was unenthusiastic about Rich as a department head, instructing the search committee to continue its deliberations. The result was a standoff: no department head was chosen for the duration of the war.

In the fall of 1946, the search committee was reconstituted, chaired by E. Kennerly Marshall, Jr., with Bard, Blalock, Chesney, and Harvey as members. A few months later, this committee recommended that Arnold Rice Rich be made director of pathology, a member of the Advisory Board, and pathologist-in-chief to the Johns Hopkins Hospital.

When he assumed the directorship, the fifty-four-year-old Rich was one of the leading pathologists in America. He had published some fifty valuable papers, covering the formation of bile and

bile pigments, the role of allergy and immunity in tuberculosis, and the role of humoral immunity in certain bacterial infections (see chapter 11).

Greatly admired by his colleagues and students, Rich led a small research discussion group that provided the testing ground for a whole generation of younger faculty members. He was also interested in medical education and curricular arrangements, and he was a loyal supporter of the *Bulletin of The Johns Hopkins Hospital.*

Rich was more than an inspiring teacher, a meticulous worker in the laboratory, a generous counselor, and a ruthless critic: time has shown him to be a wise man. He saw the growing federal support of medical research as an intrusion that would destroy the quality of academic life. He worried about the expansion that federal dollars brought, and he himself refused to apply for government grants.

To Rich, the academic life was everything, as his vivid description of that milieu reveals:

The attraction of an academic life in medicine consists, of course, in the character of the opportunities that an academic environment provides, and in the leisure for the satisfying enjoyment of these opportunities—leisure for trying to know one's field well, and opportunities for using that knowledge helpfully; leisure for trying to decrease the vast area of the unknown in health and in disease; leisure for association with the fresh young minds of students; and leisure for the enjoyment of one of the great charms of academic life—communion with one's colleagues young and old, in all fields, who are animated by these same pleasures and are interested in each others' interests. For the enjoyment of these leisures the 1920s and 1930s, like the decades immediately preceding them, were halcyon days in academic medicine, days when in most university medical schools there were few of the encroachments upon scholarly leisure that one hears so much about today, and which tend to increase with an increase in institutional size and organization. It had not yet become necessary to think seriously about the far-sighted concern of Daniel C. Gilman, the wise first president of Johns Hopkins, who, early in the present century, warned universities against the danger of losing the elements of repose, the quiet pursuit of knowlege, the friendship of books, the pleasures of conversations, and the advantages of solitude.[49]

Despite his many activities and his intense devotion to his work, Rich was always able to find time for any of his colleagues, young or old, who wanted to discuss their problems. These sessions were always brisk, with ideas tossed about, dissected, and synthesized so that all came away with a clear understanding of the problems and a firm idea of the first step necessary for solving them. This was Rich's gift, and the reason for the stimulating influence he exercised in the Johns Hopkins Medical Institutions throughout his career.

Rich was succeeded by Ivan L. Bennett in 1958. From 1969 to 1988, Robert H. Heptinstall was director of the department.

The Department of Pharmacology

When E. Kennerly Marshall, Jr., retired as director of pharmacology in 1955, he was succeeded by Gilbert H. Mudge. Mudge was an associate professor of medicine at the College of Physicians and Surgeons of Columbia University, where as a fellow of the National Research Council, he had developed his interest in the physiology and biochemistry of renal function, especially in the metabolism and excretion of electrolytes. At Hopkins, he concentrated his research on the renal mechanisms for the handling of drugs and their metabolic products. Like other clinical faculty members in research-oriented medical schools, Mudge's interests reflected the increasing depth of basic knowledge in biomedical science. His predecessor, Marshall, held a medical degree but worked entirely in the laboratory. In contrast, Mudge was both an expert clinician and an investigator who conducted basic research in renal physiology and pharmacology. The presence of such broadly capable individuals widened the range of candidates for preclinical professorships, bringing Paul Talalay to the directorship when Mudge left the department in 1962.[50]

The Department of Anatomy

The most wrenching change in the preclinical departments was the departure of Lewis H. Weed, who left the Department of Anatomy in 1948 after thirty-eight years to become a full-time member of the National Research Council. Weed had collaborated on most of the decisions concerning the School of Medicine in the 1920s and 1930s. His organizational talents, his capacity for lucid exposition, and his influence with philanthropic foundations made him an influential member of the Hopkins community.

His successor, Allan L. Grafflin, took over the department in 1948. Grafflin had received both his bachelor's and medical degrees from Johns Hopkins. He had returned to Hopkins after serving as associate professor of anatomy at Harvard, medical officer in the Army, and an American Cancer Society senior fellow in cancer research. Grafflin's research interests included fluorescent microscopy and the comparative anatomy and physiology of the kidney. Not long before his appointment to the directorship, he had become interested in enzyme chemistry in relation to histology, and it was this line of investigation that he developed at Johns Hopkins.

A key factor in Grafflin's selection was his interest in new approaches to anatomical research through the technique of fluorescent microscopy. Grafflin was one of a few scientists who appreciated the rapid changes under way in the field of anatomy. He saw that it was time for a new direction in research and a new approach to teaching, one in which gross anatomy would give way to the study of the structure and function of the cell.

Grafflin resigned the directorship in 1956, to specialize in neuro-ophthalmology. Coming from the school of hygiene to replace him as department head was David Bodian. Bodian had obtained the doctoral degree in anatomy and the medical degree from the University of Chicago; he had been an assistant professor of anatomy at Western Reserve University before coming to Johns Hopkins as an associate professor of epidemiology in the school of hygiene. Because of his varied research contributions, a colleague referred to Bodian as one of the "anchor men" in the development of the polio vaccine (see chapter 11). He was also known as an engaging teacher throughout his twenty-year directorship.

The Department of Physiological Chemistry

William M. Clark retired from the Department of Physiological Chemistry in 1952 and was succeeded by Albert L. Lehninger. Lehninger had received his doctorate from the University of Wisconsin in physiological chemistry and was involved in research on plasma protein substitutes at Wisconsin during World War II. He continued his career at the University of Chicago, remaining there until he accepted the chair at Hopkins at the age of thirty-five.

At Hopkins, Lehninger built up a distinguished faculty and an excellent graduate program. He was a gifted teacher, interested in conveying biochemical knowledge to general readers as well as to graduate students. His seven books were enthusiastically received, particularly *The Mitochondrion* and *Bioenergetics,* the latter a word that was quickly accepted as the name of an entire area of biochemistry.

Lehninger's own scientific work was characterized by great inventiveness and versatility. He made many fundamental contributions to the understanding of the biochemistry of energy capture, mitochondrial calcium transport, and associated hydrogen ion movements (see chapter 11).[51]

Lehninger was succeeded in 1978 as department director by M. Daniel Lane (see chapter 11).

The Institute of the History of Medicine

Henry E. Sigerist left his post as head of the Institute of the History of Medicine in 1947, in what was described as an atmosphere of mutual disillusionment.[52] Sigerist began his career at Hopkins with brilliance and enthusiasm, but he gradually abandoned his emphasis on medical history to concentrate on contemporary events. Sigerist's praise of medicine in the Soviet Union while most

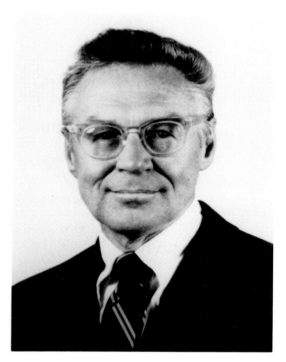

Albert L. Lehninger

of his colleagues were serving in the armed forces during World War II alienated him even further from the Hopkins medical community. His zeal for socialized medicine, particularly as practiced in the Soviet Union, was anathema to most American physicians, and his position at Johns Hopkins became increasingly uncongenial.

Sigerist's successor, Richard Harrison Shryock, was a general historian with a particular interest in the social history of medicine. He came to Baltimore from a professorship of American history at the University of Pennsylvania. Shryock expanded the reach of the institute to encompass all of the history of science; when a history of science department was established in the Faculty of Arts and Sciences in the early 1960s, however, the institute returned to an emphasis on the history of medicine.

Owsei Temkin, Sigerist's protégé, became head of the department in 1958. He was succeeded by Lloyd G. Stevenson in 1968. Since 1984, the director of the department has been Gert H. Brieger.

Established Specialties and the Full-Time System

The specialization related to the explosion of bio-medical knowledge was aided by federal funds in the 1960s. Until the rise of federal support, the Department of Medicine had not had the funds to permit the creation of full-time units. The desirability of making the subdepartments of neurology and dermatology into independent departments, for example, had been discussed even before World War II, but the reorganization had been delayed because ample facilities and basic budgetary support were lacking.

The "specialization" in the clinical departments that took place at Johns Hopkins soon after World War II was, however, the fruition of plans developed earlier. Unlike the Department of Medicine, the Department of Surgery had been able to use the fees from Alfred Blalock's private patients to place several of its divisions on a full-time basis in the years immediately following the war.

Alfred Blalock had returned to Baltimore as chief of surgery in 1941, succeeding Dean DeWitt Lewis, who had resigned because of ill health. A graduate of the Hopkins medical school in 1922,

Blalock had not been an outstanding student, and his postgraduate training had been a patchwork: a year as a house officer in urology under Hugh H. Young, followed by a year's residency in general surgery, and then a year as a fellow in otolaryngology. He moved to Vanderbilt University in 1925 as chief resident in surgery (see chapter 9); after completing his residency, he joined the faculty and began his investigation of shock in dogs. To continue these experiments at Hopkins, Blalock had brought with him Vivien Thomas, his valued associate, and George Duncan, an assistant resident in surgery at Vanderbilt (see chapter 11).[53]

Blalock's varied residency training must have contributed to his interest in the surgical subspecialties. He had accepted the department directorship at Hopkins on the condition that he be permitted to execute his plans for strengthening the special areas of surgery. The war had delayed his efforts, but in the immediate postwar years, the Department of Surgery had acquired the funds to put several of its divisions on a full-time basis. The full-time Department of Radiology was created in 1946; it was followed by the full-time Divisions of Urology (in 1947), Neurosurg-

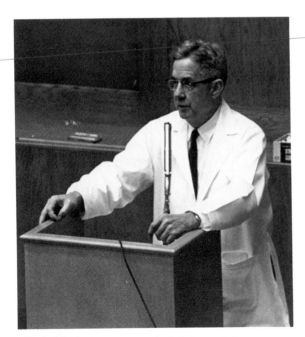

Alfred Blalock. (*Source:* J. Michael Criley, M.D.)

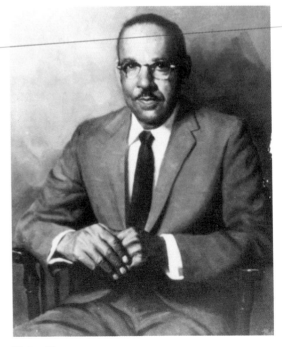

Vivien Thomas

ery (in 1947), Anesthesiology (in 1947), Oto-laryngology (in 1952), and Orthopedic Surgery (in 1953) (see chapter 8). In each instance, the change to full-time status was linked to the arrival of a new department or divisional director.

Blalock's tenure as department director lasted twenty-three years. Thirty-eight of his residents went on to important academic appointments; ten became department heads themselves. One of his first chief residents was Mark Ravitch, called by one colleague "Blalock's alter ego."[54] It was Ravitch who helped Blalock to organize the first intensive care unit for children, on Halsted 3. Here former "blue babies" were brought immediately after surgery. Throughout his career, Ravitch maintained his interest in both surgery and pediatrics, following a Halsted internship with an internship at the Harriet Lane. He was elected to important national posts in both fields, as surgeon-in-chief at Baltimore City Hospitals, chief of pediatric surgery at the University of Chicago, and, in 1970, surgeon-in-chief at Montefiore Hospital in Pittsburgh.

The success of many of his residents attests to Blalock's special interest in pediatric surgery. At Hopkins, he gave much attention to the development of a children's surgical unit. This dream culminated in the Children's Medical and Surgical Center, which was dedicated in 1964, the year in which he retired.

Alfred Blalock was succeeded by George D. Zuidema, a graduate of the Hopkins medical school and associate professor at the University of Michigan.[55] Zuidema's youth—he was thirty-six years old—was squarely in the Hopkins tradition, as was his importation from another university. Zuidema had gone to Boston for his residency in general surgery. He was legendarily prolific, by 1964 the author of more than 200 articles, many of which were of seminal importance; and he had received half a dozen prestigious scholarships and awards.

Pediatric surgery was also one of Zuidema's particular interests. When the Children's Medical and Surgical Center was completed soon after he arrived, space became available to make pediatric surgery a separate division. Zuidema appointed

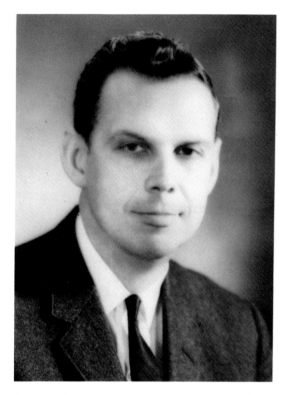

George D. Zuidema. (*Source:* Alan M. Chesney Medical Archives, The Johns Hopkins Medical Institutions.)

its first director, David C. Sabiston, Jr., from within the department, but Sabiston left a year later to head the Department of Surgery at Duke University. As the next division head, Zuidema brought J. Alex Haller back to Hopkins from the University of Louisville, where he was assistant professor and chief of the section of pediatric surgery.

The Division of Pediatric Surgery was unique in requiring its residents to have completed a general surgical residency—including board qualification in general surgery—before entering the program. This stipulation was a harbinger of changing policies in surgical training: in 1965, pediatric surgery was the only surgical specialty with this requirement, but over the next two decades, other specialties adopted the prerequisite.

Zuidema's enthusiasm for transplantation studies spanned several areas of medicine. The earliest such program at Johns Hopkins antedated his arrival, as George Santos had brought his interest in bone marrow transplantation to Hopkins immediately after the Korean War. This effort was directed particularly toward patients with leukemia, but it was later used successfully in individuals with aplastic anemia and in those with certain genetic disorders. When Zuidema arrived, kidney transplantation was well established in a number of centers, and he wanted Hopkins to enter the field. Norman Anderson, who had just finished his year as chief medical resident, went to work with Rupert Billingham at the Wistar Institute in Philadelphia for two years; upon his return, Anderson established a laboratory of transplantation immunology within the Department of Surgery.

The development of transplantation at Hopkins was impeded by the absence of a chronic renal dialysis unit. Although W. Gordon Walker, head of the Renal Division in the Department of Medicine, had expressed a willingness to operate a unit, he didn't have $30,000 to buy the necessary hardware. Zuidema's department had just been given $10,000 by a grateful patient, and Zuidema approached Thomas B. Turner, the dean, with a proposal: if the medical school would contribute another $10,000, Zuidema would approach the hospital for the final third. All parties agreed, and within the space of half a day, the sum was raised. Walker set up his chronic dialysis unit, and Hopkins was in the transplantation business. The first successful kidney transplant was performed at Hopkins by Harvey Bender in 1968. The following year, G. Melville Williams was recruited from the Medical College of Virginia to head a program in transplantation and vascular surgery.[56]

The Departments of Gynecology and Obstetrics

Complicating the administrative arrangements of the Department of Gynecology was its ambiguous relation to the Department of Obstetrics. The choice of Richard W. TeLinde as successor to Thomas S. Cullen in 1939 reflected a victory for the separatists—those members of the Advisory Board who favored independent departments of obstetrics and gynecology. The committee empaneled to appoint Cullen's successor included

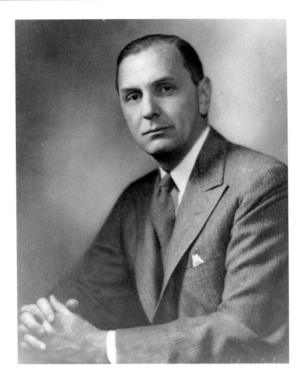

Richard W. TeLinde

Winford H. Smith, the hospital director; Alan M. Chesney, the dean of the School of Medicine; Nicholson J. Eastman, professor and director of the Department of Obstetrics; and Edward H. Richardson, Sr., part-time associate professor in the Division of Gynecology.

At the committee's first meeting, Eastman nominated Richardson for director of gynecology—a Machiavellian move, as Eastman was hoping to become head of a combined department of gynecology and obstetrics himself, and knew that Richardson's tenure would be limited. The motion was seconded at once—by all except Richardson himself, who asserted that he was too old and too involved in other activities to take on the directorship.

Next, Richardson nominated TeLinde, who was opposed to a merger between obstetrics and gynecology; the chief opponent of this nomination was Eastman, who continued to urge Richardson to take the post. When Richardson proved inflexible, Eastman backed another candidate, Houston S. Everett, an associate professor of gynecology.

The committee's deliberations then became a struggle between Eastman and Richardson. Eastman was anticipating Richardson's early retirement and was counting on his own ability to influence Everett, who seemed to offer the smallest obstacle to Eastman in his efforts to become head of a joint department. Richardson was well aware of Eastman's ambitions and persevered in his support of TeLinde, whom he viewed as best able to preserve the independence of gynecology.

TeLinde eventually won the committee's unanimous approval. Richardson was then able to suggest that gynecology be given independent status as a major clinical department and to ask for research funds for the specialty. The committee granted both requests, and the new department was given $100,000 from the medical school's annual budget.

TeLinde foresaw the role of gynecology in the investigation of endocrine functions and created a subsection of reproductive endocrinology. Georgeanna Seegar Jones was chosen as head of this division, which was a joint project of the Departments of Gynecology and Obstetrics. TeLinde was also a pioneer in the use of estrogen in menopause, and his other research interests included the management of urinary stress incontinence and the early diagnosis of cancer of the cervix.

Even after assuming the directorship, TeLinde retained his part-time faculty status. In 1956, gynecology became the last Hopkins department to be placed on a full-time basis (see chapter 8).[57]

The relationship between the Departments of Gynecology and Obstetrics was resolved a few years later. When head of obstetrics J. Whitridge Williams died in 1931, John MacFarland Bergland was asked to serve as acting chief of obstetrics and obstetrician-in-chief of the hospital. He was succeeded by Nicholson J. Eastman. The tone of the next three decades was set by the search committee, which advocated a continued link between gynecology and surgery and set out to find a head of obstetrics who would not meddle in surgical matters.

Coincidentally, TeLinde and Eastman retired in the same year. The time was right to unify the two specialties under one leader, and in 1964 Allan C. Barnes was appointed director of the Department of Obstetrics and Gynecology. Most medical centers had combined departments; since gynecology and obstetrics were the only specialties dealing exclusively with the medical problems of women, a combined approach seemed appropriate. At Johns Hopkins, the "new" departmental structure represented a return to the institution's earliest days, when Howard A. Kelly was both chief gynecologist and chief obstetrician.

Along with his considerable skills in teaching, research, and patient care, Barnes brought social activism to the department. "Society's problems are the prime concern of the university," Barnes said,[58] and his public stand in favor of fertility control was controversial for the time. He gave his services to many nonmedical organizations, advising the Ford Foundation (on population control), the World Health Organization (on maternal and child health), and the Center for Reproduction and Sexual Health. Barnes remained at Hopkins for six years, leaving to become a vice-president of the Rockefeller Foundation.

His successor was Theodore M. King, who remained as director until 1984, when he was succeeded by Edward E. Wallach.

Psychiatry, Neurology, and Neurosurgery

Some of the "new" specialties that arose at Johns Hopkins after World War II were not new areas of knowledge but segments of departments that could not develop independently until federal and private funding became available. A separate department of neurology had been under discussion since the 1920s, but money had not been available to cut neurology loose from its parent department, medicine. The best home for neurology, moreover, was a matter of continuing debate. Some felt that it belonged in the Department of Psychiatry; others believed that it should be an independent department, containing a division of neurological surgery. At one time, advocates of a separate neurological organization made an unsuccessful effort to secure funds for a center similar to the Wilmer Ophthalmological Institute. When the question arose again after World War II, however, the Advisory Board recommended that neurology remain a part of the Department of Medicine. Like many leading medical schools in the late 1940s, Hopkins was not prepared to commit any general funds for an independent department of neurology, nor were any other funds or facilities available for the purpose.

By 1966, however, the Division of Neurology at Johns Hopkins was lagging behind other divisions. Research programs were few, and Johns Hopkins was not training many leaders in the field. Part of the problem was a simple lack of space. Beds for neurology patients were scattered through the medical (and in some cases, surgical) wards, making it difficult for students, house officers, and faculty to care for patients and maintain contact with other members of the division. Research space was also in short supply, as was administrative office space.

Several events during Thomas B. Turner's deanship rekindled interest in a separate department of neurology. Across the country, scientists were turning to the study of the brain as one of medical science's great unsolved problems. A new facility encompassing pediatric neurology, the John F. Kennedy Institute for the Rehabilitation of the Mentally and Physically Handicapped Child, had been created on the East Baltimore campus. Furthermore, the person in charge of pediatric neurology at Johns Hopkins, David Clark, had departed for the University of Kentucky, and the neurology faculty had been further depleted by Orthello Langworthy's move to the Department of Psychiatry in 1944 and the retirement of Frank Ford in 1958. On the positive side, endowment funds were available for two professorships, sponsored by the Joseph P. Kennedy Foundation and the Cerebral Palsy Foundation. Finally, space could be had in the planned Traylor Building for research, and beds were available in the hospital for the care of patients with neurological disorders.

Even after the official decision to form a separate Department of Neurology, two years elapsed before the department had a director. Not until

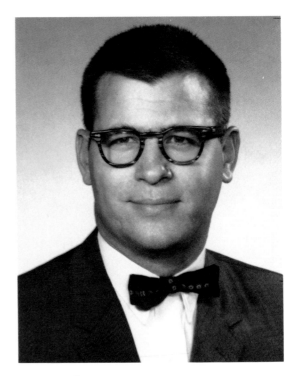

Guy M. McKhann

the spring of 1968 was Guy M. McKhann appointed head of the department. A graduate of Yale Medical School, McKhann had spent a year at Hopkins as a resident in pediatrics. He had also trained in neurology and pediatrics at New York Hospital and at the Massachusetts General Hospital, and he came to Hopkins from Stanford.

It was essential for McKhann to recruit outstanding faculty for the new department. The two endowed professorships represented extraordinary financial strength in a new department, but little additional money was available to back them up. The financial strength of the new department would therefore depend on faculty members who could command substantial research and training grants. McKhann recruited talented young investigators in the neurosciences. The first to arrive were Daniel Drachman and Richard Johnson. Robert Herndon followed, and John Freeman joined the faculty to head the Division of Pediatric Neurology.

Space for the department turned out to be a patchwork arrangement. Offices, clinical activities, and research laboratories were scattered through several buildings, wherever rooms or beds were available. Neurology's first offices were situated outside Osler 5—in space given up by the Department of Medicine—and laboratory space was made available by Joel Elkes, director of the Department of Psychiatry, who relinquished half a floor in the Traylor Building. McKhann remembers his shock at seeing the original location for neurology patients, Brady 2. Having come from a relatively new hospital at Stanford, he had not realized that such primitive wards still existed. Brady 2 was soon remodeled to become the new department's first clinical base.[59]

The Department of Neurology developed its closest relationship with the Department of Neurosurgery in the late 1960s. Head of neurosurgery at that time was A. Earl Walker. As a member of the NIH's Advisory Council concerned with neurology, Walker was able to guide the department of neurology into areas of research of particular interest to the NIH. Walker's advice was very helpful to McKhann in planning for the department of neurology as well as in solidifying the department's relations with the NIH. Walker had visions of a combined neurosciences center, but he did not remain to see it develop. When Walker retired, he left Johns Hopkins for a visiting professorship at the University of New Mexico in Albuquerque.

Donlin Long was Walker's successor as director of neurosurgery. Shortly before Long's arrival from Minnesota in 1973, the division had been given departmental status. Long expanded many of the facilities begun by Walker, including the Pain Clinic, which had been established in 1970. Long also continued the close connection between neurology and neurosurgery, so much so that in 1987 McKhann characterized them as "virtually a single department, sharing clinical space (both inpatient and outpatient), administrative staffs, nursing staffs, and teaching activities."[60]

The third member of the clinical neurosciences triumvirate is the Department of Psychiatry and Behavioral Sciences. The history of this department reflects the tradition of interest in psychobiology instituted by Adolf Meyer and continued by his successor, John C. Whitehorn, and

the other members of the department. A biologist by training, Whitehorn focused on the nature of human communication, the psychiatric interview, and the place of empathy in psychiatry. Through the work of Jerome Frank, "the faith that heals" became a respectable subject for scientific inquiry, and in parallel, Eugene Meyer studied the effects of short-term psychiatric therapy on patients attending psychosomatic clinics. Horsley Gantt, another member of the department in the 1950s, was well-known for his work on the conditioned reflex, the predecessor to biofeedback techniques. Curt Richter, the world's expert on "biological clocks," directed the Laboratory for Psychobiology (see chapter 11).[61]

The department drifted for several years after Whitehorn's retirement in 1960. Frank served as acting head until the arrival of Seymour Kety in 1962, but Kety remained at Hopkins for only a year, realizing that he preferred work in the laboratory to the combination of teaching, laboratory work, and administration that the directorship required. Kety's successor was Joel Elkes, whose particular interest was psychopharmacology.

Even before his arrival at Hopkins, Elkes had formally outlined his hopes for the department—which included changing its name to the Department of Psychiatry and Behavioral Sciences. Elkes believed that a purely clinical name, "Department of Psychiatry," did not do justice to the department's panoply of activities. These included the department's neurocommunications laboratory, directed by Richard Chase and run jointly by the Department of Pediatrics; an extension of the animal behavior studies in Gantt's Pavlovian Laboratory; the new Division of Clinical Psychology; and the beginnings of a small social psychology unit. Moreover, Elkes intended to make human development, human learning, and human communication the core themes of the department.

During Elkes's tenure as department head, the Department of Psychiatry and Behavioral Sciences emphasized the study of biological influences on mental illness, the introduction of the social sciences in the department, the development of an M.D.-Ph.D. program in the behavioral sciences and a master's degree program in mental health counseling, important research in psycho-pharmacology, the development of psychiatric services for adolescents, and the introduction of programs in drug and alcohol dependency in the hospital.

Elkes stepped down as director of the department in 1973, wishing to devote more time to the laboratory. Again the department drifted, until the arrival of Paul R. McHugh as department head in 1975. Under McHugh's leadership, the department has emphasized the study of motivated behavior, psychiatric epidemiology, and neuropsychiatry.

Dermatology

Like neurology, dermatology was one of the weaker areas at Johns Hopkins until it was given departmental status and a full-time director with the rank of professor. Primarily an outpatient division, it began as part of the Department of Surgery but moved to the Department of Medicine in 1928. The dermatology clinic failed to attract graduate students because there was no organized program, and the medical school administration was reluctant to encourage graduate students to attend clinics as informal observers for fear they would return to their communities after brief periods of insufficient training and claim that they had done postgraduate work at Johns Hopkins.

Lloyd Ketron, who served as Hopkins' principal dermatologist on a part-time basis from 1929 until his retirement in 1956, believed that establishing a formal training program was an impossible task. Such a program would require the approval of Warfield T. Longcope, the head of the Department of Medicine, who had denied Ketron's requests for additional appropriations and equipment. Longcope was satisfied with the instruction medical students were receiving in the dermatology clinic. He also saw no reason to divert funds to dermatology because Ketron had obtained substantial donations from his private patients to support the dermatology clinic and his laboratory of dermatohistopathology.

Ketron's successor, Maurice Sullivan, was a part-time faculty member as well, an internist

with three years of additional training in dermatology. The limited facilities at Hopkins made it difficult to recruit a first-class investigator and clinician from outside the institution, so the Advisory Board had decided to use the tactic that had worked so well for Halsted: they selected a well-trained internist from within and hoped that he could increase the department's academic stature. Sullivan was already on the scene as a private practitioner of dermatology and a part-time investigator of nutritional problems in E. V. McCollum's laboratory. On his retirement in 1959, he was replaced by Ernest W. Smith, a full-time faculty member who shifted his interest from hematology to dermatology. Smith left in 1964 to enter private practice.

The rapid turnover in directors of the subdepartment led the Advisory Board to reconsider its strategy. When Smith departed, funds were allocated for a full-time position in dermatology. Robert G. Crounse was recruited from Yale to head the Subdepartment of Dermatology as associate professor. Crounse was one of the first dermatologists with substantial research training, and he intended to pursue that aspect of the discipline himself. To cover the department's clinical activities, Crounse brought first Alan Schragger and then George W. Hambrick, Jr., to Hopkins. With the devoted assistance of part-time department members already in place, such as Francis A. Ellis, Maurice Sullivan, and Isadore Zeligman, Crounse was able to provide good instruction for residents and good care for patients.

Crounse left in 1969 for a full professorship at the University of Georgia and was succeeded by Hambrick, who was promoted to full professor. Hambrick also presided over the subdepartment's elevation to departmental status, a change recommended by A. McGehee Harvey, director of the Department of Medicine, before his retirement in 1973. Adequate space had become available in the Blalock Building for laboratories and offices. Although there would be no discrete dermatology inpatient unit, beds were available on the medical service. Most important, the members of the Advisory Board agreed that the dermatology program would not be able to attract first-class residents or faculty unless it was a full department. It was Hambrick who established outposts in dermatology at Good Samaritan Hospital and at the Baltimore City Hospitals. Under his direction, the Department of Dermatology trained a significant number of residents and acquired a well-trained professional staff.[62]

Hambrick was succeeded in 1976 by Irwin M. Freedberg, who remained in the directorship until 1981. His successor was Thomas T. Provost.

The Extension of Barker's Three Clinical Research Divisions

The creation of the Division of Psychiatry in Medicine in 1947 fulfilled one of Lewellys F. Barker's long-time dreams. Barker, who established the three research divisions in the Department of Medicine (see chapter 3), had hoped for a fourth —a link between medicine and psychiatry—but had been forced to abandon the plan for lack of funds.

An informal "fourth research division," spe-

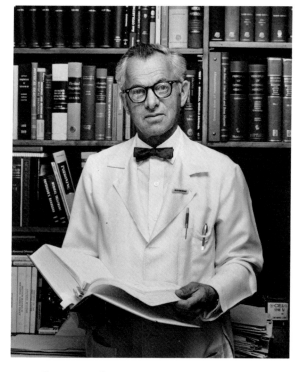

Maxwell M. Wintrobe

cializing in hematology, had been created in the 1930s, when Maxwell M. Wintrobe arrived to take charge of the course in clinical microscopy and to supervise the hospital's hematology laboratory. Outpatient activities in hematology were conducted in the gastroenterology clinic, a situation that reflected Wintrobe's interest in nutrition. The "hematology division" had no other full-time members, however, except Alan M. Chesney, who, in addition to serving as dean of the medical school, assisted in the teaching of clinical microscopy.

Barker's dream had to wait until the postwar years, when A. McGehee Harvey and John C. Whitehorn established a Division of Psychiatry in Medicine even without federal funds. It was headed by Theodore Lidz, who was trained in both fields and who later became professor of psychiatry at Yale.

True additions to the full-time complement of specialty divisions in the Department of Medicine did not come into being until the late 1940s, when the rise of the NIH and the interest in categorical diseases made funds available. Until then, specialties in the Department of Medicine had been represented mostly as separate clinics in the outpatient department and were supervised by part-time internists with an interest in a particular area.

This system worked well enough for the time: patients received specialized care, and some excellent clinical research was done. As biomedical knowledge grew in the postwar period, however, and new technical approaches became available, clinical knowledge began to expand and research opportunities increased. The availability of research and training grants in certain specialties led to their reorganization on a full-time basis. The process was augmented by the falling away of the part-time consultant staff, whose time was now being taken up with postgraduate residency training programs at other hospitals. Among the specialties to be granted full-time divisional status were the following (directors' names are given in parentheses): medical genetics (Victor A. McKusick), clinical pharmacology (Louis Lasagna), oncology (Albert H. Owens, Jr.), renal disease (W. Gordon Walker), allergy and clinical immunology (Philip S. Norman), rheumatology (Lawrence E. Shulman), pulmonary medicine (Joseph L. Lilienthal, Jr.), and gastroenterology (Thomas R. Hendrix).

New Departments in Fields Related to Medical Research

Biophysics

A separate department of biophysics in the School of Medicine was originally proposed by A. McGehee Harvey and Samuel A. Talbot in 1946 and considered by a joint committee of the graduate school of arts and sciences, the medical school, and the school of hygiene. Matters had progressed as far as a search for the head of the proposed new department when the plan was derailed by the impending arrival of Detlev Bronk, the university's new president. Bronk intended to continue his studies in biophysics, which were under way at the University of Pennsylvania. Biophysics therefore became a university department—a joint department spanning both the School of Medicine and the Faculty of Arts and Sciences. The primary base of the department was located not in East Baltimore but on the Homewood campus; and it was staffed by individuals from Bronk's staff at the University of Pennsylvania, even though it was supported in part by the Jenkins Fund, originally intended for the School of Medicine.

Biophysics remained a university department even after Bronk's departure in 1953, and through the short tenure of his successor, Lowell Reed. When Milton S. Eisenhower became the university's president in 1956, however, the Department of Biophysics was removed entirely from the medical school, relinquishing its status as a joint department to become part of the Faculty of Arts and Sciences.

This change prompted W. Barry Wood, vice-president of the university and the hospital, to use the medical school's portion of the Jenkins Fund to establish a separate Department of Biophysics at the medical school. A separate building for the department, funded in part by a donation from the Rockefeller Foundation and a grant from the National Institutes of Health, was erected on the site of the old Physiology Building. An alternative was to add two floors to the new Basic Science Building, but a separate building gave the department more flexibility and provided underground space for shielding against radiation effects.

Howard M. Dintzis, who had been senior research associate in the Department of Biology at the Massachusetts Institute of Technology, became director of the Department of Biophysics in 1961. His new department was intended to complement the biophysics department at Homewood; as a preclinical department, it would provide a base for the more applied biophysics to be used in clinical departments in both the medical school and the school of hygiene.[63]

Biomedical Engineering

The Division of Biomedical Engineering, part of the Department of Medicine, was reassessed in 1965 because of the impending retirement of its first director, Samuel A. Talbot, who had led the division since 1946. Talbot's retirement coincided with an upsurge in the application of engineering sciences and technology to medical and biological research. Members of the Advisory Board and the Department of Medicine believed that this field was in a position to apply its powers to the research and educational programs throughout the school of medicine. Furthermore, the division had won national prestige: its graduate training program, run by Moise Goldstein, was one of the three research training programs in biomedical engineering supported by the NIH. The division's expertise spanned the entire university, as Goldstein held appointments in both the Department of Medicine and the Whiting School of Engineering, and the division helped other university departments with problems in design and planning. Its research was as strong as its graduate training—an NIH grant supported such projects as the development of methods and hardware for analog-to-digital conversions and the development of new techniques in computation. The present and future importance of these activities required their coordination by a single individual, who would direct a semiautonomous subdepartment. Furthermore, the administrative shift from division to subdepartment was seen as only a stop on the way to full departmental status.

The director of biomedical engineering would be responsible for the graduate, research, and service programs, as well as the Computer Center. Established in 1960, the latter unit had been run by Richard Shepard, associate professor in the Department of Medicine. The medical institutions needed their own large, general-purpose digital computer, the Advisory Board believed. A mainframe computer would free the Computer Center from its data link to the Applied Physics Laboratory and enable the center to meet the greatly increased needs that the Advisory Board saw just around the corner.

Chosen to head the new Subdepartment of Biomedical Engineering was Richard J. Johns, a 1948 graduate of the Johns Hopkins medical school. Johns's entire career was spent at Johns Hopkins, from internship to assistant deanship In 1966, he was promoted to full professor, shortly before being named head of biomedical engineering.

Departmental status came only four years later. Under Johns's leadership, the department has expanded to encompass research in speech and hearing, cardiovascular control, and myocardial mechanics, as well as the development of hardware as diverse as a battery-powered upper-limb prosthesis and an argon-laser photocoagulator for repairing torn blood vessels in the retina.[64]

Supporting Departments

Laboratory Medicine

The clinical laboratories at the Johns Hopkins Hospital, part of a pioneering tradition begun by Osler within the Department of Medicine, had

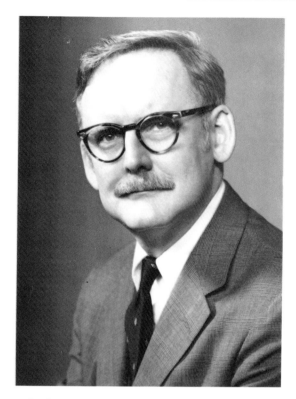

Richard J. Johns

come under great strain by the 1960s. The volume and complexity of laboratory work necessary for the practice of medicine required a separate administrative unit, and decisions about the nature and location of this unit occupied the Advisory Board for most of 1967. Was clinical pathology a distinct discipline? The Advisory Board was divided: some believed that the subject required only technical talent grounded in a good knowledge of biochemistry; others, that the subject was a true academic discipline. Should clinical pathology become a separate department, or should it be subsumed under the Departments of Medicine or Pathology, or under the Division of Biomedical Engineering? Moreover, if clinical pathology warranted departmental status, was it the department most urgently needed by the medical school? What would be the source of its financial support? And should it be represented on the Advisory Board—thereby undesirably increasing the Board's size?

The compromise that resolved the polar differences between members of the Advisory Board was the creation of a Subdepartment of Laboratory Medicine within the Department of Pathology—a subdepartment being more autonomous than a division but less independent than a separate department. A Department of Laboratory Medicine would be established simultaneously in the hospital, and in the Hopkins tradition, one person would be appointed head of both. Because laboratory medicine was a supporting department in the hospital rather than an independent clinical department like medicine or surgery, its director would have voting privileges only on the Medical Board of the hospital and not on the Advisory Board of the medical school.

The new director was Rex B. Conn, Jr., recipient of the M.D. degree from Yale, the B.Sc. degree in biochemistry from Oxford, and the master's degree in anatomy from the University of Minnesota. Conn trained in both internal medicine and laboratory medicine in Minnesota. He came to Hopkins in 1968 from a post as professor of pathology and director of the clinical laboratories at West Virginia University.[65] Conn left in 1978, and a new director of laboratory medicine, Robert C. Rock, was appointed in 1981.

Comparative Medicine

A singular consultant department links veterinary and human medicine. The Division of Comparative Medicine, founded in 1962 as the Division of Animal Medicine, is the embodiment of what Osler called "one medicine." It comprises two distinct areas: professional (pathology, clinical veterinary medicine) and animal services (complete care of experimental animals). The division is responsible for the care of more than 29,000 animals. Primates represent one-third of the division's cases requiring clinical veterinary attention, although they represent less than 1 percent of all the research animals at Hopkins; more than 90 percent of Hopkins's research animals are rodents, but these account for only 12 percent of the division's caseload.

Many of the faculty members in comparative medicine also hold appointments in other departments, and their research activities span neuropathology, immunopathology, virology, and toxicology. The division's physical facilities include medical, surgical, and pathological diagnostic and research laboratories (located in the Traylor Building), as well as a research farm.

Setting the stage at Hopkins for a strong division of animal medicine were Osler and Welch's intense interest in comparative medicine, and their work in zoology and parasitology. Osler had lectured at veterinary schools in Toronto and Montreal and had often visited veterinarians in connection with his studies of animal parasites. During the 1870s and 1880s, he published numerous articles on comparative pathology, dealing with such subjects as nematodes in dogs, hog cholera, echinococcus, bovine tuberculosis, and the parasites in the Montreal pork supply. Welch, who had studied in the laboratories at the Munich Veterinary School, reflected the common idea among physician-investigators of the time that research veterinary medicine had implications for human medicine. The Johns Hopkins University School of Hygiene and Public Health was one of three preeminent institutions fostering cross-professional cooperation among veterinarians, zoologists, and physicians in the United States. A primate colony for fundamental research was established at Hopkins in the 1920s under the auspices of the Carnegie Institution of Washington.

Until the arrival of Edward C. Melby, Jr., in 1962, however, animal medicine at Johns Hopkins was concerned entirely with routine animal services. Melby, a veterinarian, was responsible for introducing modern clinical laboratory animal services for all divisions using experimental animals. The Division of Animal Medicine, which had been created in the Department of Pathology, became an independent Division of Laboratory Animal Medicine reporting directly to the dean.

In 1966, a grant from the NIH allowed Johns Hopkins to establish a formal training program in comparative pathology; that year, too, an NIH grant provided for a unique joint program with the New York State Veterinary College at Cornell University—a three-year residency in animal and human pathology. Running the program at Hopkins was Robert A. Squire, a Cornell graduate with a joint appointment in human and animal pathology. Until 1966, animal research at Hopkins had been limited to smaller laboratory specimans, but the joint program pointed up the need for facilities to house larger animals. As a result, in 1967 Hopkins obtained a ninety-acre farm outside Baltimore to serve as a breeding, holding, and long-term care facility for research animals.[66]

Collaborative Departments

Accompanying the process of specialization after the war was intensified collaboration between departments. Faculty members held joint appointments that bridged many combinations of disciplines. The Division of Clinical Pharmacology, for example, one of the first full-time divisions of clinical pharmacology in the nation, was a joint effort of the Departments of Medicine and Pharmacology. Louis Lasagna came to Johns Hopkins in 1954 to head this division, seizing on the NIH's interest in the chemotherapy of leukemia. Lasagna was a key participant in the NIH's cooperative study groups and helped to develop the protocols used in the NIH's controlled clinical trials.

Collaboration between the Departments of Medicine and Pharmacology also resulted in the establishment of the Oncology Center. As chemotherapy joined radiotherapy and surgery in the treatment of cancer, A. McGehee Harvey decided to carve out another new specialty, one that would profit from having access to the well-trained clinical investigators who populated departments of medicine. Albert H. Owens, Jr., was chosen to head the new oncology division, and he prepared for his post by spending two years with E. Kennerly Marshall, Jr., in the Department of Pharmacology.

Upon completion of this fellowship in 1956, Owens was faced with formidable administrative problems. Johns Hopkins lacked adequate space for a separate ward for oncology patients, and in 1961 Owens therefore moved a large part of his inpatient, clinical, and research activities to the Baltimore City Hospitals. His early efforts to

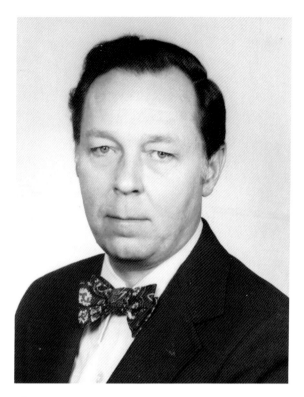

Albert H. Owens, Jr.

obtain NIH grants were hampered by his background. Because he had not trained as an oncologist in one of the recognized cancer centers, such as Sloan-Kettering, the members of the NIH's peer-review committees were reluctant to give him funding. Eventually, in 1973, Johns Hopkins was awarded funds to establish one of the newly authorized National Cancer Centers, and in 1977 Owens and his group moved back to the Hopkins hospital.[67]

The Growing Bureaucracy

The tone of the administrative arrangements at the Johns Hopkins Medical Institutions had been set in 1893, when the trustees of the Johns Hopkins University created the Advisory Board of the School of Medicine as the principal policy-making body of the medical institutions. It was charged simply "to report to the trustees from time to time their suggestions and to prepare and to carry forward the proper arrangements for the instruction and graduation of medical students."

The Advisory Board consisted of the president of the university, the dean of the medical faculty, and the heads of the major departments in the medical school. (A "major subject" was defined as one in which the students were required to pass a final examination in order to receive the M.D. degree.) Also present at monthly board meetings were the director of the hospital and the dean of the school of hygiene. It is perhaps significant that the monthly meeting of the Advisory Board customarily takes place one week before that of the Medical Board.

The Advisory Board had no bylaws, but its sense of custom and procedure were ingrained. In general, substitutes for board members at meetings were not permitted, and as a result, attendance by the regular members was high. The board considered all matters relating to the School of Medicine except the budget, which was controlled by the dean. In every other respect, though, the dean was essentially the servant of the medical faculty, carrying out the wishes of the board—and, by extension, of the trustees, to whom the board's decisions were sent for approval.[68]

The Medical Board of the hospital was the counterpart of the Advisory Board, to govern the medical staff and advise the hospital trustees. Essentially the same individuals served on both, since its principal clinical services corresponded almost exactly to the clinical departments of the medical school. The responsibilities of the Medical Board, spanning medical education and research as well as patient care, reflected the place of the hospital as part of the university.

The medical institutions enjoyed a simple, nonbureaucratic administrative structure until the mid-1950s, when the influx of financial support from the federal government drastically altered the character of the two governing boards. The membership of both boards began to grow when increasing specialization increased the number of department and division heads. More persons were attending the monthly meetings, particularly administrators, but more important, the boards acquired more voting members. In 1957, the Advisory Board's members comprised 16 department heads and administrators; by 1969, the board had 18 voting and 7 nonvoting members. This seemingly insignificant rise was actually the beginning of a continuing increase: in 1987, the Advisory Board had 29 voting and 12 nonvoting members, for a grand total of 41.

Other stresses on the triangular structure of hospital, medical school, and university came from within. In 1962, a simple change in a title threatened to alter the traditional balance of power. The hospital director, Russell Nelson, became the hospital president and was given a voting membership on the hospital's Board of Trustees. The structure mandated by Johns Hopkins and the original Board of Trustees—university president at the top, hospital director and dean of the medical faculty at equal levels below—was threatening to topple. Opponents of the change felt that the hospital had come to be equated with the whole university, not just with the medical school.

Although the traditional decentralized, laissez-faire approach to the routine affairs of the hospital and medical school had served these institutions well, pressure to centralize the interlocking activities came from within and without. During the 1950s, the increased size of the medical institutions made some standardized procedures necessary, although the strength of the individual departments was a countervailing force. Particular conflicts between administration and department heads centered on salary limits, number of faculty members, and the increasing need for research space. Not until 1959 was there an agreed-upon and published schedule of normal working hours and vacation allowances for nonprofessional employees; previously, each department had its own rules. Common supervision of research animal facilities was not inaugurated until 1962, and a system of central purchasing was not begun until 1966.[69]

Moreover, the university's spread to four campuses—the Homewood campus, housing the Faculty of Arts and Sciences and the Whiting School of Engineering; the Johns Hopkins Medical Institutions in East Baltimore; the Applied Physics Laboratory in Howard County, Maryland;

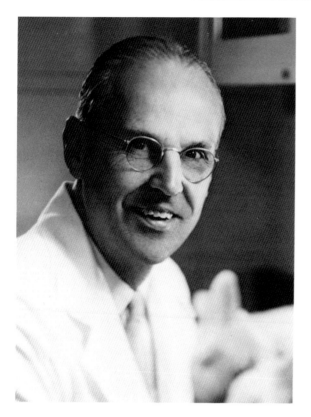

W. Barry Wood. (*Source: Modern Medicine,* copyright © 1966 by the New York Times Media Company, Inc. Reproduced with permission.)

and the School of Advanced International Studies in Washington, D.C.—imposed administrative difficulties, which were augmented by federal pressure to centralize administrative activities. University authorities were reluctant to impose such centralization, citing the diversity of projects and outlooks across the university, especially in the medical institutions. The real question was not how to centralize the university's activities but how to encourage fruitful divisional relationships, particularly between the preclinical sciences and the science departments at Homewood.

Increased administrative responsibilities brought with them the need for an augmented staff. In 1938, Chesney took W. Halsey Barker onto his staff as the first assistant dean and later added William Grose. Bard was aided by three associate deans (George W. Dana, Kenneth W. Blanchard, and R. Carmichael Tilghman).

W. Barry Wood was appointed vice-president of the university and hospital midway through Bard's deanship, in 1955. This new position was created to bring the components of the medical institutions closer to their parent university.

Wood remained in the post for five years. Under his direction, the medical school curriculum was substantially revised, salaries in preclinical departments improved, and initial funds for a new basic science building obtained. Wood relinquished the vice-presidency for the directorship of the Department of Microbiology in 1959, two years into Turner's deanship.[70] A new vice-president was not appointed because the structure of the medical institutions established by Johns Hopkins—the strength of the deanship and departments—made the post largely superfluous. After Wood's departure, university president Milton S. Eisenhower became the link between university and hospital by taking what Turner characterizes as "a direct and immediate interest in the Medical Institutions to a degree that no other president since the first, Mr. Gilman, had done."[71]

Turner had also assembled a cast of supporting deans, each of whom eventually presided over a particular aspect of medical school administration. In the first year of his deanship, Samuel P. Asper and Robert R. Wagner were associate and assistant dean of the medical faculty, respectively. In 1961, Turner added to his staff Palmer H. Futcher as assistant dean and Gilbert H. Mudge as associate dean for postdoctoral education.

Mudge's resignation the following year led to a reassessment of the staffing pattern in the dean's office. Asper was moved to the directorship of postdoctoral education. Taking his place as head of the admissions committee was Richard J. Johns; as director of the student affairs committee, Wagner was succeeded by Julius R. Krevans. Turner brought various others, including Joseph E. Johnson III, William R. Milnor, Joseph F. Sadusk, Jr., and John H. Mulholland, to part-time positions in the dean's office, but it was not until 1963 that the office acquired a full-time administrator, Douglas Walker. Walker brought a medical rather than an administrative background to his position as assistant dean, having left the private practice of pediatrics to come to Baltimore.

Department heads also needed more administrative help as their responsibilities and the size of their departments grew. In 1964, the first departmental administrative assistants arrived at the medical institutions, in the Departments of Medicine and Surgery. In the ensuing years, the success of these assistants depended not only on their own skill but also on the ability of the individual department heads to cope with administrative burdens. If a department chief was a strong administrator, he was unlikely to need—or attract—a similarly strong assistant. If, on the other hand, the department head paid relatively little attention to running the department, he needed a particularly competent assistant to keep the department on course.

The number of committees grew as well. The substantial number of junior faculty members populating the medical institution in the 1960s demanded representation, and during Turner's years as dean, the junior members of the faculty participated more in vital decisions than they had since its founding. This participation reached its apex during the last two years of his administration, when the medical faculty became involved in the problems of community medicine—a strongly debated area of interest (see chapter 10). Efforts were made to include all faculty members in the process of decision making: small faculty committees, which included junior as well as senior members of the Hopkins community, discussed most of the issues that came before the Advisory Board. Students were included in 1963, when representatives elected by each class became members of a joint student-faculty committee that initiated changes in the curriculum and in other facets of student life.

One relatively new group became a powerful force during this decade. This was the Medical Planning and Development Committee (MPD), founded in 1949. MPD became the principal clearinghouse for all matters affecting two or more components of the medical institutions. Its members were the deans of the medical school and the school of hygiene, the director (later president) of the hospital, and the president of the university, who chaired the committee. MPD reported to a joint committee of trustees—four university and four hospital trustees—with the president of the university serving as chairperson. Its most important function was to work out the budgetary agreements between the medical school (or the school of hygiene) and the hospital. In other matters, it had an advisory role, mediating between the three parts of the medical institutions. MPD's responsibilities were originally administrative, but its role gradually became advisory. When it became heavily involved in planning the future of the medical institutions, a full-time director of planning, David Price, was appointed.[72]

Several new committees reflected the federal interest in categorical research. The Joint Committee on Cardiovascular Research drew its membership from the School of Medicine and the School of Hygiene and Public Health; its purpose was to exchange and assemble information, stimulate and obtain funds for research, and advise department heads and administrative officers. The Committee on Atypical Growth, a standing university-wide committee, was empaneled at the suggestion of Lewis Weed to initiate a broad program of research in the field of growth, particularly in relation to cancer. It proved unwieldy, however, and was replaced by a Joint Committee on Cancer Teaching and Research, intended to echo the purposes of the already existing cardiovascular committee. An Inter-Institutional Committee on Venereal Disease Control was also established, with representatives from the medical school, the hospital, and the school of hygiene.

Two other groups were forerunners of the Joint Committee on Clinical Investigation (the group concerned with experimentation using human subjects) later mandated by the NIH: the Therapeutic Trials Committee, which spanned the hospital, the medical school, and the school of hygiene, enabled more systematic testing in patients of new drugs and of old drugs used in a novel way. A subcommittee, the Panel for Clinical Testing, arranged for clinical testing and collection of data. In these early days of concern with the use of experimental subjects, however, faculty members were not required to follow the committees' recommended procedures.

As the size of the full-time staff grew and many outstanding scientists populated both the basic science and clinical departments, the number of faculty members receiving attractive offers from other institutions increased. It was difficult to retain faculty and recruit replacements in view of the original tradition that there be only a single full professor in each department—the director of the department. The medical school therefore abandoned this tradition in the mid-1950s, falling in line with other universities. The new policy also allowed many of the institutions' distinguished part-time faculty members to be promoted to full professorial status.

The first non–department head to be promoted to full professor with no qualifying title attached was C. Lockard Conley, who became a professor of medicine in 1956. He had come to Baltimore ten years earlier as Emanuel Libman fellow and assistant in the Department of Medicine; since 1947, he had been physician-in-charge of the Hematology Clinic and director of the Hematology Division of the Department of Medicine. Conley's new responsibilities included the directorship of the hospital's diagnostic laboratories.

The full-time system also gained greater acceptance as young physicians hoped to continue the salaried status they had enjoyed in the armed services, and as funds from the federal government permitted a dramatic increase in the number of full-time faculty members. The concomitant expansion in the size of the house staff and in the number of postdoctoral fellows after the war rapidly changed the environment for teaching, medical research, and patient care.

Unfortunately, the NIH's policy of awarding grants to the investigator rather than to the university tended to drive a wedge between the scientist and the parent institution. Many members of this expanded faculty wore two hats: they were on the staff at Johns Hopkins, but a number were also members of NIH study sections, and a much larger number were grant recipients. Each faculty

member, therefore, was trying to secure money for his own investigative work. Moreover, the NIH tended to see the university as the potential exploiter of its grant recipients. Since the NIH was "buying" programs, it wanted the investigator to spend his time on research, rather than on teaching or other university responsibilities. The system of awarding grants thus forced prospective recipients to look out for themselves rather than working solely toward common goals for the university, and establishing consensus on matters of academic importance became increasingly difficult.[73]

Buildings

The two decades after World War II witnessed a building boom at Johns Hopkins. Its changing physical plant in these years reflected the growth of medical specialization, the advance of technology, and the particular requirements of the medical school and hospital. New departments and divisions needed new facilities for both research and teaching; furthermore, the opening of the new residence for medical students was important to the full implementation of the new curriculum (see chapter 7).

Between 1945 and 1968, the medical institutions added over 500,000 square feet of teaching and research space. The influence of the federal government was pervasive, as it contributed to every building constructed at Johns Hopkins after World War II. Federal money permitted construction of the buildings, while concomitant federal requirements shaped their design and function. Yet despite a federally encouraged emphasis on research, Hopkins also managed to replace or remodel the site of every one of its original inpatient beds. The physical plant at Hopkins thus remained a balanced expression of its original commitment to research, teaching, and the care of the sick. All three components—research, teaching, and patient care—were growing, and all three needed additional space. Individual buildings constructed during this time were therefore designed to serve multiple purposes.

In June 1948, ground was broken on the hospital lot for the first unit in the medical institution's postwar building program. The trustees of the hospital had embarked on a campaign for $3 million to provide two new buildings—one for the Departments of Surgery and Radiology, and one for semi-private patients—and the university trustees agreed to underwrite one-half of any difference between the amount of money collected and the total sum sought. First, a temporary building was constructed to house the Department of Radiology. The old Surgical Building, which had housed the radiographic facilities, was then demolished to make room for the Clinical Science Building, renamed the Blalock Building in 1964. The National Heart Institute gave $485,000 to support construction of facilities for cardiovascular research, and the National Cancer Institute provided $750,000 toward facilities for cancer research. A rise in building costs made even these two large grants inadequate, and not all of the building's planned fourteen stories were completed by the time it was put into use. A sufficient number of floors were completed to house the outpatient surgical clinic; the Department of Radiology; a new accident room; offices, laboratories, and animal quarters for the Departments of Medicine and Surgery; and a new classroom on the basement and corridor levels.

The Octagon Ward, which had housed private patients, was torn down to make room for the Children's Medical and Surgical Center; additional semiprivate patients were housed on a floor added to both the Halsted and Osler Buildings.

The Women's Fund Memorial Building (the anatomy building) was also renovated after the war; the comprehensive remodeling included replacement of its laboratory fixtures, which dated from 1894 and had become completely inadequate for either research or teaching.

The Basic Science Building was completed in 1959. Ten stories tall, it adjoined the Physiology and Hunterian Buildings. Its ground and first floors contained lecture rooms, student lounges, and administrative offices, including the office of the dean of the medical school; the upper nine floors provided space for research and graduate teaching in the preclinical Departments of Physiology, Pharmacology, Physiological Chemistry, and Microbiology. The building cost $5 million, of which the Public Health Service contributed $1.5 million. It was later named after W. Barry Wood, director of the Department of Microbiology.

Housing for medical students became increasingly problematic in the mid-1950s, when all houses on the west side of Broadway between Orleans Street and Hampton House were razed to accommodate the redevelopment plan, proposed jointly by Hopkins and the City of Baltimore, for nine blocks on the west side of the hospital. The first building constructed was a student dormitory to house 220 men and 30 women, with dining and recreational facilities. The dormitory, Reed Hall, was completed in 1957. A government loan contributed to the construction of garden apartments for house staff—the so-called Compound, first occupied in 1957. A second building to house medical students, a second Reed Hall, opened in 1966. Its fourteen floors contained two-, four- and ten-bedroom apartment units for 200 persons, and it made housing available for all Hopkins medical students. The redevelopment plan also included construction of a hotel for out-of-town patients and families, and a shopping area.

Construction that emphasized the burgeoning postwar interest in research continued into the 1960s. The entire Hunterian II Building was renovated for modern research in 1961, and additional space was provided for the Departments of Anatomy, Pediatrics, and Gynecology and Obstetrics. The Biophysics Building was completed in 1963, and one year later, a six-story research wing of the Wilmer Institute that was characterized as the largest unified center in the world for research on the eye. Work on all three buildings depended heavily on matching grants from the National Institutes of Health, but contributions from foundations and individuals were also crucial to their financing.

Federal grants also supported research facilities in the Children's Medical and Surgical Center (CMSC), which opened in 1964. An NIH grant allowed the construction of four additional floors for surgical research (including research in orthopedics) and research on mental retardation. The building also contained facilities for the care of children, and its basement housed a variety of support services for the medical institutions.

Only a few months after completion of the CMSC, the dean of the medical school announced the award of a construction grant of $2.378 million by the Public Health Service and a matching grant from the Ford Foundation, which would permit work to begin in the fall of 1965 on the Traylor Research Building, a $5-million facility for postdoctoral research. Ongoing research programs in many areas had been hampered and new projects deferred for lack of space. The new facility was planned to promote interaction and cooperation across interdepartmental lines. Clinical departments would investigate fundamental biological problems in human reproduction, human communication, biomedical engineering, neurobiology, behavioral sciences, medical biochemistry, physiology, and biophysics. Work concerned with the potential effect of the mathematical and physical components of biology on clinical problems was expected to have great influence on the current and future approaches to important medical problems. The facility would also provide training and experience in basic medical research to young postdoctoral fellows and graduate students, who would profit from intimate exposure to closely interrelated, coordinated, and sophisticated programs under the direction of skilled investigators. Finally, the building would house a central facility for the Department of Comparative Medicine, which would also allow basic investigation into animal medicine.

The Traylor Research Building was completed in 1968, along with the adjacent Turner Auditorium complex, which housed two auditoriums, conference and seminar rooms, the Alan M. Chesney Medical Archives, offices for Continuing Education and Audiovisual Programs, a

medical bookstore, a computing center, and other administrative offices.

Declining federal allocations after 1968 marked the end of this building boom. In the decade after Turner's deanship, the face of the Johns Hopkins medical campus changed scarcely at all. The past influence of the federal government became even more apparent as, without federal funds, the hospital and medical school undertook no new buildings or major renovations.

The postwar rise of federal support changed not only the size of the Johns Hopkins Medical Institutions but also their character. For its first fifty years, Johns Hopkins had been an intimate place, where everyone knew everyone else, and a faculty member who wandered down the hall could converse with a colleague working in an entirely different field. Talk of research swirled through the Doctors' Dining Room, whose demolition to make room for the Children's Medical and Surgical Center in 1964 removed an important center for communication. As the faculty spilled over into new buildings, federal support became a centrifugal force, posing a challenge to communication within the hospital and medical school that would continue into the succeeding decades.

The decline in federal support after 1968 required Hopkins' leaders to find new sources of funds. Construction began again in the mid-1970s when the State of Maryland's new Health and Higher Education Act allowed the hospital and university to issue bonds, enabling Hopkins to borrow money for building at reasonable rates. Foundations and other private donors also became increasingly important in sponsoring facilities. The patterns of construction, communication, research, education, and patient care in the next two decades would reflect the efforts of the medical school and the hospital to maintain their traditions in financially difficult times.

CHAPTER 5

RENEWAL AND REDIRECTION, 1968–1989

It is mandatory that we seek means to stabilize our institutions, continue the provision of a reasonable mix of resources for the biomedical sciences (for manpower, facilities, and materials), and provide a set of reasonably enduring principles as guides to the more effective operation of our biomedical establishment. If we do not achieve such reasonable objectives, then the divisive struggles of the special interest groups will surely devour much of the substance of our programs. Money in the form of support dollars may be important; of course it is. However, in the long run the nature and quality of our programs will be as much or more important than the level of their dollar support.

—James A. Shannon, 1982

The years after 1968 were confusing and difficult ones for American medicine. As in the preceding two decades of expansion, academic medical centers were heavily dependent on the federal government, which itself reflected public perceptions of medical practice, teaching, and research. "Not enough" and "too much" were the prevailing public complaints of the late 1960s and early 1970s. The perception was that there were not enough physicians, particularly practitioners of general medicine; not enough blacks and women in medical schools; not enough access to medical care, particularly for the poor. In contrast, too much money was being spent on biomedical research, and medical students were forced to spend too much time in laboratories, gaining knowledge not directly related to medical practice. Medical care—indeed, good health itself—became a right, as "health care" superseded "medical care" in the language. By the 1980s, the public was more concerned with the cost of medical care

than with its availability, quality, or continuing progress.

American medicine has been hard pressed to keep up with these public demands. It was Walsh McDermott who said that the survival of an institution as an effective force depends on very much the same sort of process as survival of a species, namely, the development of appropriate adaptations. (Indeed, McDermott pointed out that Darwin originally named his great concept "survival of the adapted" and used that term in the first four editions of *On the Origin of Species*.) Medicine as a profession adapts to change through its institutions, McDermott said—the organizations, accepted practices, and colleges that have grown up for the expansion and application of the body of medical knowledge.[1]

McDermott identified Banting's discovery of insulin in 1922 as the benchmark in the history of medicine, for it marked the beginning of the time when physicians could intervene predictably to help the individual patient. Nothing was the same thereafter, but the medical profession was slow to adapt to the rapid growth of medical knowledge. Continuing technologic and therapeutic advances were not matched by a delivery system that could accommodate the changing needs of medical practice. Instead, the new technology was simply engrafted on a centuries-old system designed to handle a population with an average life span of less than fifty years, a population whose principal contact with medicine was the individual personal physician. Hospital functions expanded, for patients now went to hospitals not only for treatment but also for new types of laboratory studies essential to the diagnosis and management of their diseases.[2]

By the 1970s, even the nature of common illness had changed. The growth of medical knowledge had increased physicians' ability to treat many of the acute, formerly life-threatening illnesses, and now physicians were faced with an entirely different pattern of disease. Most prominent were the chronic diseases—such as diabetes, arthritis, atherosclerosis, and chronic pulmonary disease—that could result in severe loss of function and restriction of activity but were long-term in their course. Burgeoning new technology also led to greater specialization, and physicians could remain up-to-date only in restricted sectors of medical knowledge. In the midst of this great technologic era of medicine, the public viewed doctors as less caring than in the past, and believed that with the great advances in medical science, the Samaritan aspects of medicine had been submerged. Moreover, the public's overriding concern with cost led to major alterations in the organization, financing, and delivery of medical care.

Medical institutions were under attack from all sides. Student unrest manifested itself in criticism of the medical school curriculum and demands for representation on decision-making bodies. The leveling off in federal funds for medical research, superimposed on these other changes, strained the finances of the medical schools. The rise of the Civil Rights Movement led to the inclusion of more blacks in the medical community;

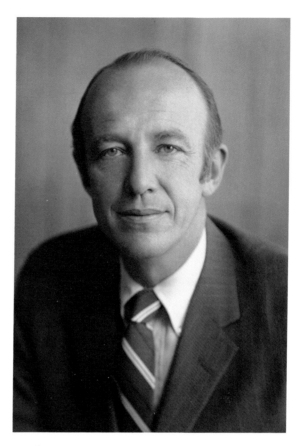

David E. Rogers. (*Source:* Orren Jack Turner.)

but with the death of Martin Luther King, Hopkins—and other urban medical schools—were caught up in the ensuing riots of 1968. The hospital and medical school's decision to remain in East Baltimore bespoke their responsibility to the neighborhood, and Hopkins' leaders worked with community leaders to reverse the decline of the surrounding area.

David E. Rogers presided over the first three years of this tumultuous time. Rogers left a position as head of the Department of Medicine at Vanderbilt University to become dean of the medical faculty when Thomas B. Turner retired in 1968. A graduate of the Cornell University School of Medicine in 1948, Rogers spent two years on the Osler Medical Service at Hopkins before returning to New York to work in the laboratory of Walsh McDermott. This postdoctoral fellowship was followed by a chief residency in medicine at

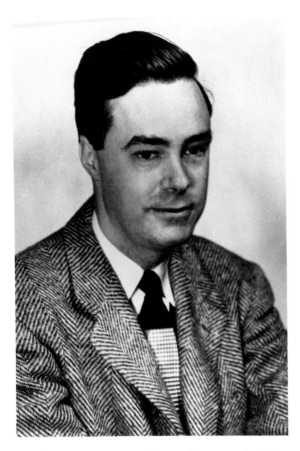

Russell H. Morgan. (*Source*: Alan M. Chesney Medical Archives, The Johns Hopkins Medical Institutions.)

studies also related image formation, visual perception, and physiologic optics to roentgenographic and fluoroscopic systems, and applied computer methods and data-processing systems to medicine. When Morgan became head of the school of hygiene's Department of Radiologic Science in 1960, he developed a vigorous multidisciplinary program in radiological medicine. Morgan remained in the deanship until 1975, when he was succeeded by Richard S. Ross.

Like his immediate predecessor, Richard S. Ross was a long-time member of the Hopkins faculty. A graduate of the Harvard Medical School in 1947, Ross served his medical internship and residency at Johns Hopkins on the Osler Medical Service. After a fellowship in physiology at Harvard, Ross returned to Hopkins as chief medical resident in 1953. When he assumed the deanship, Ross was professor of medicine and director of the Cardiovascular Division.

During the deanships of these three men,

Cornell, two years in the Navy, and a year as visiting investigator at the Rockefeller Institute. In 1955, Rogers returned to Cornell as chief of the Division of Infectious Disease, moving to Vanderbilt four years later.[3]

Rogers remained in the deanship until 1971, when he was succeeded by Russell H. Morgan. Morgan had been a Hopkins faculty member since 1946, when he became the first director of the Department of Radiology in the medical school. As a radiologist, he was renowned for some of the most important technological advances in diagnostic radiology, including the development of photoelectric timing mechanisms for automatic control of x-ray exposures, the perfection of image intensification in radiology, and the application of television techniques in clinical fluoroscopy and cinefluorography. His landmark

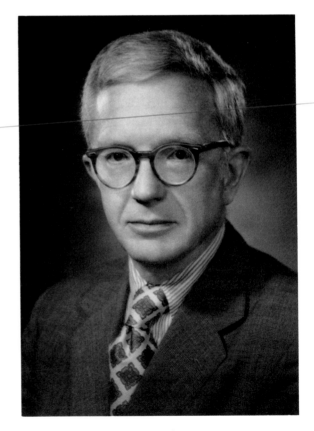

Richard S. Ross. (*Source*: Bachrach.)

Johns Hopkins preserved its traditional values in medical practice, teaching, and research. The particular accommodations of the Johns Hopkins Hospital and the School of Medicine to the vexing problems of the time reflected the fit between its traditions and current public demands. Some changes were thus less wrenching at Hopkins than elsewhere.

The Vanishing General Physician

The "vanishing general physician," for example, had never vanished from Johns Hopkins. Fewer physicians were practicing general internal medicine in the mid-1960s, as the process of increasing specialization lured physicians into ever-narrower fields. The generalist in medicine was, however, an Oslerian tradition at Hopkins. By personal example and by precept, Osler had instilled in the teaching and training program at Johns Hopkins the importance of the physician's ability to manage all his patients' problems. Osler was himself a generalist: a consummate neurologist, cardiologist, endocrinologist, and even a pediatrician. Some might call him a panspecialist rather than a generalist, but most of all, he was an internist. Osler's influence remained an important feature of teaching at Johns Hopkins after his departure for Oxford. It was carefully preserved by his successors as the best approach to the training of the physician.

This continuing insistence on the practice of general internal medicine at Hopkins contrasted with the practice in some schools. Patients at the University of Chicago hospital, for example, were placed in beds segregated by diagnostic category.[4] The Johns Hopkins Hospital eventually had seven inpatient units for general internal medicine, only one of which had any particular aggregation of patients: patients with cardiologic problems were placed in the same ward because they needed special monitoring equipment and nursing care.

This emphasis on general internal medicine delayed the development of specialization in Hopkins' Department of Medicine. For half a century, the department had only three general research and clinical divisions—the Biological, Physiological, and Chemical Divisions created by Lewellys Barker after Osler's departure in 1905. In the mid-1950s, the creation of subspecialty divisions was stimulated by the availability of federal money for research and research training, the growth of new knowledge in the individual fields, and the need to use this knowledge to provide up-to-date medical care and to stay on the frontier of progress.

The members of these subspecialty divisions nevertheless remained generalists first. They still taught and supervised the house staff on the general wards, and when patients were presented at the weekly staff rounds, the subspecialist was expected to lead the discussion regardless of whether or not the patient's problem fell in his chosen area of interest. This practice was considered a key pedagogical principle, for teaching medical students as well as for training good internists in the medical residency program.

The chief of medicine also tried to integrate the subspecialties into the department's teaching and training programs. Many departments of internal medicine appeared to be merely loose consortia of subspecialty divisions, but the image of a homogeneous department comprising a coordinated group of special areas of internal medicine was better preserved at Hopkins than in many other research-oriented medical schools.

Care of the ambulatory patient was assuming greater importance, however, and specialists were not equipped either by training or by interest to handle these patients' general medical problems. Nor did they have the time to serve as primary physicians: with the explosion of biomedical knowledge in the 1960s and 1970s, the majority of the specialty-oriented fellows had to confine their clinical activities to their chosen specialty. Even fewer fellows became available to outpatient clinics when the Welfare and Personnel Health Clinics were phased out in 1967 with the advent of Medicare and Medicaid. Not only did young men and women in specialty training want to diminish their participation in general medical care in the outpatient department—full-time members of the specialty divisions were also unwilling to give any significant part of their time to the general medical effort. The faculty's attitude was justifiable. Keeping up with their own fields was increasingly time consuming, and they were also beset by demands from an increasing number of patients in their specialties, and facing increasing difficulty in competing for research funds.

At some medical institutions, the problem of the disappearing generalist was solved by creating a department of general practice or a department of family medicine. A national organization of general practitioners sprang up shortly after World War II, and there were strong pressures to institute such training programs in all medical schools. This move was resisted at Hopkins, but a residency program for general practitioners was started at the Hopkins-affiliated Baltimore City Hospitals. The program lasted from 1960 to 1969. It consisted of two years of training in general medicine, including gynecology and obstetrics, psychiatry, and pediatrics. Moreover, to compensate for the shortage of role models and teachers in this area, the Department of Medicine at Hopkins planned to increase the number of full-time faculty members primarily interested in general practice by creating a separate division of general internal medicine.

The idea of a division of general internal medicine was strengthened by a grant in 1968 from the Commonwealth Fund's Clinical Scholars Program, which emphasized the delivery of medical care.[5] Promoted at Hopkins by Julius R. Krevans, professor of medicine, the program was intended to stimulate the young internist to enter the field of general internal medicine and emerge as a uniquely trained individual: clinically based, sponsored by a department of medicine, but concerned with the organization, assessment, and cost-effectiveness of medical care. This new general internist would be clinically competent to assess quality in medicine and would receive special training in biometrics and clinical epidemiology that would enable him or her to seek more effective procedures in health care delivery at the lowest possible cost.

A division for generalists within the Department of Medicine was successfully organized in 1973 by Victor A. McKusick, who in that year succeeded A. McGehee Harvey as department head. At the suggestion of some of the part-time members of the faculty, including William Speed, it was designated "the Division of Internal Medicine" to avoid confusion with general practice and to bolster the concept that internal medicine is in itself a specialty. In the mid-1970s, a grant from the Robert Wood Johnson Foundation, which had assumed responsibility for the Clinical Scholars Program, further supported the division's clinical practice. Research efforts in clinical epidemiology were developed through the work of Thomas Pearson and Paul Whelton, and through collaborative efforts with Leon Gordis, head of the Department of Epidemiology in the School of Hygiene and Public Health. The cross-fertilization in the important area of clinical epidemiology avoided duplication of effort in instruction and provided the basis for significant collaboration between the two schools in teaching and research.[6]

Also during the mid-1970's, geriatrics became recognized as a separate specialty. The Department of Medicine at Johns Hopkins had a long-standing interest in this area, encouraged by the presence of an extramural NIH research center for the study of aging at the Baltimore City Hospitals, under the direction of Nathan Shock. The Department of Medicine at Hopkins had proposed the creation of a separate division of geriatric medicine in the early 1960s but had not been successful in finding the right person to lead such a division. In 1981, the idea was taken up again by William R. Hazzard, the department's new associate director, who established an institution-wide program linked to facilities at the Baltimore City Hospitals.[7]

Advance of the Surgical Subspecialties

The importance of the generalist permeated other clinical departments at Johns Hopkins. In the Department of Surgery, the Halstedian tradition required that a specialist must be a good general surgeon, fully trained in the principles of general surgery, before branching out into areas such as cardiovascular or thoracic surgery. Yet the surgical world, like other spheres of medical practice in the late 1960s, was feeling pressure from the increasing trend toward specialization and the depreciation of surgical education's prestige in the undergraduate medical curriculum. From 1970 to 1975, the American College of Surgeons and the American Surgical Association therefore conducted a self-study intended to estimate the future of surgery in the United States.[8] Leading this study was the head of surgery at Hopkins, George D. Zuidema, who was also contending with the trend toward specialization in his own department.

Reorganization of the Department of Surgery

In 1972, Zuidema reorganized the surgical residency program to accommodate to the proliferation of surgical subspecialties. The five surgical divisions that Zuidema had inherited—anesthesiology, neurosurgery, orthopedics, otolaryngology, and urology—either had existed when Blalock became chief or were carved out by him in the 1940s (see chapter 4). Over the next twenty years, these divisions developed somewhat independently of their parent department. In the 1940s, the specialties of surgery had been represented by only a few individuals, most of whom had developed their interest in their specialty through an apprenticeship in general surgery. By 1963, the specialties (excluding anesthesiology and plastic surgery) handled one-half of the patients admitted to the surgical services and more than one-half of the surgical outpatients. Professional fees and research grants for the subspecialties constituted one-half of the total monies earned by the Department of Surgery, and the subspecialties were responsible for half the surgical teaching time for undergraduates and perhaps more than half for residents.

Within the Department of Surgery, division heads felt that they did not have enough authority to conduct the affairs of their own provinces. The solution was not to make each division into a new department; rather, the existing department needed reorganizing to resolve the conflicts between its component parts.

Under Zuidema's direction, several proposals were considered and rejected. One suggestion would have created a department of basic surgery, which would teach the aspects of surgery common to all the specialties and supervise the surgical operating rooms and the departmental research laboratories. In parallel, a clinical surgical specialties department would comprise anesthesiology, general surgery, neurosurgery, orthopedics, otolaryngology, and urology. Another plan advocated the formation of a departmental committee, chaired by the head of the Department of Surgery, that would have the final say in settling jurisdictional problems, distributing hospital beds and laboratory facilities, allotting operating room time, and planning the curriculum for medical students. A third plan would have given the division heads independent budgets and membership on the Advisory Board.

Under the plan adopted in 1972, the Department of Surgery was renamed the "Section of Surgical Sciences." The plan elevated what is now called general surgery to full-time, departmental status, along with neurosurgery, orthopedics, urology, and otolaryngology. It also gave formal status to services in transplantation and vascular surgery, cardiac surgery, plastic surgery, dental and oral surgery, and pediatric surgery. Overseeing this expanded organization were a director (Zuidema) and an associate director, who would be elected from among the heads of the surgical departments for a two-year term.

Zuidema remained on the Advisory and Medical Boards as director of the department and as director of the new Division of General Surgery. The directors of the four new departments were given places on the Medical Board of the hospital but not on the medical school's Advisory Board. Instead, the section's director and the first associate director (Robert A. Robinson, chief of orthopedic surgery) represented surgery on the Advisory Board.

The four specialty departments were not initially added to the Advisory Board because Zuidema feared upsetting the balance between basic and clinical scientists in the governance of the medical school. In the 1980s, however, John Cameron, who replaced Zuidema as chief of surgery, came to see this augmented representation as an important step in the continued development of his department, since a place on the Advisory Board was also an indication of the value Hopkins placed on its surgical specialties. Representation was granted, and the institution was able to recruit and retain exceptionally capable surgeons as directors of these specialties.

In neurosurgery, George B. Udvarhelyi remained as acting director until 1973, when he was succeeded by Donlin M. Long. Robert A. Robinson was director of orthopedic surgery until 1979; his successor was Lee H. Riley. The director of urology was William Wallace Scott, who was succeeded in 1974 by Patrick C. Walsh. Otolaryngology was chaired by George T. Nager until 1984, when Michael M. E. Johns assumed the post. John E. Hoopes has been the long-time head of plastic surgery. J. Alex Haller, Jr., has been the director of pediatric surgery, and Donald M. Tilghman has been the head of oral surgery.

The plan for reorganization also recommended that anesthesiology be elevated to departmental status, a change put into effect in 1975. Anesthesiology's first director was Eugene Nagel, who remained as department director until 1979. He was succeeded by Mark Rogers, head of the Pediatric Intensive Care Unit, and the department's name was expanded to Anesthesiology and Critical Care Medicine. Rogers brought in Richard Traystman from the School of Hygiene and Public Health to direct the research program, and the new department was able to attract excellent residents.

Residency Training

The revamping of the Department of Surgery included formal and informal changes in the surgical residency. The traditional Halsted residency was a pyramidal program: of the twelve interns in general surgery, only two were chosen to complete their training at Hopkins. These two spent an additional five clinical years and two research years at Hopkins and at the end of the process were fully trained in both general and thoracic surgery. The sharply pyramidal aspect of the program was softened in the 1970s, as many prospective residents would not apply to a training program that they probably would not be able to complete. During the 1970s, the number of surgical interns was increased, with the expectation that half of these house officers would enter training programs in one of the surgical specialties at Hopkins. The top of the pyramid was also expanded, from two chief residents to five. This was somewhat more tolerable than the previous arrangement, but the department still faced the annual need to turn away very well qualified residents and find opportunities for them to complete their training in other university programs. Soon after becoming chief of surgery in 1984, John Cameron decided to restrict the number of general surgical interns accepted into the first year of the program, so that this number became approximately equal to the number of openings available in the senior years.

A more formal change in the residency program took place in 1969, in response to a change in policy by the American Board of Thoracic Surgery. The board had begun requiring two years of training solely in its specialty, and it would no longer approve the mixed kind of experience that Hopkins offered, despite the fact that no Hopkins candidate had ever failed the cardiothoracic board examinations. The department's response was to cut back on general surgery training for house officers in surgical specialties but to continue to provide a core of general surgical training. Before entering their specialty training, all beginning house officers intending to practice a surgical specialty were required to spend one or two years (depending on the specialty) in general surgery.[9]

Special Intensive Care Units and Collaborative Units

Acronymic specialty units proliferated in the late 1970s: the PICU (Pediatric Intensive Care Unit) was accompanied by the NICU (Neonatal Intensive Care Unit), the SICU (Surgical Intensive Care Unit), the MICU (Medical Intensive Care Unit), and the CCU (Coronary Care Unit). These units began to grow in the mid-1960s, when the advent of many new diagnostic and therapeutic technologic advances gave rise to specialization in intensive care.

Special intensive care units had actually been part of the Hopkins scene since 1923, during Warfield M. Firor's residency in neurosurgery, when Walter Dandy set aside several beds to provide for the intensive care of neurosurgical patients in the immediate postoperative period. In the late 1950s, a recovery room was created near the operating rooms. There, patients would regain consciousness after operation, or remain for longer periods if they required intensive, specialized nursing care. This new unit also facilitated frequent examinations by the surgical staff, who found it convenient to have these patients near the operating rooms. The "Tet" room (an abbreviation of "tetralogy of Fallot") was the first cardiac surgical intensive care unit, located in Halsted 3. In the early days of the Blalock-Taussig operation, children with congenital heart disease were placed in this room for special nursing, special monitoring, and many other special services.

The first complete intensive care units at Hopkins were organized in 1967 by a small committee headed by Gottlieb Friesinger, a member of the Department of Medicine. The medical and surgical intensive care units and the General Recovery Room, which together occupied the entire seventh floor of the Osler and Halsted Buildings, opened in May 1971, although the service facilities for the two units, located on the Osler-Halsted bridge, were not yet complete. Several smaller intensive care units had gone into operation earlier. The coronary care unit, which contained a myocardial research unit, opened with four beds in 1968; the cardiac special nursing unit opened the following year; and the intermediate cardiac surgery care unit opened early in 1971.

The changing nature of hospital practice, as well as advancing technology, led to the proliferation of these intensive care units. As an increasing number of patients could be cared for on an out-patient basis, inpatient care became more intensive. This shift created problems in the training of house staff and in the teaching of medical students, forcing medical educators to create a broader exposure to medical practice than the previous inpatient setting had allowed.

Technologic and social forces also led to the increasing development of categorical units created to unite several clinical specialties in a collaborative approach to patient care. The largest categorical unit at Johns Hopkins is the Oncology Center, which combines almost all of the clinical disciplines. With the development of this center, the facilities for radiation therapy were greatly expanded and the services increased, under the direction of Stanley Order. Other categorical units linked the cardiovascular interests of medicine, pediatrics, and surgery in adjacent areas on the fifth floor of several contiguous buildings; connected allergy and immunology with rheumatology at the Good Samaritan Hospital; and connected the unit in renal disease with the dialysis unit. The Meyer Center was constructed to house the Departments of Neurology, Neurosurgery, and Psychiatry and Behavioral Sciences in adjacent quarters; and the disciplines of medical gastroenterology and surgery were combined in the Meyerhoff Clinic for Inflammatory Bowel Disease.

Another type of categorical unit reflected the growing interest in transplantation. Vincent Gott, professor of surgery, had presided over the Division of Cardiac Surgery since its formation in 1974. The advent of cyclosporine allowed the development of a program in heart and lung transplantation, and Bruce A. Reitz, a former intern in medicine who had trained in transplantation surgery at Stanford, returned to Baltimore in 1982 to head the division of Cardiac Surgery when Gott retired as its director.

Emergency Medicine

As part of the reorganization of the Department of Surgery, a separate Emergency Medical Service was created in 1973. The immediate care of emergencies had naturally been a part of the hospital's responsibilities since its opening in 1889, when its first facility was a sixteen- by twenty-foot accident reception room. In an appended room of a large amphitheater was a two-bed facility, the precursor of a modern emergency room, where patients could be kept overnight.[10]

Traditionally the "accident room" has been a part of the outpatient department at Hopkins, which in the early days was called the hospital "dispensary." In 1890, the work of the accident room was confined to injuries occurring in the immediate vicinity of the hospital, since the large railway stations and manufacturing establishments were far away and relatively inaccessible over the area's unpaved dirt roads.

In its first four years, the hospital had no ambulance and was forced to rely on a roofless police patrol wagon for the transportation of accident cases and patients with severe illnesses. The first Hopkins ambulance was a horse-drawn wagon, specially built for the hospital. It had room for a stretcher and for a few friends of the patient. Even after this acquisition, the police paddy wagon re-

mained the chief ambulance service of the city. The horse-drawn wagon was replaced in 1913 by Hopkins' first emergency automobile, which was designed to avoid the appearance of an ambulance and looked instead like a private limousine.

The facilities for accident room patients at Johns Hopkins were considerably expanded in 1927 when the Carnegie Dispensary was opened. The term "emergency room" (possibly coined by H. L. Mencken) was expanded to "emergency medicine" in 1973, when a new division of surgery was created, with Donald S. Gann as its head. With a joint appointment in surgery and biomedical engineering, Gann remained at Hopkins until 1980. A new emergency facility was completed in 1981 to serve as part of Maryland's state system of trauma care.[11]

Hubert T. Gurley was Gann's successor. Gurley was in turn succeeded in 1984 by Keith T. Sivertson.

Development of the Neurosciences

The Department of Neuroscience, created in 1980, was the first new basic science department in the School of Medicine in twenty years. Its first director was Solomon Snyder, who had arrived at Johns Hopkins in 1965. Having been a research associate in the laboratory of Nobel laureate Julius Axelrod at the NIH, Snyder was expecting to move to Stanford to undertake residency training in psychiatry, but his source of funding did not materialize. He had by that time written some thirty articles elucidating histamine metabolism and the functions of the pineal gland, and a place for him was found in the Hopkins residency program in psychiatry. During the last two years of his residency, Snyder held a concomitant Hopkins appointment as assistant professor of pharmacology and experimental therapeutics. When he finished his residency, in 1968, he was named associate professor of pharmacology and experimental therapeutics and associate professor of psychiatry. Two years later, at age thirty-one, he was promoted to full professor.[12]

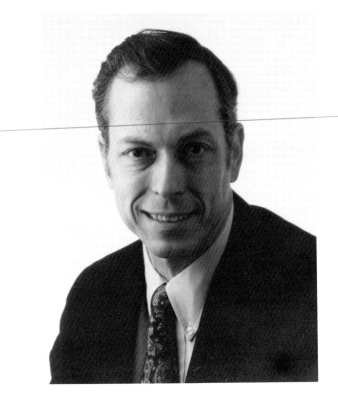

Solomon H. Snyder. (*Source*: Nova Pharmaceutical.)

Snyder took charge of a department that blended many fields previously without a common focus. Studies of the brain's activities, including neuroanatomy, physiology, pharmacology, and chemistry, typically had taken place in separate laboratories. The fundamental questions of brain function could be attacked most successfully, however, by combining these and other disciplines into an integrated approach (see chapter 11).

The department's faculty included Joseph T. Coyle, Jr., professor of neuroscience, pharmacology, and psychiatry, who developed the first animal model of Huntington disease through his studies of neurotransmitters. Coyle was a 1969 graduate of the Hopkins medical school. Also a member of the team was Michael J. Kuhar, who held a joint professorship in three departments: neuroscience, pharmacology and experimental therapeutics, and psychiatry. A recipient of the doctoral degree from Johns Hopkins, Kuhar was the first to visualize the brain's neurotransmitter receptors under a microscope.[13]

The new knowledge of receptors had obvious practical applications. Snyder was soon sought out as a research consultant by several pharmaceutical companies. He describes the development of his collaboration with one company, Nova:

Almost immediately after identifying the opiate receptor, I decided that similar techniques might enable us to label receptors for most of the neurotransmitters in the brain. As it turned out, each receptor was rather different and posed sometimes recalcitrant challenges, but within two or three years we were able to monitor the major neurotransmitter receptors in the brain and thereby work out actions of many psychotropic drugs. I was asked to serve as a consultant to drug companies to apply this technology as a means of facilitating the drug discovery process. In general, I was frustrated that the large companies seemed full of inertia. Even though the Vice-President for Research and Development, who would typically hire me, was enthusiastic, pharmacologists at lower levels were reluctant to alter their time-tested ways of screening drugs first by experiments in intact animals. Accordingly, I was re-

ceptive when, in December 1982, David and Isaac Blech phoned and then visited with me over lunch . . . to discuss a research company based on receptor technology. David was then twenty-six and Isaac thirty-two years old. In 1980 they had, with few resources, founded Genetic Systems, one of the first monoclonal antibody companies, which in 1985 was acquired by Bristol Myers for about three hundred million dollars. At the time of our first meeting, David and Isaac were puzzled by the fact that, of the roughly one hundred biotechnology companies, half did genetic cloning and the other half did monoclonal antibodies. They wondered whether there was any new area of biomedical research with potential for product development and had been told about receptor technology as a means for conducting initial screens of promising drugs. Within a month following our lunch date, David and Isaac had recruited Donald Stark, former President of Sandoz and Sterling Pharmaceuticals, as the President of Nova. I recruited David U'Prichard, a former postdoctoral fellow of mine, as the full time Scientific Director. Nova went public in August of 1983, renting about a thousand square feet of laboratory space in the Maryland Psychiatric Research Center at Spring Grove Hospital. In September 1984, Nova moved into new laboratories, about twenty-five thousand square feet, at the Francis Scott Key campus.[14]

New Sources of Funding for Research

Although Johns Hopkins continued to rank near the top of all medical centers in total funding by the NIH, the leveling-off of federal support in the early 1970s, which included the discontinuation of research training grants by the Nixon administration, required academic medical centers, including Hopkins, to turn to private foundations for funds for research.[15] Hopkins had enjoyed unusual opportunities to expand its research facilities since World War II, but in the late 1960s and early 1970s, its interest in private funding and collaborative arrangements with other hospitals intensified. It also developed new methods of obtaining internal funds for research. Space permits only a few illustrations of each type of funding.

Links with Other Hospitals

The creation of the O'Neill Research Laboratories at the Good Samaritan Hospital in the late 1960s used a university-associated hospital as the setting for the study of chronic diseases. In 1927, the trustees of the O'Neill Trust asked Dean Alan Chesney for advice about creating a program that would use their money in a medical context. Chesney suggested that they build a special hospital affiliated with Hopkins for the study and care of certain types of patients. Not until 1968 did the Good Samaritan Hospital open. Chesney's model had been the hospital associated with the Rockefeller Institute, but what emerged fifty years later was a church-affiliated hospital with special strengths.

The O'Neill Research Laboratories housed those clinical specialties with a research tie to basic immunology. The number of basic and clinical scientists located there represented a critical intellectual mass, which allowed research to progress despite the laboratories' distance from the Johns Hopkins Medical Institutions. Two of the first appointments were Kimishige and Teruko Ishizaka, who were already well known for their discovery of the immunoglobulin IgE.

This association with the O'Neill Research Laboratories allowed the Department of Medicine at Hopkins to develop categorical centers for clinical care, research, and teaching in specialty areas related to immunology. The Division of Rheumatology expanded into beds and research laboratories at Good Samaritan, with Mary Betty Stevens in charge. Collaborating closely was an orthopedics unit run by David Hungerford. The Division of Allergy was expanded, becoming the Division of Allergy and Clinical Immunology; its patient care and research were directed by Philip S. Norman and Lawrence Lichtenstein. W. Gordon Walker established a dialysis center and research laboratories as part of his Division of Renal Medicine. The Pulmonary Division was started in 1969 by Peter Luchsinger, whose ambulatory care center was one of the first to provide portable oxygen for patients with obstructive pulmonary dis-

ease. In 1970, Arthur Siebens came to Hopkins to establish the Division of Rehabilitation at the Good Samaritan Hospital. This division has since expanded in concert with facilities across the city.

The connections between Johns Hopkins and the Good Samaritan had come under strain in the mid-1970s. The Good Samaritan Hospital was labeled a hospital for chronic diseases, and state reimbursement for chronic care was not sufficient to cover the costs of operation. "Good Sam" was also maintained by the Catholic Archdiocese of Baltimore, whose point of view and that of the Johns Hopkins School of Medicine sometimes diverged. An affiliation endured between the Hopkins medical school and the Good Samaritan Hospital, however, and the special clinical and research divisions continued to flourish.[16]

Links with Philanthropic Foundations

Research at Johns Hopkins has been a major beneficiary of support from the Howard Hughes Medical Institute (HHMI), one of the world's richest philanthropies.[17] Four of the top five floors of the Preclinical Teaching Building are occupied by Hughes investigators, and the institute pays their salaries, the salaries of their support staffs, and most of their research costs. In 1987 alone, HHMI spent nearly $5 million at Johns Hopkins in support of its two research units, one in molecular genetics and the other in molecular neurobiology.

In accepting the two Hughes-supported units, the medical school became an essentially risk-free partner in a program to encourage creative research without demanding short-term gains. Scientists in this program were free from the usual concerns about funding connected with NIH grants. It was hoped that this freedom would also influence the substance of their work, since scientists totally dependent on NIH support tend to propose a continuation of previous work rather than a fresh approach that might not meet the approval of a peer-review panel. A more open policy might encourage bolder solutions to critical biological problems and might give young scientists the opportunity to try less conservative scientific approaches.

The connection between Hughes' medical philanthropy and Johns Hopkins began in the early 1950s, when a Hopkins graduate and former Osler house officer, Verne Mason, administered Hughes' funding for medical research. One of Mason's close friends was J. Earle Moore, who helped Mason to identify candidates at Hopkins for Hughes' support. "Support," at that time, consisted exclusively of salary money; no funds were given for supplies or other research needs. From the 1950s through the 1970s, a number of distinguished Hopkins investigators, including Norman Anderson, Samuel H. Boyer IV, Paul Lietman, Simeon Margolis, and David Sabiston, received support from Hughes.

Mason died in 1965, but the administrative tie between Hopkins and Hughes continued Mason's successor was George Thorn, a former associate professor of medicine at Hopkins; and in 1967, Victor A. McKusick became a member of the Hughes medical advisory board.

The pattern of HHMI support changed in 1976, when Howard Hughes died and federal tax law intervened. The trustees of the institute decided to formulate a comprehensive plan of research support, rather than continuing to give awards to people and projects piecemeal. Genetics, immunology, and metabolic regulation were the first scientific disciplines chosen for concentration; neuroscience was added later. One of the first "batch" awards at Hopkins went to Samuel Boyer, then codirector with Edmond A. Murphy of the Medical Genetics Division of the Department of Medicine. Over the next decade, HHMI funds supported eight scientists in Boyer's laboratory, who pursued the answers to some of the most important questions in genetics.

The first of the two HHMI-funded units at Hopkins began to take shape in 1982, when Daniel Nathans, director of the Department of Microbiology, became an HHMI senior investigator and began to organize a HHMI research unit in molecular genetics at Hopkins. Nathans believed that the Department of Microbiology should be expanded to include molecular biology and genetics, and that his HHMI unit should work closely with the corresponding department in the medical school. The time was right for him to step down as director of microbiology, Nathans thought, and he looked forward to collaborating with Thomas Kelly, Jr., his successor as director of the newly renamed Department of Molecular Biology and Genetics. Since winning the Nobel Prize in medicine in 1978, Nathans has turned to the study of the genetic events that regulate cell growth (see chapter 11).

The second HHMI unit, the Laboratory of Molecular Neurobiology, is also housed in the Preclinical Teaching Building, on the new floors constructed in 1986 with HHMI funds. Five neuroscientists have been brought to the new laboratory, and two more will eventually complete the laboratory's senior staff.[18]

There is close collaboration between the Laboratory of Molecular Neurobiology and the Department of Neuroscience. Collaboration in general is encouraged by the physical proximity of Hughes investigators to other Hopkins faculty members with similar interests. The HHMI laboratories are contiguous in one direction with those of the Department of Molecular Biology and Genetics, and in another direction with those of the Department of Neuroscience. This contiguity also facilitates sharing of equipment and services, daily mingling of students and fellows, and interdisciplinary research seminars.

Hughes investigators are virtually indistinguishable from their Hopkins colleagues. In addition to Hughes funding, each investigator is expected to have partial support for his research from NIH or other granting agencies, and the investigators' research progress is evaluated at three- to five-year intervals by an HHMI committee before renewal of the Hughes appointment. Investigators must also qualify for regular faculty positions at the School of Medicine, sharing in the teaching of medical students and graduate students on an equal basis with other Hopkins faculty. This smooth blending of the investigators' two roles—Hughes-supported scientist and Hopkins faculty member—has been essential to the success of the collaboration between the institute and the university.

The Medical Practice Plan

The practice of applying income obtained from medical practice to support teaching and research began informally in the 1940s, when Dean Alan M. Chesney transferred some of the practice income from the clinical departments to the preclinical departments. The funds involved were not great, however, and with the rise of federal support for research in the 1950s and 1960s, this policy had little impact on the medical school's budgetary arrangements.

Academic salaries began a steeper rise in the 1960s, however, and with federal cutbacks in funding, by the 1970s medical schools were hard pressed to meet all their expenses. Few sources of income could be augmented sufficiently to cover the greater costs; for most schools to survive in the new economic environment, they had to increase the income they received from the practice of medicine.

Medical school budgets from 1939, 1969, and 1979 reflect changing sources of income. In 1939, income from investments accounted for almost 50 percent of the budget, private gifts and grants for about 30 percent, tuition for about 15 percent, professional fees for only 3.5 percent, and government grants and contracts for only 1.5 percent. In 1969–70, tuition and investment income had both dropped to less than 5 percent of the budget. Income from professional fees had remained stable, but income from grants and contracts (both private and government) had increased to more than 70 percent. By 1979–80, grants and contracts had dropped to less than 50 percent, but income from professional fees had increased by a factor of six, to 21 percent of the total.[19]

The problem was to use this income fairly and advantageously while preserving the fundamental principle of the full-time plan—that no faculty member should receive payment from patients. Many faculty members, however, believed

a practice plan to be incompatible with the full-time system. In 1974, an "experimental clinical practice plan" was established in the Department of Ophthalmology and extended to some other departments. When this plan was presented to the Advisory Board later that year, the board expressed great concern, and one senior professor stated that Dean Morgan was "in the process of abolishing the full-time system." The board was assured that the plan was intended as a trial, an effort to discover whether clinical revenues could be increased without impairing educational programs, and that full-scale adoption of incentive programs by other clinical departments would take place only after discussion with the board.

Given these assurances, in January 1975 the board instructed Dean Morgan and the dean-elect, Richard S. Ross, to begin formal planning for a medical practice plan. Joined by George Zuidema (head of the Department of Surgery) and Daniel Nathans (head of the Department of Microbiology), they prepared a proposal that was discussed, modified, and finally approved by the Advisory Board in January 1976.

Under the new plan salaries were set by the departmental directors and approved by the dean. The criterion that was used to determine each faculty member's salary was that individual's contribution to the institution in teaching, research, and patient care. Marketplace adjustments in salaries were necessary, however, to maintain strength in the clinical departments, particularly in the surgical specialties. The marketplace, in this case, was not private practice but other academic medical institutions. As a result, not all faculty of the same rank were paid alike. For example, discrepancies occurred between the salaries of an assistant professor of ophthalmology and an assistant professor of physiology; but a hard fact countered the argument that all assistant professors should be paid the same amount: the marketplace created a difference that Hopkins would have to recognize in order to preserve the quality of its clinical staff.

Compensation was nevertheless a function of overall productivity, and there was no mathematical relationship between salary and the department's total earnings. This was a distinguishing feature of the Hopkins plan. In most other institutions, the individual practitioner kept a certain fixed proportion of collections. At Hopkins, total compensation was independent from the income generated from practice, grants, and the like.

The practice plan had several distinct benefits besides facilitating the recruitment of clinical faculty. The steadily rising income from professional practice in the hospital bespoke the clinical faculty's increased interest in patient care. It also kept the hospital full, an essential economic benefit and one that provided the best possible setting for the training of the medical students, residents, and fellows.

In the plan's first fourteen years, practice income grew twenty-five-fold. In 1973, gross clinical practice earnings were $4 million. In 1987–88, the total exceeded $100 million. The composition of the medical school's budget reflected this growth, as in 1987, almost one-third of the income came from practice, one-third came from government grants and contracts, and one-third came from all other sources. The practice plan thus provided the means for the school to maintain its leadership in medical education, research, and research training.

Eighty-eight percent of the professional fee income was returned to the departments that earned it. Departments with surpluses placed the money in a "Unit Executive Fund," which the department director could use, with the dean's approval, for projects such as recruiting division heads. In departments with deficits, the money would be applied to reduce the shortfall.

The remaining 12 percent was placed in an "Institutional Stabilization Fund." One-quarter of that 12 percent, or 3 percent of the practice plan's total income, was allotted to the basic science departments—a resource that added tremendous strength to these departments in the 1980s. Fifty percent of the so-called Basic Science Reserve was placed in a fund for use by the dean, with the approval of the department heads, for the benefit of the entire basic-science community. The remainder was divided among the preclinical de-

partments and could, with the approval of the dean, be used for whatever purpose each department director wished. Money remaining in the Institutional Stabilization Fund was disbursed by the dean at his discretion.

This discretionary money gave the dean great flexibility in fostering important needs of the school—start-up money for new programs, and provision of new space and buildings. Four to five million dollars per year could be provided as a supplement to the budget for general teaching and research. A significant amount was also placed in a reserve fund, which by 1987 had grown to almost $20 million. The minimal amount available from endowment income and the fact that government funds provided no flexibility in their use emphasized the importance of the reserve fund to the maintenance of the School of Medicine's position of leadership and to its future welfare. Consequently, the availability of the Institutional Stabilization Fund derived from clinical practice has given Johns Hopkins a distinct advantage over other private medical schools that do not have this important source of income.

In 1987, a bonus plan was superimposed upon the basic skeleton of the practice plan. Bonuses, which in total amounted to 3 percent of the gross collections of the practice, could be proposed by the department director and approved by the dean. They constituted only a small percentage of the total practice income, but they were important in keeping total compensation competitive with that of other academic institutions.

In sum, the medical practice plan maintained the fundamental principle of the full-time system in the medical school: no full-time faculty member received direct payment from patients for delivery of medical care. All monies paid to clinical faculty for the delivery of services to patients reverted to the practice plan and were distributed in accordance with written rules and agreements. Compensation to clinicians took the form of a set salary, which was proposed by the department director and approved by the dean; a few faculty members received a performance supplement or bonus, which was also proposed by the director and approved by the dean. Furthermore, no bonuses could be awarded unless a department had a surplus balance.

Many deans in other schools praised this practice plan as probably the best in the country because it separated collections from compensation. It was possible to establish such a plan only because of Hopkins' long adherence to the full-time system, in which fees for service did not revert directly to the physicians, and salaries were determined without regard to clinical earnings. Schools that began at the other end of the spectrum, with faculty who treated patients only at the school's hospital but retained their fees (the "geographic full-time" system), had difficulty approaching the middle ground, as these faculty were loath to support a plan that would diminish their personal income.

A liability of the practice plan in recent times is that it makes the medical school appear rich in comparison with other divisions of the university, an alluring target for a central university administration that needs money for less fortunate divisions and for shoring up venturesome but financially insolvent projects.

One endeavor supported by the medical practice plan is the Clinician-Scientist Program, which encourages the academic development of the physician-scientist at Johns Hopkins. The decline in the proportion of M.D. recipients of NIH research grants has led to the perception that clinician-scientists are an endangered species. Many educators believe that the day of the renaissance physician is over, for physicians can no longer care for patients, teach, and master the advanced research techniques necessary to pursue an investigative career. The Clinician-Scientist Program, initiated by Dean Richard S. Ross, enabled the medical school to buy the time of certain of its clinicians for research. One million dollars per year from the Institutional Stabilization Fund was allocated to provide salary support for research by young clinical faculty.

The clinician applying for this internal source of funds must simultaneously prepare a grant application to the National Institutes of Health. A committee of Hopkins faculty members with experience on NIH study sections gives the request a priority score. Funding through Hopkins moves more rapidly than NIH review and allows the faculty member to begin research while awaiting a response from outside agencies. Hopkins' approval requires that at least 75 percent of the applicant's time and effort be devoted to research. If the internal application is approved, up to $50,000 of salary support for two years can be awarded. Any NIH funding received subsequently is added to the internal award.

Reform of Promotions Policies

Until 1980, no rules existed governing appointment or promotions to the medical faculty, nor was there a tradition of "tenure" at the Hopkins medical school. Instead, every faculty member was evaluated yearly and either reappointed or not. It was theoretically possible to remain an assistant professor, for example, for one's entire career, without any prospect of advancement.

With the substantial increase in the size of the faculty over the past thirty years, formal regulations have become necessary to ensure that every faculty member receives fair consideration for promotion. The policies instituted during the deanship of Richard S. Ross forced department directors to evaluate faculty and either recommend promotion or encourage the faculty member to find a position elsewhere. A contract to retirement, or the equivalent of tenure, is associated with the rank of full professor. No one can remain for more than a total of fifteen years in the combined ranks of assistant and associate professor. After that time, the individual has to be proposed for promotion, given a contract to retirement (at the level of associate professor), or given a two-year terminal contract.

Despite the apparent stringency of these new regulations, a study of the promotions system at Hopkins from 1979 to 1985 revealed that 93 percent of candidates for associate professor and 79 percent of professorial candidates were promoted.[20]

Changes in Medical Education

Increases in Class Size

A perceived shortage of physicians in the 1960s led the federal government to institute the first direct aid to medical education: capitation funds intended to stimulate an increase in the numbers of medical students.[21] The size of the medical school class at Johns Hopkins was increased accordingly. Classes had comprised 70 to 75 students during the 1950s and around 90 students during the 1960s. With the capitation grants, class size grew to 100 students in 1970 and finally, in 1972, to 120—the level at which it has remained.

Enrollment of Minority Students

Efforts were also made to increase the enrollment of minority students, but these attempts were unsuccessful at first. The best black students wanted to attend medical school in Boston or New York, cities with a more sympathetic atmosphere. The first two black students were admitted during Turner's deanship. Both graduated in 1967 and became practicing neurosurgeons, one in Washington, D.C., and the other in Canada.[22]

During the deanship of David Rogers (1968–72), the few blacks accepted at Hopkins often did not graduate, a circumstance that had a circular effect, antagonizing many black students who felt that they would have graduated had they gone to other, less prestigious medical schools. The strategy employed later, during the middle and late 1970s, relied on an enlarged pool of black applicants coupled with a special effort to persuade well-qualified students to matriculate at Hopkins rather than at competing institutions. One effective tactic was the recruitment of black students by black members of the full-time faculty, particularly surgeon Levi Watkins and ophthalmologist Earl Kidwell.

By 1987 the medical school had four black Rhodes Scholars, one of whom has joined the faculty in the Department of Pharmacology. Among the black students graduating in 1984 was one born in the Hopkins neighborhood in East Baltimore.

The Decline in Laboratory Instruction

The anti-intellectualism associated with the era of the Vietnam War reverberated throughout the nation's medical schools in the 1970s. Students demanded (and in some cases, obtained) control of the curriculum, deciding what was "relevant" to their future as physicians. In most schools, students turned away from the basic sciences, and laboratory instruction declined. Medical students' time in the laboratory also diminished at Johns Hopkins, but to a lesser degree than elsewhere. The trend toward spending less time in the laboratory was largely related to the problems associated with the increase in basic biomedical knowledge and the complexity of firsthand participation in certain types of laboratory exercises.[23]

In 1975, a committee chaired by Vernon B. Mountcastle reviewed the basic science program, concluding that the concept of "learning by doing"—traditional at Hopkins since the opening of the university—was still useful and should be retained. The subsequent revision of the curriculum ensured the student's firsthand participation in the learning process, but less time was devoted to laboratory instruction than in the 1950s (see chapter 7).[24]

The most recent curriculum review committee, empaneled in 1986 and chaired by Gert H. Brieger, director of the Institute of the History of Medicine, presented its report eighteen months later.[25] The committee advocated an emphasis on laboratory experience and the integration of small seminars into all four years of medical school. Once again, "learning by doing" was confirmed as the guiding principle of a Hopkins medical education.

The FlexMed Program

A national committee chaired by Steven Muller, president of the Johns Hopkins University, in the early 1980s reaffirmed the importance of a liberal education for matriculating medical students.[26] The committee's report was hardly startling, as committees for the past half century had published similar findings. In 1983, a new plan was instituted at Hopkins to advance the concept of the broadly educated physician. A flexible admissions program (FlexMed) informed students of their admission to medical school after two years of college. They were then free to concentrate on the depth and breadth of their education, to study for two years (or even beyond the baccalaureate degree) without the pressure of total attention to preparation for medical school. The students maintained continuing ties with faculty advisors at Johns Hopkins in order to ensure the pursuit of a worthwhile educational program. Characterized by early admission and delayed matriculation, FlexMed differed significantly from the Year V Program of the 1950s, which featured early admission and early matriculation and therefore shortened the undergraduate experience (see chapter 7).[27]

The M.D.-Ph.D. Program

Although a formal M.D.-Ph.D. program was not instituted at Johns Hopkins until 1975, many medical students obtained both M.D. and Ph.D. degrees in earlier years. In this they emulated notable members of the Hopkins faculty, from John J. Abel to E. Kennerly Marshall, Jr. In 1961, the burgeoning federal support for basic science training had allowed A. McGehee Harvey, with the help of Kenneth L. Zierler, to obtain an interdepartmental training grant from the NIH. This award enabled house officers and fellows in clinical departments who chose a career in medical science to pursue the doctoral degree. The training of M.D.-Ph.D. medical scientists became a stated goal at Hopkins in 1968, when the Advisory Board mandated that the increased number of entering medical students include at least 10 percent prospective medical scientists.

The NIH had instituted its Medical Scientist Training Program in 1964, but problems in complying with federal regulations (see chapter 7)

prevented Hopkins from obtaining a federal award until 1975. In that year, Paul Talalay, former director of Hopkins' Department of Pharmacology and Experimental Therapeutics, became the head of the program at Hopkins. Its success is due largely to his efforts. The first two graduates on the Medical Scientist Training Program (MSTP) at Hopkins received their degrees in 1980. Between 1975 and 1988, 95 students pursuing combined M.D.-Ph.D. programs were graduated. M.D.-Ph.D. training at Hopkins now encompasses several programs in a number of disciplines; however, not all students receive funding from the NIH. Of the first thirty-eight fully trained participants in the NIH Medical Scientist Program at Hopkins, twenty-nine are now faculty members in clinical departments and nine are faculty members of basic science departments. The program is thus filling its mandate to prepare future faculty members for academic medical centers.[28]

The Firm System

When the increasing cost of medical care in the late 1960s moved the practice of medicine from the hospital to the outpatient setting, the traditional pattern of residency training in medicine at Hopkins had to change accordingly. It was no longer practical to maintain two separate medical residencies, one for private and one for ward patients, because the number of patients who populated the ward service had declined as Medicare and Medicaid enabled them to have private physicians. The Marburg (private) and Osler (ward) Medical Services were therefore gradually integrated between 1967 and 1970.

Other changes in the hospital population also affected the Hopkins residency programs. Medicare and Medicaid regulations required every patient to have a physician of record other than a resident physician. In addition, patients who in earlier times would have been hospitalized were receiving outpatient treatment. The in-hospital population now comprised a growing number of elderly patients, and many residents found geriatric medicine not to be a particularly rewarding area of study. The cost of hospital care and more rapid cures of many illnesses led to a reduction in the average length of stay in hospital and a concomitant rise in the number of primary admissions. As a result, more house officers were needed, and the size of the house staff gradually became unmanageable.

In the Oncology Center, for example, protocols for treatment diminished the traditional responsibility of the trainee for making decisions about the management of patients. Many patients were admitted to the center simply for diagnostic or therapeutic procedures; without the opportunity for preadmission planning for his or her own patients, the trainee was deprived of the responsibility necessary for professional growth.

In 1975, a new residency system was instituted in the Department of Medicine, under the leadership of Victor A. McKusick, director of medicine. The Medical Service was divided into four equal units, known as "firms." The idea of the firm system had emerged through the faculty exchange program with Guy's Hospital in London, which used a similar plan. Each firm—Barker, Janeway, Longcope, and Thayer—had its own chief resident, known as the "assistant chief of service" (ACS), its own house staff, and its own space in the hospital. The four firms divided the Medical Service into units of manageable size for teaching, clinical care, career guidance, and the many other tasks of the chief residents.

The system was designed to accommodate residency training to the changing pattern of medical financing while preserving the degree of responsibility characteristic of the traditional residency program. The resident physician and the resident surgeon had long had faculty appointments and a key role in teaching medical students as well as junior house officers, but the new system made the chief residents in medicine, and later in surgery, members of the "active staff" and physicians (surgeons) to the Johns Hopkins Hospital. The primary innovation of the firm system was that it delegated as much responsibility to the chief residents as to the other members of the active staff—all the duties and privileges of "physicians of record." The system also improved the

continuity of care (and the educational benefits of long-term follow-up) by specifying that patients remain with the same firm for both inpatient and outpatient care.[29]

Administrative Restructuring

Early in his deanship, David E. Rogers reviewed the governance of the medical institutions, including discussion of such items as fixed periods of tenure for department directors and more democratic decision making. To give all segments of the medical institutions a voice, a new group, the Medical School Council, was established in 1971. Composed of students, house officers, and junior faculty, it makes recommendations to the Advisory Board and through it to the trustees of the medical institutions.

One of Rogers' most significant actions was the recruitment of Robert M. Heyssel. Heyssel came to Johns Hopkins from Vanderbilt in 1968 and was made director of the new Office of Health

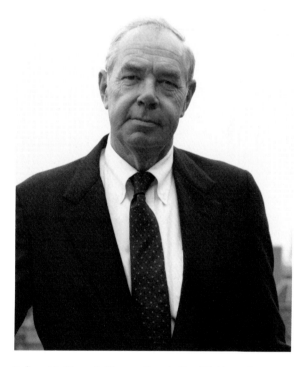

Robert M. Heyssel. (*Source:* Dennis Caudill, Visus Commercial Photography, Inc.)

Care Programs, created to oversee the ambulatory care activities at the Johns Hopkins Hospital and the medical care programs in Columbia and in East Baltimore (see chapter 10). Heyssel became executive vice-president and director of the hospital in the fall of 1973. In that post he inaugurated, as well as presided over, fundamental and far-reaching changes in the traditional administrative structure and programs of the Johns Hopkins Hospital.

Hospital Decentralization and the Development of Functional Units

A decentralized administrative structure had always been characteristic of the Johns Hopkins Medical Institutions, but in the 1970s the old way of doing business had come under strain. The dual responsibility of the department director— as head of the medical school department as well as head of the corresponding department in the hospital—was now subjected to a distressing imbalance. Although the director of a medical school department reported to the dean, the director had total responsibility for the day-to-day activities in his department, the appointment of staff members, control of the budget, and the employment of nonprofessional personnel. On the hospital side, however, there was another bureaucratic layer: nonprofessional personnel and budgets were not the responsibility of the department head but of administrative personnel reporting to the hospital director.

As the hospital grew in complexity, these problems deepened. Staffing and operation of the outpatient clinics and nursing on the inpatient service suffered particularly. Perhaps the most difficult situation occurred in the Department of Medicine, which was also coping with the departure from its outpatient clinics of NIH-supported fellows and an increasingly specialized faculty. These problems of professional staffing led to increasing confrontations between the director of the medical school department and the administrative staff of the hospital. University teaching functions thus suffered along with patient care.

Weekly meetings of the chiefs of the clinical services during the early 1970s exposed these problems to discussion. The Department of Medicine had become familiar with the decentralized system in effect at Temple University Hospital, a system that might solve the administrative difficulties at Hopkins. This system made each hospital department responsible for developing its own budget and for planning and carrying out all aspects of inpatient and outpatient care.

As director of the hospital, Heyssel recognized the value of this idea and developed a system of budgeting and accounting that would balance maximal responsibility for each department against the needs of the hospital as a whole. The measurement of agreed-upon objectives along the way was also an important part of Heyssel's adaptation of the decentralized system. Most important to the clinical chief was the ability to meet responsibilities in patient care, research, and medical education. From the hospital's point of view, the important factors were cost control and more efficient management techniques to reduce expenses. Both sides agreed, however, that to survive in the 1970s, teaching hospitals had to look for innovative approaches in both medical care and management practice. The key to cost saving was involving physicians in management practices, since most of the costs associated with hospital care resulted from decisions by physicians. It was the physicians, for example, who ordered the tests and decided on the length of hospitalization. The traditional organizational system of the hospital—central supervision of costs but little control over the decisions that affected them—was no longer working well, and a new approach was very attractive.[30]

The new system involved the heads of clinical units in management decisions for the first time, as Hopkins shifted operating responsibilites and financial accountability to the clinical departments. The hospital as a whole thus became a holding company for a series of specialty hospitals, or so-called functional units.

Each functional unit was headed by a "functional unit director," a physician who was also the director of the corresponding department in the medical school. Superficially, this arrangement represented only a change in title, as Hopkins tradition specified that the same individual head the corresponding hospital and medical school departments. Under the new system, however, a nursing director and an administrator reported directly to each functional unit director. These three individuals were a team, accountable for all direct costs associated with the operation of their department, including services acquired or purchased from other departments, such as laboratory medicine or radiology.

Although the directors of the functional units reported directly to the president of the hospital, they made most of the decisions in their special areas. Regular meetings took place between the corporate officers of the hospital and the functional unit directors, to ensure a broad understanding of policies and decisions, and to provide a routine forum for discussion. Each unit was required to operate within general guidelines that reflected hospital policies relating to overall institutional goals, allocation of capital resources, personnel policies, and rate setting. Salary guidelines were established centrally to ensure uniformity throughout the hospital.

Decentralization was an obvious financial success. Within the state's rate-setting guidelines, and despite the capital expenses of a massive rebuilding campaign, the hospital was nevertheless able to maintain a positive operating balance beginning in 1976. While holding unit cost increases below state and national averages, Hopkins continued to grow. Its overall budget increased, along with its ability to support new programs, make use of technologic advances, and construct new buildings.

Before 1973, more than 80 percent of the hospital's costs had been allocated by central administration. By 1983, the pattern was reversed. Clinical departments directly controlled 51 percent of their expenditures, with departmental purchase of ancillary services such as laboratory tests and radiologic services accounting for an additional 20 percent. Overhead expenses and institutional costs amounted to 22 percent and 7 percent, respectively.

The process of turning physicians into managers was not easy, however, for the administration or for the physicians themselves. A key factor in the plan's success was the willingness of the hospital's corporate officers to delegate decision-making authority, as had already been done in the medical school. The central administration now turned to developing policy and monitoring the performance of the functional units, since it could no longer control performance directly through administrators reporting to a central authority.

The transfer of responsibility and decision-making authority cast the directors of the clinical departments in a new role. Before the advent of decentralization, physicians were reluctant to become directly involved in hospital administration. Previously, the primary commitment of chiefs of service was to teaching and research. Now, departmental administration joined these traditional academic pursuits as a primary activity, and management skills became a requirement. Attention to hospital economics became normal procedure rather than a peripheral concern.

Each functional unit eventually acquired a financial manager and support staff, as directors found that nonphysician staff members could assume many of the time-consuming bureaucratic responsibilities. The larger departments had enjoyed administrative support since the 1960s, but decentralization required a more encompassing and more sophisticated type of assistance. The expanded team provided financial expertise for both the hospital and the medical school, alleviating the need for a large centralized administration.

In the Department of Surgery, for example, the surgeon-in-chief (the functional unit head), with the unit director of nursing, managed what was in effect a 250-bed hospital with an annual operating budget of more than $20 million. When the responsibility for the medical school department's budget was added, the total operating budget approached $40 million, and the unit head's supervisory responsibility encompassed 1,000 employees. As Heyssel and his colleagues pointed out, the team concept enabled the surgeon-in-chief to assume this kind of responsibility and resulted in an organization that was more flexible and accessible than a central bureaucracy.

The professional role of nurses was also strengthened through decentralization. Nursing directors assumed more departmental responsibility for staffing and budgeting. As strong managers placed in a collegial forum among administrators and physician chiefs of service, nursing directors were better positioned to promote the professional practice of nursing. The decentralized system attracted nurses who could manage large numbers of people, budget resources appropriately, develop strong leadership teams, and evaluate the capacity of nurses for advancement. The hospital's vice-president for nursing participated in all key decision making and set the tone for nursing practice throughout the hospital.

Decentralized management worked because it gave the institutional responsibility to those who made the decisions—the physicians. They knew that controlling expenses and reducing unnecessary treatment would be translated into support for clinical programs, new technologic procedures, and higher-quality patient care. Strategies aimed at reducing the length of hospital stay and controlling the use of ancillary services were then more likely to be successful because they were directed by physician-managers who could influence the behavior of their colleagues.

Organizational Rearrangements

The appointment of Steven Muller as president of both the Johns Hopkins Hospital and the Johns Hopkins University in 1972 was a highly significant development, a return to the system of the past. The precedent for having a single person as head of both hospital and university had been set almost a century earlier: before Henry M. Hurd's appointment in 1890 as the first superintendent of the hospital, Daniel Colt Gilman filled both roles for a short time. Muller's dual appointment reaffirmed the equality of hospital and medical school, as the president of the hospital was the administrative equal of the president of the university, and both were *ex officio* members of the Boards of Trustees. Similarly, the counterpart to the dean of the medical school was the hospital's superintendent or director.

Muller continued in this dual role until 1985, when he stepped down as president of the hospital. Robert Heyssel, the hospital's director and executive vice-president, then assumed the hospital presidency. As in 1962, when hospital director Russell Nelson assumed the hospital presidency, medical school faculty and administrators were concerned that the change in administrative structure might lessen the dean's authority, but this change was shown not to diminish the dean's authority in matters of education and research. Moreover, no single person could easily serve as an operative director of both university and hospital: the responsibilities—academic, financial, ceremonial, fund-raising and other—became too great and too diverse.[31]

Yet as Dean Richard S. Ross said, until Muller resigned the hospital presidency, no one apparently realized how important this joint presidency had been in holding the institutions together.[32] A joint presidency added symmetry to the organization, as the dean and the hospital director reported to the same individual.

With Heyssel's appointment, a joint committee of trustees was empowered to serve as a coordinating mechanism between hospital and medical school. A committee of trustees from the two boards was also appointed to reassess the organization of the institutions, looking toward the time when the president of the hospital and the dean of the medical school would retire. The most obvious solution had been suggested for many years: merging the two institutions so that a single chief executive officer—perhaps a chancellor—would control both hospital and medical school. This suggestion would have had the advantages of reestablishing the joint presidency, but the idea was not approved.

According to Heyssel, the single greatest issue that led to rejection of the idea was the merging of the authority of the hospital and university boards. The composition and responsibilities of the two boards were so different as to be incompatible. Furthermore, the question of how a "chancellor" or "super-president" would be selected by the two boards was a major consideration. Finally, the merger of the two corporations would have run counter to national trends, which encouraged the separation of hospitals from direct university governance and ownership.[33]

What is crucial to the most effective system of governance is the ability of both leaders—the dean of the medical school and the hospital's president—to work independently in their own spheres, yet cooperatively when problems overlap. Each position must be designed so that the most capable candidate can also be recruited to hold it. A balanced system will reconcile the complex, conflicting, and rapidly changing requirements of the hospital and the medical school. The hospital's president must have the power to offer the best care possible while still protecting the hospital's economic base, but decisions made to improve patient care could seriously hamper the dean's ability to carry out the medical school's most important purpose: undergraduate and postgraduate education. The relationship between president and dean must therefore be one that enhances cooperation and diminishes divisive influences.

The Johns Hopkins Health System

By the early 1980s, the Johns Hopkins Medical Institutions regarded the future with some equanimity. As Robert Heyssel described the mood at the hospital:

> We had rebuilt the institution with what looked like very cheap money in relation to prevailing rates of inflation, and future debt service was not a problem. We had mainly new facilities; much expanded parking; were at peace with the state rate-setting commission; and, in general, looked like we were set for the '80s and beyond with only some minor tuning here and there. At the same time, the Johns Hopkins

Medical School was prospering and, given our mutual interdependence, that was equally important to our sense of well-being.[34]

Some members of the faculty and several key trustees nevertheless recognized that the nation's health-care system was changing. Across the country, for-profit organizations were increasingly taking control of facilities for medical care, and increasing numbers of patients were enrolling in health maintenance organizations (HMOs) and their variants. Admittedly, the Baltimore region was relatively untouched by such HMOs, and businesses interested in developing their opportunities in the field of medical care were not very active. This was the time, the trustees believed, to study the situation thoroughly in order to ensure that plans for the future of the medical institutions would enable Hopkins to meet potential threats to its traditional patient base. No new facilities had been created for ambulatory care at Hopkins, despite a shift toward more outpatient care that was part of a general effort to reduce medical costs.

Within a year, the trustee and faculty committees appointed to study the problem had a view and a plan: to provide effective community medical care and to preserve Hopkins' well-known referral specialty practice, the hospital would have to reorganize its ambulatory care services and concentrate particularly on maintaining facilities for the institutions' strongest clinical specialties—the neurosciences, cardiology, oncology, and ophthalmology.

The outcome of these plans in 1986 was the conglomeration of institutions that make up the Johns Hopkins Health System. The Board of Trustees of the health system elects and appoints the board of the Johns Hopkins Hospital, as well as the boards of the Francis Scott Key Medical Center, Homewood Hospital (formerly North Charles General Hospital), Homewood North Hospital (formerly Wyman Park Medical Center), and the Johns Hopkins Health Plan. The trustees of the health system also approve each component institution's budgets, capital expenditures, programs, and selection and compensation of chief officers before these items are finally adopted by the individual institution's board.

At the time of transition in July 1986, the Johns Hopkins Hospital Board of Trustees incorporated itself as the Johns Hopkins Health System board and elected itself the Johns Hopkins Hospital board as well—avoiding, at that time, the need to decide which trustees would be members of the health system board and which would be only on the hospital board. It was unlikely, however, that the membership of the two boards would remain identical.

The president of the Johns Hopkins Hospital is not a member of the board of the Johns Hopkins Health System. The president of the health system is, however, a member of the board of all constituent hospitals and is responsible for overseeing all the institutions in the health system, including the Johns Hopkins Hospital. He thus has prior approval of the latter hospital's budgets, capital financing, and planning.

In addition, the Joint Committee of trustees is now legally composed of health system trustees (now Johns Hopkins Hospital trustees) and university trustees. The president of the Johns Hopkins Health System and the dean of the Johns Hopkins University School of Medicine thus have similar relationships to the president of the Johns Hopkins University.[35]

Physicians who participate in the Johns Hopkins Health System are given credentials by the health system but are not in many instances faculty members of the School of Medicine. Although the head of the health system did not intend to label all participants "Hopkins physicians," many members of the Hopkins faculty feared that bestowing the Hopkins name on non–faculty members amounted to "back-door accreditation." Others believed that this concern was inappropriate. The standard, academically trained Johns Hopkins physician would not have the interest or the talents to serve as a general physician in a health maintenance organization, nor would all of the physicians serving in an HMO have the qualifications to teach or to do research, the traditional pursuits of most Hopkins faculty

members. A two-track system for physicians was, therefore, a necessary facet of this large institutional program for patient care.

One proposed solution was the separation of the Hopkins Health Plan—the prepaid, managed clinical operation—from the rest of the Johns Hopkins Medical Institutions. Without this disjunction, some feared that the academic programs would be in danger of dilution and the standards of the university and its institutions diminished. They drew a comparison with other Hopkins divisions: just as the Johns Hopkins Applied Physics Laboratory did not compete with the Department of Physics on the Homewood campus, the Johns Hopkins Health Plan should not enter the domain of the Johns Hopkins Hospital or the School of Medicine, except to contract for specific services. With proper organization, the university and hospital could contribute to the development of new patterns of medical care without diluting traditional standards of care or infringing upon traditional academic goals.

Others felt that the medical school had much to gain from an association with a Hopkins HMO. Because health maintenance organizations had become an important part of modern medicine, they believed that all medical students and house officers should be instructed, firsthand, in this kind of care. The staff of a Hopkins HMO should include not only capable physicians but also, among them, well-qualified teachers.

From the health system's point of view, the HMO was required to be cost competitive, as efficient as competing organizations. The teaching function in the HMO setting might impair such efficiency. Furthermore, the requirement that the physicians be teachers posed difficult constraints in staffing. Some saw these problems as amenable to solution through compromises that would not remove teachers and practitioners from the medical school.

Some of the medical school faculty and some administrators feared that the health system would further diminish the traditional parity between hospital and medical school—in a relationship already strained by changes in the structure of the governing bodies. As Thomas B.

Turner wrote, "Without the Johns Hopkins Medical School, the Johns Hopkins Hospital would be just another community hospital. . . . The two were great centers of gravity in East Baltimore, had their own special problems, involving operation of a successful hospital in a medical care system on the one hand and conservation of the massive intellectual thrust of the great medical faculty on the other."[36]

In the midst of a conflict that touches so many Hopkins traditions, spokespersons for both sides have looked back to the words of Johns Hopkins to support their respective positions. It is remarkable that even today, the wishes of the founder continue to guide the actions of Hopkins' leaders. In this case, the founder's written record is open to interpretations that reflect the advocacy of both hospital and medical school. Medical school dean Richard S. Ross quoted Johns Hopkins' letter of instruction: the hospital should be "made available for the educational and other academic programs of the university and its school of medicine."[37] This emphasizes the key role of the School of Medicine. At the same time, expressing the position that the hospital is a vital part of the medical institutions, the president of the Johns Hopkins Health System, Robert Heyssel, recalled Johns Hopkins' statement that "the primary mission of the Johns Hopkins Hospital is patient care."[38] Clearly, both were correct. The two institutions had a coordinate relationship, and each was greatly dependent upon the other.

All agreed that the Johns Hopkins Health System was important to the future of the Johns Hopkins Medical Institutions. For its success, teaching and research had to be considered along with patient care in all the decisions involving hospitals, health plans, and the Johns Hopkins name. Effective communication between the leaders of the two organizations would be a primary ingredient in the future success of the Johns Hopkins Medical Institutions during this period of dramatic medical and social change.[39]

Buildings

The demolition of the Harriet Lane Home in 1974 to make way for the Nelson and Oncology Buildings marked the beginning of the most extensive construction and remodeling program in the history of the medical institutions. Several new buildings replaced older structures. The Meyer Building was constructed on the site of the Woman's Clinic; the construction of both the Maumenee Building and the Oncology Center required demolition of the old Nurses' Home.

The pattern of construction differed from that of earlier periods. Between 1910 and 1930, the structure of the hospital had required separate buildings for medicine (the Osler Medical Clinic), for surgery (the Halsted Surgical Building), for pediatrics (the Harriet Lane Home), for psychiatry (the Henry Phipps Psychiatric Clinic), for ophthalmology (the Wilmer Institute), for gynecology (the Woman's Clinic), and for urology (the Brady Institute). Construction after World War II had also met the needs of the time: facilities for a growing patient population and an expanding faculty with many different research interests. The new buildings of the 1970s and 1980s were also designed to meet the needs of the time for teaching, research, and patient care, by physically linking departments with overlapping concerns.

In connecting all the new buildings either to existing buildings or to each other, this newest building boom marked the end of the pavilion system used by Billings. Isolated buildings no longer sufficed, as the integration of associated services for patients required as much floor space as possible on the same level. The need to move large numbers of patients with minimal reliance on elevators made a horizontal orientation much more practical than the old vertical system. Consequently, the Russell A. Nelson Patient Tower extends south from the end of the Halsted Building; the Oncology Center, an L-shaped structure of three floors, extends from the end of the Nelson Building; and the Harvey Teaching Tower bridges the south ends of the Osler and Halsted Buildings. The Maumenee Building, which opened in 1982, was connected to the main corridor of the hospital.

The Adolf Meyer Center, opened in 1982, represented the single largest financial commitment by the university and hospital to any group of departments in Johns Hopkins' history. The building was a physical realization of Adolf Meyer's belief that mind and organic brain are integrated elements. With the advent of molecular biological approaches, the study of the neurosciences was able to profit from the proximity of psychiatry, neurology, and neurosurgery under one roof. Psychiatry, neurology, and neurosurgery, therefore, each occupied three floors of the nine-story building. The building incorporated ninety beds for neurology and neurosurgery and eighty-eight beds for psychiatric inpatients, as well as operating suites, faculty offices, laboratories, clinics, and other outpatient programs, including a day hospital for psychiatric patients. By eliminating duplication of expensive facilities, equipment, and personnel, the Meyer Building allowed Hopkins to emphasize breadth of service and research.

In the Osler, Halsted, and Nelson Buildings, the horizontal reorientation of obstetrics-gynecology, medicine, and surgery brought them into a layered pattern, one in which each department occupied two or three floors of these three adjoining buildings. All the hospital's imaging resources—x-ray, computerized tomography, and magnetic resonance—were located at basement and sub-basement levels. The intensive care units were located on the seventh floor of these three buildings, at the same level as the operating room.

Renovation of existing buildings accompanied the new construction. The Osler and Halsted Buildings, as well as the Children's Medical and Surgical Center, were modernized. The Marburg Building provided a home for the Brady Urological Institute and the Renal Division of the Department of Medicine, bringing medical and surgical problems of the urinary tract together. When the Department of Psychiatry and Behavioral Sciences moved into the Meyer Building, the Phipps Building was converted into offices for the Johns Hopkins Health System, administrative offices for the newly constituted School of Nurs-

ing, administrative and teaching facilities for the Department of Obstetrics and Gynecology, and offices for the plant management services. The Henry Phipps Building was renamed the Houck Building in honor of Frank Houck, a Hopkins alumnus, former assistant director of the hospital, and hospital benefactor.

Even the traditional entrance to the hospital was changed. Patients and visitors used to enter through the domed building facing Broadway, with its statue of Christ. In 1979 the main entrance was moved to face Wolfe Street, and the new lobby occupies the first floor of the Nelson Building.

The medical school's facilities were also increased by several buildings. Construction of the Preclinical Teaching Building, dedicated in 1982, required the demolition of the historic Women's Fund Memorial Building. Two floors of the Preclinical Teaching Building were added by the Howard Hughes Medical Institute, as described earlier, to house the Hughes institutes of genetics and neuroscience.

A second major piece of medical school reconstruction was the replacement of Hunterian II with Hunterian III, a laboratory building providing temporary housing for the research programs of the Department of Medicine until facilities could be provided closer to the hospital. Extensive refitting of the Physiology Building, the Biophysics Building, and the Wood Basic Science Building also took place.

These research buildings joined the Traylor Building as the main research facilities of the medical school. The School of Medicine Administration Building was added to the Traylor-Turner complex in 1975 and greatly enlarged a decade later. Additional administrative offices and the computer facilities for both hospital and medical school were housed at 1830 East Monument Street, a nine-story building completed in 1988 at the northwest corner of Monument and Wolfe Streets.

As in the previous two decades, decisions at academic medical centers in the 1970s and 1980s were often controlled by social forces. Now, however, the direction of these forces had changed. Research had been the focus of public attention during the 1950s and 1960s, but now medical care became the area of greatest public concern. Nationwide, the growth brought about by the federal largesse became difficult to support in the face of financial stringency. Moreover, the cost of health care became the center of public attention, overshadowing the availability and quality of treatment—and the continuation of medical progress. Contributing to the problems of academic medical centers were the proprietary organizations that were now offering medical care, encroaching upon the medical centers' traditional patient base.

The leveling-off of federal monies for research and the threat to the teaching hospitals' income led to a search for new sources of funds. At Hopkins, the most important innovations were the increase in the full-time staff's clinical practice, and the organization of the Johns Hopkins Health System, which competed for patients with for-profit organizations. Medical schools nationwide established better cooperative relationships with industry. Foundations and industry became an increasingly important potential source of support. Substantial funds for research at Johns Hopkins came from the Howard Hughes Medical Institute, an organization that, since its founding, had close ties to the medical institutions. Together with funds allocated from the clinical practice plan, money from external sources—both foundations and industry—ensured the continuing development of clinical science at Johns Hopkins by providing support for promising young clinical scientists who had not yet obtained other funding for their studies.

The Howard Hughes Medical Institute created a program in molecular genetics and one in molecular neurobiology. The choice of these two fields reflected the pervasive influence of molecular biology on medical research in the 1980s. At Hopkins, some of the preclinical departments were renamed, and the latest research in molecular and medical genetics affected all of the clinical departments. The rise of neurobiological research led to the creation of the Department of Neuroscience, the first new basic science department in the school in over twenty years.

The diversification of medical care in the 1970s also led to reorganization of the medical and surgical residency programs at Hopkins and elsewhere. The "firm system" gave increased responsibility to the assistant chiefs of service and made them eligible to receive the fees to which the responsible physician was entitled. The firm system also reduced the size of the clinical units, a change that gave house staff more continuity in their training by allowing them to spend more time in one place.

In addition, hospital departments at Hopkins were reorganized into "functional units," giving department directors more control over expenditures and enabling them to run their departments more efficiently in the face of rising costs.

The problems of the Johns Hopkins Medical Institutions in the 1970s and 1980s were not unique, nor were its solutions extraordinary. The unusual administrative structure at Hopkins—the link between hospital and medical school—put in place at its founding, coupled with conservative adherence to its early principles, enabled Hopkins to cope with the vicissitudes of the later years. Although it is now one of many academic medical centers in the United States, Hopkins combines flexibility in adapting to change with a respect for its traditions in medical education, care, and research.

Part II

CHAPTER 6

WOMEN AT THE MEDICAL SCHOOL

This Board, if it accepts the funds thus raised, shall agree, by resolution, that, when its Medical School shall be opened, women whose training has been equivalent to the preliminary medical course prescribed for men, shall be admitted to such school upon the same terms as may be prescribed for men.

—Minute adopted by the Board of Trustees,
the Johns Hopkins University, October 28, 1890

Without the financial contributions of the Women's Fund Committee—particularly Mary E. Garrett's donation of $300,000—and the accompanying stipulation that the medical school admit women, the Johns Hopkins medical school would not have opened in 1893, nor would women have been among its first students. After this dramatic event, the fortunes of women at Hopkins changed in accordance with the changing perceptions of women nationwide. Recent interest in the history of women in medicine has produced a vast literature on this subject, ranging from the polemic to the statistical. This chapter is not, however, concerned with the general history of women in American medicine. Instead, it places in a national context the story of women at the Johns Hopkins University School of Medicine.

The Response to the Women's Fund Committee

The Women's Fund Committee had to contend with opposition not only from the Hopkins faculty and administration but also from its allies. Even some of the committee's supporters doubted that its scheme would work. "Our Women's Club has been urged to contribute to assist the Medical School of the Johns Hopkins University," wrote a woman from Worcester, Massachusetts, to a prominent woman physician in 1890:

with the idea that women shall have there all the advantages which men have, and as I have seen your name with other well-known names, I desire to ask if you really think that they will act in good faith if the $100,000 should be given them.

We are told by parties in Baltimore who ought to know that the whole policy of Johns Hopkins is conservative in spite of its high rank, and that women would never be admitted on the same terms as men.

. . . Will you be so kind as to tell me what you think of the scheme? If the money is raised and offered on condition that women shall be so received, we are told that it will be refused. In that case, it would not seem worth while to give anything towards it.[1]

The success of the tactic was unique, but the tactic itself was not. Since the 1860s, women's groups had been well known for their futile attempts to secure admission to medical schools by offering large sums to the schools. In 1865, women in New York and Boston were prepared to give $50,000 in scholarship money to schools that would admit women. No schools accepted. Fifteen years later, Marion Hovey promised Harvard Medical School $10,000 of her inheritance if it would admit women on the same terms as men. After much debate, Harvard's Board of Trustees demurred. Johns Hopkins thus became the first school to agree to such a financial arrangement.[2]

The unusual tradition enabled and specified by Mary Garrett was not the admission of women to medical school but the combination of women's acceptance "on the same terms as men" and an insistence on academic excellence. Women physicians were not uncommon in the late nineteenth century. In Europe, women routinely graduated alongside men from medical schools of high quality. Moreover, the United States census of 1890 counted 4,557 women physicians, 4.3 percent of the nation's total.[3] When the Hopkins medical school opened, its 3 women students joined 275 women medical students in seventeen other coeducational "regular" (as opposed to homeopathic) medical schools across the country.[4] Almost twenty-five years earlier, the University of California's Toland Medical College had begun to admit women "on equal terms in all respects with young men."[5] In the same city as the Johns Hopkins University, the Baltimore University School of Medicine declared itself to be a coeducational institution. Although it purported to admit women on the same terms as men, few women attended or graduated.[6]

In 1893, more than half the women enrolled in regular medical schools across the nation attended all-female institutions.[7] One such school was the Women's Medical College of Baltimore, founded in 1882 by a group of female philanthropists with the help of seven male physicians, including Dr. Richard Henry Thomas, the uncle of M. Carey Thomas. The school's standards were relatively high, and Abraham Flexner found it no worse than many of the other schools then in existence.[8] It evidently produced some creditable physicians, for two of its graduates, Drs. Claribel Cone and Flora Pollack, obtained internships at the Philadelphia Hospital (Blockley).[9]

The Women's Fund Committee at Hopkins denied any competition with the Women's Medical College, stating, "It is not expected that the Medical School of the Johns Hopkins University will take the place of the medical schools for women now in existence, but rather that it will afford to women in America those opportunities for advanced medical training which they are at present compelled to seek in the great foreign schools of Vienna, Paris, and Switzerland."[10] For its part, the administration of the Woman's Medical College of Baltimore accepted the new medical school graciously:

> Frequently have the questions been asked, "What effect will the admission of female students to the school of the Hopkins Hospital (as has lately been agitated) have upon *this* school?" and "Will not the result be disastrous to the Woman's Medical College?" Our reply has been that it would have no such dire consequences.
>
> We even hope that by making this city more of a medical centre we may be greatly benefited. The Hopkins School ought not to have any more deleterious effect upon the Woman's Medical College than upon the several *male* colleges; as its students have heretofore been and probably will *always* be to the greatest extent post-graduates.[11]

The writer concluded, "The Woman's Medical College has, we regret to say, been overlooked by those who have been endeavoring to give women the benefit of the Hopkins, and we cannot but feel that if these same, or other friends of women, would lend some of their aid and interest to the institution, which already in their midst, has for years been in operation for the benefit of the sex, they would not find such attention misplaced."[12]

None of the medical schools in existence in 1893, however, had Hopkins' stringent requirements for admission: knowledge of the sciences, proficiency in French and German, and a bachelor's degree. There were opportunities for women to go to school and emerge able to present themselves as "doctresses," but no medical school besides Hopkins offered women (or men) a graduate medical education.

These requirements were not the invention of the Women's Fund Committee but had been set forth by Welch some years earlier, in a document prepared for Gilman and the trustees. Mary Garrett had obtained a copy of the document, and, as Welch wrote:

> she naturally supposed that this was exactly what we wanted. It is one thing to build an educational castle in the air at your library table, and another to face its actual appearance under the existing circumstance. We were alarmed, and wondered if any students would come or could meet the conditions. . . .[13]

Garrett may indeed have been trying to win favor with the trustees. Four of the five members of the original Women's Fund Committee were daughters of trustees, and the women were privy to many of the board's deliberations. The intellectual prerequisites for admission that the Women's Fund Committee forced on William H. Welch and the Hopkins Board of Trustees were, however, also a form of insurance: well-educated women were not likely to perform poorly—and the failure of women students would have embarrassed the Women's Fund Committee and might have led to the later exclusion of women from Hopkins. These requirements may also have been a tool to give Hopkins women an advantage over male physicians graduating from other schools.

Mary Garrett and M. Carey Thomas appear to have considered the admission of women the more important part of their proposal. Mary Garrett told the Board of Trustees that her interest in Hopkins derived largely from her interest in the medical education of women,[14] and testifying to Thomas' priorities, Mary Gwinn wrote, "both of us were innocent, I think, of having liked at any time a class-room or a lecture-room. . . . Neither at Cornell nor yet at the Johns Hopkins—nor at Leipzig subsequently, for that matter—was Carey [Thomas] seeking scholarship or culture or even pleasure; she was seeking simply a degree, for feminist, careerist and financial reasons."[15]

Public opinion at the time concentrated on the feminist benefits of making a Hopkins medical education available to women, although James Cardinal Gibbons discussed the beneficial influence of coeducation upon men.[16] The opening of the Hopkins medical school was "the long-awaited breakthrough that would open the prestigious medical schools to women," proclaimed an editorial in the Nation, which went on to explain the importance of graduation from a "prestigious" institution:

> The secret of women's rank in medicine, *as women,* depends upon the ability of the best women to hold their own by the side of the best men; when that is gained, the women of humble talents will fall into rank beside the men of humble talents, and it will be a question of the skill of a particular practitioner, and not, as now, of a particular sex. . . . It is, therefore, for its effect upon the position of women in medicine in general, even more than for its effect upon the knowledge of the women who shall enjoy its unapproachable facilities for instruction, that the opening of the Johns Hopkins Medical School forms an era in the progress of women towards the assumption of their natural responsibilities and duties.[17]

Even publications that supported the admission of women differed in their reasons. The Springfield, Massachusetts, *Republican* took a broader view than the Nation: "The more they [the Women's Committee] obtain, the nearer the goal of their desire for the benefit of their sex (and therefore of their country and the world) will be approached."[18] The Denver, Colorado, *Rocky Mountain News* said: "The prosperity, the stability and real worth of a nation is conditioned largely upon the health, the intelligence and the virtue of the women who are to be the mothers of children. The better educated the mother, the better and more useful will be the child."[19]

Other publications disapproved of the trustees' decision to admit women. An editorial in the *Medical Record,* "The Temptation of Johns Hopkins," accused Hopkins of "selling its privileges" and predicted that the best male applicants would choose medical schools "equally well, or better equipped, in which they can pursue their studies without the disillusioning propinquity of lady medicals. . . ."[20] (Dr. Emily Blackwell's disingenuous rebuttal denied the relation between the Women's Fund Committee's gift and the decision to admit women. She chastised the journal for insinuating that the Hopkins trustees were bribed or cajoled "into a course so deliberately adopted.")[21]

Unlike Blackwell, the Hopkins faculty were not squeamish about regarding the money as a bribe. As Osler wrote years later to the university's president:

> We are all for sale, dear Remsen. You and I have been in the market for years, and have loved to buy and sell our wares in brains and books—it has been our life. So with institutions. It is always pleasant to be bought, when the purchase price does not involve the sacrifice of an essential—as was the case in that happy purchase of us by the Women's Educational Association. . . .[22]

It is difficult to determine the true attitudes of Welch, Gilman, and Osler toward the admission of women because their expressed views sometimes contradicted their actions. Welch refused to sign the hospital staff's petition recommending that the trustees accept the committee's contribution, telling his sister that he would make no pretense of liking coeducation.[23] In 1897, he advised against accepting a scholarship exclusively for women, saying that the coeducation was not an asset to the medical school.[24] Yet he said that once the trustees had decided to accept the women's money, he did not wish to be regarded as an obstructionist.[25]

Welch also perceived a distaste for coeducation at the highest level of the university, commenting that Gilman and some of the trustees really did not want the Women's Fund Committee to succeed.[26] During Gilman's presidency at the University of California, however, women studied alongside men; and his overt response to the proposal of the Women's Fund Committee was noncommittal.[27]

As for Osler, he wrote that he was opposed to coeducation "on principle" but that he was warmly in favor of it "when the ladies came forth with half a million dollars."[28] Yet an encounter with Dorothy M. Reed hardly reflects even this ironic enthusiasm. As Reed described her meeting with Osler on her first day in Baltimore in 1896,

> There was only one passenger in the [street]car besides myself. . . . My appearance seemed to interest him for he literally stared at me out of countenance—seeming to go over me from head to foot, as if he were cataloguing every detail for future reference. . . . When the car stopped at Broadway I hopped out first, and walked quickly in the direction of the hospital gates a block away. He soon caught up with me, and walking along side of me, said very casually, "Are you entering the medical school?" I managed to gasp out that I intended to. "Don't," said he, "go home." And to my amazement without another word walked on ahead of me and went up the long flight of steps leading to the hospital door.[29]

Reed was shocked to learn the stranger's identity when she returned to the medical school for an interview the next day.

Although it was Osler who said that humanity is divided into three classes: men, women, and women physicians,[30] he could also be an advocate for women medical students. He did support the proposal of the Women's Fund Committee. And despite Dorothy Reed's initial dismay, in her memoirs she spoke of Osler as a friend, "to all of us an unfailing guide," who treated his women students, once they had arrived at Hopkins, with scrupulous integrity.[31] Osler also provided concrete support for women medical students: a few years after the school's opening, he contributed generously to a fund for a woman medical student who needed the money to continue her studies.[32]

These contradictions may reflect the pressures that beset the faculty and administration. Gilman and the trustees were anxious for the medical school to open, as the clinical professors were receiving offers from other medical schools, and further delays might cause them to leave. In the end, the administration and the faculty were eager enough for the opening of the medical school to accede to the women's demands. Welch commented that the faculty deserved very little credit for opening the doors to women.[33] Yet once the doors were open, Osler and other faculty members put aside their antipathy, for the welfare of the fledgling institution.

Some faculty members actually became enthusiastic about the admission of women when the experience of instructing a coeducational class proved less repugnant than they had expected. A few years after the medical school opened, Welch wrote that the faculty had come to regard coeducation as a success.[34] Even previously unsympathetic faculty members (himself included) were now sympathetic and friendly. Not only had the predicted embarrassments not materialized, but the presence of women had had a civilizing effect on both students and professors. Two decades after the medical school had opened, Dean David L. Edsall of the Harvard Medical School asked J. Whitridge Williams, professor of obstetrics, whether the inclusion of women medical students had been advantageous or detrimental to Hopkins. Williams replied that most of the faculty had initially been opposed to the admission of women, but the consensus of opinion after twenty-five years was that it had done no harm and in certain ways had elevated the character of the teaching. In particular, he said, it forced the faculty to restrain their use of *double entendres*.[35]

The initial aversion of the Hopkins faculty to the admission of women reflected the tenor of the times. Disdain toward women physicians was the attitude of the day. Landlords were even chary of renting offices to them. Many women at the turn of the century chose a career over marriage, but the most sympathetic public presumption was that a woman who chose to be a physician was suffering from a deep emotional disturbance or a secret grief, possibly a disappointment in love.[36]

"Women doctors were in 1892 in Baltimore somewhat of a curiosity," recalled Lilian Welsh, a graduate of the Women's Medical College of Pennsylvania in 1889. Welsh was a friend of Howard A. Kelly, and a physician then in practice in Baltimore with another woman, Mary Sherwood, who had obtained her medical degree from the University of Zurich. "We early learned not to presume that an acquaintance made in a professional capacity assisting Dr. Kelly or in our own offices entitled us to any recognition in a social way, even as one passed in the streets. Dr. Sherwood's sister-in-law at a large afternoon tea was asked by her hostess whether she was related to Dr. Mary Sherwood. She answered with some pride that Dr. Sherwood was not only her sister-in-law, but her

cousin as well. Her hostess rather frigidly replied that she knew Dr. Sherwood professionally but, of course, it would not be possible to know her in a social way."[37] "Being South for the winter" was the only way an aunt of Dorothy M. Reed, a member of the Class of 1900, could bring herself to refer to her niece's presence at Hopkins.[38]

Although public opinion made Lilian Welsh and Mary Sherwood feel "a class apart," Welsh recalled that

> we never had any reason to complain of the treatment we received from our male colleagues. Those whom we knew were uniformly courteous and friendly and helpful in a professional way. . . . The Hopkins laboratories and clinics were a medical Mecca for both men and women physicians throughout the United States. Dr. Osler, Dr. Welsh [*sic*], Dr. Kelly, Dr. Halstead [*sic*] and Dr. Hurd saw to it that the women who came found their way to Dr. Sherwood and me. These women invariably told us that they found nowhere else conditions so favorable for the study of medical science and for stimulating interest in medico-social problems.[39]

The Medical Students

Fear that the medical school would not attract a sufficient number of students led President Gilman and the faculty to seek applicants of both sexes. In the spring of 1893, they visited the Woman's College of Baltimore, whose president, John Franklin Goucher, had indicated his "hearty approval" of the trustees' decision to admit women. He was receiving numerous inquiries from women who wanted to prepare themselves to enter the new medical school, Goucher wrote, and he proposed to offer the prescribed work at the required standard.[40] The result of the Hopkins committee's visit was a mutually beneficial agreement. A memorandum printed in the Woman's College catalog assured students graduating from the college of admission to the Johns Hopkins University School of Medicine after they had completed the courses in French, German, physics, chemistry, and biology. Furthermore, "ladies from a distance who may not be quite prepared for admission to the Johns Hopkins Medical School" could study those subjects at the Woman's College.[41]

The first three women students at Hopkins—Mabel S. Glover, Cornelia O. Church, and Mary S. Packard—had bachelor's degrees from Wellesley, Smith, and Vassar, respectively. Glover dropped out after the first year to marry Franklin P. Mall, the professor of anatomy. Two years later Church left, after becoming a Christian Scientist—a conversion she attributed to Osler, whose methods of treatment reminded her of Mary Baker Eddy's.[42] Packard graduated in 1897 and then became one of the first group of medical interns at the Johns Hopkins Hospital. "There is a little feeling about Miss Packard, but fortunately she behaves sensibly and I think it will disappear," wrote Henry M. Hurd, the hospital's superintendent, to Howard A. Kelly.[43] After her internship, Packard spent two years as physician to a college settlement house and a year as a pathologist at a hospital in Boston. Packard, who did not marry, practiced medicine for the next decade and then retired, perhaps to care for the child she had adopted.[44]

Although the next seven years were a time of progress for women at the new medical school (by 1900, fourteen of forty-three graduates were women), the number of women at Hopkins soon began to decline, and the percentage of women graduating in 1900 was not equaled again until 1983. Nationwide, the number of women in medical schools also declined; except for an increase during World War I, the number of women graduating from medical schools remained relatively small until the mid-1940s.[45] The reasons are unclear. Some historians have interpreted the decrease as a byproduct of the Flexner Report of 1910, which led to a reduction in the number of medical schools and thus to the total number of places available for students nationwide.[46] Others, including Flexner himself, noted a drop in the number of female medical students before his report was published.[47] Some identify as the cause of the decrease a wave of antifeminism that was sweeping the nation's medical schools.[48] Paradoxically, another cause may have been the passage of the Nineteenth Amendment in 1920, which gave women the right to vote and which reassured many of them that emancipation was a *fait accompli*.[49]

It is ironic that another cause of the decline was the opening of the Johns Hopkins medical school to women. The standards set by Hopkins were expensive to meet. By 1903, fourteen of the seventeen women's medical colleges had closed, unable to keep up with the increasing costs of medical education in the new scientific age. Of the seventeen women's medical colleges in existence before the Johns Hopkins University School of Medicine opened, only the Woman's Medical College of Pennsylvania survived past the second decade of the twentieth century. (The Women's Medical College of Baltimore closed its doors in 1910.)

Few women regretted the demise of the single-sex school at the time, as even most female medical educators looked upon the women's schools as temporary expedients, useful only until coeducation would prevail. Supporters of the women's schools were excited and hopeful about opportunities at excellent coeducational institutions like Hopkins. These opportunities did not materialize on a large scale, however, and the end of the women's medical colleges left even fewer opportunities for women than before.[50]

Hopkins itself mirrored the national trend, as the percentage of women students gradually decreased from 1900 until the first World War. The Hopkins medical school nevertheless almost always graduated more women than the national norm. Women represented only 4 percent of medical school graduates in the United States in 1905, a figure that dropped to 2.6 percent in both 1910 and 1915.[51] At Hopkins, however, the average percentage of women graduates between 1905 and 1915 was 7.5, and in only one year (1908) was the percentage of female Hopkins graduates below the national average.

A small surge in the number of women medical graduates nationwide during and after World War I (to 5.4 percent in 1926) made women less of a rarity during the 1920s.[52] This trend was exaggerated at Hopkins, where women represented an average of 15 percent of each graduating class from 1919 to 1926.

The passage of the Nineteenth Amendment had thrown the issue of women's rights into relief, and during the 1920s both men and women struggled to adjust to the new balance of power. At Hopkins, the women's male colleagues were unhappy with them, J. Whitridge Williams said, because "the women insist upon all the rights of men and still demand the privileges accorded to women under the old regime."[53] Yet, as Lilian Welsh pointed out, the prevailing attitude toward women had changed since the 1890s: "The word lady has largely disappeared from our vocabulary as a designation for young women, and no one assumes today that there must be some peculiar underlying reason for a young woman choosing a professional or business career as an outlet for her energies."[54]

The early women graduates were "wonderful role models" in some ways, recalled a graduate of the Class of 1950. "We used to have biennial teas for the alumnae at 800 North Broadway when I was a student, and I used to laugh—although not without respect—to see these substantial women talking in their brisk and forthright way. I was amused, but I was also impressed."[55] Other students could not reconcile the early graduates' achievements with the price some had to pay. A graduate of the Class of 1922 remembered Florence Sabin as a superb teacher and lecturer, but

she had apparently sacrificed all of her personal social relationships for her work, and for her it had apparently been a completely satisfying life. My ideas were different. I felt, and still feel, that a woman in any profession should, of course, try to do her best and achieve her ambitions, but to me the woman comes first and the profession second. Dr. Sabin was a great feminist and had experienced the difficult struggle which was common to all women in the medical field at that time. This, of course, colored her attitude. She cared nothing for dress or personal appearance. She seemed remote in her relationships and always appeared a little impatient, as though she were wasting time unless she was working.[56]

One of these "substantial women," a classmate of Sabin, was Dorothy Mabel Reed. Reed's classmates at Smith College had characterized her as "brilliant" and "forceful," and when she was given the part of queen of the Amazons in the class play, her contemporaries applauded the choice.[57] Reed herself, however, believed that her years at Hopkins gave her "an independence, even an arrogance, which was foreign to my original nature. I was distinctly not such a 'nice' person, but a stronger one, after Johns Hopkins."[58]

An example of the problems Reed experienced as a medical student was this encounter with a lecturer in laryngology, who spent an hour comparing the cavernous tissue present in the nasal passages with the corpus spongiosa of the penis:

We [Reed and the only other woman present] sat just opposite the speaker and the chairman, so that the flushed, bestial face of Dr. MacKenzie, his sly pleasure in making his nasty point, and I imagine the added fillip of doing his dirt before two young women, was evident. I knew that we could not go out—not only should not, but I doubted that I could make the distance to the door without faltering. . . . I cried all the way home—hysterically. . . .[59]

Although social censure of women physicians was relaxed after World War I, pre- and postwar women came to medicine from similar backgrounds. Lilian Welsh described herself and Mary Sherwood as "two ordinary women who had looked forward from early girlhood to the possibility of self-support, who had gone into teaching because it was the only profession with any intellectual outlook which promised self-support and who had, following our intellectual bent, gone into medicine because we were interested in science and in human nature."[60] Like Welsh and Sherwood, many women entered medical school some years after receiving the bachelor's degree, and the relatively advanced age of women medical students represented a national trend until World War II.[61]

Women delayed their entrance into medical school for a variety of reasons. Some women undertook graduate study in the basic sciences after college, and some taught at the high-school or university level. Some women worked after college as laboratory assistants—a choice that persists to this day. Jobs in Hopkins laboratories were particularly prized. Looking back to the early days of the Johns Hopkins Hospital, Lilian Welsh wrote, "When one considers the profound influence made upon the lives and work of the men who had the privilege of those early associations of the Hopkins Hospital in its pre-medical-school days, one can easily understand how a woman with education, understanding and ideals was willing to make any personal sacrifice to enjoy the opportunities to be found at that time in no other medical atmosphere in the world."[62] Some sixty-five years later, a member of the Class of 1959 echoed Welch's feelings, as she remembered the years spent in a Hopkins laboratory before entering medical school.[63] Often prospective students had to overcome opposition from parents who felt that a medical career was too demanding for a woman. The father of one member of the Class of 1923 hoped that a year of teaching physics would dissuade her from coming to Hopkins, but after that year, "my father said that since I was still interested, I could go to medical school."[64]

From 1920 to 1945, the proportion of women medical school graduates in the United States ranged between 4 and 6 percent;[65] but during the same period, women averaged 12 percent of the graduating classes at Hopkins—despite Hopkins' decision in 1921 to limit the size of its entering class rather than to admit all qualified applicants.

The increased number of women and the relatively relaxed social attitude alluded to earlier may have encouraged a particular self-perception among the women medical students of Hopkins' first half-century. "We thought we could do anything," said a member of the Class of 1930. "The women in my class came from good women's colleges and I think that had something to do with our self-confidence, too. Also, we were older, more experienced—some of us had taught after finishing college, or done other kinds of graduate work. We knew what we wanted. The faculty had

softened up by then, too."[66] Most women medical students during these years were also graduates of women's colleges, and the combination of relatively advanced age and a particular type of educational experience may have produced women who entered medical school with feelings of eagerness and freedom rather than apprehension.[67]

These women were undaunted by the more hardened faculty members. Even in classes taught by unsympathetic professors, the women didn't sit together but spread out over the classroom. Confidence thus came largely from the individual, not from membership in a group. There was nevertheless great camaraderie among the women, all of whom, like their male counterparts at the time, were unmarried. Friendships also extended to house officers and young faculty: one graduate, then teaching pediatrics, recalled a camping trip with two students taking an elective in her field, who had planned the trip and invited her along.[68]

This feeling of fellowship continued through World War II, when the proportion of women in medical school increased, both nationwide and at Hopkins.[69] The seventy-five students who entered as the Class of 1950 included nineteen women, one of whom recalled the collegiality of women students that smoothed the way for her:

The men had to struggle along by themselves when they came to Baltimore—finding a room, finding places to eat—but the women could live at 800 North Broadway or nearby and had a ready-made network of people who could show them the ropes.

It wasn't just the large number of women that made it so easy to be a woman medical student here. It was the whole Hopkins tradition. Women weren't a novelty—they had been around so long that they were just accepted at face value.

When I was applying to medical school, I never even considered Harvard. It had only its second class of women medical students, and I wasn't going to fight a battle of the sexes. I just wanted to study medicine.[70]

A decline in the number of women medical students followed the post–World War II increase.[71] At Hopkins, between 1951 and 1973, women accounted for an average of 8 percent of medical students. At the time, women in the professions were often denigrated, and because of so-cial pressure, some women hesitated to commit themselves to medicine. One Hopkins graduate recalled her reluctance to apply to medical school:

> After having spent five years in close association with the medical profession, and an equally long time trying to convince myself that I wouldn't be a good physician, I gave in! The role of women in the professions is a much disputed one, and I lacked the conviction that I could play the dual role of woman and physician as well. When, at last, I gained the maturity necessary to see that I would be able to do so, or at least to try my best, I applied to the Johns Hopkins and was accepted.[72]

During the early 1960s, the perception of a nationwide dearth of physicians caused attention to be focused on women as a group that could fill the gap.[73] An article in the *New York Times* in 1961 reflected the national attitude: in light of the shortage of physicians, it said, women should be encouraged to go to medical school.[74]

It was not until the mid-1970s, however, with the recurrent rise of the feminist movement, that the national percentages caught up with Hopkins' production of women physicians.[75] By then, a kind of complacency had set in at Hopkins. Faculty and administration did not realize that Hopkins was lagging behind other medical schools—some of which had begun only recently to accept women students—in the number of applications received from women. The lag was only temporary, however. From 1975 to 1984, women represented between 16 and 32 percent of medical school graduates, both at Hopkins and nationwide, and the percentage has continued to rise.

Dropping Out

Pressure on women to terminate their medical studies has come from different sources during different decades. Custom rather than formal pro-hibition kept all medical students at Hopkins—men and women—unmarried until the 1920s. House officers at Hopkins were not permitted to marry, however, so that a married medical stu-dent would not have been able to apply for a

Hopkins internship. Not until 1923 was this rule rescinded.

For women in particular, the choice between spouse and career was often agonizing. "[You will] apparently abandon all for me," wrote Franklin P. Mall to his beloved "Mablets." "Why should you not go through a thinking stage; one moment su-premely happy, and the next angry at yourself for abandoning all your ambition."[76]

Yet new privileges created new problems for women medical students. After the passage of the Nineteenth Amendment in 1920, the central issue was the need to balance professional, political, or other activities with marriage and family. Many women who were attracted to medicine ruled out a career as a doctor because the work appeared too strenuous and inflexible to combine with per-sonal responsibilities.[77] Those who entered med-ical school, however, tended to cope. In a group of 121 women who attended Hopkins from 1948 through 1964, 40.5 percent married before or dur-ing medical school, and most of these graduated from medical school and began their careers.[78]

Across the country, attrition among medical students has fluctuated significantly since 1920. Nationwide, between 1949 and 1958, 8 percent of men and 16 percent of women medical students left school without graduating.[79] At Hopkins, a smaller but proportional number of male and female medical students dropped out during those years.

Nationwide, more students left for academic than for nonacademic reasons, although these reasons were often intertwined. A similar propor-tion of men and women left because of academic failure, but nonacademic problems were the cause of attrition in significantly more women than men.[80] At Hopkins, women were more likely to leave for personal and family reasons than for academic ones. Yet because the numbers of women at Hopkins were relatively small in the 1950s, the percentages represent few individuals. Indeed, the attrition rate at Hopkins has always been so low that the medical school has not kept statistics on attrition. A comparison of men and women in eighty-five consecutive classes at Hop-kins shows that 97 percent of male students and

94 percent of female students graduated. When the number of men and women in each entering class is compared with the respective number in the graduating class four years later, the difference in the two attrition rates is not statistically significant.

One of Hopkins' most celebrated dropouts was Gertrude Stein, whose ambivalence about medical school culminated in her departure in June of her senior year. Stein successfully completed her first two years at Hopkins, but the clinical years of medical school she found "boring." By the last semester of the fourth year, her academic standing was tenuous. She was failing four courses: laryngology and otology, ophthalmology, dermatology, and obstetrics. In June 1901, on the recommendation of William Osler, the Advisory Board decided not to allow Stein to graduate.

J. Whitridge Williams, the professor of obstetrics, had voted to deny her the medical degree, but Franklin P. Mall wanted to give her another chance, and he persuaded the board to allow Stein to salvage her degree. He gave her a problem similar to one Florence Sabin had completed successfully in her fourth year. Stein worked for several weeks on the project, which involved the sectioning and reconstruction of a human embryo brain. Her results perplexed Mall. He took them to Sabin, saying, "Either I am crazy or Miss Stein is. Will you see what you can make out of her work?" Sabin concluded that Stein must have embedded the cord when it was turned back under the embryo brain instead of extended from it. So flawed was Stein's model that Mall threw it in the wastebasket. When Stein was refused her degree, she left for Europe.[81]

Stein's failure remains a paradox. Florence Sabin thought that she had no flair for science. Dorothy Reed found her clumsy, untidy, careless, and "very irritating in her attitude of intellectual superiority." Stein was intelligent enough to have completed her four years of medical school and her remedial project successfully, had she wished, but other pressures besides "boredom" may have led to her departure. A passionate attachment to another woman caused Stein great emotional turmoil during her fourth year of medical school, and during that same year, her beloved brother, Leo, decided to abandon his graduate studies at the university and leave Baltimore. In later years, she wrote of her "gratitude" for having been forced to leave Hopkins, as she felt that the study of medicine was not equal to her talents.[82]

Other students left for reasons as varied as their personalities. Some entered other professions; some married and became housewives; some married and completed medical school elsewhere. A special category comprises the students who dropped in again. One member of the Class of 1907 began her medical studies at Hopkins in 1900; particularly in the early 1900s, some students simply took longer than four years to graduate.

After Graduation

Until the 1970s, opportunities were relatively scarce for the new women physicians once they left the Hopkins nest. Indeed, even the original members of the Women's Fund Committee did not intend that the school's female graduates take their place beside men in the professional world. The chairwoman of the Baltimore Committee of the Women's Fund wrote to the Board of Trustees, "There is little doubt that a sufficient number of women ought to be educated and trained in such manner as to be fully able to care for sick women who may wish or ought to be treated by women. We have devoted ourselves to the furtherance of this object."[83] The trustees responded:

This board is satisfied that in hospital practice among women, in penal institutions in which women are prisoners, in charitable institutions in which women are cared for, and in private life when women are to be attended, there is a need and place for learned and capable women physicians, and that it is the business and duty of this board, when it is supplied with the necessary means for opening its proposed medical school, to make provision for the training and full qualification of such women for the abundant work which awaits them in these wide fields of usefulness.[84]

Even M. Carey Thomas saw these constraints as progress, characterizing the board's "cordial words of acceptance" as "especially significant, in that there is as yet no legal provision made for women physicians in the asylums and penitentiaries of Maryland."[85] (A minority opinion came from James Cardinal Gibbons, who believed that female physicians should have the same right as female nurses to care for male patients.)[86]

University positions for women were particularly scarce. Of the 302 medical appointments and residencies—government, municipal, and hospital—open to women physicians in the United States in 1901, fewer than three dozen were located in university-affiliated or private hospitals.[87] Facilities for women and children, state hospitals for the insane, women's departments of prisons, and homes for "incurables" or, specifically, tuberculous patients provided the rest of the opportunities available to women medical school graduates at the turn of the century.[88]

At Hopkins, the first attempt to place women physicians in a residency at the hospital was sabotaged from within. The Baltimore Women's Fund Committee put forth two candidates, Drs. Alice Hall and Mary Sherwood, and pressured faculty and administration to appoint them as residents. Osler gave Sherwood a place, and Kelly accepted Hall on his staff; their appointments were to begin in the fall of 1891. During the summer, however, Hall announced her marriage—thus relinquishing her residency (because house officers were not allowed to marry) and disqualifying Sherwood (because hospital authorities would not sanction the appointment of only one woman). Sherwood was bitterly disappointed, and the members of the Women's Fund Committee were furious.[89]

House officers were necessarily taken from other institutions until 1897. Once Hopkins students were available, the first choice of internship was offered to the Hopkins graduate with the best academic record, the second choice to the next on the list, and so forth. In 1900, neither of the top two graduates, both men, chose to undertake a medical internship at Hopkins, leaving two of the four places open for the next two graduates—Florence R. Sabin and Dorothy M. Reed. They be-

came the first pair of women to choose Hopkins internships in medicine, but they had to struggle to obtain the posts. If both interns were women, one would have to work on the "colored wards" with both men and women, and this seemed "unwise" to Hurd and the other members of the selection committee. The committee in charge tried to force one woman or the other to relinquish her post, but after Reed protested, both women were allowed to take the internships.[90]

Many women graduates stayed on to train at Hopkins, in straight or rotating internships in medicine, pediatrics, psychiatry, or gynecology and obstetrics. The Department of Surgery, however, did not accept a female intern until 1947, when Hopkins graduate Rowena Spencer persuaded Alfred Blalock to give her a place.[91] Shortages of qualified physicians during both world wars permitted some women to move into positions previously reserved for well-trained men. Some department heads were also known for their willingness to accept women interns. In the 1930s, for example, the Hopkins department of pediatrics had an unusually large number of female house officers, in part because department head Edwards A. Park was known to be sympathetic to the idea of women doctors.

Although there were plenty of women in internships, residencies were much harder for them to obtain, even at Hopkins. "The department head with the courage to keep a woman intern on, he was a rare bird indeed!" recalled one member of the Class of 1925.[92] Several department heads told women straightforwardly that they could not advance beyond internship or assistant residency.[93]

Women took one or two of the dozen available training positions at Hopkins annually until 1912. During the next forty years, the number of positions available for interns, residents, and fellows rose to more than 70, but women accounted for no more than 17 percent, and often the percentage was much smaller. (With one-quarter of the faculty in the army during World War I, the proportion of women doubled; however, the percentage declined to prewar levels—as did the percentage of women medical students, interns, and residents—when the men returned.) The number of postgraduate positions rose substantially between the mid-1950s and the mid-1980s, but the number of women occupying those positions did not rise until the 1980s. Of 209 positions at Hopkins in 1954–55, only 6 percent were filled by women, but in 1985–86, women occupied 21 percent of the 1,161 available places.

What careers, if any, did women pursue when they had finished their training? A common choice during the early twentieth century was a missionary career.[94] Later, pediatrics was the most popular specialty for women nationwide, followed by psychiatry.[95] At Hopkins, in contrast, almost twice as many women graduates between 1948 and 1958 chose internal medicine as chose either pediatrics or psychiatry.[96] Most women went into clinical practice, in part because academic positions were difficult for women to obtain. Women married to physicians with academic appointments had a particularly difficult time, as rules against hiring both spouses eliminated the wives from consideration.

Most women graduates did practice medicine: nationwide studies from the 1960s showed that more than 91 percent of women physicians had part-time or full-time careers, and a Hopkins survey of women graduates from 1897 to 1948 produced a comparable figure.[97] Of the Hopkins graduates, 331 had worked or were working full-time; 38 abandoned medicine after internship; 9 worked part-time; 8 died or became chronically ill shortly after graduation; 4 retired after a few years of practice; and the remaining 4 were unaccounted for.[98] A later study revealed that more than 23 percent of the Hopkins women graduates between 1948 and 1958 were in academic or research medicine, as compared with 10 percent of the women in a national survey.[99]

On the Hopkins faculty, women were not prominently represented until the 1980s. Elizabeth Hurdon, assistant in gynecology, was the sole woman faculty member from 1898 to 1903, when she was joined by Florence R. Sabin as assistant in anatomy. Until World War I, only 6 percent of the Hopkins faculty were women, clustered in the lowest positions. In 1917, Sabin became the first female full professor at the medical school—but her colleague George W. Corner stated in print that she was denied the directorship of her department because she was a woman.[100] A second female full professor was not appointed until 1959, when Helen B. Taussig was promoted to professor of pediatrics. Hopkins has been criticized for failing to promote Helen Taussig to a full professorship until relatively late in her career, but promotions to the highest academic level were rare for men as well as women. Until the 1950s, with few exceptions (Florence Sabin being one), Hopkins policy permitted only the department head to hold the rank of full professor.

The size of the entire faculty more than doubled between 1959 and 1972, and by 1965 the representation of women on the faculty had crept up to 14 percent. During the 1970s, three women were promoted to full professor in clinical departments. The basic sciences remained without a female full professor until 1980, when Teruko Ishizaka became the first since Florence Sabin. By 1985, the wave of women medical students encouraged by the women's movement and federal legislation in the 1970s had reached the Hopkins faculty: only 9 of 161 full professors but 17 percent of the total faculty at the medical school were women.

Notable Women Graduates

Two of the most eminent women graduates of the School of Medicine were members of the Class of 1900: Florence Rena Sabin and Dorothy Mabel Reed.

During her medical internship at Hopkins, Sabin found that she preferred research and teaching to clinical practice. Franklin P. Mall, director of the Department of Anatomy, arranged for the Women's Fund Committee to provide a fellowship for Sabin, and within four years, she had received the prize of the Naples Table Association, had published a classic series of papers on the development of the lymphatic system, and had been promoted to associate professor of anatomy (see chapter 11).

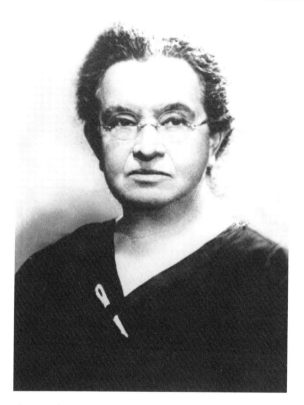

Florence R. Sabin. (*Source:* Alan M. Chesney Medical Archives, The Johns Hopkins Medical Institutions.)

Of her research, Mall wrote: "I think Miss Sabin's discovery regarding the growth of lymphatics is one of the greatest importance, for it allows us to separate most distinctly lymph spaces from tissue spaces. It is an extremely small point, but it has caused an immense amount of trouble for the past two hundred years."[101] Nor did George R. Minot regard Sabin's finding as trifling: in 1913, he included it in his list of the five most significant developments in biology in the preceding quarter century.[102]

As department head and as Sabin's mentor, Mall must have sponsored her promotion in the spring of 1917. She was appointed full professor of histology on June 5, 1917, becoming one of the few full professors at Hopkins who was not head of a department. The date on which the university trustees approved her appointment is crucial, because the promotion has at times been characterized as a consolation prize given to Sabin instead of the anatomy department's directorship.

In fact, the director was alive and well until six months after Sabin's promotion: Franklin P. Mall died suddenly on November 17, 1917, following an operation for gallstones. Hopkins cannot be criticized, therefore, for having discriminatory intentions in its appointment of Sabin as full professor.

Sabin was not, however, considered as a potential replacement for Mall after his death, even when eighteen months of negotiations between the search committee and Ross G. Harrison fell through. She was saddened when the post was eventually given to one of her students, Lewis H. Weed, and privately criticized the choice. She nevertheless remained at Hopkins until 1925, when, at the age of fifty-four, she took a post at the Rockefeller Institute.[103] The reasons for Sabin's decision to leave Hopkins remain unclear. Six years elapsed between Weed's appointment as director and Sabin's departure—a long time for as eminent a scientist as Sabin to remain in an unsatisfying position. Perhaps the most pressing reason for her move to the Rockefeller Institute was a purely professional one: at the Rockefeller Institute, Sabin was able to spend her time on pure research, unburdened by teaching.[104] Her interest in tuberculosis continued after her retirement, when she returned to Colorado, her home state, and became a prominent reformer of the public health laws. Sabin was the first woman to become a member of the National Academy of Sciences, president of the American Association of Anatomists, and full member of the Rockefeller Institute for Medical Research.[105]

Dorothy M. Reed's most significant contribution was a detailed description of what are now known as Reed-Sternberg cells, a discovery made in Welch's laboratory during a pathology fellowship only two years after her graduation from medical school. Although these cells had been recognized some twenty-five years earlier, it was Reed who described them accurately and linked them with Hodgkin's disease. The studies of Florence Sabin on the development of the lymphatic glands helped Reed to interpret her findings, a key element of which was the description of microscopic changes. A striking feature of Reed's

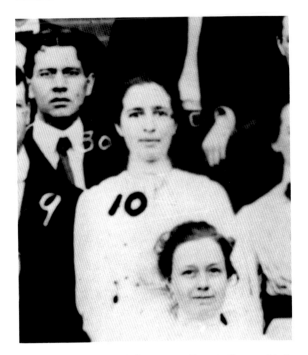

Dorothy Reed Mendenhall. (*Source:* Alan M. Chesney Medical Archives, The Johns Hopkins Medical Institutions.)

specimens was the presence of "giant cells"; they were usually free in the interstices of the tissue but were occasionally seen in the reticulum, and characterized by irregular protoplasmic processes. These cells occurred in great numbers in the large lymph sinuses of the node and occasionally appeared in the blood vessels.

Reed's pathology fellowship was followed by a three-year residency at Babies Hospital in New York. In 1906, she married Charles E. Mendenhall (a physics professor at the University of Wisconsin), moved to Madison, and retired from the practice of medicine for the next nine years. When her children were in school, Reed did not return to the laboratory but chose instead to study infant mortality. She worked through the new United States Children's Bureau, attempting to reduce the death rate of mothers and infants at childbirth, and her "weighing and measuring test" was used nationwide as a guideline for identifying healthy babies. It is generally agreed, however, that she did her best work early in her career.[106]

Another preclinical scientist was Gladys Rowena Henry Dick (Class of 1907), who with her husband made important contributions to the prevention and treatment of scarlet fever. The Dicks were responsible for the human-inoculation experiments proving that a streptococcus causes the disease, and their observations on soluble toxins in scarlet fever were also of fundamental importance. It was the Dicks who first prepared a usable "toxin" from filtrates of cultures of streptococci obtained from patients with scarlet fever. They showed that an intracutaneous injection of this filtrate practically never produced a skin reaction in people convalescing from scarlet fever or with a history of a previous attack, whereas persons who had no previous history of scarlet fever had a positive reaction. This was the basis of the Dick test.[107]

An account of the achievements of Hopkins women could become an unmanageably extensive roll call of awards, publications, and titles. More than thirty Hopkins women have become full professors at medical schools nationwide, and the professional accomplishments of women graduates have spanned all of medicine.[108] For example, one of the first physicians to investigate the sexuality of women was Clelia Duel Mosher (Class of 1900). Esther Rosencrantz (Class of 1904), an associate professor at the University of California Medical School, was a specialist in the treatment of tuberculosis and a member of the Red Cross Tuberculosis Commission during World War I; for her work on the commission she was decorated by the American and Italian governments.

Notable contributions to the understanding of experimental syphilis, the chemotherapy of African sleeping sickness, and the genetic constitution of rabbits were made by Louise Pearce (Class of 1912), who joined the staff of the Rockefeller Institute after her internship at Hopkins. Esther Loring Richards (Class of 1915) became psychiatrist-in-chief of the Psychopathology Division at the Baltimore City Hospitals. Ruth E. Fairbank (Class of 1916) was a psychiatrist and professor of hygiene at Mount Holyoke College; her classmate Edith Maas Lincoln was head of the children's chest clinic at Bellevue Hospital Center and a pioneer in the use of streptomycin, promizole, and isoniazid in the treatment of tuberculosis. Martha

M. Eliot (Class of 1918), a pediatrician, was the first woman president of the American Public Health Association and associate director of the World Health Organization. Ella Oppenheimer, also a 1918 graduate, was director of the Maternity and Infancy Division of the United States Public Health Service. Ella Oppenheimer Miller (no relation), Class of 1924, was one of the first pathologists in the country to specialize in pediatric pathology. A long-time member of the Department of Pathology at Hopkins, she was known as a superb teacher and was recognized for her research on cystic fibrosis. A pioneer investigator in the inheritance of disease was Madge Thurlow Macklin, a graduate of the Class of 1919.

A graduate of the Class of 1925, Harriet G. Guild was a recipient of the Elizabeth Blackwell Award for her work on pediatric nephrosis and kidney disease. Helen B. Taussig, a 1927 graduate, was best known for her part in developing the Blalock-Taussig procedure for the treatment of congenital heart disease (see chapter 11). Sarah S. Tower Howe (Class of 1928) taught in the Department of Anatomy before becoming a psychiatrist and psychoanalyst at Hopkins.

Graduates of the Class of 1930 included Car-

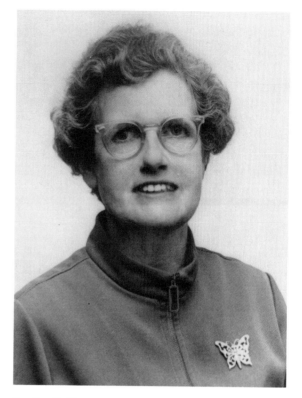

Caroline B. Thomas

oline Bedell Thomas, who pioneered the use of sulfanilamide to prevent recurrences of acute rheumatic fever, for which she received the James D. Bruce Memorial Award in Preventive Medicine from the American College of Physicians. Later, her work in preventive medicine concentrated on identifying the precursors of hypertension and coronary artery disease through long-term observations of Hopkins medical students and physicians. Hattie E. Alexander developed a serum for the treatment of infants with influenzal meningitis.

Others in the Class of 1930 were Ann G. Kuttner, associate professor of pediatrics at New York University, known for her research on streptococci and rheumatic fever; and Miriam E. Brailey, who obtained a doctorate in public health at Hopkins; taught in the Department of Pediatrics at the Johns Hopkins medical school; and served as director of the Bureau of Tuberculosis of the Baltimore City Health Department until 1950, when she was fired for refusing to sign a loyalty

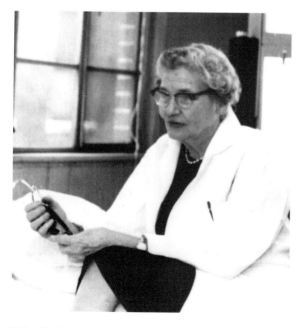

Helen B. Taussig

oath. (The Society of Friends, of which she was a member, forbade the taking of oaths). Hopkins nevertheless retained her on the faculty for the next nine years, until she left to join a religious community.

The Class of 1936 included Georgeanna Seegar Jones, who has broken new ground in the treatment of infertility; Anne M. Bahlke, who investigated the use of gamma globulin in poliomyelitis and the epidemiology of pneumococcal pneumonia; and Dorothea Cross Leighton, a psychiatrist who, with Clyde Kluckhohn, studied the Navajo Indians. Katherine H. Borkovich (Class of 1939), a cardiologist on the faculty at Hopkins, was the first woman president of the Baltimore City Medical Society.

Jessica H. Lewis (Class of 1942) studied the coagulation and proteolytic enzyme systems of the blood. Julia Tutelman Apter (Class of 1943) became professor of surgery at Rush University in Chicago, with a particular interest in medical engineering, computers in patient care, and mechanical properties of tissues and organs. Graduates from the 1940s contributing to pediatric cardiology were Ruth Whittemore (Class of 1942), who studied the etiology and prevention of congenital heart defects; Mary Allen Engle (Class of 1945), whose particular interest was congenital malformations of the heart and great vessels; and Eugenie F. Doyle (Class of 1946), who concentrated on the treatment of acute rheumatic fever, rheumatic heart disease, and the natural history of congenital heart disease, especially aortic stenosis and the types of congenital cardiovascular defects associated with intrauterine infection with rubella. Janet Jordan Fischer (Class of 1948) has investigated pyelonephritis, bacterial endocarditis, and antibiotic sensitivity testing. Dorothy H. Clark Henneman (Class of 1949) performed clinical investigations of the biochemistry and physiology of metabolism, and of anesthesiology.

Graduates of the School of Medicine during the 1950s included Carol Johnson Johns (Class of 1950), a specialist in sarcoidosis at Hopkins who took a leave of absence to serve as acting president of Wellesley College. Elizabeth Dexter Hay (Class of 1952), professor of anatomy at Harvard and a

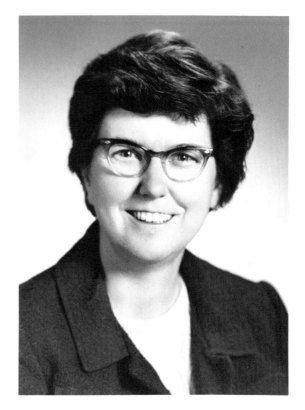

Mary Ellen Avery

member of the National Academy of Sciences, is known for her research on hormones in regeneration; on autoradiographic studies of protein and nucleic acid synthesis in embryos; on the fine structure of developing muscle, cartilage, skin, and eye; and on collagen synthesis by epithelium and embryonic induction. Classmate Patricia A. McIntyre specializes in hematology and nuclear medicine. Mary Ellen Avery (also a member of the Class of 1952), became the first woman chief of pediatrics at Harvard and physician-in-chief at the Children's Hospital Medical Center in Boston. In her studies of hyaline membrane disease, she and her co-workers discovered the source of lung surfactant and found that steroids accelerate surfactant production. Genevieve Murray Matanoski (Class of 1955) has studied the epidemiology of streptococcal infections, the risks of occupational exposure to radiation, and the etiology of oral cancer. Mary Betty Stevens, also a 1955 graduate, served as the director of the Connective Tissue

Division at Hopkins and is a full professor of medicine.

Buildings and Solidarity

Despite Gilman's insistence that faculty were more important than the structures that housed them, buildings at Hopkins have played an important part in the history of women at the medical institutions. Mary Garrett and M. Carey Thomas considered bricks and mortar an extension of their influence. They feared that what they had accomplished would be lost, and insisted on physical reminders of their cause. Carefully placed plaques and carefully worded descriptions kept the presence of the Women's Fund Committee alive at Hopkins. Garrett and Thomas' constant threat—during their lifetimes and even afterwards, when the provision was incorporated into Thomas' will—was that if any of several conditions were breached, Bryn Mawr College would supersede Hopkins as the beneficiary of the funds.[109]

The most important of these conditions, not surprisingly, concerned the admission of women to Hopkins. In the letter of transmittal to the trustees that accompanied her gift in 1891, Garrett specified that she would take back her donation if Hopkins treated women unfairly; but Thomas would sometimes convey her displeasure obliquely, as in a 1925 letter to Dean Lewis H. Weed from the president of the John Price Jones Corporation, a company in New York:

> Here is some information that has come to me from a reliable source, quoted almost from the lips of Miss Thomas herself:
> "By the way—inform your Hopkins friends that Bryn Mawr and M. Carry [sic] Thomas in particular believe Hopkins is discriminating against women in admission to the Medical School. This is against a definite stipulation made by Miss Thomas in one of her donations. Miss Thomas is a trustee of Hopkins and holder of the Garret [sic] millions. They are quietly collecting evidence to this fact."
> It is important enough to receive your consideration.[110]

Mary Garrett was more direct, even about trivial matters. She got her way when she insisted that the plaque on the Women's Fund Memorial Building be placed outside, not inside as President Gilman wanted, and when the building was referred to as the "Anatomical Laboratory" in a university circular, she sent Gilman a letter: "I judge that I am correct in inferring from your note that you will at once have a new issue of the Directory printed and sent out and destroy what remains undistributed of the present one?"[111]

To Thomas, buildings were not only memorials, they were also contributions to the solidarity of the group of women medical students and to their individual comfort. After Mary Garrett's death in 1915, Thomas gave the hospital the funds to build the Mary Elizabeth Garrett Memorial Room for the women medical students. The "room" was actually an entire one-story building, attached to the hospital. Thomas maintained it sumptuously: the bookshelves in the main room were filled with leather-bound classics, and bronze sculptures rested on the broad window sills. The walls were covered with grass cloth and the tiled floors with oriental rugs.[112]

Outside the hospital, the medical school administration's laissez-faire policy toward housing left the women on their own in an often unfamiliar city. Like their male colleagues, the first women medical students rented rooms from local families, particularly on Broadway and in Jackson Place. The Women's Medical Association was founded to meet a common need for a suitable eating place.[113] In 1918, alumnae and students raised enough money to rent a house at 410 North Broadway. The seven bedrooms were let to students, and the entire ground floor was used as a dining room by about thirty women. At first, the manager of a teahouse prepared the food, but the next year a second-year student took charge, beginning a tradition of student-run housing that endured until the 1940s.

The arrangement at 410 North Broadway was so successful that in 1920 the group that had convened to rent it became legally incorporated, as "the Women's Association of the Johns Hopkins Medical School." All women medical students automatically became members. There were no dues, as the organization relied upon voluntary contributions.

The association's first formal act was the purchase in 1920 of the house at 800 North Broadway. It contained three full floors and a basement and included eight bedrooms; two bathrooms, one with a tub and one with a shower; a small dining room; and a large living room.[114] Some of the women medical students earned their room and board by cooking and maintaining the house (known by the male medical students as "the Henhouse"). Although the building on North Broadway was legally owned by the student group, support for the residence also came from individual alumnae, from the Women's Fund Committee, and from M. Carey Thomas.

When M. Carey Thomas died in 1935, the residence and the Mary Elizabeth Garrett Room lost an important source of help. A group of women led by Caroline B. Thomas (whose husband was M. Carey Thomas's nephew) decided that the women alumnae, who by then numbered over 200, should assume responsibility for the residence. The alumnae formed the Johns Hopkins Women's Medical Alumnae Association, which over the next forty years paid off the mortgage on the house and assisted with its maintenance. It also established the Florence Rena Sabin and Dorothy Reed Mendenhall scholarship funds for women medical students and helped the hospital with the relocation and redesign of the Mary Elizabeth Garrett Memorial Room. When construction plans in the 1960s called for tearing down the original Garrett Room, the hospital administration questioned the need for a replacement. Various unsatisfactory locations were proposed, but when Caroline Thomas reminded the university administration of the 1916 agreement between M. Carey Thomas and the university that established the original memorial to Mary Garrett in perpetuity, the hospital found an equivalent amount of space for a new Garrett Room.

With the construction of university-owned housing for students, the residence at 800 North Broadway difficult to maintain and somewhat superfluous. The alumnae association arranged for its sale in 1957 when Reed Hall, the student residence named after Lowell J. Reed, was completed. The following year, for tax purposes, student and alumnae organizations merged.[115]

The Women's Medical Alumnae Association now collects biennial contributions, keeps alumnae informed about one another, and continues to maintain its scholarship funds. Since women are part of all professional activities at Hopkins, the alumnae association is more charitable and collegial than educational. It has also absorbed the informal functions of the Women's Advisory Committee, a group of six women formed in response to another of Mary Garrett's original stipulations to the trustees. This group was intended both to advise the women students about lodging and other practical matters, and to advise the medical school about the character of applicants and other nonacademic disciplinary issues. The committee is listed in the medical school's circular to this day, in accordance with the provisions of Mary Garrett's original donation, but it was never a powerful influence on either the students or the administration.

The strength of the committee's relations to the medical students has varied. In the 1970s, at the height of the feminist movement, some students wanted to turn it into a political and educational organization, but that attitude has now faded. In the 1980s, women students are so numerous that many do not feel the need to participate in a separate group based on gender.

Means and Ends

The history of women at the Johns Hopkins University School of Medicine reflects the institution's independence as well as its response to prevailing ideas of the past century. As consequential as its opening was for the history of American medicine, its willingness to admit women on the same terms as men was, in the words of one historian, "an even more crucial event for the history of women in the profession."[116] The university's decision to admit women to its medical school was also the beginning of an institutional tradition.

Like the school's policies toward other aspects of medicine, the expression of this tradition has been altered over the years by social change.

In their response to the idea of women physicians, Americans reflected the particular prejudices of their day. Objections over the years have included the fear that women would take jobs away from men;[117] women's purported physical, mental, and emotional defects;[118] the traditional view of women's domestic obligations; and the dreaded possibility of "feminization," a term connoting the antithesis of all that leads to achievement in a field.[119] Behind these reasons, said feminist historians of the 1970s, are a fear of female sexuality, the perception of a threat to the traditional masculine role, and a backlash against the reforms prompted by the women's rights movement itself.[120] To counter this opposition, women have used a variety of tactics to achieve equal opportunity at all levels of the profession.

While their goal has remained unchanged through the decades, the best means of attaining it has often been in dispute. Women's efforts to achieve equality of opportunity have been, in the words of one historian, "riddled with tension between separatism and assimilation, femininity and professionalism."[121] Women have been forced to decide whether to band together or blend in, and supporters of schools for women continue to disagree with advocates of coeducation about the relative benefits of each.

Similarly, some awards have been endowed solely for women. The Stetler Research Fund for Women Physicians, for example, was established by Pearl M. Stetler, a 1913 graduate of the Johns Hopkins University School of Medicine. Finding a career in research closed to her, she became a surgeon, practicing in Chicago for almost fifty years. Through her will, she has given other women the opportunity that was denied to her. Her fund supports six or seven postdoctoral fellowships for women each year, at three medical schools: the Universities of Illinois and Wisconsin, and Johns Hopkins.

The benefits of separatism and assimilation are not always clear. What some see as assistance, others interpret as paternalism. Mary Garrett's creation of the Women's Advisory Committee, which was intended to reinforce the presence of women at the medical school, brought a strong protest from the Boston and Salem women's fund-raising committees, which feared that "conditions . . . which permit extra-academic surveillance of the women" would be "ruinous to the School."[122]

Progress was thus hampered not only by outside forces but also by the attitude of the women themselves. The attitude of male physicians, which was the attitude of the larger society, placed women physicians at the margin of their profession, and this attitude was both resisted and internalized by women doctors themselves.[123] The tension has persisted through the past century, as prejudice and discrimination have often turned apparent progress into something more superficial than real.[124] The most striking example is the passage of the Nineteenth Amendment, which failed to eliminate the roadblocks to equality. On the contrary, women lost ground professionally over the next fifty years, as women born in the two decades after 1920 were lulled into believing feminism a concern of the past.[125] The opening of the Johns Hopkins medical school to women, heralded as the beginning of the genuine assimilation of women into the medical profession, led instead to the closing down of other medical schools and a consequent decrease in the total number of places available for women.

Many women, especially successful ones, have believed that advancement is solely the responsibility of the individual. Florence Sabin wrote in 1933, "Concerning the opportunities for women, I do not think that they need consider any longer that opportunities are closed to them in practically any field of endeavor, because with requisite ability, I believe that women can make places for themselves to do the things they most earnestly want to do."[126] The work was the important thing, not the recognition: "Dr. Mall used to say to me humorously as he always put things, Women can get what they want in the way of opportunities to work if they will give up the chance to walk in processions."[127] Even when women obtained that chance, however, academic rank did not guarantee power. Although Sabin was a full professor, she was not part of the voting faculty that shaped the policies of the school.[128]

Advancement for women has come to be seen as a political, not an individual, problem. As one historian summed up, "The continued absence of effective solutions to the private and personal dilemmas of those young women who wished to combine marriage with gainful employment outside the home obscured the fact that the problems they encountered in fulfilling those intentions resulted not from some personal inadequacy, but from a fundamentally inegalitarian social structure which persevered despite the enormously compelling but ultimately cosmetic changes which the 1920s had wrought."[129]

The changes of the 1970s, which brought large numbers of women into medical schools across the nation, appear to be more than cosmetic, although these changes have not eradicated what one woman faculty member called "the classic conflict": the pressure to choose between family and career. When to have children? How to meet one's own professional expectations and those of one's colleagues? Women physicians are still forced to consider the answers not solely as individuals or professionals, but as women. Yet the diversity of their choices provides a spectrum of role models for the next generation, as women physicians now have a wide range of new opportunities to make important contributions to medicine.

As other features of the Johns Hopkins medical school were emulated nationwide, the practice of educating excellent women also spread across the country. The large number of highly educated, highly competent women who populate the nation's medical schools today, as students and as faculty, reflects Hopkins' part in leading the way for the many other schools that now offer an education for women "on the same terms as men."

CHAPTER 7

"LEARNING BY DOING"

What more than anything strikes the student at Baltimore is the atmosphere of activity and ambition in things intellectual. There is no mental laziness nor deadness. The student is treated not as a bucket for the reception of lectures, nor a mill to grind out the due daily grist of prepared text-book for recitation, but as a being in search of truth, which he is to discover for himself, the proper encouragement and advice as to means and methods being furnished by the instructor.

—John Dewey, 1885

The phrase "learning by doing" is most closely associated with John Dewey and his followers, the proponents of "progressive education," whose tenets dominated American schooling in the early 1900s. Yet before Dewey promulgated his educational philosophy, "learning by doing" was a hallmark of the new Johns Hopkins University School of Medicine, a curricular feature that set the school apart from most other medical schools of the time.[1]

The proximate source of the policy at the School of Medicine was the Johns Hopkins University. Its leading proponent was university president Daniel C. Gilman, supporter of so many other bold ideas.[2] Gilman's guiding principle was his intention to make Hopkins the first true university in America, an institution dedicated to "the most liberal promotion of all useful knowledge; the special provision of such departments as are neglected elsewhere in the country . . . the encouragement of research; the promotion of young men; and the advancement of individual scholars, who by their excellence will advance the sciences they pursue and the society where they dwell."[3]

These goals implied a particular method of education: the student would have to seek knowledge rather than passively receive it. When the university was founded in 1876, however, "learning by doing" was simply a method; not until the early twentieth century did it take on the weight of a philosophy. Nor did Gilman define his method with the words "learning by doing"—the idea was simply inherent in his hopes for the new university.

The introduction of "learning by doing" into the Johns Hopkins University was part of Gilman's general enthusiasm for what he called "hand-craft." This he contrasted to "rede-craft," which he defined as "the power to read, to reason, and to think." Both were necessary for progress, Gilman said: rede-craft and hand-craft were not opponents but brothers. Although in 1886 rede-craft held the place of honor at all educational levels, Gilman was hopeful that hand-craft was gaining in importance: "In universities, the highest of all schools, work-rooms, labour-places, laboratories, are appreciated as book-rooms, reading-rooms, libraries; they show that a liberal education means skill in getting and in using knowledge; that wisdom comes from searching books and searching nature; that in the finest human natures the brain and the hand are in close league."[4]

The moment was right for the inauguration of "learning by doing" in the new university. Education seemed to be a solution to the social problems of the Industrial Revolution, and the common assumption was that the values and guides formerly imparted by the family and church, but now lacking in this unstable society, should be supplied by the school. The primary school was, however, unready to assume this responsibility, for the culture that it communicated had become entirely detached from its students' experience—not through forces peculiar to education, but because of the rapid social changes of the time.[5] Americans began to adapt to their own needs the ideas of three European educators—Friedrich Froebel and Johann Friedrich Herbart of Germany, and Johann Heinrich Pestalozzi of Switzerland—and to see education as a process of individual development rather than the inculcation of information.[6]

Accompanying this pressure on the American educational system in the 1870s was the ferment caused by the ideas of Charles Darwin. *On the Origin of Species* had been published in 1859, and Thomas Huxley, one of the best-known teachers of biology in the English-speaking world, was a leading disseminator of Darwin's principles. His course in zoology for prospective elementary school teachers deemphasized formal lectures; students spent much of their time performing dissections and making drawings. Huxley began his course with three assistants; he later took on a fourth, Henry Newell Martin, who brought this method of teaching to the Johns Hopkins University.[7]

So important did Gilman consider Darwin's ideas that he invited Huxley to give the principal address at the opening of the university. Moreover, Martin was only one of several faculty members who shared Gilman's enthusiasm for Darwinism. Gilman had also appointed Granville Stanley Hall, whose explicitly evolutionary theory of psychology had a fundamental effect on

pedagogy, to serve as professor of psychology.[8] At its opening in 1876, therefore, the Johns Hopkins University had acquired a faculty in the forefront of educational reform.[9]

When the Johns Hopkins University School of Medicine opened in 1893, it incorporated the principles Gilman had instituted so successfully in the Faculty of Philosophy seventeen years earlier. Interest in science had risen throughout the nation, and the rapid scientific advances during those seventeen years gave even greater weight to Gilman's idea that students should be taught to create new knowledge, not inculcated with a fixed body of information. In planning the new medical school, John Shaw Billings had also been a key proponent of learning by doing. "An important part of the higher education of modern times," he said, "is the teaching how to increase knowledge; and the best way of teaching this, as of many other things, is by doing it, and by causing the pupils to do it."[10] In both the basic and the clinical sciences, "doing" required the use of all the senses; to "learn by doing," medical students left the lecture halls for the laboratories and wards.[11]

Many of the curricular techniques employed at Hopkins were also used at other American medical schools. Beginning in 1835, for example, ward visits formed part of the instruction at the Harvard Medical School.[12] Furthermore, the method of bedside teaching turned into a routine by Osler and Halsted was already being discussed and probably carried out in other medical schools two decades before the Hopkins medical school opened. Yet Hopkins was the first medical school to make the principle of learning by doing a matter of stated policy and then to carry that policy out. Other schools offered bits and pieces of the method; still others recognized the importance of clinical and laboratory experience but, lacking control of a teaching hospital, were unable to execute it.

At Johns Hopkins, change in the medical school curriculum, and consequently the degree of adherence to the principle of learning by doing, has been cyclical over the past century as new curriculum committees have rediscovered old ideas. Even a century ago, William Henry Welch commented that the rapid growth of scientific information precluded students from digesting all of medical knowledge during the four years of medical school. It was better to teach students how to learn, he said, and how to continue the process of self-education after those four years were over.[13]

"Learning by Doing" in the Laboratory

The first two years of the original curriculum at the Hopkins medical school were occupied by study of the laboratory sciences: anatomy, physiology, and physiological chemistry in the first year; and anatomy, pharmacology, pathology, and bacteriology in the second year. Elsewhere, these subjects had been taught mostly by textbook, a system that Welch termed "very defective."[14] Here was a striking justification for the link between medical school and university, Welch believed, because only in universities, such as Johns Hopkins, did the laboratory sciences receive proper recognition. Welch's method of teaching pathology, revolutionary in the United States, resembled instruction in the other preclinical sciences at Johns Hopkins. It was based on the German model and emphasized the use of the laboratory rather than the traditional lectures and recitation based on texts.

"In the laboratory," Welch said, "the student learns the fundamental importance of accurate observation and experiment, here he finds that only that knowledge is living and stays by him which comes from direct contact with the object of study, and not from being told about it, or reading about it, or merely thinking about it, and here he becomes acquainted with methods and instruments essential for diagnosis, and, therefore, for intelligent treatment of disease."[15] "The medical student must acquire power rather than information," said William T. Porter of Harvard; in the laboratory, the students gained more than mere physiological or anatomical knowledge, they acquired a conceptual tool necessary to order the body of information they needed to master.[16]

Welch was giving the horses water, but he was also concerned with getting them to drink. Arousing the student's interest was so important a part of "learning by doing" that the medical school instituted a system of electives spanning all four years. The curriculum should not be too crowded, Welch said, for the student should be allowed time to read, exercise, and digest knowledge. Instead of filling the students' hours with required subjects, Welch asked: What is the irreducible minimum in a subject without which one cannot let the student receive the degree?[17]

The best method of arousing the students' interest—and of implementing "learning by doing"—was left to the discretion of each teacher. John J. Abel, the professor of pharmacology, transformed his subject from a descriptive study of drugs to an experimental course on the drugs' mechanisms of action.[18] Instruction in pharmacology, Abel believed, should consist mainly of extensive demonstrations bearing on the action of a given substance. "These demonstrations constitute the best introduction to pharmacology. . . . In this way the beginner receives ocular proof of the fact that an intoxication, whether acute or chronic, is as complex a matter as any of the clinical conditions that he will later study in the hospital. . . . In short, an interest in the manifold problems of medicine can here be aroused."[19]

Abel recommended "brief lectures" in pharmacology to complement the extensive demonstrations, but Welch saw no point in imposing pedagogical rules on the faculty: "If a teacher is convinced that didactic lectures are useless, it is not likely that his lectures will be of much value, and it may be as well for him to dispense with them."[20] Abel also believed that students should be allowed to skip lectures and recitations and that only laboratory sessions and demonstrations should be required. Teachers, moreover, should not be so petty as to mind if students did not attend their didactic sessions, he said, as "the head of the department and his corps of assistants will surely be above any small resentment when the student accepts this permission in good faith."[21]

Nor were demonstrations the very essence of learning by doing. Under Abel's guidance, each student performed at least half a dozen laboratory experiments—not manufactured exercises, but original experiments on matters of interest to the professor, investigations that tested the theories of the day. Students were also encouraged to undertake small pieces of original or advanced work. A rare individual, such as John B. MacCallum, would reveal a genuine talent for laboratory investigation (see chapter 11), but the Hopkins faculty believed in the educational value of this type of endeavor for all students, not only the gifted few.

G. Canby Robinson, Class of 1903, described his first assignment under William G. MacCallum, John's brother and one of three young instructors in Welch's pathology course:

> He [MacCallum] gave me a specimen of an unusual tumor that had been removed from the neck of a recently autopsied subject, suggesting that I describe it, study it microscopically, and make drawings of it. I devoted many hours to this task, including efforts to make sketches of the specimen. When I had done my best as an artist, I took my drawing to Max Brödel, who even then was recognized as one of the greatest medical artists. He viewed my drawing from various angles, upside down and sideways, and then said: "What is this, a hunting scene?" In spite of this initial discouragement, my crude first attempt as an illustrator was, with his help, made presentable. MacCallum assisted me in reviewing the foreign literature, and it was found that the tumor was a cyst originating from the thyroglossal duct, of which only one case had been fully described in Germany. This little piece of work was published, with the drawings, in the *Bulletin of The Johns Hopkins Hospital* in 1902 as my first medical publication. Pathology was the study that especially awakened my interest in medicine, and it was a great privilege to have had William H. Welch and his brilliant associates as my teachers.[22]

Despite the emphasis on laboratory work, the aim of the school was to educate medical practitioners. As Welch said, "The aim of the School will be primarily to train practitioners of medicine and surgery, that is to qualify persons to take care of diseased and injured conditions of the human body."[23] Professors in the preclinical sciences therefore took pains to relate their subjects to clinical medicine. Abel even wanted to defer the study of pharmacology until the third year of medical school, when the student began his clinical studies:

> [I]t is impossible to avoid reference to diseases and their symptoms. In the interest of the student, by way of lightening his work and making it more profitable for him, it is imperative to teach pharmacology hand in hand with the early clinical work. For now he begins to see drugs used; he notes, for example, how a patient behaves under ether; for what conditions the clinician prescribes iron, quinin, mercury, salicylic acid, codein, digitalis, potassium iodid, amyl nitrite and the like; what antiseptics and local anesthetics are used by the surgeon. . . . Though only a beginner, he meets at every turn with some practical application of the articles of our materia medica. Drugs now have some significance for him, an interest is aroused in their action, important data and conceptions are gathered by actual experience.[24]

Therapeutics was the province of clinicians, Abel believed, and the clinical work of the third and fourth years of medical school offered abundant opportunity for training in this area. Abel nevertheless gave third-year students a special course in practical therapeutics. Linked with toxicology and pharmacology, this course was an early attempt to bridge the gap between clinical and preclinical medicine.

Perhaps the most extreme proponent of "learning by doing" was Franklin P. Mall, the professor of anatomy, who considered even brief lectures too didactic. Mall gave no lectures at all, leaving that part of the instruction to his subordinates. His course consisted of independent laboratory work, and he required students to thrash about until they discovered for themselves the principles of anatomy.[25]

Mall considered the teaching of anatomy in the United States to be generally inferior.[26] Since the Civil War, anatomy had been the servant of surgery, and it was frequently taught by young surgeons awaiting a faculty position in surgery. Progress in anatomy was consequently "practical" rather than theoretical. In medical schools, dissections were carried on mostly by professional prosectors, not by the students themselves. These prosectors were usually young men who planned

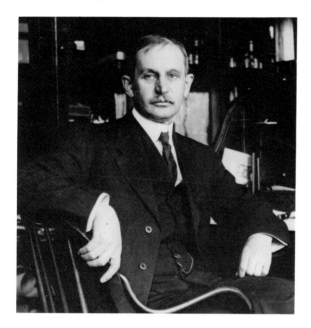

Franklin P. Mall. (*Source:* Alan M. Chesney Medical Archives, The Johns Hopkins Medical Institutions.)

to be surgeons, and their demonstrations naturally applied to the surgical operations of the day. It was not unusual for anatomy classes to consist of 500 students seated in an amphitheater, watching a prosector dissect. Examinations were similarly standardized, a course of quizzes given by former prosectors.[27]

Mall intended to change the teaching of anatomy by reviving the inductive method of education. Instruction in anatomy had a long and honorable history, he said, mentioning such great predecessors as Vesalius and John Hunter. Mall's own training had taken place in Europe, where as a student in the laboratories of His and Ludwig he was an active participant in experimental research.[28] Mall's recent experience had not included the standard anatomical dissections supposedly familiar to a professor of anatomy, but he was not dismayed by his own lack of knowledge. Indeed, Mall believed that professors should be students themselves, an attitude described by Charles R. Bardeen, a member of the first graduating class at the Hopkins medical school and later professor of anatomy at the University of Wisconsin:

In November of 1893, the first class of The Johns Hopkins medical school came into Mall's dissecting room. So far as I can recall, there was no formal meeting of the class. Each student was assigned to a part of a cadaver and told to go to work. Most of us had little idea how to begin. Some were more intelligent or lucky than others in their first attempts at unraveling the secrets of human structure. These students received praise. Others were less fortunate and had the deficiencies of their work more or less caustically called to their attention. Quality of work, not learning lessons, was emphasized. From the start he was essentially a fellow with his students, never a task master, but as a fellow student he never hesitated to be frank as only members of the family are as a rule frank to one another.[29]

The results varied. Some students never caught on, but others flourished. As Lewellys F. Barker, Mall's first assistant said:

The method was drastic, and some, I fear, never understood its purpose. For most students with good natural endowment, however, the compulsion to realization of the fact that on entrance to the medical school the period of spoon-fed education was over and that the time for acquiring the power to work more independently had arrived, though abrupt and perhaps painful, was most salutary, and I have heard many a student admit that he owed to Mall's method his intellectual awakening and his first arousal of desire to become an independent scientific worker.[30]

Those who never caught on thought that Mall was lazy and uninterested in teaching. Alan Gregg recalls his first encounter with Mall—and one of Mall's students:

On arrival at the Hopkins I wandered into the anatomy building. I saw a very sharp looking person with very intelligent eyes there in the hall, and he came over to me. . . .

This individual was Franklin P. Mall, whom I didn't know from a hole in the wall. He gave me about fifteen minutes of talk about what Johns Hopkins was. I left in a perfect storm. I wanted to sign on so much. I went out into the street and I saw . . . a fellow I had been a counselor with up in a YMCA camp in my freshman year. He looked at me with astonishment and said, "Why Alan Gregg, what the hell are you doing here?"

I said, "Why, I am trying to make up my mind what medical school to go to. . . . "

He said, "You come here. You won't make any mistake. We have wonderful professors. In physiology there is Howell. Popsy Welch is in pathology. Then there is Thayer in medicine." He was all enthusiastic, and then he added, "All except one son of a bitch."

I said, rather guardedly, thinking that it would be a good thing to know early on, "And who is that?"

"He thinks he's our professor of anatomy. His name is Franklin P. Mall. I'll just tell you what he did to us. The first day he met us in anatomy he said, 'Gentlemen, the dissection room will be open from nine o'clock in the morning until ten at night except on Saturday afternoon when you ought to go out and get some exercise anyhow. Up until six o'clock there'll always be somebody to get you out of any tangles you get into. I can recommend the three following textbooks, and when you are ready to take the examination let me know.' Now," said my young friend, "if you can beat that son of a bitch of laziness in a professor you're going some."

Mall has stayed in my mind as a good example of excellent teaching completely wasted on a badly prepared student mind. This boy I spoke of just missed Franklin Mall by yards and yards and yards. I privately think that Mall's teaching was designed for and appreciated by A No. 1 students, but that Mall had an appalling mortality because so many of his students thought, "Well, he must be interested in golf or something. He isn't teaching."[31]

Mall was far nearer to being the core of Hopkins, Gregg said, than many people realized.

Mall applied his enthusiasm for active learning to both general and specific aspects of the medical school curriculum. A college should cater to the interest of its students, he believed, but in a university, the student was important only insofar as he contributed to the institution's intellectual life.[32] The key to medical education was, therefore, to establish conditions in which everyone from faculty to students could contribute to scientific medicine. As Mall had suggested, students at the School of Medicine immersed themselves in one subject—or at most, two—at a time. Anatomy occupied all their time for the first two trimesters of the year; half was devoted to gross anatomy and the other half to histology.

Laboratory periods occupied three consecutive hours. Similarly, instructors taught only two terms a year, and for only a half day at a time; they thus had available large chunks of time for research.

Mall was also eager for Johns Hopkins to adopt a liberal elective system, so that students could follow their own interests:

> We all know that students are very unequal in ability, as well as in capacity for work, and why should they all pursue the same course of study? It is certainly very injurious for students to repeat courses with which they are familiar, feeling at the time that they do not grow from day to day. Furthermore, it is not beneficial to the true student to study with a whip over him, and we know only too well that this weapon is more often used by a poor instructor upon a good student than by a good instructor upon a poor student.[33]

Mall pointed out that electives were in vogue in the leading medical schools of Europe and that President Eliot had instituted them at Harvard College as well. Allowing students to choose their courses of study, Mall said, would correct the deficiency of the present system, in which the weak were cast out, the mediocre continued along the trodden path, and the strong were retarded.[34]

Mall's examinations were as unorthodox as his educational theories. As his student Florence R. Sabin remembered, his first aim was to eliminate fear, and he did this by asking some startling question that often set the student's mind working, allowing him to relax in a stressful situation. "The question might not be on anatomy at all, as for example 'How can you ride downtown [on a streetcar] and back on one fare?'—for which he had found a method that would work."[35] Examinations were less a test of the student than of the teacher, Mall felt, and he ridiculed the pedantic instructor who tested only memory, not intelligence.[36] His specific recommendation was later adopted in the Johns Hopkins curriculum reform of 1927: the examinations given were reduced to two sets, one at the end of the preclinical and the other at the end of the clinical years.

More important for the student than success in examinations was competence in original research, which gave the student "a standard by which he weighs all things later in life, and enables him with much more certainty to separate the real from the bogus in our superabundant medical literature. . . . So much am I in favor of students of medicine undertaking scientific work that I would require for the degree of M.D. a dissertation of some merit from each candidate."[37]

"Learning by Doing" in the Clinical Years

The Johns Hopkins Hospital and the School of Medicine paved the way for the development of the modern teaching hospital across the country. Their opening coincided with the floodtide of natural science. New discoveries in biology, physics, and chemistry were waiting to be applied to the study of disease in human beings and to the training of more scientifically oriented physicians. At Hopkins, the instructors in the preclinical sciences were themselves investigators, scientists who were devoting their careers exclusively to research and teaching. The resources of the basic sciences were the foundation upon which the great superstructure of clinical science was built. "There is or should be no real distinction in the spirit and methods of study between the laboratories of medical science and the hospital wards," said Welch.[38] Indeed, the clinical subjects—medicine, surgery, and gynecology and obstetrics—were taught at Hopkins with the same attention to "learning by doing" as the preclinical subjects.

The original Hopkins curriculum introduced students to clinical medicine near the end of the second year, in a physical diagnosis course designed to prepare them for the third year's clinical work. In the last two years of medical school, the dispensary and wards occupied the same relative position as the laboratories in the first two years. Third- and fourth-year students at Hopkins also participated in clinical laboratories, in which they were trained to apply microscopic and chemical procedures to the diagnosis and clinical study of disease. "These technical procedures can be taught best by those frequently engaged in using

them," said Welch, "and at a time when the student can appreciate their importance."[39]

A hospital setting was necessary to solve the particular problems inherent in teaching the clinical sciences, for large group demonstrations are less valuable than in the preclinical sciences. It is useless for students to watch operations, said Howard A. Kelly, chief of gynecology, as they can normally see little of what is happening—and in a deep, abdominal, or vaginal operation, they can see absolutely nothing.[40] Even seeing and hearing is not enough, as only practice in performing operations teaches the student to carry out the measures that distinguish this branch of medicine. Observing surgery is useful only to those who have already performed operations themselves.[41]

By the turn of the century, medical educators recognized the importance of the Hopkins approach to teaching in the clinical years.[42] As an editorial in the *Journal of the American Medical Association* in 1900 stated, "Indeed, to a large extent, the hospital, with its wards, its outpatient department, its operating-rooms, its dead-house, and its laboratories, is the medical school."[43] Welch narrowed the AMA's sweeping definition, identifying the hospital as the laboratory for the clinical branches of medicine, "where the results of nature's experiments are to be studied and alleviated by the methods of science."[44]

The Medical Clinic of William Osler

Osler's medical clinic was one of the most important facilities for "learning by doing" for students in the clinical years of medical school.[45] It combined, for the first time, a variety of diverse elements into a harmonious whole: the welfare of the patients, the education of undergraduate and graduate students, and the advancement of knowledge in internal medicine. In the six years that elapsed between the opening of the Johns Hopkins Hospital and the use of its facilities by the first class of students of the School of Medicine, the operation of the Medical Clinic—the organization of the wards, the outpatient department, the laboratories, the staff, the record keeping, the library, the hospital, the medical society,

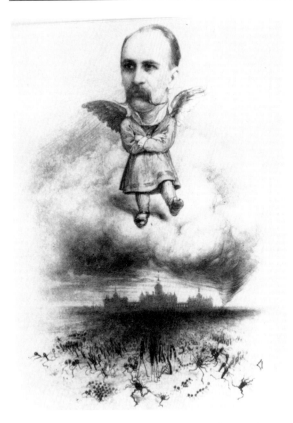

"The Saint of the Johns Hopkins Hospital," drawing by Max Broedel. (*Source:* Robert Austrian, M.D.)

and the care of patients in the hospital—had been polished and perfected. By the time the medical students arrived, therefore, they benefited from an effective system that was firmly in place.

Work in Osler's clinical laboratories taught third-year students to apply the laboratory methods of chemistry, physics, and biology to the study of patients. Instruction in the theoretical basis of these methods was followed by drill in their application two or three afternoons a week. By the end of the course, each student was skilled in clinical examination of the blood, the stomach juice, the feces, the urine, and the cerebrospinal fluid. In this course, Osler said, students began to regard the microscope as "a clinical tool and not a mere toy."[46]

Percy M. Dawson, a member of the Class of 1898, recalled participating in Osler's "infant clinics," "we juniors being the infants referred to":

The procedure involved the whole class. . . . When we were comfortably seated, with pen or pencil ready, the patient was brought in. Then Osler would call upon one of us to make the examination. The "Chief" drilled us in orderly procedure: Inspection, palpation, percussion, auscultation. Until we had gained all the information possible by one method, we were forbidden to pass on to the next. And to begin with, for inspection the patient *must* be in the best light possible. "Mr. ———, what do you see?" Mr. ——— would describe what he saw. Perhaps another would be called upon to examine and to verify or contradict Mr. ———'s findings, and so the examination continued to completion. "Now, Mr. ———, what is your diagnosis and why?" The class had heard by this time all the results of the examination and a discussion might arise. Says one, "His head vibrates in unison with his heart beat. It must be an aneurysm?" "An aneurysm of what?" asked the "Chief." "His foot goes the same way," said another student. "Has he two aneurysms?" asked the "Chief." "What did you say about his pulse, Mr. ———?" "It's very strong, oh very, very strong." Following this clue, the case turned out to be a leaking aortic valve. Then the "Chief" told of a clinician passing down a ward and, seeing a patient's foot sticking out, caught his big toe playfully as he was passing and stopped short. "Hello," he said, "When did this aortic case come in?" Osler then said, "Mr. ———, that pulse is known as the Corrigan or Water Hammer pulse, after [Sir Dominic John] Corrigan, a Scot, who died while I was at McGill. Will you please read Corrigan's description of aortic regurgitation and report on it next week. It's in the *Edinburgh Medical and Surgical Journal* for 1832. Miss Thies will help you find it. And bring the volume with you. Mr. X, do you know what a water hammer is?" "Yes, Sir, it's a thing we had in physics." "Well, Mr. X, will you please go to Dr. Jones's laboratory and tell him you want to make a water hammer and he will let you have the glass tubing. Then bring the water hammer for the class to see."[47]

Another distinctive feature of instruction in medicine was the involvement of the medical student in the day-to-day care of patients. After receiving instruction in history taking and elements of clinical diagnosis, each third-year student was required to assist in recording histories and performing physical examinations in the outpatient department. By the end of the third year of medical school, therefore, students entered the medical wards armed with a thorough education in clinical and laboratory work.

The culmination of everything the students had learned in the medical clinic was the clinical clerkship. All fourth-year students spent three months in the medical clinic, giving their whole time to the medical wards. Under the eye of the resident staff, they took the histories of all new patients, assisted the interns in performing the first physical examination and all the clinical laboratory tests on these patients, and accompanied the chief on morning rounds. At rounds, the clinical clerk gave an oral summary of the findings regarding the patient, watched the process of examination used by the professor, and participated at the bedside in discussing the case. Students looked up recent articles on the subject, reporting them at later ward rounds. They followed the patient to the operating room if surgical procedures were indicated, watched the effects of the treatment employed in each patient assigned to them, and kept in touch with the patient during convalescence at home.[48]

The main group teaching event of the week in medicine was the Saturday morning clinic in the Amphitheater, where all the third- and fourth-year students, the entire resident staff, physicians of the hospital, physicians of the town, and physicians from a distance were assembled. The clinical clerk was asked to tell the audience briefly, from memory, the main points of the patient's history and to report upon important laboratory findings. This pedagogic technique was simple but significant. The student had to know all the aspects of the patient's illness thoroughly in order to give—without notes—a concise and well-organized summary, so that the professor would immediately be able to think clearly about the possible diagnosis and treatment. The student thus grew accustomed to facing a large audience and to thinking and speaking off the cuff. This latter skill would be useful in later professional life, when the practicing physician would need to call in a consultant with special knowledge of a primary aspect of his patient's illness. The best use of the consultant's time and knowledge would rest

on the physician's ability to present the important facts concisely.[49]

Osler's clinical clerkships for medical students extended the principle of preceptorships, which themselves developed from the apprenticeships of medieval times. Early clinical instruction in the United States derived largely from the Scottish model, in which the professor, followed by an entourage of students, stopped successively at the bedsides of several patients. The professor questioned the patient in a loud voice, and a senior student chosen for the purpose repeated, in an equally loud voice, the patient's answers. The professor commented on diagnosis, prognosis, and treatment before moving to the next patient. A student of the time complained that being the chosen student was no easy task. It required considerable exertion to convey the conversation between physician and patient to the more distant members of the class, who were completely dependent on their ears for information because they were too far away to see the patient.[50] When classes grew in size, this "walking round" was replaced by lectures in the amphitheater. Neither method allowed the student to touch the patient.

In devising a new system of clinical education, Osler showed the influence of intellectual antecedents in Germany and France. Medical students in Germany were required to examine ambulant patients in a daily teaching clinic, and by the mid-1800s, this practice had found its way to the United States. Osler's belief in the importance of research could also be traced to the German laboratories, but the most important influence on his practice of medicine was the great French physician Pierre-Charles-Alexandre Louis.[51]

Louis' methods formed the basis of modern techniques for gathering information from the patient, and they are still in use. He was probably the first full-time clinical investigator, even though his principal tools were observation and numerical analysis rather than the use of the experimental method. His techniques included physical examination by eye, hand, and ear; obtaining a thorough history of the patient; and determination of the anatomical site of a lesion. As one student said, Louis' notes did not state opinions but facts, because he described specific changes in color, consistency, firmness, and so forth rather than relying on general terms such as "inflamed" or "cancerous."[52]

Through the students who traveled to his school in Paris in the first half of the nineteenth century, Louis is said to have created the American school of clinical medicine. Osler was one generation removed from the American physicians who studied with Louis, but he knew several of Louis' more eminent students from his years in Philadelphia. In perpetuating the ideas of Louis at Hopkins, Osler applied the contributions of an early proponent of "learning by doing" to the current training of medical students.

As American antecedents for Osler's clinical clerkship, there were programs at the Medical College of Ohio in Cincinnati, Harvard Medical School, and the University of Michigan, which incorporated ward work for medical students into the curriculum. Most important in the mid-1800s was a course at the New Orleans School of Medicine. There, each student received a list of questions to ask patients and a printed ticket with spaces on which to record clinical information. From this information, the student was expected to write a "connected narrative" about each patient, to be read to the professor on rounds. Furthermore, every member of the faculty gave bedside instruction, and lectures were subordinate to clinical activities.[53]

It was not until Osler reached Johns Hopkins, however, that he found an environment where classes were small enough for him to establish a clerkship system. Classes at the University of Pennsylvania, where he taught from 1884 to 1889, comprised about 130 students; early classes at Hopkins, about 25. "Though the clinical clerkship may not have been Osler's idea," says Edward C. Atwater, "it was he who established it firmly in the American scene. . . . Medical school endowments made it possible to pay professors, restrict class size, and establish clinical facilities under faculty control. Johns Hopkins was the first school to do all these things."[54]

The Hopkins system was unique in that it was more than a teaching device. Unlike ward classes, Osler's clinical clerkships constituted what Welch called a part of the regular, orderly machinery of the hospital. Students did work important for the interests of the patient, work that, if not done by the students, would have had to be done by others. The students' knowledge that the histories they registered and the results of the laboratory tests they made would become part of the hospital's permanent records, the students' feelings of responsibility upon realizing that the facts they had collected had contributed to the patients' diagnosis and treatment, the personal relationships established between students and professor—all were important to the students' development as physicians.

Equally important was the ineffable part of the student's education: the art as well as the science of treating patients. Osler had moved to Oxford eight years before George Corner became a medical student at Hopkins, but he had left behind him well-trained associates and pupils. Corner recalled with admiration the clear, wise, humane Oslerian discourse of teachers like William S. Thayer, Louis Hamman, Thomas R. Boggs, and Charles R. Austrian. On one occasion, Lewellys F. Barker was discussing the illness of a young woman with a chronic degenerative disease of the nervous system. Wishing the students to observe her peculiar gait, he helped her out of bed and walked with her along the ward. Corner remembers the ill-formed, stumbling girl in her wrinkled hospital gown, the tall, handsome, elegantly dressed professor at her side, guiding her with great courtesy, and the riveted attention of the medical students.[55]

Osler's approaches to instruction in medicine were unusual at the time. The importance of careful history taking and accurate physical examination had been generally recognized, but Osler's was one of the first systematized courses of instruction. That his methods continue to be used in medical schools worldwide attests to his brilliance as a medical educator.

Instruction in Surgery and the Hunterian Laboratory

The curriculum of the third and fourth years featured no systematic lectures in either surgery or medicine. The core of the instruction in surgery was Halsted's weekly clinic, given throughout the year. At each session, students examined four to six patients; their examination was followed by a question-and-answer period.[56] Two similar clinics were given weekly by one of the associate professors. Students presented weekly "recitations on assigned subjects," with Halsted presiding. In the third year, minor surgery was taught in the outpatient department twice weekly, to small sections of the class. In the final year, students were placed on the wards, where they watched and assisted at operations and acted as surgical dressers. They also performed minor operations themselves.

A course in surgical pathology was required one afternoon a week; students with a particular interest could take an additional, elective, course in this aspect of surgery. Instruction was given in clinical pathological diagnosis, illustrated by pamphlets, photographs, museum specimens and microscopic sections; and demonstrations were given of fresh material received in the Surgical Pathological Laboratory.[57]

One of the most innovative teaching devices in surgery—the Hunterian Laboratory course in experimental surgery—was introduced by William Halsted in 1895 and later expanded by Harvey Cushing. (Halsted offered to transfer the course to Cushing as an inducement for him to return after a period of study abroad.)

Cushing recalled the course's beginning:

The delightful feature of the J[ohns] H[opkins] H[ospital] organization in those days was the absence of any obvious departmental machinery and I hope it may always stay so. The Professors' junior associates practically agreed among themselves as to what they would teach, and they were allowed to go about it in their own way. Dr. Finney had for many years given a course in operative surgery on the cadaver and this he relinquished in order to give me something to do. Though untrained in laboratory methods except for my short period abroad in the physiological laboratories of Kronecker and Sher-

rington, I had been introduced to some experimental work on animals by Dr. Halsted, through an investigation we started together on parathyroid extirpations. . . . The third-year students occasionally attended these experiments as onlookers, but I always felt that they did not profit much thereby. The experience . . . sufficed to make me think that something might be done with a course on animals at which the students should do their own operations. . . . The course was offered as an optional exercise for third-year students, and . . . during the first year I took only two groups, with two tables of five men each—only 20 men in all.[58]

Previously, students' major contact with operative surgery had been as part of a large audience. Under Cushing's direction, students now performed operations on anesthetized dogs using techniques of strict asepsis. The revolutionary feature of the course was its simulation of surgery on a hospitalized patient. Students noted the "patient's" history, kept an anesthesia chart, wrote operative and postoperative notes, and performed a complete postmortem examination. Working on living, anesthetized animals required students to learn and observe the principles of surgical cleanliness. They had to develop the ability to dissect and gently manipulate living tissues without damaging them. They also had to learn proper control of hemorrhage. After participating in the course, students were more useful as assistants in the operating room, and they learned more from watching surgical procedures. Additional benefits, Cushing pointed out, were that students learned to keep proper records and to appreciate the risks of anesthesia.[59]

The first classes in operative surgery were held in the corner room on the first floor of the Women's Fund Memorial Building (anatomy building), which later became Florence R. Sabin's laboratory. Mall needed this room for the Anatomy Department, however, and in 1903 Cushing asked the medical school's trustees to provide the funds for a small, inexpensive building in which he could conduct his classes. Cushing's timing was unfortunate, however. The financial losses suffered by the university in the Great Baltimore Fire of 1904 forced the trustees to deny his request. Cushing then raised $5,000 from friends, but the trustees declined this offer, believing that the sum was insufficient for construction of a building in conformity with those already in existence. A further appeal late in 1904 by William G. MacCallum and Cushing produced positive results; the trustees voted to provide $15,000 for the construction of the building, which was completed in the summer of 1905. Half of its space was allotted to pathology and the other half to surgery. The laboratory was used for the teaching of medical students, the practice of veterinary medicine, and the performance of research.[60]

The name of the building was a source of puzzlement to many local residents. Cushing had favored naming the laboratory after Magendie, the famous French physiologist, but Magendie's name was anathema to the antivivisectionists in Baltimore. Welch suggested John Hunter's name, and the laboratory became known as the Hunterian Laboratory for Experimental Medicine. As one former student in the Hunterian recalled, "It was a good solution to the problem of a suitable name, but it mystified Baltimoreans who thought the term had reference to pointers, retrievers, and setters."[61]

The Hunterian did provide a haven for dog fanciers who brought their pets to it for treatment. Observations of disease in these dogs led to attempts to reproduce the disease in normal animals, as a foundation for the study of analogous diseases in humans. The operation developed in the 1940s for mitral stenosis can be traced to the Hunterian Laboratory. In an article published in 1908, Cushing and J. R. B. Branch commented on "the possibilities of future surgical measures in man directed toward the alleviation particularly of the lesion characterizing mitral stenosis" and mentioned the Hunterian as the site of their investigations.[62] The Hunterian was also the location of essentially all of Cushing's experimental work on the pituitary gland, carried out in collaboration with Samuel J. Crowe and others. It was also in the Hunterian that MacCallum and Voegtlin performed their pathbreaking experiments on the parathyroid gland and its relation to calcium metabolism.

Instruction in Obstetrics and Gynecology

During the late 1800s, the teaching of obstetrics and gynecology was obstructed by prudery. Despite the pioneering and controversial introduction of demonstrative midwifery in the 1850s, teaching continued to consist of little more than didactic lectures. Gynecology was, as a rule, very badly taught, remarked Howard A. Kelly in 1900. In contrast, in Kelly's courses at Hopkins, "the history-taking, the ward-work, the touch-course, all of which demand personal instruction, [were] the most valuable methods, bringing student and patient together, as they must meet in the natural course of events after graduation, and carrying the student up to the point beyond which he will not be apt to go, that is, up to the point of deciding upon the line of surgical treatment to be followed."[63]

Similarly, J. Whitridge Williams, professor of obstetrics, supplemented theoretical teaching with practical instruction, including weekly clinical case conferences and practical work in the lying-in ward. Williams asked rhetorically, "How can we expect, for example, the student to have a definite conception of the changes in the endometrium, which result in the formation of the decidua, if he has not carefully studied and drawn sections of the normal endometrium and decidua, instead of hearing them described by a lecturer, who has obtained his knowledge from the meager descriptions of the text-books?"[64]

"Manikin work" was another important aspect of the instruction in obstetrics. If enough patients were available, techniques of abdominal palpation, vaginal touch, and internal pelvimetry could be better taught on the living woman; but "if the clinical material is limited in amount," wrote Williams, "we consider it advisable that the students be taught the rudiments of palpation, touch, and pelvimetry upon the manikin, so that they will know exactly what they are to do when they examine the patients in the wards, whereby clinical material is economized, and the patients saved considerable annoyance."[65]

The obstetrical manikins, made of metal and rubber, were the shape and size of a pregnant woman's lower abdomen and pelvis, and each contained a dummy leather baby in its simulated uterus. One morning, Williams was showing the medical students the use of the obstetrical forceps of the formidable axis-traction type. He inserted the forceps, placing its curved blunt blades on the fetal head, and began to deliver the leather baby with a firm pull. The handles of the forceps suddenly came off, and the professor was thrown off balance, falling backwards so that his shoulders struck the floor with a thud. Undaunted, but muttering a curse, he got up and repeated the performance, only to have the handles give way again. Over he went once more, but he scrambled to his feet and exclaimed, "Obstetrics is a dangerous specialty!"[66]

The students at Hopkins were required to do laboratory work in obstetrics during their clinical years, since, as Williams pointed out, the immense sweep of the first- and second-year courses in histology and pathology precluded attention to more than the salient points of obstetrics, "which are soon forgotten. It is therefore necessary that this field should be gone over again more in detail and with especial reference to the practical side of obstetrics, and this can only be done by one, who is particularly interested in this branch of medicine."[67]

The Spread of "Learning by Doing"

Although teaching in the preclinical sciences was flourishing by the early 1900s, instruction in the clinical sciences lagged behind. Most medical students had little or no hands-on contact with patients.[68] Welch asked:

> Do the methods of teaching the clinical subjects generally adopted in our medical schools at the present time bring the student sufficiently in that intimate, prolonged, personal contact with the object of study, in this case the living patient, which secures that abiding, vital useful knowledge, the possession of which alone is power for good, and the lack of which is helplessness and even power for harm? As I have intimated, I believe that the clinic falls behind the laboratory in this regard, and that the greatest

strength of the curriculum is not where it should lie.[69]

This type of contact, Welch said, presented difficulties only in medical schools not closely affiliated with hospitals. Such schools lacked the authority to place students on wards as clinical clerks, and the permission of hospital boards was difficult to obtain. Clinical research in such medical schools was hampered by the same difficulties.[70]

After 1910, however, the principle of "learning by doing" became enormously popular in medical schools, largely because of the Flexner Report and the coincident national enthusiasm for "progressive education," the realization of John Dewey's pedagogic philosophy. Flexner's advice to medical schools in the early twentieth century emphasized "learning by doing," not simply because it was part of Hopkins, the school he had set before medical educators as a model, but also because he was a strong advocate of Dewey's tenets. The issues that Dewey addressed were basic to medical education: the content and methods of education, and the social responsibility of schools.[71]

To Flexner, "learning by doing" was the best way to master scientific knowledge. It also taught the student the scientific method—without which, Flexner believed, the student could not handle experience critically.[72] Although he acquires a vast amount of knowledge in medical school, Flexner wrote, the student armed with the scientific method "will still be ignorant of many things, but at any rate he will respect facts: he will have learned how to obtain them and what to do with them when he has them."[73]

Not only did the progressive education movement affect medical education, but when Flexner inspired the establishment of a school affiliated with Teachers College of Columbia University, medical education also influenced the course of the progressive education movement. "Mindful of the tremendous influence on medical education exerted by one modest but sound institution, the Johns Hopkins Medical School," he wrote, "I had long cherished the notion that a model school, quite modern in curriculum and discipline, might play a similar role in general education."[74]

The popularity of Dewey's ideas derived partly from their accessibility. Dewey's brand of education was perceived as the answer to the social problems brought on by industrialization. Progressive education brought the school into the "real world," enabling it to impart the information and values necessary for changing times.[75] Pragmatism and progressivism became part of the national culture, and philosophy was a subject for popular discussion. Charles S. Peirce's article entitled "Why I Am a Pragmatist" appeared in *Harper's,* and philosophical points were discussed in the Letters column of the Baltimore *Sun.*[76] So well known was Dewey himself that Flexner's reports to the Carnegie Foundation, *Medical Education in the United States and Canada* and *Medical Education in Europe,* refer to him simply as "Professor Dewey."[77]

Consequently, like Molière's Monsieur Jourdain, who discovered that he had been speaking prose his entire life, Hopkins found that it had been pursuing the ideas of John Dewey since its inception. Yet rather than absorbing Dewey's ideas, Hopkins had helped to generate them. John Dewey had enrolled at Hopkins as a graduate student in philosophy in 1882. Although his first specifically pedagogic writings were not published until the late 1890s, the seeds were planted in Baltimore—and the man responsible for this influence was Daniel C. Gilman. What convinced the young John Dewey to study at Hopkins was Gilman's controversial invitation to Thomas Huxley, the defender of Darwinism, to speak at the opening ceremonies of the Johns Hopkins University in 1876, and Gilman's reply to his critics. At Hopkins, Dewey was exposed to the best of Gilman's faculty, even taking a course in animal physiology with H. Newell Martin.[78] His central intellectual experience in graduate school, however, was his association with two men, George Sylvester Morris, who taught him philosophy, and Granville Stanley Hall, who taught him psychology.[79]

Dewey reconciled and transformed Morris's and Hall's seemingly antithetical ideas about the nature of knowledge as he incorporated them into his pedagogic philosophy.[80] Morris's emphasis on the subjective was reflected in Dewey's perception of education as a "continuous process of reconstruction of experience"[81] and in his ideas about the unity of the individual mind and the social milieu, but Dewey also believed, like Hall, that "the scientific method is the only authentic means at our command for getting at the significance of our everyday experiences of the world in which we live."[82]

Dewey's description of the ideal progressive education matched the intent of the Johns Hopkins medical school:

> If one attempts to formulate the philosophy of education implicit in the practices of the new education, we may, I think, discover certain common principles amid the variety of progressive schools now existing. To imposition from above is opposed expression and cultivation of individuality; to external discipline is opposed free activity; to learning from texts and teachers, learning through experience; to acquisition of isolated skills and techniques by drill, is opposed acquisition of them as means of attaining ends which make direct vital appeal; to preparation for a more or less remote future is opposed making the most of the opportunities of present life; to static aims and materials is opposed acquaintance with a changing world."[83]

The words of John Shaw Billings—the Hopkins ideal of "giving to the world men who can not only sail by the old charts but who can make new and better ones for the use of others"—are brought to mind by Dewey's translation of a passage from Rousseau, who compared his "ideal" student, Emile, with other children: " 'See what a difference there is between the knowledge of your pupils and the ignorance of mine. They learn maps; he makes them.' To find out how to make knowledge when it is needed is the true end of the acquisition of information in school, not the information itself."[84]

The popularity of Dewey's ideas inevitably led to their misinterpretation. The importance of arousing the learner's interest was distorted to mean that the child should decide what to study. Dewey, however, insisted that the content of the curriculum was the teacher's decision: in planning the curriculum, the teacher must consider the essentials first and the refinements second.[85] In fact, Dewey identified the matter of selection and organization of intellectual subject matter as the weakest point in progressive schools.[86]

Similarly, some educators interpreted Dewey's words to mean that activity or experience in general was educationally beneficial.[87] Yet Dewey referred to the phrase "learning by doing" as a "slogan," albeit a useful one.[88] He also used the phrase "learning by experience," and his definition of experience was detailed and precise. It encompassed active and passive elements, meaning, and growth. "The belief that all genuine education comes about through experience does not mean that all experiences are genuinely or equally educative. Experience and education cannot be directly equated to each other. For some experiences are mis-educative. . . . Activity that is not checked by observation of what follows from it may be temporarily enjoyed," he said, "But intellectually it leads nowhere. It does not provide knowledge about the situations in which action occurs nor does it lead to clarification and expansion of ideas."[89]

The distortion of Dewey's tenets was never part of the Hopkins curriculum: "experience" never superseded the "respect for facts" that Flexner identified as the hallmark of a Hopkins medical education.[90] Learning by doing at Johns Hopkins implied only one type of experience: instruction that met the faculty's high standards of educational worth. The quality of the instructor was also a matter of great concern. For example, most schools that involved students in obstetrical work sent them to perform deliveries alone. At Hopkins, in contrast, students received supervision and instruction when they participated in home deliveries.[91] Even some opportunities for "learning by doing" were rejected as an insufficiently valuable use of the student's time: in making recommendations for the teaching of pharma-

cology, John J. Abel wrote, "It is unnecessary for the student himself to perform the many simple experiments to which he is equal, but which can be more quickly performed for him."[92]

As the influence of Flexner's recommendations and the progressive education movement increased during the 1920s, even Hopkins, a medical school pioneer in "learning by doing," instituted a sweeping curriculum reform that accentuated the principles of progressive education.

The Curriculum Revision of 1927

The medical curriculum had been gradually altered during Hopkins' first three decades, mainly by accretion. As medical specialties developed, the curriculum was stretched to accommodate them. As a result, the crowded curriculum left students little free time, particularly in the clinical years. Students spent at least eight hours a day in classes five days a week, with seven hours of classes on Saturdays.[93]

British physicians who visited Johns Hopkins in 1920 noted the curriculum's flaws; their criticisms prompted hospital superintendent Winford Smith to suggest that Hopkins reassess its educational program. The outcome was the establishment of a permanent committee to ensure that the medical school curriculum would come under continuous scrutiny. The Curriculum Committee was inaugurated in 1921, with the director of pediatrics, John Howland, at its head. Its five members were broadly representative of the medical school, spanning the basic and clinical sciences: W. W. Palmer (Department of Medicine), Winford Smith (superintendent of the hospital), Lewis Weed (Department of Anatomy), and J. Whitridge Williams (Department of Gynecology and Obstetrics).

Recognizing that medical knowledge would continue to increase, the committee members hoped to establish a structure that could weather the years to come. The committee's report, issued in 1921, advocated striking changes. First, electives should be given a prominent part in the curriculum, and students should be required to take only the minimal number of courses in major subjects. Second, heads of departments should personally take charge of basic introductory courses in their field of interest.

Much of the committee's report concerned the responsibilities of the faculty. Current instruction in the Dispensary and on the wards was less than ideal, the committee members believed, largely because many of the Dispensary's departments were staffed almost entirely by outside or part-time physicians. Because they had no intimate connection with the hospital service and were consequently ignorant of its needs, the instruction they gave was casual. These deficits reinforced the importance of the full-time system, the committee report said, as the performance of scientific investigation was essential for the best teaching. For the proper conduct of each service, the committee members believed, the inpatient and outpatient services of each department had to be conducted as a single unit, in a new building constructed for the purpose. This proposal was a forerunner of the firm system instituted by the Department of Medicine in 1975 (see chapter 5). Similarly, the committee proposed reducing the number of part-time instructors of fourth-year clerkship students, as the demands of these physicians' private practices often superseded their commitment to teaching.[94]

The facilities of the hospital were inadequate to support the recommended fusion of the inpatient and outpatient departments. A new system of medical records was needed, so that the entire record of each patient in all inpatient and outpatient departments of the hospital would be readily available at all times. A suitable library was also essential, they said, to replace the fragmented system in effect at the time. It was difficult to find books because part of the library was then housed in the hospital and part in the medical school—and both facilities were overcrowded.

The committee was also dissatisfied with the quality of the medical students. They recommended a reduction in the number of students in each class, from ninety to seventy-five. This step

would weed out the weaker applicants, while giving the remaining students more intensive experience on the wards. Efforts to improve the quality of matriculating students began right away. The catalog for 1921–22 contained the daunting statement:

> The seventy-five students entering the first year class are admitted with the understanding that only the sixty-five having the highest standing at the end of the year will be advanced to the second year, and that only sixty of the original seventy-five students will be advanced to the third year. This means that, even though they may not have failed in any subject, a certain number of students will be obliged to withdraw at the end of the first and second years respectively, and an attempt will be made to fill the vacancies thus created by admitting to advanced standing desirable students from other schools.[95]

A qualifying phrase was added the next year: " . . . but no student will be dropped whose standing averages seventy-five or more."[96] In the following year, 1923, the criteria were softened still further, as a specific qualifying average was abandoned, and promotion now depended on "the understanding that only those who, in the opinion of the Committee on Instruction, give promise of being a credit to themselves and the School will be advanced."[97] Promotion in the subsequent years would also depend on the judgment of the committee.

In fact, although the number of entering students was reduced (from ninety-one in 1921 to seventy-nine the next year), only the entering class of 1921 suffered the kind of attrition described in the catalog. Seventy-nine of the first-year students remained for the second year, and sixty-six of those continued to the third year.

No changes were made in the curriculum as a result of this first committee's recommendations. Instead, in 1923, the new dean, Lewis Weed, organized a second committee on educational policy. John Howland again chaired the committee, but it was co-chaired by a representative of the basic sciences, pathologist W. G. MacCallum. This committee labored for five years, and its report proposed changes even more extensive than those recommended by its predecessor.

The study of medicine was a professional venture, the new committee stated, and the courses in the School of Medicine should reflect the graduate status of medical education, to a degree compatible with training students for a profession. It was proposing, in effect, a curricular clean slate.[98]

Although the revised curriculum put into effect in 1927 was far more flexible than the system it replaced, the alterations hardly represented new ideas. Instead, they reaffirmed the approach to medical education propounded by Franklin P. Mall when the medical school was founded. Like the committee members, Mall also believed that lock-step curricular requirements were incompatible with the Johns Hopkins ideal of self-education under guidance. Consequently, the redesigned curriculum kept required courses to a minimum. In the major departments, the student was required to satisfy only basic requirements, referred to by Weed as the "skeletal basis of instruction."[99] The committee even recommended that the medical degree be given to students who had not completed these courses but had instead devoted four years of study to a particular subject within the course of instruction.

The new approach would remove all distinction between required courses and free time. Students would be held responsible for information at the time of the group examination. Only two sets of examinations would be given: knowledge of the preclinical subjects would be tested at the end of the second year, and knowledge of the clinical subjects at the end of the fourth. Furthermore, students should be allowed to interrupt their scheduled courses at Hopkins to investigate a special subject or to study elsewhere.

Some changes were introduced in 1926. In particular, one-third of the third year and one-half of the fourth year of medical school were set aside for electives. Heretofore, the third year had consisted largely of obligatory courses, and unassigned time had occupied only one trimester of the final year.

In 1927, the trimester system gave way to a quarter system, permitting more diversity and, in some cases, shorter courses. Required courses now occupied only half the students' time during the four years of medical school. The student was expected to use the remaining time for additional work based on individual interests. This plan afforded great opportunity for students pursuing so-called departmental programs, since a student who had already chosen a career in any branch of preclinical or clinical medicine could arrange with the department head a program that would incorporate studies in that department into all four years of school.

The provisions of the new system profoundly changed the experience of medical school. The student had fewer classmates, as the number of students in each class was reduced from ninety to seventy-five. Grading on required courses was only "pass" or "fail." Examinations continued to be held at the end of the second and fourth years, but even the type of examination was different: after 1927, examinations were comprehensive and general, in contrast to the detailed tests that had previously been given at the end of each major course of instruction.

Under the new system, the amount of "free" time increased through the 8-week quarters of medical school. In the first year of medical school, free time was confined to the last quarter. The entire fourth quarter of the second year was elective, except for one half day in the Pharmacology Laboratory and two lectures in pharmacology. In the third year, the student could schedule his or her own blocks of courses. All afternoons were free during the second and third quarters; and, again, one quarter was entirely free. Fully half of the fourth year was free, and scheduled classes in the final year occupied only two quarters, which were devoted mainly to medicine (including pediatrics) and to surgery (including ophthalmology and some exposure to the surgical specialties).

The deficiencies of the new system began to emerge over the next few years. From the students' perspective, the main problems concerned the examinations and the elective courses. Students disliked taking only two sets of examinations, since they had to wait until the end of their second year of school to learn their standing. It was evidently difficult to prepare for such comprehensive examinations: a significant number of students failed their examinations in 1934. Students also tended not to use their elective time effectively, particularly early in medical school. Furthermore, the number of elective courses offered in the third and fourth years seemed insufficient, and the physical facilities—particularly the number of inpatient beds and the number of outpatients—were inadequate for some of the desired work.[100]

Nor was the faculty content with the revised curriculum. After the program had been in effect for four years, Arnold R. Rich, a member of the Department of Pathology, set forth his objections in an article published in the *Bulletin of The Johns Hopkins Hospital*.[101] Throughout his long career, Rich was regarded as one of Hopkins' statesmen, a faculty member with the gift of balancing tradition and innovation. His penetrating criticisms of the new curriculum honored the past while pointing the way to the future.

Education in medical school was strictly an undergraduate process, Rich believed, since graduate education requires that the student complete preliminary work in the basic principles of the field. Medicine required mastery of enough basic material to fill many required courses in medical school, material important to every student, regardless of his or her choice of career. Elective courses should not be included in the curriculum at the expense of elementary training. Moreover, early and intensive specialization would restrict the individual's breadth of outlook. Surely there was enough time for specialization after medical school, he believed. In short, students could best develop their individual interests after graduation by pursuing a broad educational program before: "a more thorough grounding for each student in the general principles of pathology, for example, is more valuable in the long run than is a hurried general course which must be skimped by the entire class in order to leave free time for an elective course concocted for a few students on, say, the pathological changes occurring in the spleen."[102]

Like Franklin Mall, Rich believed that all students were accountable for their own medical education. Students were responsible for absorb-

ing the basic principles of medicine and determining their particular field of interest as quickly as possible, so that "the period of passive absorption of information may give place as soon as possible to that active acquisition of information which, alone, constitutes experience in the true sense."[103]

For this reason, students who chose a medical career early in college should not be required to spend four years in the passive acquisition of knowledge for medical school. The amount of cultural information acquired in present-day colleges was too slight to justify the insistence that students spend four years there, Rich said. The undue extension of formal education sapped students' enthusiasm, energy, and confidence, and neat schemes for "freedom of learning" at the college level were no antidote. College students who had fulfilled the premedical requirements in languages and in the fundamental sciences should therefore be encouraged to enter medical school at once.

In scrutinizing the curriculum, Rich echoed Welch's belief that it should be planned not for the exceptional, highly gifted student, nor for the group of poor students at the bottom of the class, but for the average, good student. The proper sequence of courses was crucial, but the present curriculum lacked a good sequential design. It contained too many fragmented, required courses, which gave the student a smattering of unconnected information. The accretion of barnacles on the basic curriculum was justified by some who cited the rapid, continuing development of knowledge. Rich, however, pointed out that a large mass of new facts did not necessarily require the student to master a larger body of information. Rather, the faculty was responsible for structuring courses in a more concise and simple manner than the theoretical dogmas of a previous age had permitted. It is a mistake, he said, to assume that each new discovery results in an addition to the total quantity that the student has to learn.[104]

Although the responsibility for obtaining a medical education was primarily the student's, the role of the faculty—and not just the organizers of the curriculum—was crucial. Rich enunciated the same precepts that Billings had brought out years earlier: The first function of a university faculty was to keep alive and pass on to succeeding generations the best of accumulated knowledge. The second function was to improve or add to this store of knowledge. Departments that overemphasized the second at the expense of the first would become mere research institutes—and research institutes, however important their work, are not universities.

Specialization by the faculty could be as dangerous as specialization by the students, Rich believed. A department that produced contributions to the general body of knowledge would be a failure from the university standpoint, he said, if its senior faculty did not have a breadth of knowledge that spanned their entire field. The presence of many such professors in the university would demoralize the younger faculty, who would conclude that mastery of a subject was held in less esteem than the writing of papers about a restricted corner of a field. In contrast, if mastery was encouraged by example, the university would be safe in its primary function, and properly educated young people with the talent and inclination for research would find their way easily into it. Research had become a fetish in many universities, Rich believed, and this attitude was forcing many young physicians into an area of medicine for which they had no aptitude—to the detriment of the individual and of the clinical departments.[105]

Despite his criticisms, Rich applauded the drastic action of Weed's committee. It had cleared away the tangled thickets of required courses and electives, leaving a free space on which to build afresh. Rich's recommendations for further curricular change included lengthening some of the required courses; providing an ample, but not superfluous, amount of free time in the curriculum; structuring the curriculum so that the required courses would be completed by the end of the third year, without prolonging the academic year or sacrificing any courses called for by the present calendar; and consolidating all the student's free

time, currently scattered throughout the four years of medical school, into the final year, which the student would spend as an apprentice in one or several departments. Thus, at the end of the third year, the student would have completed every required course, in an orderly way. Having studied each of the main preclinical and clinical divisions of medicine, students would be ready to decide what elective training would be most helpful to them and what branch of medicine appealed to them most. A prolonged medical education had been a useful experiment, Rich believed, and it was now time to promote the earlier development of intellectual independence.[106]

One of Rich's suggestions was acted upon soon after his article appeared: examinations were rescheduled, taking place first at the end of each year and later at the end of each course. Other recommendations were included in the changes made after a review of the curriculum in 1936. For example, the Curriculum Committee decided that the reduction in required hours in the preclinical years had been too severe. Despite Rich's criticisms, however, the curriculum underwent no major revision for the next thirty years. Changes during that time were gradual, as the amount of time allotted to required courses crept upwards. By 1936, two-thirds of the medical curriculum was taken up by such courses; and the amount of free time in the final year diminished from one-half in 1936 to one-quarter in 1951. Another of Rich's ideas took more than twenty-five years to reemerge: the Year V Program, inaugurated at Hopkins in 1959, reflected Rich's wish to shorten the college years for students planning a medical career.

The Year V Program

The Year V Program followed in the wake of a pioneering effort in curriculum reform supported by the Commonwealth Fund at Case Western Reserve University. By the mid-1950s, the topic of medical education was again in the air, as many faculty members believed that medical education had become piecemeal, lockstep, and constricted. The program at Case Western Reserve was thus intended to revitalize the curriculum. Theoretical work, laboratory work, and contact with patients all moved forward together in a sequence that fitted the student's learning process, so that a growing understanding of people and an increasing sense of clinical responsibility were the strongest motives for mastering the necessary scientific underpinnings. Laboratories in separate departments were abandoned, as were departmental lectures. Instead, teaching and laboratory work were combined to facilitate the study of physiological systems. Students were exposed to patients in their first years of medical school, rather than solely during the clinical years.[107]

At Hopkins, a committee headed by professor of psychiatry John C. Whitehorn took a new look at the curriculum during the mid-1950s. The committee's study coincided with the return of W. Barry Wood in 1955 as vice-president of the university and the hospital and professor of microbiology. Wood's ideas about medical education echoed those of Arnold Rich, and he proposed major changes intended to solve not only the particular problems of the present Johns Hopkins curriculum but also some of the problems of American medical education in general. These were perceived as an excessive number of years of formal schooling required to train a physician, the "iron curtain" between the liberal arts and medical science, and the decline of faculty strength in the basic medical sciences.[108]

Johns Hopkins' solution was the Year V Program, a flexible course of medical education that was in effect for twenty years, from 1959 to 1979. The Commonwealth Fund was eager to fund progressive educational programs at medical schools nationwide, and it gave the Year V Program substantial support. The purpose of the program was to attract a greater number of talented students to the study of medicine by shortening the course of training by two years, thus cutting the cost of their medical education and emphasizing creative and independent study. It was intended to break the barrier between the liberal arts and the medical sciences, broadening the training of medical stu-

dents while bringing the School of Medicine into close collaboration with the Faculty of Arts and Sciences. Duplications of courses in undergraduate and medical school were eliminated, and the academic standards of premedical science courses were raised. The program stressed the application of the social sciences to the humanistic and sociological problems of medicine, while encouraging more students to pursue careers in the basic medical sciences.[109]

Year I was a transition year between college and medical school, as students continued their study of the liberal arts and natural sciences needed for medicine. The Year I class thus comprised students who had completed either the sophomore or junior year of college. The conventional first year of medical school was renamed Year II, and only college graduates were admitted to this year of the program. Years I and II emphasized the unity of the educational process, as Year II students took an intensive course in the history and philosophy of medicine and science. Responsibility for teaching organic, physical, and analytic chemistry was shifted from the college to the Department of Physiological Chemistry in the medical school, and the basic science department consequently took on additional faculty.

Distinctions between the preclinical and clinical years were abolished. Year II was devoted to the study of the structure and function of the normal human body and mind; Year III to changes in structure and function induced by disease, and to the action of drugs, antibiotics, and vaccines; and Year IV to the study of health and disease, carried out in the various clinical departments of the Johns Hopkins Hospital. Year V students spent three-quarters of the year as apprentices on the hospital wards.

The school year was lengthened from thirty-six to forty weeks; as a result, the total number of elective hours remained about the same as previously, while the number of required hours actually increased. Although acceleration attracted the most public attention, it was only a minor part of the Hopkins program. A limited number of students in each class could complete their medical training in three years by taking required courses during elective periods and summers. The Johns Hopkins program succeeded in turning some students toward the basic sciences, as its block system permitted clustered time for intensive study and research.

Changing Student Attitudes, 1950 to 1975

The changing interests of medical students contributed to the acceleration of curriculum reform nationwide during the 1950s and early 1960s. Subspecialty medical practice was still popular, but it was combined with a desire to be associated with an academic medical center on a part-time or full-time basis. In a study of the career choices of medical students, Daniel Funkenstein, a dean at the Harvard Medical School, categorized medical students as either "bioscientific" or "biosocial."[110] By the late 1950s, admissions committees emphasized scientific preparation, and the proportion of bioscientifically oriented students increased accordingly. Both types of students were less interested in primary care. Ambulatory medicine was less appealing to the medical students than medicine on the wards, which the students considered the most exciting milieu.[111]

Similarly, changes in the medical curriculum nationwide during the early 1960s reflected the more "scientific" orientation of medical schools, with a corresponding emphasis on academic medicine. Pathophysiology became an important part of the introduction to clinical medicine, and as a result, full-time clinical faculty were heavily involved in the teaching of what had been considered preclinical subjects. The more that molecular and cell biologists became the popular recruits in basic science departments, the more medical schools had to depend on full-time clinicians to share the teaching of organ physiology, anatomy, bacteriology, and pharmacology. Exposed to teaching by clinicians even before they entered the clinic, medical students were impressed by the physicians' theoretical as well as practical knowledge of the basic sciences. Full-time physician-scientists provided a very visible and popular role model, that of the "renaissance" physician

—compleat clinician, stimulating teacher, and successful clinical investigator.[112]

At Johns Hopkins, the medical student's traditional participation on the ward team yielded new enjoyment, as technologic advances were put to use by a patient-care team that included a member of the full-time clinical faculty along with a mature, knowledgeable resident staff. The year 1965 was the peak of the "scientific era" of medical student interest, an era when the best students at all levels across the country looked upon full-time academic medicine as the most prestigious career.[113] Not only had Johns Hopkins provided the early model of medical education for the nation, but as one educator said, "Medical education in the United States became so standardized during the half century between the Flexner Report and the 1960s that students could transfer from one school to another and hardly know they had moved."[114]

Only a few years later, the entire atmosphere in medical schools had changed. Nationally, it was a time of ferment, with controversy over the Vietnam War and cutbacks in federal funding for medical research. Students demanded "relevance" in the curriculum, and faculties were responsive to their demands. In the words of one medical educator, medical school faculties "recognized" that "what is relevant for the man preparing for a career in surgery is not necessarily appropriate for the embryo psychiatrist"[115]—a perception that might have elicited some disagreement from William H. Welch. In contrast to Rich's belief that a crowded curriculum is an inevitable result of scientific progress, medical educators in the 1960s called the system "overloaded" and advocated vast changes in the curriculum to accommodate the flood of new scientific information.

By 1968, 80 percent of AAMC member schools had instituted or were developing new curricula. Following the example at Case Western Reserve, the traditional division of the curriculum into two years of preclinical followed by two years of clinical sciences was replaced by interdisciplinary instruction, a combination of clinical instruction with work in the basic sciences, and courses that would encourage the student to develop insight and compassion. Instruction in the basic sciences was reduced, largely through elimination of laboratory work in gross anatomy, biochemistry, and pharmacology. Schools introduced an extensive elective program: in some schools, the entire fourth year contained only elective courses. Although the concept of "learning by doing" was undergoing extensive modification, the expansion of elective time, at least, represented the rediscovery of a curricular concept from the past.

The number of medical school graduates seeking postdoctoral research training peaked at 5,419 in 1968, but a decade later, the number had fallen to 1,883.[116] This striking change illustrated the new student activism that began to replace students' commitment to scientific medicine during the late 1960s. (Other medical schools felt the change more than did Johns Hopkins, although a certain level of anti-intellectualism was apparent at Hopkins as well.) A more constructive part of this activism was a concern with "the needs of the people." Many more students chose a family practice residency; students who might have become psychiatrists in earlier years now leaned toward careers in public health.[117]

Attitudes toward other aspects of American medicine changed as well. Group practice became a popular idea, as did national health insurance and the abolition of fee-for-service. By 1971, 86 percent of the graduating class at the Harvard Medical School professed unhappiness with the delivery of medical care in the United States. This unhappiness was pervasive. The public also perceived the nation's system of medical practice as insensitive to the need for primary care. To counteract the disappearance of the family physician, Congress funded a series of health manpower acts, beginning in 1968, that provided medical schools with powerful incentives to increase the number of medical students enrolled and encourage a more general type of medical practice; it also abolished certain incentives connected with research fellowships leading to academic careers in the medical subspecialties.[118]

As Congress gave proportionately larger amounts of money for primary care, the nature of "learning by doing" changed as well. Although the

dollar support of research continued to increase during the 1970s, the percentage of support that this represented fell from a high of 55 percent in 1965 to less than 30 percent by the end of the 1970s. The number of full-time clinical faculty continued to grow, largely because they brought money into the medical schools through faculty practice plans. The division between clinical and research faculty widened as research became more technically complex, and the faculty became separated into those who received their support largely from research grants and those who generated support from the practice of medicine.[119]

The role model of the 1950s and 1960s, the renaissance-type academic clinician who could participate with equal facility in research, teaching, and patient care, was disappearing. Clinical faculty were more likely to be interested in the fellows in their own subspecialties than in the residents or in the medical students. Now students were more likely to be directly supervised by a resident or a fellow than by a member of the faculty. As the complexity of inpatient care increased, it became more difficult to teach at the bedside. As a result, the immediate supervisors—the residents and the fellows in the medical subspecialties—were an increasing influence on medical students in the 1970s.

The Curriculum Revision of 1975

The Curriculum Revision of 1975 addressed not the prevailing social upheaval but a particular scientific phenomenon—the rapid growth of molecular biology since the 1960s. This growth had blurred the boundaries between the traditional basic science departments: anatomy, biochemistry, physiology, and pharmacology. In 1975, Dean Richard S. Ross appointed Vernon B. Mountcastle, director of the Department of Physiology, to chair a committee that would consider the effects of this change on the medical school curriculum.[120]

Mountcastle's committee intended to create a new approach to basic science education without altering the existing framework of instruction. Their plan was to shift instruction in the basic sciences away from blocks of courses in separate disciplines to a more cohesive, cross-disciplinary approach—a change that would take advantage of the natural and obvious paths of study that cut across traditional departmental lines. For example, the first-year student would immediately be exposed to new courses in cell biology and biochemistry. The relation between these two fields would become obvious, and the student would be fortified with information about the molecular level before going on to a course in gross anatomy. At the same time, students would study ethical and social issues in health care and would observe emergency room procedures and the day-to-day functioning of a physician's office. Later in the year, a course would be added that stressed the link between the behavioral sciences and the neurosciences.

The committee also believed that the curriculum should preserve Hopkins' unique emphasis on laboratory experience. This aspect of instruction in the preclinical sciences had been the traditional parallel to bedside teaching on the clinical side. Retaining time in the laboratory for students proved to be difficult, however, as the increasingly technical nature of laboratory work, along with other constraints, combined to reduce the number of hours that students spent in this type of "learning by doing."

The Human Biology Program

Three years after the changes suggested by the Curriculum Committee of 1975 were put in place, the Year V Program gave way to the Human Biology Program.[121] The new program, which was also sponsored by the Commonwealth Fund, was intended to eliminate one year from the conventional eight-year course of study for the bachelor's and medical degrees and to increase all students' interdivisional access to the various courses relating to the study of human biology. The regular medical curriculum was retained in parallel with this university-wide effort. Students in the Hu-

man Biology Program spent their junior and senior years of college studying human biology, liberal arts, and some preclinical subjects usually taught in the first years of medical school. Consequently, the Faculty of Medicine and the Faculty of Arts and Sciences collaborated to develop joint courses in biochemistry, genetics, physiology, neurobiology, and cell and developmental biology. Biochemistry, long needed at the undergraduate level, was offered at both the college and the medical school, with an advanced medical school course available for students who had completed the undergraduate course.

The pool of applicants for the accelerated program remained small, however, despite strenuous efforts to attract students. The admissions committee was accepting 100 of 4,000 aspirants for the standard medical school program and 25 of 300 for the Human Biology Program. Moreover, although the pool for the accelerated program contained excellent students, they were not the superstars that Hopkins had anticipated. When the Commonwealth Fund's grant ended in 1981, the Human Biology Program was discontinued. The effort to offer a broad range of educational choices to prospective medical students reemerged in the FlexMed Program, which was inaugurated in 1983 (see chapter 5).

The Curriculum Review Committee of 1987

Although the idea of "learning by doing" was a hallmark of Johns Hopkins medicine at its inception, the school needed reminding of the fact a hundred years later. As pointed out in the widely heralded Report of the Panel on the General Professional Education of the Physician (GPEP) in 1985, medical faculties once again needed to reduce the number of scheduled lecture hours in order to curtail the passive form of medical education.[122] The committee that produced the report, chaired by Steven Muller, president of the Johns Hopkins University, devoted over two years to studying all phases of medical education. Partly in response to the GPEP report and partly in recognition of the medical school's impending second century, a Curriculum Review Committee was empaneled. Composed of seven department directors and four members of the dean's office, the committee submitted its report at the end of 1987.

The report looked back to the words of John Shaw Billings, who in 1875 had urged the Johns Hopkins School of Medicine to prepare its students so that they would know "how to begin the study of some of the many problems still awaiting solution." The goal of the school, the recent committee said, "is to prepare physicians to practice compassionate clinical medicine of the highest standard and to identify and solve fundamental questions in the pathogenesis and treatment of disease, in health care delivery, or in the basic sciences."[123]

The committee proposed that the medical school curriculum be restructured so that time would be available for all students to carry out a research project, and that a series of seminars or small group meetings be instituted during all four years. The aim would be to provide an educational setting offering more active learning and a closer relationship between students and faculty.

Training Medical Scientists at Johns Hopkins

The tradition of training medical scientists at Johns Hopkins, a tradition as old as the medical school itself, was for many years embedded in the granting of the medical degree. Before World War II, Hopkins medical school graduates were implicitly assumed to have acquired the knowledge and skills necessary to conduct research in the basic sciences. Yet since its inception, the medical school has opened its resources to students other than those working toward the M.D. degree. In 1896, the Department of Pathology gave physicians the opportunity for "advanced work and special research." By the 1930s, clinical departments were offering individualized programs to physicians who wished to extend their knowledge by "assisting in the care of outpatients and performing a certain amount of laboratory work," but graduates of these programs received no formal recognition by certificate or diploma. Although

Ph.D. degrees were given before the late 1950s, it was not until 1959 that doctoral students in other branches of the university and from other universities were invited to study in the medical school's preclinical departments. In the following year, six departments—anatomy, biophysics, history of medicine, microbiology, physiological chemistry, and physiology—began to offer formal programs to award the doctoral degree.

These early programs were sparsely populated. A few maverick students obtained both medical and doctoral degrees from Hopkins during the 1950s, but on their own initiative, and usually at considerable financial sacrifice. Although Hopkins sponsored a Post-Sophomore Research Program, it was a desultory effort, suffering from an informal structure and a paucity of participants.

Federal interest in training medical investigators began to increase during the late 1940s, owing to the widespread perception in the postwar years that "something was drastically wrong" with the education of biomedical scientists.[124] Medical education was not providing the scientific rigor that would permit physicians to pursue a successful investigative career, and graduate education did not encourage biological scientists to participate in research concerned with problems of human disease.[125] With the logarithmic growth of knowledge and the concomitant trend toward specialization in medicine, many medical school graduates felt inadequately prepared for medical investigation, and an increasing number of science graduates were becoming involved in medical research.

The pioneering force in graduate training at the Hopkins medical school was Albert L. Lehninger, who in the early 1950s used newly available federal training grants to build a graduate program in physiological chemistry. Burgeoning federal support of basic science training in the early 1960s allowed A. McGehee Harvey and Kenneth L. Zierler to obtain an interdepartmental training grant from the National Institutes of Health. This grant, awarded in 1961, enabled house officers and fellows in clinical departments to pursue advanced scientific training and the doctoral degree. Participating departments were, in the School of Medicine, the Departments of Pharmacology, Physiological Chemistry, Physiology, Microbiology, and Biophysics; in the School of Hygiene and Public Health, the Departments of Biochemistry and Pathobiology; in the Faculty of Arts and Sciences, the Departments of Biology and Biophysics; and, after 1965, the university-wide Subdepartment of Biomedical Engineering.

Although the program represented progress in the formal training of investigators, not many participants actually received the Ph.D. degree, and some did not continue their careers in scientific research. Between 1957 and the end of the Harvey-Zierler training grant in 1976, sixty-four young physicians had received advanced training in the basic sciences, either through the training grant or with other funding.

The federal government's largesse raised ambivalent feelings throughout the university. President Milton Eisenhower was concerned that the "forced feeding" of research would lead to an imbalance in the activities of the medical school and hospital, to the detriment of teaching and patient care.[126] The School of Medicine needed to exercise closer surveillance and control over its own postdoctoral activities and a greater degree of autonomy in administering its own programs. In 1961, therefore, the university decided to remove the M.A. and Ph.D. degrees from the sole jurisdiction of the Faculty of Arts and Sciences and transfer it to a university-wide board, known as the Graduate Board. The Faculty of Arts and Sciences would still retain control over the basic policies in the award of these degrees, but the Graduate Board would carry forward the detailed arrangements. The counterpart of the Graduate Board in the medical school was the Committee on M.A. and Ph.D. Programs, which began as an *ad hoc* committee in 1963 and attained formal status the next year.

Extensive as these federal training grants were, the NIH considered them no more than a pilot effort. Recognizing that medical and graduate education had been kept in separate compartments in a way that served neither the education of the physician nor the purposes of medical re-

search, NIH director James A. Shannon devised and implemented far-reaching programs for the training of medical scientists.[127] As a result, a variety of grants were superseded in 1964 by the NIH's Medical Scientist Training Program (MSTP), for medical students who intended to obtain both medical and doctoral degrees.

Although Hopkins continued to receive other types of training grants, it was relatively late in perceiving the trend toward M.D.-Ph.D. training and was not able to modify its way of doing business sufficiently to obtain these federal dollars. The medical school committed itself to offering research training in 1968, when in deciding to increase the number of medical students, the Advisory Board mandated that M.D.-Ph.D. students make up 10 percent of each class. Yet Hopkins' first two applications for MSTP grants, in 1969 and 1971, were not funded. The school may have been hampered by its traditional adherence to the full-time system; although the NIH wanted a permanent program director in charge, Hopkins asked its existing department heads, who were already overburdened, to coordinate the M.D.-Ph.D. program. Most important, the NIH was looking for evidence of the school's commitment to training medical scientists—in particular, a director who would devote most of his academic time to the program—and a willingness on the part of the institution to use its own endowment dollars to support M.D.-Ph.D. students.[128]

Paul Talalay, who had recently relinquished the directorship of the Department of Pharmacology, took on the responsibility as "a sort of crusade." Like motherhood, Talalay has said, an M.D.-Ph.D. program was widely approved, but it was difficult to find someone who would accept the program as his major academic responsibility, as the NIH expected. Hopkins' third application convinced the NIH that the university would provide a hospitable and encouraging environment for this type of training, and in 1975 Hopkins' proposal for a Medical Scientist Training Program (MSTP) was accepted and funded. It has continued to enjoy high-priority funding and is one of the larger programs in the United States.

This grant enabled Hopkins to create an in-

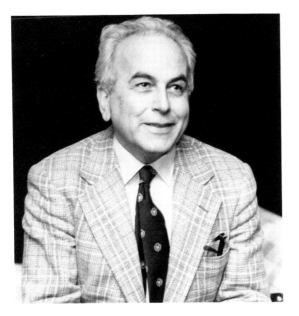

Paul Talalay. (*Source:* "W" Magazine, Women's Wear Daily, 11 April 1980.)

The inauguration of the NIH-financed Medical Scientist Training Program at Hopkins was not met at first with unqualified enthusiasm from the medical school community. Some believed that students should be admitted to the program no earlier than the third year of medical school, not as entering freshmen, since early bloomers did not always prove to be the best candidates. Clinical faculty members worried about "doctoral students mucking about in the clinics." Objections to the single-committee system for admissions reflected a perception of the M.D.-Ph.D. program as a special constituency. The temper of the times was also discouraging: the program was seen as an "elitist" endeavor, and the idea that these special students' full tuition throughout their training would be paid by the government met with disapproval.

A decade of experience seems to attest to the program's success. The M.D.-Ph.D. students have been characterized as extremely intelligent, and their ability to care for patients and their performance in the laboratory have both been superior. They are very much accepted as part of the student body and house staff. Furthermore, the number of M.D.-Ph.Ds on medical faculties is increasing dramatically.

Most M.D.-Ph.D. programs have had to adapt to vast changes since their inception. As the interests of the Departments of Physiological Chemistry, Microbiology, and Biophysics began to merge, their combined efforts formed the Program in Biochemistry and Molecular Biology (BCMB). These three departments were joined by the Department of Pharmacology and Experimental Therapeutics in 1976, the year in which the program also incorporated the doctoral program in microbiology/immunology. In 1978, the Department of Cell Biology and Anatomy joined the BCMB. Three years later, the Department of Neurosciences began to participate, dropping out in 1984 to form its own doctoral program. The five departments currently contributing to the BCMB are the Departments of Biological Chemistry, Biophysics, Cell Biology and Anatomy, Molecular Biology and Genetics, and Pharmacology and Molecular Sciences.

terdisciplinary program in which students would no longer be selected by and isolated in individual departments but would be exposed to the variety of the medical school's resources. Most joint-degree students are identified on admission to the medical school, but some are admitted to the program during the first two years of medical school. Initially, the Year V Program provided even more flexibility: some students were selected before receiving a bachelor's degree.

Twelve courses of study based in the School of Medicine are now offered to students in the MSTP: biophysics; cell biology and anatomy; physiological chemistry; molecular biology and genetics; neurosciences; biomedical engineering; physiology; history of medicine; pharmacology and experimental therapeutics; human genetics; immunology; and biochemistry, cellular and molecular biology. In the School of Hygiene and Public Health, the biochemistry and epidemiology departments sponsor joint-degree programs; and MSTP students can also obtain doctorates from the graduate departments of biology, chemistry, biophysics, the Carnegie Institute of Embryology, and the McCollum-Pratt Institute. In principle, a student can prepare his or her dissertation in any department, or even off-campus.

The M.D.-Ph.D. program has benefited from the enduring Hopkins tradition of decentralization. Programs have moved fluidly from department to department, school to school. Individual department heads have been free to alter or even eliminate programs that did not fit their professional viewpoint. Students can work toward the M.A. degree in medical illustration (a program begun in 1959) or in the history of medicine, the M.S. in clinical engineering, the Ph.D. degree, or both M.D. and Ph.D. degrees. Some departments (such as physiology) conduct only one doctoral program; others (such as biophysics) offer a doctorate only under the umbrella of an interdisciplinary effort (such as the Biochemistry, Cellular and Molecular Biology Program); still others (such as cell biology and anatomy) offer both types of doctoral programs. In sum, the MSTP has revitalized graduate training in the medical school.

Residency and Fellowship Training

Since the opening of the hospital and medical school, the residency and fellowship programs at Johns Hopkins have been intertwined with the education of medical students, and Hopkins' commitment to "learning by doing" has been manifest at the postgraduate level. Residents advanced through a graded period of training that ensured that they would assume appropriate levels of responsibility and master all the elements of caring for patients, and fellows spent years in the laboratory acquiring the knowledge and skill necessary for independent scientific investigation.

The residency and fellowship programs in the early years of the medical school were the basis of Johns Hopkins' success in training investigators and teachers to populate other developing universities. These postdoctoral physicians —both residents and fellows—bridged the gap between the faculty and the medical students, forming a continuum that connected the care of patients, the advancement of medical knowledge, and the perpetual education of all three groups. Some fellows became full-time bench scientists.

Others received clinical training in a specialized area of medicine or surgery while engaging in clinical investigation.

The School of Medicine perpetuated the fellowship arrangement already in use in the university's Faculty of Philosophy.[129] The university's fellowships were intended to give promising young graduate students a means for further study and an avenue to university careers in literature or science. In its first year, 1876, the university's fellowship program drew 152 applicants, of whom 107 fulfilled the eligibility requirements. To accommodate this unexpectedly large response, the trustees increased the number of fellowships from ten to twenty. For its part, the university would benefit from their presence, and Gilman intended to draw permanent members of the faculty from this group. His hope was soon fulfilled: three of the fellows in the early years— John J. Abel and William H. Howell (who worked with Martin), and Franklin P. Mall (who worked with Welch)—became the first professors of pharmacology, physiology, and anatomy, respectively, in the School of Medicine.

The medical school's policies toward scientific investigation emerged in meetings held in 1884 between Martin and the other two professors appointed to the founding faculty of the medical school, Ira Remsen and John Shaw Billings. While considering the organization and policies of the medical school, they emphasized the importance of encouraging research in what they called "the scientific branches of medicine," including pathology, pharmacology, anatomy and histology, and physiology.[130] Laboratories in these fields should be open to medical students, they said, as well as to those who wished to become experts in these sciences or to complete their professional education. Medical school graduates in particular should be admitted, and this group of students should receive fellowships for study.

Adapting Gilman's objectives to the medical institutions was John Shaw Billings, who specified that the medical institutions must do more than care for the sick and educate medical personnel. "In this country," he said, "it is too much the case that scientific and medical men who are qualified and have the desire to make original investigations, and thus increase our stock of knowledge, want either the means or time to do so."[131] No medical institution in the nation was offering appropriate opportunities for research, and Billings wanted Johns Hopkins to fill the gap.

Billings' vision of medical education entailed a significant financial commitment, as the cost of creating adequate facilities for research was substantial. Educating physicians to be original investigators required not simply textbooks and lectures but also well-equipped laboratories and professors whose training and views of medical education would enhance the university's goals. As he so clearly said in a lecture on medical education delivered at the Johns Hopkins University in 1877:

> I am of the opinion that the Diploma of Doctor of Medicine from this University should be restored to its old meaning,—that the holder is qualified to teach as well as to practice. I do not mean that full blown Professors are to be produced, but that the graduates shall be men who can when occasion demands tell what they know, and why or how they know it.[132]

The first medical fellows were trained in Welch's Pathological Laboratory (see chapter 1). Fellowships were given to graduate students who had displayed special talent in the study of any area of medicine or surgery. Their holders were not permitted to engage in the practice of medicine. The income of these fellowships provided either board or lodging in the hospital, for those who wanted to pursue clinical study, or an annual stipend for those who wanted to work in the laboratories and wards in order to become experts in pathology, medical jurisprudence, hygiene, and so forth.

By the time Lewellys F. Barker's clinical laboratories opened in 1905, the rationale for training fellows had expanded beyond Billings' wish to "increase our stock of knowledge." The technological excitement of the early twentieth century offered practical justification for fellowships. As Barker said,

Technology has demonstrated how necessary it is for the promotion of the industrial arts to secure investigators trained in the so-called "pure" sciences of physics, chemistry, and biology who will devote themselves to the application of the methods and principles of these sciences to the solution of the special problems by which those who wish to advance the industrial arts are confronted. One has only to recall the tremendous advances in metallurgy, in brewing, and in electrical engineering in the manufacture of arms and ammunition, in sugar refining, and in food preservation, to realize how fundamentally significant the interesting of men trained in pure science in the solution of so-called "practical problems" has been for the extension of knowledge and practice in more strictly utilitarian domains.[133]

The practitioners of these industrial arts saw "learning" and "doing" as separate endeavors, however. Mechanical engineering, for example, was marked by a struggle between "shop" and "school"—between proponents of on-the-job training and advocates of formal, technical education.[134] At Hopkins, in contrast, clinical and preclinical laboratories in the School of Medicine merged "learning" and "doing" into a harmonious whole.

Before the opening of the Johns Hopkins Hospital, opportunities for postinternship training in specialties had been essentially unknown in the United States, as postgraduate training facilities had been available only overseas. The clinical residencies inaugurated at Hopkins were analogous to the fellowships in the preclinical fields as well as to the earlier assistantships in the graduate school. A chief resident and a number of assistant residents were appointed in each of the services. The average length of training and other features differed somewhat among the services, but the total arrangement added up to a graduate school within the hospital. Moreover, residents enhanced the care of patients as well as the undergraduate educational program. Increasing specialization in practice required extensive training under expert supervision.

Medical Residencies

It was Osler who introduced the "graded residency" used by all three clinical services, medicine, surgery, and gynecology. Like the idea of fellowships in preclinical fields, the concept of prolonged periods of training in clinical services in a university-affiliated hospital originated in Germany, and Osler's recommendations for postgraduate training in medicine acknowledged his debt to the German system. He advocated using the title "first assistant" for physicians undertaking residency training and expressed the hope that the system would be successful enough to allow for "second assistants," as in the German clinics.[135]

The residents comprised a lower resident staff (interns appointed for a single year, usually on graduation with high standing from the medical school) and an upper resident staff (the resident physician and several assistant resident physicians). Members of the upper staff were usually former hospital interns who wanted to spend several years extending their training. They were chosen partly from the lower staff, but to prevent "inbreeding," new assistant residents were imported from other teaching hospitals. The position of chief resident physician carried large responsibilities and opportunities and was given only to physicians of exceptional ability, extensive experience, and great promise.

The residents, who were salaried, were carefully selected by the staff, with the approval of the Medical Board and the Board of Trustees. They were appointed annually, and their expected tenure was indefinite. As in the large German hospitals, these highly trained physicians remained as residents for several years (see chapter 9).

For residents, "learning by doing" included a large measure of autonomy—sometimes more than they wished. George Corner, a Johns Hopkins graduate and resident in gynecology, recalled a dramatic incident in the operating room:

One morning in the spring of 1915, Dr. Kelly had finished his own operations and had gone elsewhere in the hospital to visit the convalescents while the resident's team operated on a woman from a public ward. In spite of his skill, Neel [the resident in command of the operating room] found himself in trouble. The patient's internal condition was much worse than expected; Neel had a large task of excision and repair. Two hours went by, and the patient began to weaken. The anesthetist—that was my part in the team—found it necessary to warn Dr. Neel to hurry, but Neel could not hurry. The pulse became so weak and rapid that I could not count it. The usual precautions against shock, such as we had then, were instituted, and we all worked on in grim silence broken only by Neel's worried inquiries to me about the patient's condition and my doubtful replies. The students were getting restless in the stands. In short, we were almost dangerously rattled, when the door opened and in came Dr. Kelly. "How are you getting on?" he asked. "Badly," said Neel. "I'm afraid we're going to lose her; wouldn't you like to scrub up and help me?"—a suggestion that would have cost a precious ten minutes at least. By this time Dr. Kelly was behind Neel looking over his shoulder. "Oh, no," he said. "You are doing an excellent piece of work. I can't add anything. You have a hard job there, Doctor, but that's the way I'd do it myself."

He came to the head of the table and asked me about the pulse. "One hundred and eighty," I said, "the last time I could count it." "Yes," said Dr. Kelly, taking the pulse himself, "I can barely feel it. I see you're doing all the right things," and then to the students, "The doctor is giving a very nice anesthesia; you'd do well to study the chart afterward." I don't remember that he said anything more. He remained a quarter of an hour calmly watching us work and then paid Neel the best compliment of all: he went out of the operating room and disappeared, leaving behind him five young men who felt as if they had been knighted on the field of battle. If we were to lose our patient on the table, the chief was witness that we had made a valiant fight. But we did not lose her, and a month later she was well.[136]

The resident staff was a full-time group of enthusiastic young physicians, developing under ideal conditions. They were also an excellent work force, carrying out the routine of the wards, laboratories, and outpatient departments. The faculty were therefore free to plan, supervise, control, and teach.

The medical residents all worked on the

public wards until 1915, when the private service acquired its own resident staff. The public ("Osler") and private ("Marburg") residencies maintained the graded, pyramidal system instituted in 1897, and the Osler residency in particular offered unusual responsibility and accountability. Osler residents were supervised by the full-time staff, under the close direction of Warfield T. Longcope, head of the Department of Medicine from 1922 to 1946. Visiting physicians were drawn largely from the full-time staff, especially during periods when the full-time staff was large, before the Depression of the 1930s and before the depletion of the staff during World War II. During the 1950s and 1960s, the house staff was enlarged to accommodate the increased number of patients passing through the hospital and the development of specialized areas of medicine.

As the growth of medical specialties changed the practice of medicine, the Osler residency changed accordingly, adjusting to give its residents the best patient mix, exposure to faculty, and required degree of responsibility. The Osler house staff suffered from lack of exposure to the "part-time" faculty that admitted patients to the Marburg Service. They were also relatively isolated from the recently developed research specialty divisions in the Department of Medicine. After World War II, the spectrum of clinical problems seen among Osler patients was narrowed as an increasing number of patients chose admission to the private ward. A later consideration was the advent of health insurance, which permitted each patient to have his own physician. Furthermore, the character of the chief residency had changed. By the 1960s, administrative pressures kept the chief resident away from the bedside. The chief resident's job had always been hectic, but it had now become less personally satisfying and a less satisfactory preparation for a career in academic medicine.

In 1970 some alterations were made in the medical residency—including the combining of the Osler and Marburg Services—but a broad structural change was seen as the best solution. In 1975, the Osler Medical Service (incorporating both original services) was organized into four

firms, each headed for a two-year term by an assistant chief of service who held a junior faculty position in the medical school and a post on the active staff of the hospital. His ward staff at any one time consisted of two assistant residents and three interns (who also rotated to specialty units and to the Emergency Room). Each firm contained twenty-seven beds and an outpatient clinic. Each provided comprehensive and integrated care.[137] The fundamental structure of the Firm System was preserved when modifications were made in 1988 to accommodate to the increasing emphasis on experience in the ambulatory setting.

Surgical Residencies

The surgical residency instituted by William S. Halsted was unique in American surgery at the time.[138] It developed in parallel to the medical residency at Hopkins, and like Osler's program, its pyramidal aspects were derived from the German system. No one was guaranteed regular advancement from the bottom to the top of the staff, and there was harsh competition for the top position of "house surgeon." Only the best graduating medical students at Johns Hopkins were awarded surgical internships, and three of the best interns were invited to remain as assistant resident surgeons. Candidates from any part of the country were eligible for the positions as assistant residents, and one assistant resident was eventually chosen as house surgeon. In the final selection of the chief resident, Halsted emphasized originality, a capacity for independent thinking, a real interest in teaching others, and adequate surgical skill.

The chief resident worked closely with the professor throughout his tenure. This resident was responsible for the complete care of all the charity patients, helped to teach the rest of the house staff, and participated in research.

By 1904, Halsted's surgical staff consisted of eight interns and one extern. (The extern specialized in surgical pathology, attending operations that related to this primary interest.) The training of surgeons changed little at Johns

Hopkins over the next forty years. Even as recently as the 1950s, a description of the surgical training program at Hopkins could have applied to the program a generation before, as Mark Ravitch recalls:

The two most remarkable features of the Hopkins system as we knew it were the graded responsibility of the house officers and the near autonomy of the house service, with advice and supervision readily available. The graded responsibility was strict. We knew at each level what decisions we could make alone and which required confirmation or sanction. Elevation to the status of "the operator" was long delayed. I had been in a white suit seven years before I performed my first appendectomy and eight years before I performed my first cholecystectomy. We had assisted The Resident and the visiting staff so many, many times at operation after operation, that by the time we undertook the procedures on our own, it hardly seemed as if, in fact, we were so doing for the first time. Of course, people can be taught to operate skillfully in less time than that. We accepted the fact that we were expected to emerge as polished surgeons, prided ourselves on that, but took it for granted. The big point was that we would be mature, knowledgeable, experienced, and canny clinicians as well, and have a grounding in our profession that would permit us to grow in almost any direction.[139]

Before World War II, except in the most prestigious teaching hospitals, the majority of medical school graduates did not follow the internship year with full residency training. Although teaching hospitals were the location of choice for the few medical school graduates who pursued residency training, most graduates completed only a one- or two-year internship at a community or teaching hospital. Extended residencies did not become popular until after World War II, when physicians returned from the armed forces with an interest in specialty practice. By the mid-1960s, teaching hospitals dominated both internship and residency training and fellowship training in the subspecialties. In many teaching hospitals it became commonplace to continue with a subspecialty fellowship after completing two years of the formal residency program, and then return to complete the residency years.[140]

A few residents from the most prestigious teaching hospitals could fulfill their military obligation as public health officers at the National Institutes of Health. It was not uncommon for such physicians to spend more than the required two years at the NIH. They received superb training, and assignment to the NIH became an attractive pathway into academic medicine.

The Rediscovery of Educational Ideas

Although the principle of "learning by doing" has guided medical education at Hopkins throughout the School of Medicine's first hundred years, the phrase has nevertheless been subjected to a diversity of interpretations. With each curriculum revision, ideas have emerged, submerged, and re-emerged in new guises, as succeeding generations of faculty members have struggled with the pressures of presenting too much information in too little time.

The balance between formal lectures and experience on the wards and in the laboratories has shifted several times in the past century, not only at Hopkins but nationwide. Classroom work was the mainstay of medical education before the Hopkins medical school was founded. In the medical school's early years, lectures were deemphasized in favor of experience on the wards and in the laboratories—an attitude that subsequently spread throughout the country. More recently, teaching has shifted away from the bedside and back to the classroom. A recent survey of 136 teaching hospitals revealed that only 8 percent of teaching rounds were done at the bedside alone; most were conducted at both bedside and classroom, or in the classroom alone.[141] Among the house staff, most residents surveyed believed that morning report was of greater educational value than attending or teaching rounds, and that attending rounds were conducted too often and lasted too long—a vivid contrast to the attitudes of the earlier generations who developed their clinical skills at the bedside with a compassionate and skilled physician.

Elective courses have also fallen in and out of

favor over the past century. In 1927, the curriculum was perceived as overcrowded with obligatory studies, but four years later, when the number of required courses had been reduced to a minimum, many faculty members feared that students were not being given all the information they needed in an age of rapidly expanding medical knowledge. The cry for "relevance" during the 1960s and 1970s weighted the curriculum heavily toward elective courses again, as a curriculum tailored to the individual student's interests came into favor.

Related to the balance between elective and required courses is the choice between a general and a specialized education as a preparation for medical school. Here again, the preference of admissions boards has shifted over the years from applicants with particularly strong science backgrounds (who were favored in the 1950s) to those with a broad liberal education (who were selected for the Flex/Med Program of the 1980s).

Although methods have fallen in and out of favor, the goal of the Johns Hopkins University School of Medicine has remained the same over the past century: to train scholars of promise and compassionate physicians, graduates who will maintain the highest standards of research, education, and medical care. The conclusions of the most recent Curriculum Review Committee re-emphasized the educational principles on which the school was founded a century earlier. This fact makes the point forcefully: the founders planned well, and the wisdom of their decisions still finds welcome in the beginning of Hopkins' second century.

CHAPTER 8

FULL-TIME PROFESSORSHIPS

The turning point in medicine in this country which has given rise to our leadership stems beyond question from the introduction of the full-time principle, first in the basic sciences and then in the clinical departments. Yet the straining of the finances of medical schools by the inevitable growth of medical faculties and the mounting cost of research has resulted in an alarming distortion of the principle of full-time. Full-time is retained in a number of institutions in name, but in many of these it is retained in name alone. In many institutions the so-called full-time man devotes a highly significant portion of his working hours to the care of private patients either for the purpose of earning a large part of his own salary or, yet more dangerously, to amass funds to help pay salaries and defray costs even in the preclinical departments.

—Robert F. Loeb, 1959

The "full-time system" specified that physicians and scientists in a university school of medicine should devote their entire professional lives to the work of the university. The clinicians among them should not accept fees from private patients. The university should be the sole source of income for its faculty, and it should pay them well. This system was intended to free professors for teaching and investigative work, buying them time that is not available to physicians who must depend upon private practice, even in part, for their living.

These are the bare bones of the full-time plan. As Robert F. Loeb's statement implies, however, the system has been stretched over the years, as changing social circumstances have forced its reinterpretation. Its application to the preclinical sciences in the late nineteenth century was accepted gratefully by medical scientists, who no longer had to leave the laboratory to earn a living

wage. In contrast, the expansion of the full-time system to the clinical departments was problematic, as many practicing physicians felt that the university was benefiting at their expense. The Johns Hopkins University School of Medicine was the standard-bearer for the full-time system in both the preclinical and the clinical departments. Implemented at different medical schools in different ways, and at Hopkins in different ways at different times in different departments, the full-time system has touched on the most sensitive professional issues: time, money, and prestige.

The Full-Time System in the Preclinical Departments

The full-time system in medical schools began in Boston, in the 1870s, with one man, Henry Pickering Bowditch. A former student of Carl Ludwig in Germany, Bowditch was chosen by Harvard president Charles Eliot to establish the first university facility for experimental physiology at the Harvard Medical School. He accepted Eliot's offer on two conditions: that physiology be made a separate department, and that he be included in the group of leaders responsible for running the school's affairs. Unlike other medical school professors, who divided their time between clinical and laboratory pursuits, Bowditch was paid a salary to devote his full time to teaching and research.[1]

Bowditch's affiliation with Harvard was unique for the time. In medical schools of the mid–nineteenth century, the qualifications of teachers too often comprised, in Welch's words, "a few books and some oratorical gifts."[2] Most investigators were forced to subordinate laboratory work and instruction to medical practice. They relied upon income from patients to support their medical school activities, sometimes using this income to buy equipment and supplies. Their time in the laboratory was therefore fragmented, and they were distracted from both teaching and investigation. Bowditch's laboratory at Harvard was a small beginning, but it represented the professionalization of physiology in the United States, and, more important, the beginning of university support of full-time preclinical medical scientists.

Yet the idea of full-time basic scientists did not catch on immediately. Even after Bowditch's laboratory had been in existence for twenty years, most medical schools still relied on practicing physicians to teach the preclinical subjects. Moreover, any student who elected to train under Bowditch for a career in experimental physiology had to face the possibility of being greeted with indifference upon emerging from his laboratory. As William H. Welch wrote to his sister, "I was often asked in Germany how it is that no scientific work in medicine is done in this country, how it is that many good men who do well in Germany and show evident talent there are never heard of and never do any good work when they come back here. The answer is that there is no opportunity for, no appreciation of, no demand for that kind of work here."[3]

Although in 1893 a few full-time preclinical chairs existed in medical schools nationwide, Johns Hopkins was the first medical school in the United States to place all of its preclinical departments on a full-time basis. Led by Welch, the trustees of the university implemented a novel program that gave serious attention to all the basic sciences. Anatomy, physiology, pathology, bacteriology, pharmacology, and physiological chemistry were all taught by full-time scientists. In fact, the entire faculty of these departments was salaried, and the professors, associate professors, and instructors gave all their time to teaching and research.

The policy of staffing the preclinical departments entirely with full-time faculty was decided upon—and tested—long before the medical school opened. In 1884, when Billings and Gilman were selecting faculty members for the future medical school, they hoped to hire Matthew Hay, professor of medical jurisprudence at the University of Aberdeen in Scotland, as the professor of pharmacology. Hay wanted to have the opportunity to practice medicine in Baltimore and asked to be exempted from the full-time requirement, indicating that the care of private patients would be a desirable adjunct to his teaching. The Hopkins trustees, however, rejected Hay's request, stating, "Medical education in the United States now suffers from the fact that the chairs are almost always filled by practitioners and consequently the scientific work of the Schools of Medicine has been less efficient than it should be. It is thought best here to initiate our Medical School by appointing several teachers who shall not engage in practice." Hay accepted the decision, but he resigned, for undisclosed reasons, before coming to Hopkins.[4]

In 1893 the time was ripe to replace practicing physicians in preclinical departments with salaried teachers and investigators. Knowledge in the basic sciences was expanding, and the public was becoming interested in the potential of scientific medicine to cure disease. At Hopkins, these factors, and the efforts of a few men who appreciated the value of the German scientific approach to medical education, were combined to raise the standards of teaching. Welch was one who believed that the full-time system would open the way for academic careers after the German model: "that is, if young men who do good scientific work, who publish valuable results of original investigation, and who acquire a reputation among those who are competent to judge them, [could] look forward with some reasonable assurance to securing positions in our leading medical schools."[5]

Welch's hopes were realized, as this innovative policy set new standards for medical teachers across the nation. By 1910, enough positions were available in medical schools to accommodate most of the qualified scientists in the United States. Schools and medical practitioners had accepted the idea that the preclinical sciences should be taught by persons who devoted full time to their study, and reputable medical schools no longer used practitioners for this purpose. Medical science had advanced and was continuing to advance so rapidly, particularly in anatomy and physiology, that physicians who cared for patients were unable to remain competent as teachers of the preclinical sciences, and they were often relieved to relinquish these responsibilities. Replacing practicing physicians on basic science faculties were young medical scientists who did good scientific work, published valuable results of original investigations, and earned the respect of their peers.

Welch had lived through the lean years for the preclinical sciences, years in which well-trained instructors were few, and those who were well trained had either inadequate facilities to work with or no place to go. By the turn of the century, the preclinical sciences had prospered, but the clinical sciences were still undeveloped. In 1901, a preclinical scientist could "look forward with reasonable assurance to securing a desirable position as a teacher and a director of a laboratory of his special branch of science," said Welch, but "young physicians desiring corresponding careers in clinical medicine and surgery had to face the fact that, with few exceptions, American hospitals did not offer such opportunities for training; and, in addition, the prospect of securing a stable posi-

tion to carry on their work in clinical science was poor."[6]

Given the progress of experimental science in the United States at the time, some historians have viewed the growth of the full-time plan in the preclinical sciences as predictable.[7] Its spread to the clinical sciences was far more problematic and controversial.

Full-Time Professorships in the Clinical Departments

At the turn of the century, the increasing applicability of the preclinical sciences to the problems of disease in human beings made it apparent that clinical departments in medical schools would have to adopt a similar research orientation. Research was now seen as the key to improvement in the clinical departments, but clinical professors were generally chosen from among the local practitioners, and would-be clinical scientists could obtain important academic positions only if resignation or death created a vacancy in a medical school in the city where they practiced. Moreover, they had to be successful practitioners before they could anticipate any appointment at all. No one could obtain a clinical position through pursuit of the scientific side of medicine alone. Furthermore, the pay in the clinical departments was so low that staff had to support themselves by private practice, giving only a limited part of their time to medical school activities. Clinically trained individuals interested in research thus had to work for the most part in the laboratories of the preclinical departments. Education in the clinical departments suffered as a result.

The success of the full-time system in the preclinical sciences at Johns Hopkins encouraged the professors in those fields—particularly Welch and Franklin P. Mall—to consider implementing it in the clinical departments. It was Lewellys F. Barker, however, whose 1902 address to Hopkins alumni, "Medicine and the Universities," made the question of full-time professorships a national issue overnight.[8] Barker had been a member of both Osler's clinic and Welch's Pathological Laboratory and had then joined the faculty of Mall's anatomy department. Barker was a faculty member at the University of Chicago when he delivered this address, which formally set forth a plan for instituting the full-time system in the clinical departments.

A modern university must be a center of original research as well as a place of instruction, Barker said, "made up of a group of scholars who are not only familiar with the results of previous investigations, but who, endowed with unusual capacities and skilled in the methodology of their respective sciences, invade new territories, searching diligently for new facts."[9] Although Barker believed that the services of part-time faculty were also necessary, he thought that the greatest need was for full-time physicians and surgeons trained in physiology and pathology, who, after careful observation in the wards and over the operating table, would submit the ideas there gleaned to experimental tests in laboratories adjacent to the wards.[10]

The first two years of medical school had been redesigned to encourage scientific investigation, Barker pointed out, as instruction was offered by professors who gave their whole time to teaching and research. Students consequently obtained a thorough scientific training in those branches of science fundamental to clinical work. Now, he continued, students accustomed to the well-regulated work to the first two years of medical school were exposed to the unsystematic teaching of the clinical years. Courses were poorly coordinated within and between departments, and insufficient attention was given to the sequence of subjects. Worst of all, clinical professors were usually unaware of the modern work in anatomy, physiology, physiological chemistry, and pathology.

Welch agreed strongly: "The most urgent need in medical education at the present time in this country," he stated in an address at Harvard in 1906, "I believe to be the organization of our clinics both for teaching and for research in the spirit of this modern movement and with provision for as intimate prolonged, personal contact of the student with the subject of study as he finds in the laboratory."[11]

Flexibility in implementing the full-time system was crucial, Welch believed. Fixed rules would be harassing, improper, and unnecessary, he said.[12] Salaried clinicians could be allowed to act as consultants at the hospital and to admit a limited number of patients to the private wards. The admission of such patients would be determined mainly by the scientific interest of the clinician, and the professional fees derived from such patients would accrue to the hospital or the university. Some practitioners love to teach, Welch said, and it would be detrimental to the school to lose those who could give only a part of their time to instruction. Moreover, although the head of each clinical department should be a full-time professor, the number of salaried faculty members of lower rank could vary by department.

The clinical faculty themselves had serious doubts about the full-time system. "It is an experiment I would like very much to see tried," Osler wrote, "but not at the Johns Hopkins first. It might have been different if we had started so, but I do not believe there is any possibility for success at present."[13]

Yet Osler's reservations went beyond the mere logistics of instituting the full-time system at Hopkins. As a physician who emphasized the interpretation of the manifestations of disease rather than the experimental investigation of the underlying disease processes, Osler believed that pathology was the basic science of clinical medicine and that the other preclinical sciences should be left to their practitioners in the laboratory. His attitude may be partly attributed to the lack of adequate facilities for research, but it also reflected the precepts of the French physician P.-C.A. Louis, some of whose students had been Osler's colleagues, as well as the prevailing attitudes among physicians of the day. Like most of his colleagues in America, Osler did not fully appreciate the rapid progress of physiology and chemistry, nor did he recognize their potential to form the basis for important advances in clinical medicine.

His introduction of laboratory methods at the bedside was primarily for diagnostic, rather than investigative, purposes.

Nor did the full-time clinician fit Osler's view of the ideal physician. Osler feared that the full-time system would produce "clinical prigs,"[14] laboratory workers isolated from the surrounding medical community of practicing physicians; that these full-time faculty would be out of touch with the world of clinical practice—the world in which the young residents would eventually have to live; the worst of all, that under this system, the practice of medicine might eventually be taught by laboratory workers who lacked clinical experience.[15]

The financial aspects of the system also worried Osler. Small salaries might attract good men at first, but they would soon leave. Moreover, the salaries that the trustees would have to authorize for each professor would spell ruin for the hospital. In another of Osler's scenarios, the hospital would be converted into a sanitarium—a haven for the wealthy who were not seriously ill—and a large part of the professors' time would be taken up with earning money for the hospital from private patients.[16]

Other objections from the clinical faculty mirrored the opinions of many practicing physicians nationwide. The most obvious sticking point of the full-time system was money: accustomed to augmenting their medical school salaries with fees from their private patients, clinicians were loath to eliminate this source of income. The principles behind the idea, however, were also debated. In this great age of individualism in the United States, the practice of medicine was particularly entrenched as an individual endeavor, and associations of physicians, particular the American Medical Association, were determined to maintain the status quo. The idea of clinicians without a private practice was termed by some "unethical, immoral, and illegal."[17] Patients were entitled to a private physician who would be available to the patient at all times and in turn would be paid for his efforts. The community would suffer from the full-time system, which would siphon off good physicians from outside

practice. Moreover, these physicians were unlikely to maintain their expertise. Deprived of valuable experience in caring for patients, they would become too far removed from medical practice to remain good clinicians and teachers.

Paradoxically, although they would have left the community, the community would continue to seek them out. Once these full-time physicians were identified as academic leaders, they would be besieged by a public clamoring for care by the "best physician available." The full-time system would therefore promote a hierarchy of physicians, and many patients would insist on seeing only the head of the clinic, who would have less time available for the care of patients than before.

The main objection to the full-time system raised by faculty members was the alleged difficulty of obtaining the best individuals for the positions with the salaries that Johns Hopkins could afford. Welch saw this problem as serious but temporary. The first occupants of the full-time clinical chairs should be seasoned physicians, he believed, not young physicians, however promising they seemed to be. Young physicians would lack the clinical experience and the established reputations necessary to attract the best staff. Although this stipulation restricted the field of choice considerably at first, the full-time system would soon generate its own professors, Welch said. They would have grown up within the system, enjoying its benefits and accepting its salaries because they would not have become used to living on the scale of successful practitioners.[18]

Welch believed that the rest of the faculty's objections could also be overcome. Full-time faculty would see fewer patients than physicians in private practice, but they would also have the benefit of a capable and varied staff to assist them in caring for patients and carrying out research. The members of this staff—young associate professors, associates and assistants—would themselves be in training for higher positions in other schools. These young physicians would be the embodiment of Billings' goal: well-trained scientists who would take the Hopkins system to other institutions.

In sum, Welch thought that the advantages of the full-time system would outweigh its disadvantages. The system would place before students and the profession higher ideals of the mission of the physician and of his relation to the community. It would advance both the science and the art of medicine by training investigators, by making better physicians, and by contributing to useful knowledge. The full-time system, Welch said, would initiate reform in medical education "so far reaching as to constitute a new era."[19]

This new era was a long time in coming. The debate over clinical full-time professorships extended over the first two decades of the twentieth century. So intense were the feelings aroused that William S. Thayer suggested abandoning the expression entirely, substituting "university plan" as a term shorn of emotion and more reflective of the origins of the idea. The use of "university" as a synonym for "full-time" reflected the prevailing academic system: faculty members in nonmedical fields, for whom patient fees were irrelevant, derived their entire salaries from the university.[20]

Welch was in the middle of the controversy, an advocate of the full-time system who nevertheless had to contend with the objections of the clinical faculty. Even Welch had doubts about whether the plan could succeed, and Mall had to prop him up, as Florence R. Sabin recalled:

> I remember many a time when he [Mall] came into my laboratory somewhat discouraged, his saying that Welch had gone back on the idea of the full-time and he had to begin all over again on converting him. His phrase was then: "Well, Popsy has cold feet again and I have to start anew." He took literally years to convince Doctor Welch of the value and the feasibility of the plan and then was typically happy to have the plan associated with Doctor Welch's name, with himself staying in the background.[21]

The cause of the full-time system was advanced slightly when Osler left for England in 1905. His departure opened the way for a successor who would bring the perspective of a basic scientist to a clinical department. Lewellys F. Barker was such an individual, a man whose training spanned both the basic sciences and clinical medicine.

Barker's appointment as director of the Department of Medicine and physician-in-chief symbolized of the entrance of science into clinical medicine. The contrast between the two Canadians, Osler and Barker, was striking. Osler was a great physician and a preeminent teacher, but he was not an investigator, in the present-day sense of the word. His primary interest, the study of patients, could be carried over directly into the practice of medicine outside the hospital, and, because of his experience, skill, and personality, he was constantly in demand as a consultant to practicing physicians. Barker's concept of a professor of medicine was that of a teacher involved in research, whose primary interest would not be interrupted by medical practice outside his departmental activities.

Barker accepted the professorship of medicine at Hopkins with the hope that it would be a full-time position, but a sufficient endowment was not available to support his salary. Along with the negative attitude of many members of the clinical faculty, money was the major problem. A crucial barrier to implementing the full-time system, as Osler had forecast, was the expense of paying the salaries of the clinical staff. Although Barker himself could not be a full-time chief, he did sequester sufficient funds to create three full-time research divisions in his department (see chapter 2).

Welch knew that promotion of the full-time system would be useless as long as medical endowments remained meager. He therefore waited patiently for opportunities to strike in the interest of full-time appointments. An important chance appeared in 1908, when he helped to establish the Hospital of the Rockefeller Institute, which was organized on the full-time plan. He had been chairman of the institute's board of scientific directors, and helped to obtain Rufus I. Cole as the first director of Rockefeller Institute Hospital.

Cole was Hopkins-trained, and he came to his post at the Rockefeller Institute's hospital from Barker's Department of Medicine, where he had been full-time chief of the Biological Division. Cole arrived at the Rockefeller Institute in 1910, the same year that the Flexner Report was issued.

Talk of upgrading medical schools was in the air, and Cole foresaw that clinical departments would need professors who recognized the diagnosis and the treatment of disease as inseparable from their study in the laboratory. The paucity of such individuals was widely commented upon in the wake of Flexner's report. Many agreed that a university atmosphere was necessary to train future teachers and investigators. By replicating Barker's full-time system at the Hospital of the Rockefeller Institute, Cole was able to train clinical professors for the new era, individuals who were both skilled physicians and talented investigators. Organizations such as the Rockefeller Institute could not have flourished until improved medical schools furnished an adequate supply of graduates with research training.[22]

After the Flexner Report was published, the application of the full-time concept to clinical departments gained momentum. It could be a particularly American innovation, said William Henry Howell, then dean of the Johns Hopkins medical school: "The university school which shall first establish departments on this basis [full-time] may . . . secure both reputation and students as compared with schools organized on the present system. . . . Our country is in a peculiarly favorable position to make such an experiment. Our system of medical education has heretofore simply developed along lines laid down by the experience of foreign countries; perhaps in the direction suggested . . . we may have an opportunity to take the lead instead of trailing along in the rear."[23] Although preclinical departments in Germany were staffed by full-time professors, the full-time system had not been applied to clinical departments in Europe.

When many leading educators became convinced that the possibility of full-time clinical professorships was real, the debate became intense. Mall was not averse to using *ad hominem* arguments to support the full-time system. As he wrote to Charles Minot, "The problem would be easy if the pork barrel were removed. Its removal would no doubt remove the exploiting medical professor and open the way for the real university professor of medicine. We are told that medical

and surgical professors cannot take interest in medical problems and the sick unless they are paid for each move; that the sick man is not as conducive to real science as the dead or as a dog. It falls to us to demand of the last two years of medicine what they demanded of the first two and I think that the day of reckoning is at hand."[24]

The General Education Board's Endowment

The Rockefeller Foundation's General Education Board began to promote the full-time system for clinical departments soon after Flexner's report was released in 1910.[25] Hopkins was a natural place to institute the system, given Flexner's enthusiasm for the medical school and hospital, and medical education was a particular interest of Frederick T. Gates, Rockefeller's adviser. Gates sent Flexner to Baltimore to make a detailed study of what might be done there. Mall argued eloquently that all of the money that might be obtained from the board should be spent to place the heads of the clinical departments at Johns Hopkins on a full-time basis. Flexner's report to Gates presented several alternative plans, one of which included Mall's suggestion, along with an increase in the school's endowment and a reduction of its total enrollment to 250 students (a cut of 97 students).

Welch hoped to persuade Gates to fund a fourth alternative, a sort of pilot project. Clemens von Pirquet, professor of pediatrics at Johns Hopkins, had been offered the professorship of pediatrics in Breslau, but he was willing to remain in Baltimore if his appointment was placed on a full-time basis. Welch therefore asked the General Education Board for an endowment of $200,000 to support a full-time professorship of pediatrics. He and Gates fenced about the issue in a series of letters, Gates insisting that Welch provide him with an estimate of the cost of placing all the clinical chairs on a full-time basis, and Welch demurring, saying that cost was a "perplexing" question. Gates would not yield, and Welch's request for a full-time head of a single department was denied.[26]

Welch was reluctant to inaugurate the full-time system in all of Hopkins' clinical departments because the faculty did not unanimously support such a move. For the next two years, Welch worked behind the scenes, trying to generate a general agreement that would not require the imposition of the full-time system by force. The spirit and atmosphere at Johns Hopkins were so valuable, he felt, that they should not be damaged by unnecessary haste in such an important matter.

Finally, in 1913, Welch could write to the General Education Board that "the faculty of the medical school are fully convinced of the wisdom and necessity of commanding the entire time and devotion of a staff of teachers in the main clinical branches,"[27] and that the trustees of the university and hospital had authorized him to ask for funds to place the Departments of Medicine, Surgery, and Pediatrics on this basis. Two days later the board agreed to appropriate the money, specifying that the gift be named "the William H. Welch Endowment for Clinical Education and Research."

The Department of Medicine

Although the full-time plan went into effect immediately in the Departments of Surgery and Pediatrics, finding a full-time professor of medicine took longer. Barker, a fervent advocate of the full-time system ten years earlier, declined the post.[28] Barker had become enmired in the very situation that the full-time system was trying to prevent. In the decade since he arrived at Hopkins, Barker had built up such a large clinical practice (and such an elaborate way of life) that he could no longer consider a smaller income.

The responsibilities of a full-time professorship were too onerous for one person, said Barker. The head of a clinical department had to supervise

one, the practice of medicine . . . by which I mean the actual diagnosis and treatment of disease in the patients who enter the clinic; two, the teaching in the wards, in the dispensaries, and in the laborato-

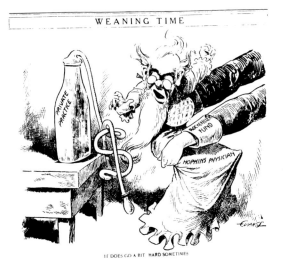

WEANING TIME

IT DOES GO A BIT HARD SOMETIMES

Cartoon printed in the *Baltimore American* on October 30, 1913. It is interesting that Lewellys F. Barker, who was an early champion of the idea of full-time status for clinical faculty but himself refused to take a full-time position, included this cartoon in his autobiography in 1942.

ries of (a) undergraduate medical students, (b) assistants and associates, (c) physicians taking postgraduate courses in the department; three, the prosecution, by professors, assistants and postgraduate students, of original "inquiries" in internal medicine, the search for new methods of diagnosing and treating disease, the attempt to advance our knowledge of the subject beyond its present boundaries. Four, the administrative duties, including the admissions, transfer and discharge of patients, interviews and correspondence with physicians who bring patients, and with the relatives and friends of the sick, the relations of the clinic to housekeeping and nursing, the maintenance of records and statistics, the arrangements for publication, the superintendence of budgets and expenditures, the making of appointments and promotions, the attendance on departmental and interdepartmental conferences, the formulation of curricula, the organization, equipment and running of the several clinical laboratories, the library, and the museum, the integration of departmental activities, the development of an esprit-de-corps, etc.[29]

As part-time chief, Barker had less time to spend on these administrative duties than he felt they deserved. As full-time chief, he said, he would not have the time to continue as a physician and an investigator unless part of the burden of running the department could be assumed by full-time assistants. Moreover, since the duties were so many and no one individual could assume them all, the directorship of the Department of Medicine should be divided.[30] Barker's version of the full-time system would have divided the responsibilities between two professors of equal status: a research professor, who would supervise the younger staff members and the postgraduate students, and a professor responsible for the care of patients and the instruction of medical students. The flexibility that Welch had attributed to the full-time system did not encompass this type of division, however, and Barker declined the post of full-time director, resigning from the Advisory Board as well. The board's next choice, William S. Thayer, a clinical professor of medicine, also declined the position.

The inauguration of the full-time system also led to a reconsideration of academic titles. As a result, the medical school faculty was divided into two parts. "University" staff, instructors who gave their entire professional time to the work of their departments, fit the standard definition of "full-time." "Clinical" staff, in contrast, were instructors engaged in private practice—part-time as opposed to full-time faculty. In the hospital, a similar distinction was made; there, part-time members were designated "visiting staff." (This distinction was abandoned in 1931.) Although Barker, Thayer, and Finney resigned from the Advisory Board of the medical school, they did not leave the Medical Board of the hospital. They remained on the hospital staff, and Barker accepted the title, "professor of clinical medicine."

After Barker and Thayer's rejections, the Advisory Board turned to Theodore Caldwell Janeway. In the spring of 1914, Janeway accepted the first full-time professorship of medicine. Janeway was the first of three men to fill the post of full-time professor of medicine between 1914 and 1946. His successors were William S. Thayer and Warfield T. Longcope. The differences in their backgrounds, expectations, and accomplishments

reflected the changes that took place in the full-time system over its first thirty years.

Theodore C. Janeway (1914–1917)

Theodore C. Janeway came to Hopkins from a professorship of medicine at the College of Physicians and Surgeons of Columbia University. Like Welch, he was a member of the board of scientific advisers of the Rockefeller Institute. The offer from Johns Hopkins was enticing to Janeway because he had found little time for experimental work as professor of medicine at Columbia. At Hopkins, in contrast, the medical clinic was organized in accord with his ideals for patient care, laboratory work, teaching, and investigation. It existed alongside similar clinics in other fields of medicine and surgery, and it was associated with strong departments in the preclinical sciences.

Janeway added other full-time members to the full-time and part-time faculty already in place within the Department of Medicine. Herman O. Mosenthal, who was interested in metabolic studies, was recruited as an associate professor in charge of the Chemical Division. Leonard G. Rowntree moved from the Department of Pharmacology to the Department of Medicine. Clyde G. Guthrie assumed directorship of the clinical laboratory, and Paul W. Clough joined the Biological Division after finishing his duties as resident physician. Arthur L. Bloomfield, later to become head of the Department of Medicine at the Stanford University Medical School, also became a full-time member of the Biological Division, as did Allen K. Krause, who had a special interest in tuberculosis. Janeway chose full-time staff members whom he expected to augment the research of the department, and indeed these men were responsible for a significant increase in research during his tenure.[31]

Janeway was not entirely in sympathy with Welch's version of the full-time plan, however.[32] Despite Welch's intention to avoid rigid rules, Janeway felt that the full-time system at Hopkins was too strict. Janeway's main disagreement with

Welch centered on the payment of fees to physicians. Janeway had himself been an unpaid instructor, a professor giving part of his time to consulting practice, and a well-paid full-time teacher. He could speak from personal experience, saying that a university professor in a medical school must give more time than any of his university colleagues to routine duties, to keeping up with an enormous literature, and to doing research work. For him to earn any considerable part of his own living by private practice is manifestly impossible. "But as well say that he must not be a good musician, or a devotee of chess, as to insist that he must never sharpen his wits on a case that has puzzled some physician outside the hospital who wishes his help." If he is to serve the profession, Janeway said, "it is unnatural and repugnant to a patient's sense of judgement that he should not receive the usual fee for such service."[33] Welch, on the other hand, believed that such fees should be turned over to the medical school.

Shortly after coming to Johns Hopkins, Janeway proposed his own version of the full-time system. It resembled the plan in effect in specifying that:

1. Clinical teachers should be chosen for the same qualities that governed choices for other university positions, absolutely without geographical limitation.

2. Adequate facilities for laboratory investigation should go hand in hand with clinical training for every member of the department staff.

3. Salaries should be sufficiently ample to make outside practice unnecessary, especially for the younger faculty who show ability as investigators. Salaries should also be proportional to the time given to teaching and research.[34]

Janeway's plan emphasized that every member of the staff should be given full freedom to develop into practitioner, consultant, teacher, or investigator, as best suited his or her individual talents. Original appointment, reappointment, and promotion should be made on the basis of true university accomplishment. Moreover, all appointments of clinical teachers should be term appointments,

Janeway said; not even professors should hold lifetime chairs.

The widest variety of interests would create the strongest department, Janeway believed, and physicians of varied interests could not be produced by any single type of training. Outside professional engagements, therefore, seemed desirable for most members of medical faculties at some period of their careers, and clinical teachers who engaged in some outside practice would be valuable to any scheme of medical education. "Uniformity of environment is not the distinctive feature of the university," Janeway said, "but unity of purpose."[35]

Janeway's modifications to the full-time system derived from his view of the hospital clinic as a monopoly, put into the hands of the professor, that contained the potential of exploitation for private gain. Life tenure for the nonmedical university professor is appropriate, he pointed out, because the older he grows in the university service and the more valuable is his devotion to his subject, the less capable he becomes of earning his living in any other way. The professor of medicine, on the other hand, is ever more able to command increasing fees. "The more illustrious he becomes, as the university should wish him to become, the greater is his potential earning power."[36]

Despite his conflict of opinion with Welch, Janeway still believed in the predominant importance of developing new knowledge within clinical departments, and the university's responsibility to nurture and encourage faculty fully engaged in such work. One hears echoes of Barker and Osler in his recommendations, but they are also not really incompatible with Welch's more stringent vision of the full-time system.

Janeway was, however, not happy in his transformation from active New York consultant and teacher to full-time university professor. Refraining from private practice as required by the full-time system created financial hardship, but equally important, Janeway was both a member of the first generation of full-time clinicians and a product of the old system. He began his career in

Baltimore during the heyday of the clinician—a time when, in one physician's description,

> physical signs were collected with less interest in their relevancy than in the virtuosity by which they were obtained. Elegance was the keynote of percussion; in vain did I try to develop the graceful wrist action that would have been more appropriate to Paderewski's piano playing. It was not sporting to look at a chest x-ray until the patient had been worn out by a tiresome period of physical diagnosis, and much time was spent on estimating the blood pressure by palpation before the sphygmomanometer was applied, although the inaccuracy of palpation had long since been proved. As I look back, I realize that it was a misuse of elegance to draw a clef and place the heart murmurs on it in absolute pitch.[37]

Janeway's scientific approach was thus not always matched by a sympathetic environment, and by 1917, a mere three years after arriving in Baltimore, he announced his intention to resign his professorship to return to New York. Before the university could act upon his formal resignation, Janeway died suddenly from pneumonia.

Although his tenure at Johns Hopkins was brief, Janeway gained the respect and esteem of his colleagues. He helped to plan a new building, the Hunterian Laboratory for experimental surgery and medicine (Hunterian II), improved the facilities for metabolic studies, fostered research in the heart station, and secured a substantial increase in the endowment for experimental studies in tuberculosis, known as the Kenneth Dow Fund. The medical department and the medical division of the hospital, with its wards, dispensaries, and classrooms, constituted a considerable administrative problem, which Janeway handled adroitly.

William Sydney Thayer (1917–1921)

William S. Thayer had refused the directorship of the Department of Medicine in 1914. When it was offered to him again three years later, he accepted reluctantly. At the age of fifty-seven, he felt that, in the Hopkins tradition, the post should belong to a younger man.

Not until 1919 did Thayer take up the post of director, for during World War I, he served as chief medical consultant to the American Expeditionary Forces in France. The full-time plan at Hopkins was temporarily in abeyance during the war, and the medical department was directed by a part-time physician, Louis Hamman.

In contrast to Barker's view of the departmental structure, Thayer envisioned a traditional pyramidal structure: a single director in charge, with a corps of associates and assistants under him.[38] Like Barker, however, Thayer felt that the administrative responsibilities of the departmental and divisional directors would not allow them time to conduct a private practice, although ideally, all would have clinical duties. Not only would it be impossible for any physician with a consulting practice to organize and direct a university medical clinic—but also, under the system Thayer outlined, consultants, practitioners, and professors would each be a separate group of physicians.

The training of these groups should nevertheless be identical, Thayer believed. Long service in institutions offering opportunities for study and research would give them valuable experience with modern methods of diagnosis and treatment, and they would efficiently accumulate the clinical experience that could be acquired only after a much longer time in independent practice. Furthermore, as the number of aspirants exceeded the number of professorships, those who were not offered a professorial post would nevertheless be well equipped to enter the practice of medicine or surgery as consultants. For those with an interest in research, a considerable number of assistantships should be available, offering salaries sufficient to enable them to continue their work for many years.[39]

Thayer retained the departmental organization already in place at Hopkins. He proved to have a talent for identifying outstanding physicians early in their careers, expanding the full-time staff with such physicians as Dana Atchley, Robert F. Loeb, Alphonse R. Dochez, William S. Ladd, George A. Harrop, Jr., Henry Jackson, Jr., and W. W. Palmer. Yet these new faculty members met with hostility from the part-time faculty, who remained an important power during Thayer's regime. The part-time clinicians were for the most part strongly opposed to the full-time system. Their hostility was directed at the new arrivals, however, rather than against Thayer, who had been one of them—a part-time clinician himself—before assuming the professorship of medicine.

So strained was the atmosphere for the full-time staff that when W. W. Palmer received offers to direct the departments of medicine at Yale, Michigan, Harvard, and Columbia, he was inclined to leave Baltimore. Thayer had already decided to resign, and Hopkins countered by offering Palmer the directorship of the Department of Medicine in 1921. Palmer nevertheless declined the offer, accepting the directorship of the Department of Medicine at Columbia instead. He took to New York a large segment of the outstanding young talent that Thayer had assembled, including Atchley, Loeb, Dochez, and Harrop.[40]

The department needed a temporary leader while it regrouped. George Canby Robinson, a 1903 graduate of the School of Medicine, was asked to serve as the chief of medicine for a year. Robinson was waiting to assume a full-time position as dean and professor of medicine at Vanderbilt University, but he was spending time in the laboratory at Hopkins while waiting for the completion of Vanderbilt's new buildings (see chapter 9). The post at Hopkins was considered excellent preparation for his new position at Vanderbilt, and Robinson accepted the offer.[41]

To fill the vacancies in the department's full-time ranks, Robinson recruited Alan M. Chesney from Washington University and William S. McCann from Cornell Medical College. Both men continued their careers within the full-time system: Chesney remained at Hopkins to become director of the medical clinic's experimental research laboratory for syphilis, and later dean of the medical school; and McCann became professor of medicine at the University of Rochester's new medical school.

By March 1922, the Advisory Board had found a new professor of medicine, Warfield The-obald Longcope, who assumed his duties four months later.

Warfield Theobald Longcope (1922–1946)

Barker had instituted full-time research laboratories, but his tenure antedated the full-time system in clinical departments. The tenures of Janeway and Thayer were relatively short. Because Longcope retained the directorship for twenty-four years, he was the first full-time professor of medicine with the opportunity to make vigorous changes in the department.

Longcope presided over five full-time divisions. To Barker's original three clinical laboratories, Janeway had added the tuberculosis research unit (directed by Allen K. Krause), and Robinson had added the syphilis division (under Alan M. Chesney). Without the unique link between hospital and medical school, it would have been difficult to finance five full-time laboratory chiefs. Because these chiefs were responsible for the corresponding routine diagnostic laboratories of the hospital, however, the hospital paid a portion of their salaries, and the combined amount from hospital and medical school was sufficient to keep the divisions on a full-time basis. The five clinical laboratories were run by full-time associate professors, each of whom was responsible for a clinic service. In addition to their ward responsibilities, each associate professor not only directed the clinical diagnostic laboratory related to his field but also conducted research in his specialty area.

Besides laboratory technicians, each associate professor had at least one instructor or fellow to assist him. The resident and one assistant resident worked especially closely with the professor, whereas each of the other assistant residents conducted his work under the supervision of the associate professor to whose ward he was assigned. Longcope gave the resident and the assistant great responsibility on the medical ward, but at the same time, they had the opportunity to carry on clinical investigation under the direction of an experienced physician.

In an era of rapid advance in medical research, specialization was on the rise. Barker's original three full-time divisions were transformed: the Physiological Division became the cardiovascular division, the Chemical Division was expanded to become the division of endocrinology and metabolism, and the Biological Division became the division of infectious diseases.

The later eminence of the faculty members whom Longcope recruited to staff these laboratories attests to the success of the full-time system. Many became notable investigators, and those who left spread the full-time system to other medical schools. Maxwell M. Wintrobe's work in hematology was largely responsible for the rapid growth of the field. Arthur L. Bloomfield led the Biological Division; when he left to become professor of medicine at Stanford, the division was placed under the direction of Harold L. Amoss. When Amoss left to become professor of medicine at Duke University, William S. Tillett took charge and performed the work that led to his discovery of streptokinase. In 1937, Tillett left Johns Hopkins to head a department at New York University. His successor as head of the Biological Division was no less sterling an investigator: Perrin H. Long, well known for his pioneer work on the sulfonamides. Long later became head of the Department of Medicine at the newly organized State University of New York, Downstate Medical Center in Brooklyn.[42]

As in the past, part-time staff dominated the activities of the outpatient department and contributed their expertise to consultations on the wards. By the 1930s, the conflict between part- and full-time staff had largely abated. Johns Hopkins erased the formal distinction in its catalog by dropping the designation "clinical" for part-time staff—a term that many had seen as connoting "second-class citizenship." The improved relationship between the full- and part-time staff reflected the final acceptance of the full-time system at Johns Hopkins, as the part-time staff realized that their place was secure.

The expression of the full-time system in the Department of Medicine changed little during the tenures of Janeway, Thayer, and Longcope. The primary changes were the growing ease of obtaining well-trained full-time investigators, and the

narrowing of these researchers' investigative targets—both effects related to the growth of medical subspecialties in the 1920s, 1930s, and 1940s. All these trends would accelerate during the years after World War II.

A. McGehee Harvey (1946–1973)

By the postwar years, there were a substantial number of well-trained physician-scientists available for export, and an equal number of positions available to receive them. Although the full-time system had been initiated in the preclinical departments earlier than in the clinical departments, by the late 1930s the clinical departments at Hopkins were growing faster than their preclinical counterparts. Enterprising members of the clinical faculty were acquiring research funds and training grants from outside the university and using income from patient care to establish formal, full-time specialty divisions in their departments.

Rapid scientific advances had greatly increased the medical profession's knowledge about certain areas of internal medicine, making it desirable to expand the Department of Medicine's facilities for research and specialty training. During Harvey's directorship, new full-time divisions joined the three major full-time divisions already in place.

The creation of additional full-time specialty divisions coincided with the federal government's growing interest in the support of medical research and training after World War II, and the divisions developed in parallel to the categorical institutes of the National Institutes of Health (NIH). With grants from the NIH and private foundations, new divisions of gastroenterology, clinical pharmacology, pulmonary disease, allergy and immunology, oncology, arthritis, medical genetics (see chapter 11), biomedical engineering, and renal disease sprang up at Johns Hopkins in the two decades following the war. A division of psychiatry in medicine had been envisioned by Barker but never came to fruition because of a lack of funds. In 1946, Harvey and John Whitehorn, director of the Department of Psychiatry, established this division jointly with a grant from the Commonwealth Fund and placed Theodore Lidz in charge. In addition, the Department of Medicine was successful in obtaining NIH funds to establish a Clinical Research Center, under the direction of W. Gordon Walker, on the fifth floor of the Osler Building. Here were housed patients who were participants in any of the numerous clinical research programs.

The foundation of the new full-time specialty divisions was already in place. Full-time faculty members with a particular specialty interest were in charge of the hospital's routine diagnostic laboratories, which were divided along divisional lines. Similarly, part- and full-time faculty headed the several specialty clinics in the outpatient department. The hospital paid a substantial portion of the salary of these laboratory directors, who were also the directors of the corresponding medical subdivisions. Part-time staff members, who concentrated on clinical work rather than laboratory investigation, found patients for their clinical research in the outpatient department and through the diagnostic laboratories, and grants from pharmaceutical firms as well as federal funds augmented laboratory research in the specialty divisions.

A. McGehee Harvey began the process of reorganizing for the postwar years even before he formally assumed the directorship of medicine. Many of the faculty members he recruited later became leaders and staff members of the department's subdivisions (for example, C. Lockard Conley in hematology). Other subdivision leaders were chosen from part-time faculty already in place: an example was John Eager Howard, who became full-time head of the Endocrinology and Metabolism Division (originally the Chemical Division). The majority of division heads, however, had grown up in the department either as members of the resident staff or as research fellows.

Specialization in the Department of Medicine was accompanied by continuing collaboration among the new divisions, and full-time status gave division heads time to pursue this type of research. When separate divisions of cardiovascular and pulmonary medicine were formed, the faculty members of the two divisions continued to work closely together. Subsequently, when Joseph L. Lilienthal, the first head of the Pulmonary Division, became director of the Department of Environmental Medicine in the School of Hygiene and Public Health, he inaugurated a close relationship between his new department and the Department of Medicine's Pulmonary Division, which he continued to direct. As head of environmental medicine, Lilienthal acquired the funds to recruit Richard L. Riley, an outstanding pulmonary physician and respiratory physiologist.

During the 1950s, it became imperative to carve out full-time divisons in medicine at Hopkins that could develop knowledge in specialties unknown a decade earlier. Money, mainly in the form of training grants and NIH awards, was available during this time to create these full-time divisions and to equip existing divisions with the newest technology. The availability of faculty members in these growing specialty areas also ensured high-quality medical care of the patients referred to the hospital by their primary physicians.

The Cardiovascular Division (Physiological Division)   Under the full-time system, the Cardiovascular Division has enjoyed a succession of strong leaders. Head of the division when Harvey became chief of medicine was Elliot V. Newman, a distinguished investigator whose particular interest was renal physiology. Newman had succeeded Edward P. Carter as head of this division after World War II. When Newman left in 1952 for a professorship at Vanderbilt, the heart station came under the direction of E. Cowles Andrus, a long-time distinguished faculty member. Working with him was William Milnor, who took over the division when Andrus retired. When Milnor moved his primary activities to the Department of Physiology in 1959, Richard S. Ross was appointed the division's director.

The centerpiece of the division was a state-of-the-art laboratory. Early in Ross's tenure, Harvey obtained 15,000 British pounds (then about $50,000) from the Wellcome Trust to build a research-oriented catheterization and hemodynamics laboratory at Johns Hopkins. This laboratory replaced the first catheterization laboratory, which had been organized by Richard Bing soon after the Blalock-Taussig operation became an established procedure (see chapter 11). The Wellcome Research Laboratory collaborated with the Department of Radiology; and Russell H. Morgan, director of radiology, developed much of its innovative equipment. Through its first seven years, the Wellcome Research Laboratory was the center of the Cardiovascular Division's research, emphasizing cineangiographic studies in valvular, congenital, and ischemic heart disease. A particularly active member of the staff during these years was J. Michael Criley, who used angiographic techniques to investigate the physiologic basis of physical findings, particularly the pathophysiology of hypertrophic cardiomyopathy.

A major project of the Wellcome Laboratory was an investigation of ischemic heart disease, directed by Gottlieb C. Friesinger. Friesinger had joined the faculty after his chief residency in medicine in 1962–63. A graduate of the School of Medicine, Friesinger remained at Hopkins until 1971, when he became director of the Division of Cardiology at Vanderbilt Medical School. In the Wellcome Laboratory, Friesinger developed the so-called selective injection method for the measurement of myocardial blood flow. Radioactive gas was injected into the coronary arteries, and myocardial blood flow was measured by monitoring the rate of disappearance of radioactivity with a detector positioned over the chest—a technique particularly useful in studies of drug action.

During the 1960s, the division became known for its excellence in clinical teaching through the efforts of such full-time faculty as J. O'Neal Humphries and Nicholas Fortuin. Humphries returned from clinical training in London in 1961 and built a strong clinical cardiology service, and Fortuin, a member of the division since 1971, developed the division's capabilities in echocardiography.

A second large laboratory, the Peter Belfer Laboratory for Myocardial Research, which opened in 1972, enhanced the division's research

capabilities. Myron L. Weisfeldt, a 1965 graduate of the Johns Hopkins medical school, was recruited from the Massachusetts General Hospital to head this laboratory, which became heavily engaged in basic studies of the isolated heart and papillary muscle preparations. Ross became dean of the medical faculty in 1975, and Weisfeldt was appointed head of the division the following year.

The Gastroenterology Division The harbinger of the full-time Gastroenterology Division at Johns Hopkins was a modestly funded effort that placed Sherman M. Mellinkoff in charge of the gastroenterology clinic in 1953. After completing his assistant residency at Johns Hopkins, Mellinkoff spent a year in Philadelphia, studying gastroenterology with Grier Miller. Mellinkoff became a full-time member of the Department of Medicine after completing his year as chief medical resident, and began to make rounds and establish a consultation service in gastroenterology.

When Mellinkoff departed for the University of California at Los Angeles in 1954, the department invoked Halsted's tradition of selecting a promising young physician to organize a new medical specialty, and Thomas R. Hendrix was chosen to develop a full-time Gastroenterology Division. Shortly after his appointment in 1954, Hendrix left for Boston for further training with Franz Ingelfinger, who had what was generally considered the best training program in gastroenterology at the time.

Ties with Sinai Hospital, one of many hospitals in Baltimore affiliated with Hopkins, facilitated the division's development. In Hendrix's absence, the Gastroenterology Division was run by Albert Mendeloff, full-time chief of medicine at the Sinai Hospital, then still adjoining the Johns Hopkins Hospital lot. Mendeloff had only to cross the street to work in his two laboratories in the Carnegie Building. During the mid-1950s, he began to conduct gastroenterology rounds on the Osler Service and to supervise the teaching of gastrointestinal pathophysiology to the second-year medical students.

Hendrix returned to Johns Hopkins in 1957.

In that year, his division received one of the first NIH training grants given in gastroenterology, enabling the new division to buy equipment and support fellows in training. Hendrix and Mendeloff ran the division jointly for the next six years. Even when the Sinai Hospital moved to a new location, more distant from Johns Hopkins, this collaboration continued. Mendeloff established a full-time research division at Sinai Hospital, and David Turner and his successor, Padmanabhan P. Nair, obtained funds from the NIH to support a lipid laboratory specializing in the methodology of investigating bile acids. The NIH funded the laboratory as a national training facility, and during its four years of existence, it provided instruction for more than 200 scientists from around the world. Mendeloff was also an associate in epidemiology at the School of Hygiene and Public Health, and principal investigator for research studies concerned with the epidemiology of inflammatory bowel disease and of cirrhosis of the liver. His joint appointment facilitated collaborative work in gastroenterology at both schools.

In 1988, Hendrix was succeeded as head of the Gastroenterology Division by Mark Donowitz.

The Divisions of Infectious Diseases, Allergy and Clinical Immunology, and Rheumatology Like the other divisions in the Department of Medicine, the Biological Division organized by Rufus Cole was expanded after World War II. Full-time faculty members George S. Mirick and Frederik B. Bang shared the directorship of the division, renamed the Division of Infectious Diseases, until 1953, when Bang was appointed professor of pathobiology in the School of Hygiene and Public Health. Ivan L. Bennett succeeded Mirick in 1954, when Mirick became the first full-time chief of medicine at the Baltimore City Hospitals.

After 1958, the division had a series of directors as its leaders moved rapidly on to higher positions. When Bennett became professor of pathology in 1958, he was succeeded by Leighton E. Cluff, who remained in charge until 1966, when he became head of the Department of Medicine at

the University of Florida at Gainesville. Cluff was succeeded by C. C. J. Carpenter, and in 1970, William B. Greenough became the division's head. The present director, John G. Bartlett, assumed the post in 1980.

Full-time faculty members Philip S. Norman and Lawrence M. Lichtenstein were particularly interested in hypersensitivity and allergy. During the 1950s, they developed this interest into a new full-time specialty, the Allergy and Clinical Immunology Division. As with medical specialties carved out previously, ties with another Baltimore hospital facilitated the development of this division. The Good Samaritan Hospital offered adequate space for research laboratories and clinical inpatient services for this specialty, and Norman and Lichtenstein developed an integrated program linked with the Department of Medicine on the East Baltimore campus.

The Department of Medicine also established a full-time connective tissue disease division in 1955, headed by Lawrence E. Shulman. Charles Wainwright remained in charge of the outpatient rheumatology clinic, but Shulman set up a special rheumatology clinic within the Moore Clinic. Mary Betty Stevens joined Shulman in the new division on a full-time basis. A training grant and several NIH research grants enabled them to enlarge the program and, like the Division of Allergy and Clinical Immunology, it was given additional space for research laboratories and an inpatient clinical service at the Good Samaritan Hospital. The Rheumatology Division was well entrenched by 1975, when Shulman left to join the National Institutes of Health and Stevens succeeded him as director of the program. The current directors are Douglas T. Fearon and David B. Hellmann.

The Renal Division The Renal Division was begun in 1957 by W. Gordon Walker, who had just completed his chief residency in medicine. The following year, chief of medicine A. McGehee Harvey diverted a generous gift for the department to the new division, enabling it to acquire one of the first hemodialyzers. By 1967, the division had helped to create a state-wide program that would provide funding for dialysis patients and license dialysis facilities. The Hopkins dialysis program also served as the model for a national program established three years later.

In cooperation with the Department of Surgery, the Renal Division developed a program that combined dialysis and transplantation. George Zuidema, head of surgery, helped Walker to obtain funds to open the first routine dialysis unit in the hospital, but it had only two stations and no room for expansion. An agreement with Good Samaritan Hospital allowed Hopkins to create a ten-station dialysis unit there—a very large unit for the time. The arrangement and the financial support that it provided allowed Hopkins to expand its dialysis facilities, increase the number of beds for patients with kidney disease, support the division's research activities, and recruit a full-time surgical staff. This staff included G. Melville Williams, a vascular and transplant surgeon who arrived in 1970.

Walker also obtained a federal grant for what turned out to be the first clinical research center in the country—a facility that was essentially an extension of the Metabolic Ward on Osler 5, which had been in existence since the 1930s and whose staff had included such notable physicians as John Eager Howard and George Thorn.

With the help of Louise Cavagnaro, vice-president of the Johns Hopkins Hospital, a regional, and then a nationwide program was established to oversee the harvesting of potential kidneys for transplantation. The federal government assumed the laboratory costs of tissue typing, and under the direction of Wilma Bias, the tissue-typing laboratory at Hopkins has played a central role in the development of the renal transplantation program.

Victor A. McKusick (1973–1985)

In considering a successor to A. McGehee Harvey in 1972, the search committee identified immunology and genetics as particularly important areas of medical research for the last quarter of the twentieth century. Its final choice was Victor A. McKusick, who combined an interest in medical genetics (see chapter 11) with broad competence

in clinical medicine. McKusick had spent his entire medical career at Johns Hopkins, graduating in the Class of 1946 and serving as resident physician under Harvey.

The divisional structure of the Department of Medicine changed little during McKusick's tenure. The Division of Internal Medicine was formally activated, with McKusick as its first head. Later, Philip A. Tumulty and then Craig R. Smith became its directors. An informal division of geriatric medicine was created in 1981 when William R. Hazzard was recruited as associate director of the Department of Medicine and associate physician-in-chief of the Johns Hopkins Hospital. Hazzard's mandate was to establish a university-wide program in gerontology and geriatric medicine, based at the Baltimore City Hospitals (later Francis Scott Key Medical Center). When Hazzard assumed the chairmanship of the Department of Medicine at the Bowman Gray School of Medicine, he left a strong program, which was carried on by John R. Burton and others.

Cross-departmental professional alliances were a conspicuous development during McKusick's tenure. The Oncology Center, which came to function virtually as a separate department, included faculty members from both clinical departments (medicine, pediatrics, surgery, and radiology) and preclinical ones (pharmacology). Cardiology developed a strong cross-departmental program based in contiguous facilities on the fifth floor of the Carnegie, Blalock, Halsted, and Children's Center buildings. Gastroenterology was allied with gastrointestinal surgery under John L. Cameron; its link with radiology is illustrated by the development of the Swallowing Center by Martin W. Donner and Thomas R. Hendrix.

McKusick also expanded the purview of some divisions; for example, the Pulmonary Division assumed responsibility for the medical intensive care unit and became identified with critical care medicine.

When McKusick announced his intention to step down, several major divisions of the department needed new heads. It was decided to allow McKusick's successor to fill these important posts. The final selection for the directorship of the Department of Medicine was John D. Stobo, an outstanding immunologist-physician who was chief resident during A. McGehee Harvey's last year as director in 1972–73.

John D. Stobo (1985–   )

John D. Stobo returned to Hopkins after nine years as chief of rheumatology and immunology at the University of California, San Francisco. In recruiting new division heads, Stobo reintroduced a principle espoused by Lewellys F. Barker when he was director of the department of medicine (see chapter 2): Stobo split the responsibility for the division in two. Research became the province of the division's director; clinical medicine and teaching the responsibility of the associate director. Exceptional credentials in research thus were the first and leading criterion in selecting a new division director; outstanding clinical competence and excellence in teaching were most important in choosing the associate director. The Rheumatology Division, for example, has had as its director since 1986 Douglas T. Fearon, a distinguished immunologist, and as its clinical director, David B. Hellmann. Mark Donowitz became director of the Division of Gastroenterology in 1988, and Theodore M. Bayless is its clinical director.

The Department of Medicine now comprises twelve divisions, three of which are shared with other departments. Those not previously mentioned are: the Endocrinology and Metabolism Division (Simeon Margolis, acting director; Paul W. Ladenson, clinical director), the Geriatric Medicine Division (John R. Burton, acting director), the Hematology Division (Jerry L. Spivak, director), the Internal Medicine Division (David M. Levine, director), the Medical Genetics Division (Victor A. McKusick, acting director), the Nephrology Division (Joseph S. Handler, director), the Cardiology Division (Myron L. Weisfeldt, director; Stephen C. Achuff, clinical director) the Infectious Disease Division (John G. Bartlett, director), the Clinical Pharmacology Division (Paul S. Lietman, director), and the Pulmonary Division (Jimmie T. Sylvester, director).

The Department of Pediatrics

The Department of Pediatrics was the first completely successful full-time department at Johns Hopkins. When director John Howland arrived in 1912, he became the leader of a new department carved out of the Department of Medicine. The Department of Pediatrics thus had no tradition of part-time leadership to overcome. This tradition had hampered Theodore C. Janeway who, as the first full-time professor of medicine, represented the end of an era. He had practiced under the old system too long to be able to adopt the new with unambivalent ease.

Howland, in contrast, was able to implement his creative ideas for the department without confronting any established traditions. He instituted a complete pediatric inpatient service and assembled an unusually talented staff of young physicians, almost all of whom later become heads of pediatrics departments in other medical schools. Howland's plan was the epitome of Barker's idea of compartmentalization. He kept the clinical and research activities of his department so separate that members of the research staff were permitted to work in the outpatient department but not on the wards. Howland considered one of his fellows, W. McKim Marriott, so essential in the laboratory that Marriott even had difficulty in obtaining permission to work in the Dispensary. Howland also took personal charge of all the children on the wards and personal charge of all private patients. He refused to allow the organization of any specialty clinics. His policy was to keep the department completely under his immediate control and to create conditions that maximized his staff's time for research.

To Howland, "research" included mastery of the nuts and bolts. He encouraged his staff members' self-sufficiency by refusing to provide technicians in the chemical laboratory. Only if his investigators became experienced and resourceful in technical procedures, Howland insisted, could they have full faith in their results.[43]

His department did not have the spirit of an autocracy, however. Edwards A. Park remembers it as a "joyous place," a happy family in which each had his duty.[44] Howland set the course for modern pediatrics by adding laboratory study to bedside observation and conjecture, by developing a model clinic, and by imbuing his students, fellows, and staff with his ideas. In so doing he embodied Billings' basic precepts: learning by doing, advancing one's field by adding new knowledge as well as by passing on existing knowledge, and training investigators who would carry the spirit of research to other developing institutions.

As Howland's successor in 1927, Park believed that research would advance more rapidly if full-time physicians concentrated on a single special area of pediatrics and that patients, particularly children with chronic diseases, would benefit most from intensive care by these specialists. Park saw the specialty divisions that he established—endocrinology, cardiology, neurology, and psychiatry—as a training ground for the next generation of leaders in pediatrics, whose experience in running specialty clinics would give them the opportunity to develop. Park had Halsted's gift for spotting promising young candidates for leadership. Three of his choices—Lawson Wilkins, Leo Kanner, and Helen B. Taussig—were themselves outstandingly successful in attracting young physicians for training, individuals who then left Hopkins to occupy important full-time posts in other medical centers (see chapter 9).

The Department of Surgery

In the Department of Surgery, what determined the establishment of full-time specialty divisions was not money (as in the Department of Medicine), but personalities. Even by the 1950s, not all the faculty were enthusiastic about the full-time system. Chief of surgery Alfred Blalock had the funds to place his specialty divisions on a full-time basis, but he was often unable to implement his plans until eminent part-time division chiefs retired.

During the 1940s, the Department of Surgery was the fastest growing of all the departments at Hopkins. Developing the surgical subspecialties on a full-time basis had been one of Blalock's main goals when he assumed the directorship, but his plans were delayed by World War II. Immediately after the war, Blalock began to staff the surgical subspecialties with full-time faculty, using income from the basic surgical subspecialties established by Halsted, and from the cardiac surgery he performed. When several faculty members left or retired soon after his arrival in Baltimore, Blalock was in a position to rebuild the department. The death of long-time faculty member Walter E. Dandy (chief of neurosurgery) and the retirement of chief of urology Hugh H. Young gave Blalock the opportunity to reorganize these divisions on a full-time basis, and similar shifts took place in other divisions when their long-time leaders departed. By 1948, radiology had become an independent department, and anesthesiology, urology, and neurological surgery had become separate full-time surgical divisions. Otolaryngology was placed on a full-time basis in 1952, and orthopedic surgery in 1953. All divisions were supported largely by their own earnings, supplemented by a portion of the parent department's professional fees, and, in some instances, by federal grants-in-aid for research.

The Department of Radiology

Radiology had been under consideration as a separate department since 1902, when radiologist Frederick H. Baetjer was appointed to the surgical faculty.[45] (Before Baetjer arrived, all the radiographs at the hospital had been taken by Harvey Cushing.) Like the heads of the other surgical subspecialties, Baetjer was a member of the part-time faculty. He was promoted to professor of clinical roentgenology in 1921. As he became a leader in his field, the Division of Radiology became an increasingly independent unit.

When candidates for director of surgery were being considered in 1939, hospital director Winford Smith urged that the Medical Board approve J. M. T. Finney's motion that radiology be made a separate, full-time department, since it served all other departments of the hospital. Under Blalock's leadership, the necessary committees were formed, and in 1944 the position of director of radiology was offered to Merrill C. Sosman, clinical professor of radiology at Harvard. Sosman declined the appointment, and it was offered to Russell H. Morgan, associate professor of roentgenology at the University of Chicago. Morgan had been one of the committee's original choices, but he was reluctant to leave Chicago. Furthermore, as an officer in the U.S. Public Health Service, he would have been unavailable until after the war. On further exploration, however, it appeared that he would be receptive to an offer from Johns Hopkins.

Before accepting the appointment, Morgan raised questions about space, equipment, and salaries for associates and staff. Only a full-time department would have the resources that Morgan required, and his concern was testimony to the spread of the full-time system's acceptance. A new surgical building was being planned; although funds for construction had not been secured, a low-rise building for radiology was eventually constructed beside the Halsted Building. The participation of both medical school and hospital has ensured the department's continued strength: at the department's founding in 1946, the hospital provided $200,000 for new equipment, and since then, the hospital has carried most of the department's budget.

Today, the department's formal name is the Russell H. Morgan Department of Radiology and Radiological Science. From 1972 to 1987, its director was Martin W. Donner; he was succeeded by William R. Brody.

The Division of Anesthesiology

As the story of the division of anesthesiology at Hopkins demonstrates, fields of knowledge developed more rapidly in full-time departments than in ones staffed by part-time faculty. By the 1940s, the full-time system was clearly the road to progress.

In the hospital's early years, general anesthesia was customarily administered by members of the surgical house staff. A few physicians such as Griffith Davis and Warren H. Buckler made a career of anesthesiology when inhalation anesthesia was induced almost entirely by ether, but nurse-anesthetists gradually took over this function.

Research in anesthesiology was vitalized at Hopkins by Austin Lamont, a fellow in surgery in 1934 who worked principally in the Hunterian Laboratory.[46] His interest in the administration of anesthetics by routes other than inhalation dovetailed with Blalock's work in cardiology. Blalock encouraged Lamont to develop a clinical interest in the field, since it was evident to him that cardiac surgery would require sophisticated anesthetic techniques. Blalock sent Lamont to the University of Pennsylvania for a year of study with Robert E. Dripps, and then to the University of Wisconsin. On his return in 1943, Lamont became head of the new division of anesthesiology.

Lamont saw many ways to develop the field at Hopkins. He wanted subdepartment status for anesthesiology, a staff of at least one full-time physician assistant and one house officer, laboratory space, technical assistance, funds for investigative supplies, liaison with the Department of Pharmacology, and some teaching time in the curriculum. Financial support should come from both hospital and medical school, he felt, and in return, his group would supply anesthesiology services to all the surgical specialties, as well as gynecology and obstetrics.

The medical school balked at contributing from its limited general funds, however, and Blalock did not give Lamont the necessary support. Lamont sent a strong letter to Blalock later in 1943, expressing his frustration and comparing the situation at Hopkins unfavorably with conditions at other university medical centers. World War II prevented the university from dealing with Lamont's complaints, but in 1946, Bowman appointed a committee to consider his suggestions. The committee agreed "guardedly" with Lamont's proposals, but that year Lamont resigned to take a post in the Department of Anesthesia at the University of Pennsylvania. He was understandably bitter about his experience at Hopkins.[47]

For five years after Lamont's departure, mention of anesthesia or anesthesiology in the medical school catalog was limited to one elective course in the practical application of basic techniques, and the so-called division was supervised by Olive Berger, Blalock's most trusted nurse-anesthetist. Donald F. Proctor, a practicing otolaryngologist with an interest in anesthesia, was appointed chief of anesthesiology in 1951, and he quickly encountered problems similar to Lamont's. Blalock would not listen to his research ideas for more than a few minutes, he complained. Proctor remained in the directorship only until June 1955. After his resignation, the division remained leaderless for six months, until the appointment of Donald W. Benson of the University of Chicago as associate professor and director of the division.

Although Blalock placed anesthesiology on a full-time basis in 1947, it remained largely a service function rather than a field of study equal to the other surgical subspecialties. Blalock probably did not fail to appreciate the field's research potential. More likely, he found it difficult to withdraw the responsibility for preanesthetic medication and anesthesia from his surgical residents and reassign it to residents in anesthesiology. Blalock's outlook, which was accepted by the Advisory Board and the rest of the medical school faculty, retarded progress in anesthesiology at Johns Hopkins for the next two decades. Even as late as the 1960s, long after other universities had thriving divisions of anesthesiology, Johns Hopkins' division was still service- rather than research-oriented. Its directors during those years were disillusioned in their belief that they had been brought in to lead a university department of anesthesiology. Blalock sought able leaders for the division, but once they arrived they did not have the facilities to fulfill their research goals. (For the more recent history of the Department of Anesthesiology, see chapter 5.)

The Division of Urology

The retirement of Hugh Hampton Young in 1942, after forty-four years as director of urology, enabled Blalock to carry out his plans for the division. Urology had been an informal part of surgery at Hopkins since 1895. Halsted had singled out Young, one of his residents, to develop the field as a subspecialty in 1898. Young became clinical professor of surgery in 1914; eight years later, he began to develop the Brady Research Laboratory, bringing in Edwin C. White and Justina Hill to conduct bacteriologic research. Although he did not originate the operation, Young was one of the pioneers in performing suprapubic prostatectomies, and his papers on the surgical treatment of hermaphroditism became classics. His reputation as "the father of American urology" rested on his ability to devise a new procedure in the midst of an operation, to operate with daring on otherwise incurable patients, and to prepare these patients to withstand the procedure. Founder of the *American Journal of Urology,* Young was an educator and scientist as well as a clinician.[48]

When Young retired in 1942, J. A. Campbell Colston was appointed acting chief until World War II was over. Colston was one of the division's senior members, a graduate of the Hopkins medical school who as a part-time faculty member had spent his entire career in urology at Hopkins. Like Colston, many of the urologists trained in Young's division stayed in Baltimore and went into private practice.

After the war ended, Blalock had to surmount serious difficulties to place the Division of Urology on a full-time basis. Young was the most prominent urologist in the United States, and the urology residency at Hopkins was considered outstanding. Yet the laboratory research program of the Brady Clinic did not meet the same standards at that time. Furthermore, the division's financial underpinnings were not strong, as it had only a meager endowment, which its staff did not supplement with large professional fees. The division's one endowment fund, named after Young, was worth only about $250,000. Another fund of about $85,000 and a few earlier bequests would eventually become available to the division.[49]

In the search for Young's permanent successor, it quickly became evident that his legacy was a division resistant to the full-time system and resistant to change. At war's end, the directorship was offered to Charles B. Huggins of the University of Chicago. Although Huggins first accepted the post, he changed his mind after visiting Baltimore. Huggins was at the height of his career, fully launched on the research program—studies of the effects of sex hormones on cancer of the prostate—that would bring him the Nobel Prize in medicine. But so hostile were the division's faculty that they petitioned President Bowman to withdraw the invitation to Huggins. Bowman declined to do so. Huggins wrote to Bowman, Chesney, and Blalock,

> I was looking for a formula by which the Institute could be run from a practical standpoint. I failed to find it. I encountered a spirit of antagonism and resistance on the part of the present faculty in Urology which made it abundantly clear that the early years, at least, at the institute would be characterized by such struggle and worrisome anguish that my usefulness to Johns Hopkins would be seriously impaired. I am emotionally unprepared for such an ordeal. The conflict is between the whole time system of a scholar with men of affairs. The present urological faculty are very successful and able practitioners of urology, long established in Baltimore where they have intricate roots in the civic body, and it would involve very serious financial and other sacrifices on their part to take up the life of a university professor, especially at their ages. The difficulty is fundamentally a conflict of ideologies.[50]

Huggins had accepted the directorship on the condition that urology be made an independent department. Now the Advisory Board rescinded its decision to elevate urology to departmental status and assembled a new search committee.

A few months after Huggins' withdrawal in 1946, the directorship was accepted by William W. Scott, a member of Huggins' staff. Scott had spend his professional life at the University of Chicago, receiving the medical degree, training as a house officer, and joining the urology division to work with Huggins. He was only thirty-three years old when he came to Hopkins, four years out of his residency, and his appointment to succeed the world-famous Young alarmed many alumni—who had forgotten that Young was only twenty-eight when he started the new specialty at Hopkins.[51]

Scott was chief of urology until 1974. Residency training and laboratory investigation flourished during his tenure. As a formal part of their training, urology residents spent a full year in the Brady Laboratory, usually during the second year of the four-year residency program. The success of Scott's students attests to the strength of his leadership: twenty-two of his sixty-five residents later headed departments of urology around the country. When Scott arrived, the Brady Laboratory was confined to the top floor of the Urology Building. The laboratory had been used mainly for bacteriologic cultures, and contained largely useless pre-Pyrex glassware and other outdated equipment. During Scott's tenure, the laboratory was refurbished and expanded into a facility suitable for the full-time division that urology had become.

In 1974, Patrick C. Walsh succeeded Scott as director.

The Division of Neurosurgery

Blalock was able to move the Division of Neurosurgery to full-time status after Walter E. Dandy died in 1946. A 1906 graduate of the Hopkins medical school, Dandy had spent his entire career at Hopkins. He was a member of the Department of Surgery for forty years and had made Johns Hopkins one of the great centers for the practice of neurosurgery. Dandy was responsible for fundamental studies spanning the range of neurological surgery (see chapter 11). He was also a master teacher. A year with Dandy sometimes convinced assistant residents in surgery to choose neurosurgery as a career.[52]

When Dandy died in 1946, Frank J. Otenasek, then only an instructor in surgery, was placed in charge of neurosurgery on a temporary basis. Later that year, Blalock suggested to the Advisory Board that the directorship of a full-time division be offered to Barnes Woodhall, a former resident in surgery at Hopkins who had become professor of neurosurgery at Duke University, but Woodhall declined the post. Blalock's next choice was A. Earl Walker—who, like Morgan and Huggins, was also a faculty member at the University of

Chicago. Walker accepted the directorship of neurosurgery early in 1947. Born in Winnipeg, Walker received bachelor's and master's degrees from the University of Alberta. He then went to the University of Chicago, where, with interruptions for fellowships at the University of Iowa and a traveling fellowship from the Rockefeller Foundation, he remained until coming to Hopkins.

Walker's main interests were the structure and function of the thalamus and the physiology of the cerebral cortex. A stimulating teacher, he established an outstanding residency program in neurosurgery and was a visiting professor at universities around the world. Walker also established the electroencephalographic laboratory and maintained an active neurosurgical pathological laboratory, which was expanded in the 1960s to include histochemistry and enzyme chemistry of the central nervous system. He also established the neurometric laboratory, which was the first such facility in the country. In 1973, Donlin M. Long became the division's director.

Although the divisions of neurosurgery and urology were well known before Blalock reorganized them, full-time status gave them another dimension. In the full-time divisions, residency training included a block of time allotted to research; as full-time divisions, they acquired the facilities and the faculty to create a proper research environment for residents and fellows who wanted a full-time academic career.[53]

The Division of Otolaryngology

The Division of Otolaryngology acquired its first full-time director in 1952, when John E. Bordley succeeded Samuel J. Crowe, who had been head of the division for forty years.

The division had been formed in the typical Hopkins manner. To organize a university division, Halsted selected a promising young man who knew nothing about the field. When Halsted asked Crowe to head this new division in 1912, Crowe abandoned his plans to accompany Harvey Cushing to Boston. Crowe's founding of an otological research laboratory, the correlations his group established between hearing defects and anatomic defects of the inner ear, his pioneering recognition of lymphoid ingrowths as a major cause of deafness in children, and his development of a method of prevention and treatment using radium—all contributed to a department that became a cornerstone of modern otology and laryngology.[54]

Bordley augmented the division with several other full-time faculty members, including George Nager, who would succeed him as head of otolaryngology in 1969. The idea of a separate speech and hearing clinic was Bordley's; it was the first such unit connected with a medical school. Bordley's clinical research included long-term studies of hearing loss. In collaboration with Curt Richter, in the Department of Psychiatry, Bordley and his associate William G. Hardy devised a method of using Pavlov's conditioned reflex and the galvanic skin response to test the hearing of small children. The expansion of the division, and its subsequent renaming as the Department of Otolaryngology, Head and Neck Surgery, was a consequence of its full-time status. In 1984, Michael M. E. Johns succeeded Nager as director of the division.

The Division of Orthopedic Surgery

The last of the surgical specialties with a completely part-time staff was the Division of Orthopedic Surgery, which did not acquire a full-time chief—Robert A. Robinson—and full-time faculty until 1953. The organizer of the first orthopedic clinic was William S. Baer, whom Halsted had appointed head of orthopedics in 1900. Baer remained in the post for thirty-one years. His two part-time successors were also drawn from the department's faculty: George E. Bennett, who directed the division from 1931 until his retirement in 1947, and Robert W. Johnson, Jr., who served as director for the next six years.

As Johnson's successor, Robinson came to Hopkins from the University of Rochester School of Medicine, where he had already carried out important work with the electron microscope on the fine structure of bone. Robinson expanded the division's residency program, adding facilities at the Baltimore City Hospitals in 1956 and at the Loch

Raven Veterans Administration Medical Center in 1970. In the 1970s, affiliated programs were established at Sinai Hospital, Union Memorial Hospital, and Howard University School of Medicine. An orthopedic program was established at the Good Samaritan Hospital in 1972, which included a combined orthopedic-rheumatology center (the only one then in existence in the middle Atlantic states) and a research laboratory. At Hopkins, Robinson presided over the opening of the pediatric orthopedic service in 1964 and an orthopedic surgery research laboratory the following year. Robinson placed in charge of all these services outstanding full-time faculty, many of whom were graduates of his own training program. One of his residents, Lee H. Riley, Jr., succeeded him as director in 1979.[55]

The Departments of Gynecology and Obstetrics

The appointment of the head of gynecology, Richard W. TeLinde, as a full-time member of the faculty in 1956 finally placed every department at the Johns Hopkins University School of Medicine on a full-time basis. The tradition of opposition to the full-time system in the Department of Gynecology extended back to Howard Kelly, the first head of the department, who kept its staff on a part-time basis throughout his tenure. His opposition nevertheless diminished his influence, and in 1919 he resigned as professor of gynecology to give more time to his private clinic.[56]

Kelly's resignation allowed the Advisory Board to restructure the department. It became a subdepartment of surgery, and Kelly's successor, Thomas S. Cullen, was appointed professor of clinical gynecology. As part-time head of a division, Cullen was given a seat on the Medical Board of the hospital but not on the medical school's Advisory Board. When Cullen retired as head of gynecology in 1939, he was succeeded by another part-time member of the department, Richard W. TeLinde.

TeLinde remained on a geographical full-time basis as director, retaining the income from his private patients but combining his practice with teaching and administrative duties.[57] Part-time status was not, however, TeLinde's choice. The directorship had been offered to him on a part-time basis, as the department's $10,000 budget did not provide for his salary. Certain privileges were denied him as a part-time faculty member: his title was "chief gynecologist" rather than "gynecologist-in-chief," the form of title for all other (full-time) department heads; and he was appointed to the Medical Board of the hospital but not to the Advisory Board of the medical school. Unlike almost any other Hopkins faculty member of the time, TeLinde brought with him a very large private practice, and his devotion to Johns Hopkins was such that he would have turned over to the institution his income according to the full-time concept—had he been asked to take a full-time salaried position.

TeLinde was finally asked, in an oddly informal way, in 1956. At a dinner given by the trustees of the hospital and university for department heads, each director spoke about his department. When TeLinde's turn came, he said that he was the only department head employed by the university on a part-time basis, and that he had never been offered a full-time position. The next morning, W. Barry Wood, vice-president for medical affairs, offered TeLinde a full-time position at the top full-time salary of $25,000, and a place on the Advisory Board. TeLinde accepted. For the next four years, until his retirement in 1960, TeLinde's earnings and those of his associate Lawrence Wharton, Jr., supported the Department of Gynecology.

In contrast to the Department of Gynecology, the Department of Obstetrics had operated on a full-time basis since 1918.[58] J. Whitridge Williams, its director, was a strong advocate of the full-time system and an advocate of the amalgamation of the Departments of Obstetrics and Gynecology. Offered a position in New York in 1918, Williams told Welch that he would remain at Johns Hopkins on three conditions: full-time status for his department, a new building, and responsibility for some of the patients then assigned to gynecology. Welch and the Advisory Board agreed, but the split between gynecology and obstetrics widened when obstetrics became a full-time department. The departments were not united until 1964 (see chapter 4).

Varied Approaches to the Full-Time System

The concept of the full-time system was malleable, and different individuals and institutions could shape it to their views. Participation in the full-time plan indicated an attitude toward the advance of clinical medicine, rather than acceptance of a rigid set of principles. The Departments of Medicine, Surgery, Pediatrics, and Gynecology of the Johns Hopkins Medical Institutions approached the full-time system from different perspectives. Once the system was broadly in place, each department's leadership and financial strength determined how the system would be applied to particular specialty divisions.

At the start, not even the definition of full-time was standardized. In the Department of Medicine, full-time associates in charge of the research divisions antedated a full-time director. When the General Education Board provided funds to inaugurate the full-time system in the clinical departments, the money was sufficient to pay the salaries of the directors of the Departments of Medicine, Surgery, and Pediatrics; and two full-time associate professors in medicine, two in surgery, and one in pediatrics. In some departments, "full-time" referred to the status of the department head, not to the rest of the department's faculty. Some departments were able to support other full-time faculty members, but many members remained on a part-time basis.

In the Department of Pediatrics, the path to the full-time system was smooth. The department was founded on a full-time basis, and its first chief, John Howland, was brought to Hopkins as a full-time faculty member. The system's growth hinged on a professorial decision, however. No specialty divisions were allowed to develop during Howland's tenure as professor of pediatrics. In contrast, his successor, Edwards A. Park, believed that, in order to increase knowledge in particular

areas, the department needed to carve out separate divisions. The full-time system was nevertheless not applied consistently. The division of pediatric cardiology, for example, was full-time from its inception, under the directorship of Helen Taussig, while Lawson Wilkins did not move from part- to full-time director of endocrinology until Francis Schwentker became director of pediatrics in 1946.

At the other extreme was the Department of Gynecology, which had no specialty divisions and whose first leader, Howard A. Kelly, disliked the full-time system. This department lingered on a part-time basis until the 1950s.

As chief of surgery, Alfred Blalock wanted to develop the surgical specialties to counteract what he saw as the domination of Hopkins by the Department of Medicine. Full-time surgical specialty divisions were instituted in the mid-1940s, when Blalock's practice of cardiac surgery generated the necessary income from his patients and Blalock was able to recruit new division chiefs.

The Department of Medicine under Osler contained no specialty divisions, as he did not believe that the department's responsibilities included application of the techniques of basic research to the study of disease in man. Osler's successor, Lewellys F. Barker, felt strongly that full-time research divisions were essential if medicine was to progress. His three full-time divisions were the foundation for research in the Department of Medicine, as the Chemical Division turned to the study of endocrinology, the Biological Division to infectious disease, and the Physiological Division to cardiovascular medicine. Later, new areas of special interest were developed, primarily in outpatient clinics supervised by part-time faculty with a particular interest in the field. Good clinical investigation was carried out in these clinics, but in general the specialty areas were not far advanced in using the tools of the basic sciences for patient-oriented research.

Unlike the Department of Surgery, the Department of Medicine was not able to generate sufficient income through patient care to support new full-time specialty divisions, and the research space available was insufficient. It is ironic that all full-time departments now depend to a large degree on income from the care of patients for full-time salaries, as well as for general purposes. Not until federal funds became available, in the 1950s and 1960s, were the divisions in the Department of Medicine placed on a full-time basis. For many years, insufficient space also prevented the elevation of the subdepartments of neurology and dermatology to full-time departmental status. Once space and funds were available, however, the growth of opportunities for research in all fields of medicine enabled the rapid advance of these specialties and their elevation to full departmental status.

The Spread of the Full-Time System

By the 1960s, the full-time system was an integral part of academic medicine. While some features of the system at Johns Hopkins were modified at other schools to fit their administrative structure, others were left intact. The unique administrative structure at Johns Hopkins, for example, facilitated the implementation of the full-time system. Since one individual was both professor in the university and director of the corresponding service in the hospital, his salary was divided between hospital and university, so that neither had to assume the full financial burden of the full-time plan. This structure became a model for teaching hospitals across the country, although schools without a single primary teaching hospital, like Harvard, had to resolve problems concerning equitable salaries and regulations that would span all the school's affiliated teaching institutions. The Hopkins tradition of allowing only full-time faculty to serve on the medical school's Advisory Board also made some questions of governance easier to resolve at Hopkins than elsewhere.

Even the issue at the core of the controversy surrounding the full-time system—the income of the physician—admitted variations. At the opening of the Johns Hopkins Hospital, professors in the clinical departments were permitted to augment their base salaries with income from private patients. This system is known today as the "geographical full-time" plan, as the faculty member spends his entire time in the hospital and has no outside office.

Johns Hopkins adopted a strict full-time plan in 1913, as specified by the General Education board. So obsessed with the full-time system was Abraham Flexner that he—and by extension, the General Education Board—made the adoption of the Hopkins version a requirement for any medical school requesting support. Some schools assented—Vanderbilt, Yale, Washington University, and the University of Rochester, for example—but others did not.

For the Harvard Medical School, the sticking point was not the idea that physicians should confine their professional activities to the university hospital. Harvey Cushing and Henry A. Christian were working out a full-time system of their own at the Peter Bent Brigham Hospital, having installed themselves as full-time teachers and investigators there. Rather, it was Flexner's insistence that fees be withheld from individual physicians that caused Harvey Cushing to advise President Lowell not to approach the General Education Board for funds:

It is my impression that the reasons for the adoption in Baltimore of the proposal from the General Education Board were based upon the feeling, chiefly on the part of the heads of the preclinical departments, that the school was getting into a rut, from which it should be extricated no matter how seriously the method adopted might temporarily wrench their machine. Unquestionably this feeling would not have arisen had the heads of the clinical departments been given the opportunity some years ago voluntarily to place themselves on a whole-service basis similar to that on which my colleague and myself now serve in the Brigham Hospital.

It seems to me that the clinical departments of the Harvard Medical School, on the other hand, by their own initiative give promise of getting out of the rut into which they had fallen, and the injection at this time of a new element into the situation might seriously complicate it. Were we at a standstill or in financial straits we might have to ask others to help pull our load, and to accept their terms no matter how experimental they might appear to be. On the other hand, were our engine moving more smoothly than it is, we might otherwise be justified in venturing to test it on an unbroken road.[59]

Lowell agreed, and despite negotiations that continued for years, Harvard never did accept the General Education Board's version of the full-time system.[60]

Later, other medical schools supported by the General Education Board were permitted to use a geographical full-time system. This system worked well from the start for Duke University, whose circumstances differed considerably from those of Johns Hopkins. Duke's medical school was not founded until 1930; it was supported generously by the Duke Endowment; and it was located in what was then a relatively rural area, forcing it to rely heavily on its local physicians. Duke's outpatient facility, known as the Private Diagnostic Clinic, was run not by Duke University but by its staffing physicians. Physicians received fees from patients, and, provided that they conducted their university duties satisfactorily, they were allowed to develop their private practices as they pleased. They could not, however, maintain offices outside the Private Diagnostic Clinic or admit patients to hospitals other than Duke's. J. Deryl Hart, chief of surgery at Duke and a former surgical resident at Hopkins, was one who considered Duke's system superior to the strict full-time plan.[61]

The full-time system was characterized by its opponents in the early 1900s as an untried experiment that might fail. As Donald Fleming points out, however, "so had been the life-pattern of Welch; and so also had been the whole conception of the Johns Hopkins University, hospital, and medical school."[62] In the end, Welch was vindicated, as the principal objections to the full-time system diminished, and increasing numbers of the nation's medical schools accepted the full-time plan.

CHAPTER 9

THE EXPORT OF HOPKINS PHYSICIANS

We have become so accustomed at The Johns Hopkins University to academic suitors for our young men that our position has been compared to that of the benignant father of a large family of girls in one of your overpopulated, feminine towns in this state, who replied to the young man who graciously requested the privilege of marrying one of his daughters: "Take her, young man, take her. God bless you. Do you know who wants another?" Whatever may be thought of free trade in other matters, free trade in the selection of those who are to fill positions of teachers in our universities is conducive to vigorous development.

—William H. Welch

The export of men and women "fitted to make research" was one of the cornerstones of the new Johns Hopkins University School of Medicine. Hopkins graduates were also uniquely qualified to teach and to practice scientifically based medicine and surgery. Rather than retaining all of the school's well-trained graduates and young faculty, John Shaw Billings and his colleagues intended that they bring the specific innovations developed at Johns Hopkins to other medical schools across the country. During the early twentieth century, Hopkins thus exported ideas and methods as well as individuals.

The success of this first outward movement helped to transform American medicine. In the process, it diminished the uniqueness of the Johns Hopkins medical school and hospital. As its graduates helped to create other strong schools, Johns Hopkins became one of many. In later years, therefore, a second type of export prevailed: the dispersal of Johns Hopkins graduates at all levels of training and experience, physicians who repre-

sented a "heritage of excellence," the legacy of their predecessors.

The spectrum of postgraduate education extended from pure "bench" science to specialized clinical training, and the residency and fellowship programs contributed substantially to Johns Hopkins's preeminence as an institution dedicated to the advancement of scientific and clinical knowledge.

The idea of exporting physicians was partly based on the principle of nationalizing medical school faculties, a novel idea in the 1890s. At that time, academic provincialism prevailed across the country, as faculty members in medical schools were drawn from the pool of local physicians, and taught the basic sciences while continuing to practice medicine. Hospitals and medical schools were responsible for appointing their own staffs, and medical schools thus found it impossible to obtain clinical professors from other communities because such clinicians would have no access to hospital beds for teaching and research.[1] At Hopkins, however, faculty were brought from around the world, and they were chosen on the basis of their qualifications alone.

From the beginning, the preclinical departments were professionalized. Their members received a salary and no longer had to earn their income by caring for patients. The clinical divisions were at first composed of part-time professors with an aptitude for teaching and medical practice. Yet even before the advent of full-time positions in the clinical departments, Johns Hopkins paid the clinical departmental directors a substantial salary, thus anchoring their professional allegiance as in the basic science departments. Johns Hopkins was also able to encourage research at all levels because of its unique administrative structure, which gave control of hospital appointments to the medical school and put a single individual in charge of corresponding medical school and hospital departments.

Fellows in the First Preclinical Laboratories

The first instruction and research in a preclinical science at Johns Hopkins was carried out not in the medical school but in the laboratory of Henry Newell Martin, professor of biology in the Faculty of Philosophy. When Martin's laboratory was organized in 1876, it was the first medical science laboratory at Johns Hopkins and one of the only two real centers of research in physiology in the United States at the time. (The other was Henry P. Bowditch's laboratory at Harvard.)[2] Martin's laboratory set the pattern for the later export of Hopkins physicians, training young scientists who became influential in disparate fields of American medicine. Four of Martin's fellows joined the first faculty of the Johns Hopkins medical school— William T. Councilman (in pathology), William Henry Howell (in physiology), John Jacob Abel (in pharmacology), and Ross G. Harrison (in anatomy). Others achieved equal eminence at leading schools across the country. Two notable examples were Henry Sewall, who went to the University of Michigan as professor of physiology, and William T.

Sedgwick, who became professor of biology at the Massachusetts Institute of Technology.

In planning the medical school, Martin, Remsen, and Billings worked closely with William H. Welch, the first appointed professor who actually served on the medical school's faculty after its opening. Welch's laboratories were not finished when he came to Hopkins in 1884, so he traveled to Europe for a second time, to study the emerging science of bacteriology. Returning to Baltimore the following year, he shared Martin's laboratory at the university for a short time until the Pathological Building on the hospital lot was completed.

Despite the inconvenience, the four-year hiatus between the opening of the hospital and that of the medical school was beneficial, allowing the school to benefit from the hospital's increasing eminence as an institution for the advancement of scientific medicine. Welch's laboratory became a mecca for young, aspiring scientists. The first professors of anatomy, obstetrics, and surgery at Johns Hopkins—Franklin P. Mall, J. Whitridge Williams, and William S. Halsted—had trained as fellows in Welch's laboratory. Welch even trained his own successor, William G. MacCallum, who became professor of pathology at the Columbia University College of Physicians and Surgeons before returning to Baltimore. Most important, however, was Welch's effect on preclinical departments in other schools, which developed independently as his students established their own laboratories elsewhere. As one of the first of the great laboratories of experimental medicine, Welch's laboratory was partly responsible for the spread of this type of facility throughout the country. Among its students were George M. Sternberg, bacteriologist and organizer of the Army Medical School; Walter Reed, professor of bacteriology at the Army school, and James Carroll, who discovered the cause of yellow fever; J. H. Wright, a pathologist at the Massachusetts General Hospital who later developed the reticulocyte count; Reid Hunt, who became professor of pharmacology at Harvard; and Simon Flexner, first scientific director of the Rockefeller Institute.

Other departments at Hopkins' School of Medicine followed Welch's example and were in turn responsible for training equally eminent physicians. Franklin P. Mall, for example, was largely responsible for elevating anatomy from its position as a handmaiden of surgery to an independent basic science. He carried on the tradition of training investigators for export: of Mall's seventeen fellows, eleven became professors of anatomy at medical schools nationwide. Walter Jones, the head of the Department of Physiological Chemistry, also had many student collaborators in his research laboratory, including future Nobelist George Whipple.

Clinical Residents

While fellows in pathology concentrated on research, residents on the clinical side were predominantly concerned with the care of patients in the hospital. On the wards, Osler's "graded residency" prevailed (see chapter 7). His system was eventually adopted throughout the country, and it may be as responsible as any single innovation for the development of America's outstanding position in the world of medicine. As in the large German hospitals, highly trained physicians remained at Johns Hopkins as residents for three, five, or even—like William S. Thayer—seven years. Some moved directly from completion of the residency to a professorship at a university medical school.

In organizing his surgical residency, William S. Halsted intended to establish a school of surgery, one that would disseminate the principles of surgery he considered essential. He hoped to develop not just surgeons, but surgeons of the highest type, who would stimulate the nation's youth to study surgery and raise the standards of surgical science. Halsted's program trained surgeons with a research spirit, many of whom went from this experience to professorships in other institutions.[3]

Despite its novelty, Halsted's program attracted little attention in its early years, largely because it was ahead of its time. Surgery in America during the 1890s and early 1900s was an unscientific profession. Any licensed doctor was allowed to operate; most surgeons were self-taught. Knowledge of anatomy, and dexterity and speed in operating were far more important than surgical technique. Good teachers of surgery were in short supply, and renowned surgeons carried on their work in hospitals unconnected with university centers. It was difficult to attract the outstanding surgeons of the era to chairs of surgery, as salaries in university medical centers were poor, and many surgeons were reluctant to pass on to others the hard-earned skills they had acquired under adverse conditions. Research and the practice of surgery were almost completely separated; practicing surgeons enjoyed little exchange of knowledge and little intellectual stimulation. The benefits of a long period of discipline and responsibility had to be demonstrated before other medical schools would adopt such a program. Halsted's retiring manner also contributed to the program's lack of renown, as despite his hopes for its perpetuation and expansion, he made little effort to promote or publicize it.[4]

As a result, the program remained unique for many years, and its goals and features were spread mainly by its original participants. George Heuer, for example, instituted a Halsted-type residency program first at the University of Cincinnati and later at Cornell Medical College, where he was chief of surgery, in 1922. Entrusting surgical patients to the care of residents was a new idea to everyone at Cornell, and the success of the program did much to help the cause of surgical training throughout the country.[5]

Over thirty years elapsed before even ten Halsted-type residencies had been established. Progress was rapid thereafter, however, and by 1939 the American Medical Association directory listed 203 surgical residencies in the United States. Eleven of Halsted's seventeen chief residents instituted training programs of their own— programs that produced the next generation of resident surgeons trained in the Halsted tradition, who in turn trained the third generation.[6]

The Reorganization of Medical Training in the 1920s

Even before the Flexner Report of 1910, many schools across the nation benefited from the presence of men and women trained at Johns Hopkins. The medical school at the University of Iowa, for example, adopted the Hopkins system of appointing one chief for the corresponding hospital and medical school departments, and inaugurated a clinical clerkship for fourth-year students.[7] At Wisconsin, Charles R. Bardeen (M.D., Johns Hopkins, 1897) obtained eight Hopkins graduates for his first faculty, including Joseph Erlanger (M.D., Johns Hopkins, 1899), whose classic studies on the diagnosis and understanding of heart block and blood pressure preceded the investigations of nerve fibers that won Erlanger a Nobel Prize.[8]

It was in the wake of the Flexner Report, however, that the export of Hopkins-trained physicians gained momentum. With funds from Rockefeller's General Education Board, medical schools across the nation were created or reorganized along the lines of the Hopkins model, and with this reorganization of medical education came a demand for physicians with Hopkins training. University presidents traveled to Baltimore to consult with Welch and other faculty members at Johns Hopkins about implementing such innovations as the full-time system in their own schools—and acquiring physicians and scientists trained at the source to put the innovations in place. Specially chosen physicians also came to Baltimore to spend one year in a residency and another in the laboratory; notable examples were Francis W. Peabody and George R. Minot of Harvard.

The flood tide of export began in 1921. William S. Thayer had assembled a skilled full-time staff in the Department of Medicine. Walter W. Palmer, who had trained under Lawrence J. Henderson at Harvard, was brought to Hopkins to head the Chemical Division. Palmer in turn recruited Dana W. Atchley, and Robert F. Loeb joined the group as an assistant resident in med-

icine. Alphonse Dochez, a Hopkins graduate, returned from the Rockefeller Hospital to head the Biological Division; and William S. Ladd was also recruited from New York to join the department. When the Columbia University College of Physicians and Surgeons and the Presbyterian Hospital collaborated in building a joint medical center in 1920, Palmer accepted the full-time professorship of medicine there, and all of these men (along with George A. Harrop, the medical resident at Hopkins) migrated to New York to staff Palmer's new department.[9]

Washington University

One of the first schools to reflect the Hopkins influence was Washington University in Saint Louis.[10] So severe were Abraham Flexner's criticisms of its school of medicine that university president Robert S. Brookings abolished it in 1909 and began over. His intention was to "Johns Hopkinize" the medical department. David Edsall had been invited to become head of the Department of Medicine, and his wife commented of Brookings and the trustees, "Their plan was to make their medical school the Johns Hopkins of the Southwest."[11]

The six executive faculty members of the new medical school included two Hopkins graduates: Eugene L. Opie (M.D., 1897) in pathology and Joseph Erlanger (M.D., 1899) in physiology. As at Johns Hopkins, the professors were young: four of the six were in their thirties. The junior faculty that they brought to Saint Louis also included Hopkins graduates and residents. Roger S. Morris, for example, became associate professor of medicine at Washington University in 1913. A student of Osler at Johns Hopkins, Morris had also worked under Thomas R. Boggs in the clinical laboratories. Farther down the ladder, many of the residents in the newly established residency program were graduates of Johns Hopkins, including Barney Brooks (M.D., 1911), who joined the surgical house staff after interning under Halsted. At Washington University, Brooks organized a surgical pathology laboratory and a course in surgical pathology that served as models for other institutions. The research interests he pursued at Washington University included studies of the regeneration of bone, intestinal obstruction, and arteriography. Morris later became professor of medicine at the University of Cincinnati and Brooks, professor of surgery at Vanderbilt.

Several key features of the new medical school reflected the Hopkins influence. The laboratories in medicine, surgery, and pediatrics were modeled on those at Johns Hopkins, and the medical school acquired Barnes Hospital as its teaching facility. Most important, the full-time system was adopted in the clinical departments.

With the full-time system in place, other Hopkins-trained physicians arrived to take faculty positions in the new medical school. W. McKim Marriott left John Howland's staff in 1918 to become professor of pediatrics at Washington University. Under his direction, scientific investigation became an important activity at the Washington University School of Medicine. Marriott's own research included significant contributions to the understanding of infant nutrition, and many of his students became professors of pediatrics at other institutions. Later, E. Kennerly Marshall, Jr., left Hopkins to become professor of pharmacology. Also joining the faculty was Herbert S. Gasser, a Hopkins graduate who was a faculty member at the University of Wisconsin. Gasser (along with Joseph Erlanger) would subsequently win the Nobel Prize for Physiology or Medicine.

George Canby Robinson (M.D., Johns Hopkins, 1903) went to Washington University in 1913 as associate professor of medicine. Robinson had trained at the Ayer Laboratory in Philadelphia, a facility directed by one of Welch's pupils, Simon Flexner. The laboratory itself was headed by a number of Hopkins graduates. When Flexner left to become director of the Rockefeller Institute, Warfield T. Longcope (M.D., Johns Hopkins, 1901), one of Flexner's students, succeeded him as director of the Ayer Laboratory. A later director, John R. Paul, was also a Hopkins graduate.

Robinson was given the responsibility at Washington University for organizing both the outpatient department and the inpatient medical service. He was also especially interested in setting up the chemical, bacteriological, and physiological laboratories of the medical department, facilities closely related to both the patients and the teaching laboratory of clinical chemistry and microscopy. Robinson's experience at Washington University gave him the background for the program he would implement several years later as dean of the Vanderbilt University School of Medicine.

Vanderbilt University

The Rockefeller Foundation supported Vanderbilt University's decision to be the site for the development of a modern medical school in the South.[12] In 1920, George Canby Robinson arrived in Nashville as the new dean and professor of medicine. Robinson gave Vanderbilt an Oslerian philosophy of medical education, specialized physical surroundings, and transplanted faculty who provided a particular climate for medical education. Unlike Washington University, which took over an already existing hospital, Vanderbilt had to build its own. Robinson therefore moved to Baltimore for several years, during which time he consulted with architects and observed hospital administration under Winford Smith, the director of the Johns Hopkins Hospital.

Robinson decided to abandon the medical school buildings on Vanderbilt's south campus, including a partially completed new hospital, and build new ones on the west campus instead. The idea, as Robinson said, was to break down the distinction between inpatients and outpatients for the staff and students. He also wanted to make the new university hospital an integral part of the medical school building. For the first time in this country, the teaching hospital and the laboratories for the preclinical departments would be under the same roof. The biochemistry, physiology, and pharmacology departments would connect directly with medical wards on two floors, and the offices for the full-time staff in medicine would be located in between. Offices for anatomy and pathology would have the same relation to the surgical wards. Laboratories, space, and facilities for research in clinical departments would be near laboratories in the preclinical departments.

To staff the hospital and medical school, Robinson imported a number of Hopkins physicians, including R. Sidney Cunningham (M.D., Johns Hopkins, 1915, and associate professor of anatomy) as professor of anatomy; Ernest W. Goodpasture (M.D., Johns Hopkins, 1912, and assistant in pathology) as professor of pathology; Paul D. Lamson (who came to Baltimore from Harvard in 1915) as professor of pharmacology; Barney Brooks (M.D., Johns Hopkins, 1911, and intern under Halsted) as professor of surgery; C. Sidney Burwell (chief resident in medicine at Johns Hopkins under Robinson) and Hugh J. Morgan (M.D., Johns Hopkins, 1918, and resident in medicine under Thayer) as associate professors of medicine; Horton R. Casparis (associate in pediatrics at Johns Hopkins, 1920–25) as associate professor of pediatrics; and John B. Youmans (M.D., Johns Hopkins, 1919) as head of the medical outpatient service.

The pediatric service in particular reflected the Hopkins influence, as Casparis brought with him Katherine Dodd (M.D., Johns Hopkins, 1921, and Casparis' assistant at Johns Hopkins, 1922–23) as an instructor. Scott Wilkinson (M.D., Johns Hopkins, 1924) was appointed one of three assistants in clinical pediatrics.

In 1925, Tinsley R. Harrison (M.D., Johns Hopkins, 1922, and assistant resident at Johns Hopkins under Warfield T. Longcope) and Alfred Blalock, a classmate of Harrison, went to Vanderbilt as residents in medicine and surgery, respectively. Extending Hopkins' influence still further, Harrison left Vanderbilt in 1941 to organize the Bowman Gray School of Medicine.

The importance of basic and clinical research was foremost in Robinson's mind as he selected the new faculty. "Research is the life-blood of science. Only when it is fostered do the sciences thrive," Robinson said.[13] Not only was practically everyone on the faculty involved in some sort of research, but house staff were caught up in it as well. Emphasizing the German model of research, Robinson sent Burwell and Casparis to study in

Germany for a year between their resignation from Johns Hopkins and their arrival at Vanderbilt.

The curriculum that Robinson put in place also resembled the one at Johns Hopkins, but it departed from the Hopkins model by transposing the clinical experiences of the third and fourth years. At Vanderbilt, the clinical clerkship, in which students served with residents on the wards, was scheduled in the third year, and the fourth year included the care of patients under supervision in the outpatient service.

The syphilis clinic at Vanderbilt was also based on the corresponding facility at Johns Hopkins. Like Osler a generation earlier, Hugh J. Morgan, the faculty member at Vanderbilt in charge of this clinic, had a deep interest in this disease. Elsewhere, patients with syphilis were treated solely for the clinical manifestations of the disease, either in the dermatologic clinic or in other departments such as neurology and ophthalmology. At Johns Hopkins and Vanderbilt, syphilis was considered a systemic disease, and patients were treated in the Department of Medicine. Even the name of the facility at Vanderbilt was taken from Johns Hopkins: the clinic was known as "Medical L," the discreet abbreviation for "lues," or syphilis. A rotation through Medical L was an elective for medical students at Vanderbilt, as it was at Johns Hopkins.

The Hopkins influence emerged at Vanderbilt in other varied ways. A small department of medical illustration was developed by a pupil of Max Broedel, and a Historical Club was modeled on the one founded at Johns Hopkins in 1889 by Welch, Osler, and Billings. The influence was an ongoing one, moreover, as 40 percent of medical resident physicians between 1946 and 1959 were Hopkins graduates.

The University of Rochester

The creation of a new medical school at the University of Rochester in 1925 was directly influenced by the effort to extend the full-time system.[14] Again, the General Education Board provided the funds. The first generation of Hopkins-influenced schools was in place, and Rochester could draw on several models for its facilities and curriculum. Rochester incorporated the same general architectural plan as Vanderbilt, for example, with medical school and teaching hospital under one roof. Related clinical departments and hospital wards were also placed on floors adjacent to the various preclinical departments.

The president of Rochester, Rush Rhees, turned to Hopkins' faculty and administrators for advice about staffing the medical school. Whoever was chosen to organize and preside over the medical faculty, he was told, should be a pathologist, because it is pathology that connects the preclinical and clinical divisions of the curriculum, and the pathologist is therefore in the best position to understand and guide the work of the school at large. Welch and Simon Flexner suggested George H. Whipple (M.D., Johns Hopkins, 1905), then director of the Hooper Foundation, an institute for medical research, and dean of the University of California School of Medicine (at San Francisco). Whipple accepted the deanship of the new medical school.

With Rhees's approval, Whipple adopted a simple administrative structure copied from Johns Hopkins. The dean, the director of the hospital, and the department heads formed an Advisory Board, presided over by the president of the university, which made recommendations to the university's trustees. At its monthly meeting all administrative affairs were discussed and voted on. The professors were each responsible for representing the views and needs of their respective junior staffs while sharing the corporate interests of the whole institution.

Whipple's faculty reflected the Hopkins influence as well. Rochester was soon perceived (with what one participant recalls as "some amusement, perhaps even a touch of disapproval, in certain circles") as a junior Johns Hopkins faculty at Rochester.[15] Another faculty member at the time remembers the benefits of the link with Johns Hopkins: "Before long, the premedical student underground had the Rochester School of Medicine tagged as a small edition of the Johns Hopkins Medical School. This was no small com-

pliment for a fledgling school and a morale lifter for us."[16]

The faculty included George W. Corner (M.D., Johns Hopkins, 1913), who went to Rochester in 1923 from an associate professorship in anatomy at Johns Hopkins; Karl M. Wilson, who had been part-time professor of obstetrics at Johns Hopkins and became full-time professor of obstetrics and gynecology at Rochester; John J. Morton (M.D., Johns Hopkins, 1913), who joined Rochester's faculty as professor of surgery; and Samuel W. Clausen (M.D., Johns Hopkins, 1915, and resident under John Howland), who became professor of pediatrics.

William S. McCann, professor of medicine, had headed the metabolism division of the Department of Medicine at Johns Hopkins. McCann met Whipple's requirement that faculty members be broadly competent, having taken a surgical internship with Cushing in Boston. McCann recalled the circumstances of his appointment:

To my surprise, I received a letter from Dean Whipple asking me to come to Rochester in consultation, as there were some problems concerning the department of medicine on which they needed my advice.

Two days were spent going over plans and blueprints, and discussing general problems of teaching and hospital organization. As the second day wore on George Whipple asked me if I would like to look at the city of Rochester, so we took a tour of the town in Whipple's car, finally pulling up to the curb on a side street looking straight ahead to a view of two tall smoke stacks emitting yellow smoke, which I learned was the main Eastman Kodak plant. There we remained in silence, which was broken after what seemed a long time by Whipple's question, "How would you like to be the professor of medicine in the new medical school?" I replied that I would, and he said "that is settled. . . ." All of the initial group (professorial team) were graduates of Johns Hopkins, except Faxon, Bloor, Fenn, Wilson, and me. Both Wilson and I had a substantial part of our teaching experience in Johns Hopkins, so it is fair to say that the new school in Rochester was formed by simple fission from the famous institution in Baltimore.[17]

Whipple brought to Rochester not only his own already famous research program but also faculty members who valued investigation as much as he did. McCann set up two good-sized laboratories in the Department of Medicine. Awaiting the completion of the hospital at Rochester, Wilson spent a year in the Baltimore laboratory of the Carnegie Institution's Department of Embryology. Corner continued his research at Rochester on the anatomy and physiology of reproduction. Clausen brought with him a knowledge of the newer aspects of pediatrics, based on biochemistry. Over the next few decades, faculty members at the University of Rochester medical school made important contributions in hematology, respiratory medicine, occupational disease, and nutrition.

Laboratory activities were the core of learning at Rochester, even in clinical departments, and the medical school adopted other policies begun at Johns Hopkins as well. An advertisement in *Science* for the new medical school in 1925 mentioned the presence of all facilities under one roof, opportunities for cooperation of school and hospital, equality of admission for men and women, small classes, and entrance requirements that included a knowledge of French and German.

Duke University

The School of Medicine at Duke University was the most complete Hopkins colony.[18] Of the original faculty of the Schools of Medicine, Nursing, and Health Services at Duke, thirty of forty-six members had trained at Johns Hopkins. In selecting the dean for the new school, all roads again led to Welch. President William P. Few of Duke asked the Rockefeller Foundation for advice; he was sent to Wickliffe Rose, promulgator of the hookworm control program in the South and a recipient of Rockefeller funds. Rose sent him to Welch, who recommended Wilburt C. Davison (M.D., Johns Hopkins 1917), then assistant dean at Johns Hopkins.

Davison had been a resident in pediatrics at Johns Hopkins under John Howland. Davison's administrative, laboratory, and clinical experience at Hopkins were at the heart of the philosophy of medical education and administration that

he brought in 1927 to Duke, where he was appointed professor of pediatrics, head of the department, and dean.

In selecting the original faculty at Duke, Davison was forced to consider whether to choose those of established reputation who had "arrived" or to gamble on promising younger physicians with a future. As Davison recalled from his visits to Osler in Oxford, "Fortunately, I had heard Osler discuss this question several times and though most people thought of the original 'Four Doctors' of the Hopkins as great men . . . they were comparative youngsters when originally appointed by President Daniel Coit Gilman. . . . Duke might not be able to find the equals of those Hopkins pioneers of modern medicine . . . but our best chance was men under forty years of age. At any rate, that explains why the average age of the original Duke medical faculty also was 35 years."[19]

Davison's first appointment was Harold L. Amoss, who left a faculty position at Johns Hopkins to become professor of medicine at Duke. Amoss in turn recommended other faculty members for the new medical school.

The Department of Surgery in particular has been a home for Hopkins-trained individuals over the years. J. Deryl Hart (M.D., Johns Hopkins, 1921) came to Duke in 1929 as the first chief of surgery. As director of the department until 1960, he developed the surgical specialties with Hopkins graduates. The first specialty division to be established at Duke was neurosurgery. For three years, funds for a neurosurgeon remained unused in the surgical budget as Hart searched for someone who had "the potential to become the best in the country."[20] In 1937, he found Barnes Woodhall (M.D., Johns Hopkins, 1930), who had just finished his surgical residency at Hopkins. In the 1940s, a plastic surgery division was developed with Hopkins-trained faculty, including the division's chief, Kenneth L. Pickrell (M.D., Johns Hopkins, 1935).

Another member of the Department of Surgery was Harold Fink (M.D., Johns Hopkins, 1928), who first became a resident and then a faculty member. The Departments of Surgery and Pathology at Johns Hopkins gave Duke its first chief of pathology, Wiley D. Forbus (M.D., Johns Hopkins, 1923), who had been surgical pathologist at Johns Hopkins. Hart's two successors as chief of surgery were also graduates of Johns Hopkins: Clarence E. Gardner, Jr. (M.D., 1928) and David C. Sabiston, Jr. (M.D., 1947). Edwin P. Alyea (M.D., Johns Hopkins, 1923) and Watt W. Eagle (M.D., Johns Hopkins, 1925) left faculty positions at Hopkins to join the Duke faculty as instructors; Alyea eventually became chief of urology, and Eagle, professor of otolaryngology. Former Hopkins residents who joined the Duke faculty were Alfred R. Shands (instructor in orthopedics), Lenox D. Baker (professor of orthopedics), and John Dees (professor of urology).

In the basic science departments, Hopkins-trained Francis H. Swett became professor of anatomy. William A. Perlzweig (chemist to the medical clinic at Johns Hopkins) was professor of biochemistry, and George S. Eadie, Ph.D. (also a faculty member at Johns Hopkins) was appointed professor of physiology.

Junior faculty members at Duke with a former Hopkins affiliation included assistant professor of medicine Oscar C. E. Hansen-Pruss (M.D., Johns Hopkins, 1924); instructors Roger D. Baker in anatomy and Frederick Bernheim, Ph.D., in physiology; surgical residents Clarence E. Gardner, Jr., and Robert R. Jones, Jr. (M.D., Johns Hopkins, 1928); pathology resident Earle B. Craven (M.D., Johns Hopkins, 1929); and anesthesiologist Mary Muller.

Other Hopkins-trained faculty came to Duke from elsewhere: F. Bayard Carter (M.D., Johns Hopkins, 1925), professor of obstetrics and gynecology at the University of Virginia, came to Duke to head the corresponding department in 1931. Bacteriologist David T. Smith (M.D., Johns Hopkins, 1922) became professor of bacteriology and associate professor of medicine. Susan Gower Smith joined Perlzweig in the Department of Biochemistry, as did Wilmer Institute chemist Haywood M. Taylor. Duncan C. Heatherington came from Vanderbilt to take charge of histology and neuroanatomy.

Policies in every area reflected the influence of Johns Hopkins. For example, departments were given maximal administrative independence. Davison advocated the full-time system, but a relatively small budget for salaries prevented him from placing all the clinical faculty on a full-time basis. Part-time clinical appointments ("geographic full-time") were therefore the rule.

Davison also consulted with Winford Smith, superintendent of the Johns Hopkins Hospital, regarding Duke's physical facilities. They agreed to follow the pattern of the Vanderbilt and Rochester schools by relating the departments to each other within the buildings according to their relationship in practice. Thus, the surgery and pathology departments were closely associated, and the x-ray department was placed as nearly as possible equidistant from medicine, surgery, and the outpatient department.

Davison's ideas regarding medical education were particularly influenced by his experience at Johns Hopkins. Success in selecting students ultimately depended, he believed, on quality rather than quantity of preparation. Statistical analyses of the performance of students at Johns Hopkins showed that only students with no major weaknesses completed the medical course in numbers that justified the school's investment in training them. The lesson for Duke was that only outstanding candidates should be admitted, even if this meant smaller classes and correspondingly higher tuition.

The chief advantage of such rigid selectivity, Davison felt, was an increase in the liberty that could be granted to the students. Johns Hopkins had liberalized its curriculum in 1927, and Davison used this revision as his model. He retained the quarter system but made each quarter eleven weeks long and offered an extra term in the summer. Students could thus graduate in three years by attending school all year round. A significant amount of time was allotted to elective courses, as Davison emphasized the Hopkins principle of self-education. "Learning by doing" characterized the entire educational process at Duke as it did at Hopkins. At every stage, from first-quarter anatomy to fifth-year senior residency, the Duke faculty trained its students for responsibility by giving them responsibility. Davison also instituted the clinical clerkship, but as at Vanderbilt, the order of the third and fourth years were reversed.

The Hopkins influence often emerged in the curriculum in subtle ways. In studying his field, Wiley D. Forbus, head of pathology, extended the basic comparative method taught to him by W. G. MacCallum at Johns Hopkins. Forbus in turn used the clinical records accompanying each set of specimens to convey a sense of the individuality of the disease in each case. A weekly journal hour in pathology for students was further evidence of the Hopkins influence on Duke's department.

The president of one southern university asked, "How are you going to get men to spend five to six years in residency training?" but the residency system was accepted by the students in the first graduating class, and the anticipated problems never materialized.[21] As at Johns Hopkins, the general surgical residency was a pyramidal program that in turn sent well-trained Duke graduates to populate other medical schools.

Davison's success in building the Duke University School of Medicine has been attributed in part to a willingness to gamble in appointing a young, Hopkins-trained faculty. This faculty was recruited from necessity, as the new school could not pay salaries large enough to attract full professors from established institutions, but Davison had confidence in this approach. Many southerners studying at Johns Hopkins came to Duke to contribute to improving the practice of medicine in their native region. By offering training based on principles proven at Johns Hopkins—including a close relation between laboratory and bedside instruction—Davison was able to provide Duke's students with a superior medical education.

The Pediatric Subspecialties and the Export of Physicians

The Division of Pediatric Cardiology and the Division of Pediatric Endocrinology illustrate the process of export from Johns Hopkins of physicians with highly specialized training. Edwards A. Park,

director of pediatrics during the 1920s and 1930s, had a gift for spotting promising young candidates for leadership. Several of his choices, including Helen B. Taussig and Lawson Wilkins, were themselves outstandingly successful in attracting young physicians for training—individuals who then left Johns Hopkins to occupy important posts in other medical centers.

Park placed the twenty-nine-year-old Helen B. Taussig in charge of his new pediatric cardiac clinic in 1930, instructing her to study each patient with the clinic's new machine, the fluoroscope, for evidence of congenital heart disease. Taussig was unenthusiastic about her assignment, as congenital heart disease did not seem to lend itself to other than anatomic research. She nevertheless studied every child referred to the cardiac clinic in meticulous detail, bringing to the task a particular capacity for correlating data and for understanding the functional circulatory changes caused by various cardiac malformations.

Taussig perceived that some cyanotic patients did reasonably well as long as the ductus arteriosus was open, but when the ductus closed, they became more cyanotic and their clinical condition worsened. She gradually understood that the basic problem was thus to reestablish the flow of blood to the lungs. She consulted Alfred Blalock about the problem, and the result of their collaboration was the "blue-baby" operation, first performed in 1944 (see chapter 11).

Between 1942 and 1962, Taussig taught 123 residents and fellows about pediatric and congenital heart disease. Many of these second-generation pediatric cardiologists developed their own programs, training a third generation—which has by now produced a fourth generation of such specialists. In the words of Taussig's student Dan McNamara, professor of pediatrics at Baylor College of Medicine, "Establishment of the sub-board of pediatric cardiology in 1962 brought official recognition to what many thought was the birth of a new discipline, but it was actually the maturation, rather than the birth of pediatric cardiology. For the preceding 32 years the acknowledged founder of the sub-board had been practicing the art and developing the science of

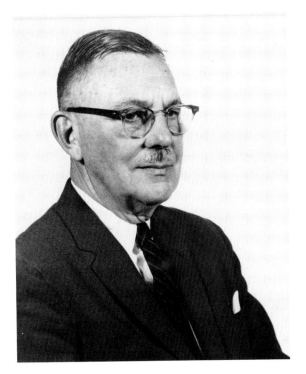

Lawson Wilkins. (*Source:* Alan M. Chesney Medical Archives, The Johns Hopkins Medical Institutions.)

pediatric cardiology."[22] Many of Taussig's postgraduate students later chose other fields of study. Leon Gordis, professor of epidemiology at the Johns Hopkins School of Hygiene and Public Health, is an example of former fellows who applied their fellowship training to a career outside pediatric cardiology.[23]

Park's decision to start a pediatric endocrinology clinic in 1935 was met with disbelief by the person he chose to head it, Lawson Wilkins. Endocrinology was considered an "unscientific" discipline at the time, and its practitioners were looked on as little better than charlatans. Wilkins was a 1918 graduate of the Johns Hopkins University School of Medicine; he had served an internship at the New Haven Hospital in Connecticut and then returned to Hopkins for a residency in pediatrics. Although he chose to enter private practice, he continued his interest in research, investigating the calcium and phosphorus metabolism of rickets. Wilkins' interest in epilepsy brought him to Park's attention, and Park invited him to join Edward Bridge in running the epi-

lepsy clinic in the Department of Pediatrics.

Park then persuaded Wilkins to relinquish his studies of epilepsy and head a new division of pediatric endocrinology. Wilkins' first investigation in this area focused on children with thyroid deficiency and resulted in his classic study of osseous and mental development in cretins and dwarfs. He was promoted to full professor in 1957. Wilkins was a leader in his methodical approach, his superb record keeping, and his broad knowledge of pediatrics. Wilkins' studies were based on the most meticulous investigations of his patients, not primarily on the literature.

One of his major contributions was the training of the next generation of pediatric endocrinologists. Students came to him from all over the world, and the list of his former pupils includes many who are now heads of departments of pediatrics or directors of pediatric endocrine clinics.

Wilkins was particularly proud of his fellows, whom he called "the boys," although a few "girls" belonged to the group as well. In the spring of 1963, only a few months before his death, Wilkins called all the "boys" to invite them to a scientific meeting in Baltimore. This was a momentous occasion, attended by the oldest "boy," Walter Fleischmann, professor of pediatrics at Hopkins, who was Wilkins' first associate in the endocrine clinic and an important contributor to his work on the thyroid. After Wilkins' death, the "boys" decided to organize a reunion along with the second generation of fellows. Beginning in 1965, these meetings have taken place at Hopkins biennially. By 1971, the group had become too large for its informal structure; thus the Lawson Wilkins Pediatric Endocrine Society came into being. A constitution for the society was written, and Claude Migeon, professor of pediatrics at Hopkins since 1971, was elected founding president.[24]

Nobel Laureates Trained at Johns Hopkins

The export of men and women who received a significant part of their training at Johns Hopkins, as medical students, interns, residents, or fellows, has continued at a vigorous pace over the years. The number who have attained the rank of full professor outside Hopkins has risen steadily, so that it is not feasible to list them all. Another distinction that illuminates the quality of the physicians and scientists who have left Hopkins to populate other medical schools is that several among them have won the Nobel Prize.[25]

The Nobel Prize has come to be viewed as the pinnacle of achievement in the various fields for which it is given. Although only Daniel Nathans and Hamilton Smith have received the coveted prize while at Hopkins (see chapter 11), a number of Nobel laureates were either educated at Johns Hopkins or served on the faculty for an extended period of time.

The first native-born American scientist to win the Nobel Prize for Physiology or Medicine was Thomas Hunt Morgan (Ph.D., Johns Hopkins, 1890). Morgan created a revolution in the study of heredity, founded a school of genetics, and trained many important students, among them Hermann Muller, who was to receive the prize in 1946. Morgan was awarded the Nobel Prize in 1933 for his discovery concerning the function of the chromosome in the transmission of heredity. Morgan received his Ph.D. at Hopkins in Henry Newell Martin's Department of Biology.

The following year, the Nobel Prize for Physiology or Medicine was awarded to George R. Minot, William P. Murphy, and George Hoyt Whipple for their discovery concerning the treatment of anemia with liver. Both Minot and Whipple had been affiliated with Hopkins. After receiving his medical degree from Hopkins in 1905, Whipple served on the faculty of the Department of Pathology at Hopkins until 1914 (except for one year spent as pathologist at a hospital in Panama). He then moved to the University of California medical school as professor of research medicine, and from there, to the new University of Rochester School of Medicine and Dentistry as professor and dean. It was while he was at Rochester that Whipple was awarded the Nobel Prize.

Whipple's major study on the influence of food on blood regeneration was begun in 1920.

He found that dogs whose anemia was created by withdrawing blood at intervals were most effectively restored by a diet consisting mainly of liver. Whipple's investigations gave Minot and Murphy the idea of feeding liver to patients with pernicious anemia.

Minot, a 1912 graduate of Harvard Medical School, spent his entire career at Harvard except for two years at Hopkins, one as an assistant resident physician under Thayer and one as a research fellow in physiology. During his stay in Baltimore, from 1913 to 1915, Minot worked in the laboratory of William H. Howell on problems regarding blood coagulation. Minot also wrote his first article on pernicious anemia while at Hopkins: "Nitrogen Metabolism Before and After Splenectomy in a Case of Pernicious Anemia."

In accepting the award, Minot credited several individuals with having taught him how science provides the means to alleviate human suffering and helped him to understand the fundamental aspects of the problem to be solved. Among them were Thayer and Howell.

The Nobel Prize for Physiology or Medicine was awarded in 1944 to Joseph Erlanger and Herbert Spencer Gasser for their discoveries regarding the highly differentiated functions of single nerve fibers. Erlanger received his M.D. degree from Hopkins in 1899 and served a one-year internship in the Johns Hopkins Hospital. He then joined the Department of Physiology under Howell, remaining until 1906, when he accepted an invitation to become the first professor of physiology at the University of Wisconsin's new medical school. Herbert Gasser was one of the first medical students at Wisconsin, and he met his distinguished collaborator when he took Erlanger's course in physiology. After two years at Wisconsin, Gasser came to Hopkins for his clinical work, obtaining the M.D. degree in 1915. It was as faculty members at Washington University in Saint Louis that Erlanger and Gasser performed their pioneering work with the cathode-ray oscillograph. Theirs was the first use of this type of oscillograph in the study of electrophysiology. They were able to demonstrate that single nerve fibers could be differentiated on the basis of their size and the speed with which they transmitted impulses.

An important contribution in the field of endocrinology was made by Vincent du Vigneaud of Cornell, who succeeded in synthesizing pitressin and oxytocin, the two polypeptide hormones of the posterior pituitary. For this work, du Vigneaud received the Nobel Prize for Chemistry for 1955. Twenty-seven years earlier, du Vigneaud had worked in Abel's laboratory at Johns Hopkins. He isolated the active principle of the posterior pituitary, and the material he obtained was so powerful that it would stimulate the uterus even in an almost infinitesimal dilution. Abel mistakenly concluded that a single hormone of the posterior pituitary was responsible for the effects on blood pressure, urine secretion, and uterine contraction. While working with Abel, du Vigneaud gained valuable experience in the synthesis of cystine peptides. It subsequently became clear that two hormones, closely related chemically, were involved and it was these two hormones that du Vigneaud succeeded in synthesizing.

Peyton Rous, who shared the 1955 Nobel Prize for Physiology or Medicine with Charles Huggins for their work in cancer research, was a native Baltimorean who received his A.B. degree from the Johns Hopkins University, graduated from the School of Medicine in 1905, and served as an intern at the Johns Hopkins Hospital. Rous then turned to medical research, becoming an instructor in pathology at the University of Michigan. He soon accepted an invitation to join the staff of the newly organized Rockefeller Institute, where he made the revolutionary discovery of a malignant sarcoma in chickens that was caused by a filterable virus.

The 1967 Nobel Prize for Physiology or Medicine was shared by H. K. Hartline and George Wald of the United States and Ragnar Granit of Sweden for their discoveries concerning the primary chemical and physiological visual processes. Hartline was a 1927 graduate of the Johns Hopkins University School of Medicine who served as professor of biophysics at Hopkins from 1949 to 1953. At the time of his award, he was a faculty member of the Rockefeller University. He

and his associates were the first to demonstrate that individual nerve cells in the retina never act independently; it is the integrated action of all units of the visual system that gives rise to vision.

David Hubel and Torsten Weisel, who received the Nobel Prize for Physiology or Medicine in 1981, had worked for several years in the Division of Ophthalmic Physiology at Johns Hopkins under Stephen W. Kuffler. Hubel received his clinical training in neurology at Hopkins with John W. Magladery and joined Kuffler's group after training at the Walter Reed Institute for Medical Research. Weisel came to Baltimore in 1955, beginning a twenty-year collaboration with Hubel. Both eventually left for Harvard, where each was for a time head of the Department of Neurobiology.

Hubel and Weisel received the Nobel Prize for their demonstration that the stimulation of sight in infancy is tied to future visual capabilities. Their twenty-year collaboration produced a breakthrough in the understanding of the brain's ability to interpret the code of the impulse messages from the eyes. They found that the capacity of the visual system to interpret images is developed directly after birth. The eyes must also be exposed to varied visual stimuli. If stimuli are dull and distorted—for example, through errors in the eye's lens system—the infant's ability to analyze visual information may be permanently impaired. They also discovered that the transmission of information from the retina of the eye to the brain involves a step-by-step process in which each step involves columns of nerve cells that receive information, analyze it according to the cell column's specific property, and pass the results along.

Stephen Kuffler had died the year before Hubel and Weisel received the Nobel Prize. Hubel commented that only the Nobel Committee's rule against awarding the prize posthumously prevented Kuffler from sharing in it.

Deans and faculty members of other medical schools—particularly new ones—had more freedom than the early Hopkins leaders to carry out Hopkins' ideals. The founders of Hopkins had broken the path, and their successors at other schools were often able to move quickly and easily. Compare, for example, G. Canby Robinson's freedom to design an entire physical facility at Vanderbilt in the 1920s with Welch's struggles at Johns Hopkins to situate his pathological laboratory close to the wards.

Hopkins-trained deans were a key influence on these new or revitalized medical schools, as they created the school's architectural shape and administrative structure and brought in faculty to implement their plans. Bardeen at Wisconsin, Davison at Duke, Robinson at Vanderbilt, Whipple at Rochester, Ross Harrison and Milton C. Winternitz at Yale—all brought the Hopkins policies to their new or reorganized schools and persuaded former colleagues to follow them to their new institutions.

By midcentury, the Hopkins model had become so successful that its daughter schools were exporting well-trained graduates of their own—some of whom returned to Hopkins. The University of Chicago was the source of so many Hopkins faculty members that one of them has referred to it as Hopkins' farm team.[26] The University of Michigan had also played a major role in planting the seed of excellence at Hopkins. Of the original faculty in Baltimore, Mall, Abel, Howell, and Hurd had been students or faculty members at Michigan.[27]

The most direct influence, however, was exerted by those who moved out from staff positions at Johns Hopkins, whether or not they were graduates. Former Hopkins faculty members transformed departments elsewhere—for example, William G. MacCallum at Columbia, and Harvey Cushing, Henry A. Christian, and William T. Councilman at Harvard. Osler's students in particular left his indelible imprint on every department of medicine they touched. The strength of this influence derived in part from the sheer number of graduates who pursued careers in academic medicine—a number that historian Richard Shryock called "phenomenal."[28] The distribution of Hopkins graduates across the country, to the faculties of strong medical schools, remains widespread today.

The vitality of Hopkins' ineffable "heritage of excellence" spans the years, from Cole's description of an early class of medical students (see chapter 2) to a recent reminiscence by John D. Stobo, current director of the Department of Medicine. Speaking of his residency at Johns Hopkins, Stobo said:

> I'll always remember my internship, residency, and chief residency as a time when I devoted my full energies to learning, patient care, and teaching. The reason for becoming totally involved in these endeavors was simple—that was the tradition, the system, and most important, preservation of the system was dependent on total commitment of the house staff to the learning and practice of medicine. . . . The system provided the structure under which responsibility for patients was given to the house staff.[29]

Stobo recalls the sense of pride attached to being a Hopkins house officer, "which derived not from merely physically being a member of the house staff, but rather from contributing to an excellence in medicine that had been present since the hospital was founded."[30]

CHAPTER 10

JOHNS HOPKINS MEDICINE AND THE COMMUNITY

The indigent sick of this city and its environs, without regard to sex, age, or color, who may require surgical or medical treatment, and who can be received into the Hospital without peril to the other inmates, and the poor of the city and State, of all races, who are stricken down by any casualty, shall be received into the Hospital without charge, for such periods of time and under such regulations as you may prescribe.

—Johns Hopkins, 1873

Johns Hopkins' letter of instruction to the trustees in 1873 stipulated that the hospital and medical school that bear his name offer service to the community. In accordance with his wishes, the Johns Hopkins Hospital assumed the responsibility for giving free medical care to the indigent. He also specified in his will that the Johns Hopkins Hospital support a Home for Colored Orphans. By "community," Johns Hopkins meant not merely the environs of the hospital, but the City of Baltimore and State of Maryland. The hospital's primary patient base has, however, always come from its immediate neighborhood. As Catherine DeAngelis, professor of pediatrics, commented: "The 'Harriet Lane Home' has served as the family doctor for children of East Baltimore from the day it opened. . . . Children and their parents waited on wooden benches for many hours until they were seen by pediatric residents. . . . The wooden benches are now modern, modular furniture. But the children's faces really have not changed, and some of the staff members who now serve these children once sat on those wooden benches themselves."[1] The larger community includes inhabitants of the surrounding area and patients who have been referred to distinguished Hopkins physicians with a national reputation. Although Hopkins established affiliations with other hospitals—such as Sinai, Baltimore City, Church Home, Good Samaritan, and Union Memorial—for teaching and research, it has reached into the community primarily through patient care.

To carry out Johns Hopkins' wish, when the hospital was established, it maintained an outpatient service, or Dispensary, which served as the local physician for the community. Most of the Dispensary staff were members of the faculty, and some of the latter were distinguished physicians and surgeons. The Dispensary was also used to teach third-year medical students the techniques of history taking and physical examination.

The Diagnostic Clinic

The Diagnostic Clinic, proposed by Winford Smith in 1921, was the first program designed specifically for the benefit of the community. It served the community in two ways. First, it was intended for individuals of modest means. Those who could not afford to pay at all were cared for in the Dispensary; those who could afford private medical treatment consulted the part-time clinical staff in their offices and were hospitalized on the private wards of the Marburg Building. Smith intended the Diagnostic Clinic to help the large group of patients who fell between the two extremes. Second, it made the full diagnostic and therapeutic capabilities of the hospital available to local physicians who had no hospital appointment, and gave them a means of keeping in touch with the best current methods of diagnosis. Smith's proposal was included in Hopkins' request for funds from the Carnegie Foundation for a new outpatient facility, and the clinic opened when the Carnegie Dispensary was completed in 1928.[2]

The Diagnostic Clinic provided diagnoses and recommendations for patients who could pay between $10 and $25 for the service. Patients were accepted only upon the referral of their physicians. Under no circumstances was treatment provided by hospital physicians. Instead, diagnostic and laboratory reports and recommendations for treatment were returned to the patient's referring physician. Nor was the clinic used for teaching either medical students or house staff. Its sole purpose was the diagnostic care of patients.

Paul W. Clough was the clinic's director throughout its twenty-five-year life-span. His staff included general internists—C. Holmes Boyd, then Harry Wasserman, and later Thomas C. Wolff and T. Nelson Carey—as well as consultants for each specialty.

The Diagnostic Clinic was an instant success. During its first year, patients had to be turned away because they could not be accommodated in its twice-weekly sessions. About 60 percent of the patients were referred by physicians in Baltimore; the remainder were sent by physicians elsewhere in Maryland or out-of-state. The most prevalent disorders identified were otolaryngological: approximately three-fourths of all patients required this type of specialty care. Dental problems were next in frequency, followed by ophthalmologic,

surgical, orthopedic, and gynecologic problems. Each patient, whatever the presenting complaint, was given a complete general medical examination, which, along with the indicated laboratory examination, was called a "diagnostic work-up."

The clinic continued to grow modestly during the 1930s; the original staff of three internists increased to six, and the number of consultants increased from nineteen in 1932 to thirty-six in 1940. It flourished during World War II, when physicians were diverted to wartime service and the nation's income was rising. Between 1940 and 1945, the number of patients utilizing the clinic rose 50 percent, from 1,879 to 2,708.

Although both fees and income rose, by the mid-1950s the $75 cost of a diagnostic survey in the Diagnostic Clinic was no longer outside the reach of most private patients. In 1953, the Diagnostic Clinic was merged with the private outpatient clinic.[3]

The Medical Care Clinic

No program specifically for patients in the surrounding community existed until 1947, when the Baltimore City Health Department created a medical care program for the city's indigent and asked the Johns Hopkins Medical Institutions to create and run one of two proposed clinics. This program was also the first program of its kind to receive financial support from outside Hopkins. The Baltimore City Hospitals received its financial support from the city, but its location on the outskirts of Baltimore was inconvenient for many poor patients. Therefore, the patients went instead to Johns Hopkins, which was carrying the burden of care for the city's indigent without financial recompense.[4]

The city's proposal came in response to pressure from the Johns Hopkins Hospital's trustees and administrators. Since 1889, the hospital had carried the full financial cost of its outpatient service, as there was at that time no tax money to support the care of the indigent. As the city's population grew, the burden had become increasingly heavy.

In addition to its financial problems, the Carnegie Dispensary lacked the prestige of the inpatient service, which housed patients with more serious and "interesting" medical problems. Enthusiasm for working on the inpatient wards was greater, particularly in departments such as medicine, most of whose patients required extensive and time-consuming examinations. In ophthalmology, in contrast, both inpatients and outpatients needed relatively circumscribed examinations, so the resistance to caring for outpatients in the specialty clinics was less.

As the clinical departments adopted the full-time system, it was mainly the part-time staff who were left to uphold the quality of outpatient medical care. This they did, with determination and pride. Despite little financial help from either the hospital or the medical school, the heads of the various specialty clinics managed to conduct outstanding clinical investigations in the dispensary.

During the 1930s, formal attempts were made to ameliorate conditions in the Dispensary. Thomas B. Turner was assigned to review the situation and formulate plans to upgrade its functions. G. Canby Robinson also tried to personalize outpatient care, studying patients whose diseases had a psychosomatic component in an effort to improve the dispensary's Samaritan aspects. The severe lack of financial support during the Depression, however, impeded attempts at improvement.[5]

When the patient load increased after World War II, existing problems were exaggerated. The staff of the dispensary changed, as much of the outpatient care was assumed by fellows involved in research training programs or by members of the resident staff. Part-time staff also had less time to spend at Hopkins. Many were also staff members at other Baltimore hospitals, as they did not have visiting privileges at Hopkins; postgraduate training programs were proliferating at other hospitals, and the staff members were forced to participate in the programs as the price for maintaining their presence at these facilities.

The Medical Care Clinic resolved many of the problems connected with outpatient care at Hopkins. It marked the beginning of the era of "programs" in community medicine, which culminated in the Johns Hopkins Health System of the 1980s.

The intent of the Medical Care Clinic, which the hospital's Medical Board termed a "desirable experiment," was not merely to set up a clinic but also to establish a model program for giving comprehensive care to Welfare Department clients, and to determine the cost of such a program. The clients fell into three groups: they received so-called old age assistance, general public assistance, or aid to dependent children.

The Medical Board set stringent limits for Hopkins' participation in the new welfare clinic. No individual department would be responsible for running it; instead, it would be under the direction of Harry L. Chant, an assistant director of the hospital. Work would be supervised by full-time Hopkins faculty, but local physicians would be paid $10 to $12 a session to carry the burden of care. Mass screening of the indigent population would include an initial examination for each client but no annual check-up. Hopkins would not assume responsibility for the hospitalization of any clinic patients, nor would Hopkins support the clinic with operating funds from either hospital or university. The city would, in fact, pay Hopkins $7 for each client, and Hopkins physicians would be paid for their services. The program was strictly for patient care; no teaching or research would be conducted in the clinic.

The Medical Care Clinic opened in August 1948 in temporary quarters in the old Surgical Building. Two months later, it moved to a permanent home on Rutland Avenue. Although progress was slow at first, by 1950 the Medical Care Clinic had registered 11,250 clients, who represented about 85 percent of the individuals assigned by the city. One hundred eighty-nine practicing physicians—136 white and 53 black—worked in collaboration with the clinic.

It quickly became apparent that the Medical Care Clinic was filling a great need. A study of initial examinations revealed that the clinic was recognizing disease in a significant number of persons who had not previously been treated. Mental or physical abnormalities were discovered in 57 percent of the clients screened, 60 percent of whom were new to treatment. As anticipated, most of these persons were elderly.[6]

By 1954, the clinic had streamlined its examination process. The preponderance of disease among elderly clients led physicians to perform a shortened examination on younger persons without a major presenting complaint. The city also wanted to expand the program to include the large group of individuals just above the poverty level, and the Johns Hopkins Medical Institutions, taking a new interest in primary care, saw the value of using the clinic for teaching home and family practice.

To implement these changes, the clinic was turned over to the Department of Medicine. John C. Harvey replaced George Dana, who was Chant's successor, as clinic director, and ten full-time clinicians, all department members, were added to the staff. Two research programs were inaugurated. One compared the effectiveness of the clinic's abbreviated examination with a standard complete physical examination, and the other investigated the effectiveness of an oral mercurial diuretic, neohydrin, in patients with congestive heart failure. Students in the department's physical diagnosis course were also brought into the clinic.[7]

By the mid-1950s, the Medical Care Clinic was financially self-supporting, for the number of patient visits had doubled between 1953 and 1954. It also operated more efficiently: 15 to 20 percent fewer patients were referred to hospital specialty clinics, and the resulting savings steadily eliminated the clinic's modest deficit. In addition, more patients were being seen by participating physicians for long-term follow-up, thus removing them from the hospital clinics' rolls.[8]

Participating physicians benefited professionally from their association with the clinic. In addition to obtaining new patients, they used the clinic as a consultation service, and their request for monthly educational meetings enhanced the clinic's *esprit de corps.*

Harvey also established an unusual fellowship program by combining clinic funds with money available from the medical institutions'

Personnel Health Clinic: postgraduate students from overseas were brought to study at Hopkins, spending half their time in the Medical Care Clinic or the Personnel Health Clinic and the other half in a specialty division of their choice. Between 1957 and 1967, the clinic trained 109 fellows from around the world, many of whom went on to distinguished careers.[9]

The Medical Care Clinic, along with its fellowship program, ended abruptly in 1967 with the advent of Medicare and Medicaid.

The Columbia Medical Plan

Johns Hopkins entered the arena of prepaid group practice in 1964, with consideration of the Columbia Medical Plan. In the early 1960s, James Rouse, a Baltimore banker and shopping center developer, conceived the idea of building a new city halfway between Washington and Baltimore. Over a period of years he purchased a tract of land the size of Manhattan Island and, with the financial backing of the Connecticut General Life Insurance Company, started to build his visionary city of Columbia. By 1980 the city would contain one hundred thousand people, who would naturally require health services. Rouse believed that this city would be the ideal setting for a prepaid health plan, and he approached Johns Hopkins for help.

The reaction at Hopkins to Rouse's proposal ranged from enthusiastic assent (largely from faculty at the School of Hygiene and Public Health) to fervent opposition (from the more academically inclined members of the clinical faculty). Dissenters on the faculty wanted to keep Hopkins' resources at home. They were concerned that Hopkins would be spreading these resources too thin and would be unable to maintain its strengths in research and teaching if it assumed responsibility for this new area of medical care. They feared that Hopkins would not be able to continue providing sophisticated hospital care to patients with complex diseases if it was also required to invest faculty time, money, and hospital beds in this ancillary venture. It would be a mistake to divert funds to a new program, they believed, when hospital facilities, such as those in radiology, needed upgrading. A new program in Columbia would also overload an outstanding faculty already overburdened with its traditional responsibilities. Moreover, the dissenters felt that the university would be unable to recruit what they considered a high-caliber faculty for the new facility, since they believed that physicians experienced in giving primary care would probably lack experience in teaching and research.[10]

Proponents of Rouse's plan thought that Hopkins was being handed a unique opportunity to develop a model health care system that could be passed on to other communities. Here was a chance to design an entire system from scratch, to control its financing and use it as a base for experimental approaches to the distribution of physicians and ancillary staff. The existence of a population of manageable size and predictable growth rate would allow Hopkins to take advantage of accumulating experience and to improve its program as each new segment of the city came into being. This venture would also broaden the experience of Hopkins' students and house staff, giving them a better understanding of the spectrum of human illness and the direction that medical care was taking. Beyond the benefits, the proponents of the plan cited the university's responsibility to examine problems related to the distribution of health care.[11]

A long and heated debate ensued. The faculty made their feelings known that if a program was to be organized in Columbia, a similar program should be launched in East Baltimore. The outcome was a decision to participate but to use only new money and additional faculty. All funds would come from newly developed resources. None would be derived from the endowment of the Johns Hopkins University or Hospital. This plan would protect the school's traditional strengths: its commitment to biomedical research and its specialized management of individual illnesses.

Negotiations with the Connecticut General Life Insurance Company made the company the major financial supporter of the Columbia pro-

gram. The company would provide all up-front capital and would bear 100 percent of the financial risk for the first five years and 90 percent thereafter. It would also provide the money for a Hopkins-owned hospital in Columbia. Approaches were also made to three foundations— the Rockefeller Foundation, the Commonwealth Fund, and the Carnegie Foundation—which together provided a total of $750,000 over the next three years. In sum, the Columbia Medical Plan would not burden the Johns Hopkins Medical Institutions with any operational financial risk.

Hopkins decided not to create a department of community medicine to run the Columbia plan, as most faculty members believed that "primary care" was a function of all existing departments. Instead, the Office of Health Care Programs was created in 1969 as part of the dean's office of the medical school. Under the direction of Robert M. Heyssel, who was appointed associate dean, the office would span the three Hopkins components involved in Columbia—the medical school, the school of hygiene, and the hospital.[12]

The Columbia program was intended to concentrate on research in medical care, primary care, "human resource utilization," and the evaluation of techniques for preventive care. The operation would also serve as a base for instruction of students in medicine, nursing, and related professions. To carry out all these objectives, a complicated system of advisory and controlling committees was formed. There was an advisory committee for the Columbia program and a separate advisory committee for the Health Services Research and Development Center, which was responsible for evaluating the Columbia project as it developed. Since this center, initially headed by Dr. Malcolm Peterson, was part of the Office of Health Care Programs, its early involvement in the Columbia and East Baltimore programs was assured. It was Dr. Peterson and his staff who undertook much of the work related to human resource utilization and use of medical services within an HMO.

A new corporation was constituted, known as the Columbia Hospital and Clinic Foundation.

A joint committee of trustees from the university and hospital became the owners and directors of the foundation. They, in turn, appointed a Hopkins-dominated board of trustees. Physicians associated with the Columbia Program would be responsible to a group of three partners, all deans in the Johns Hopkins Medical Institutions, led by the dean of the medical faculty, David E. Rogers.

This was the institutional arrangement keyed to the basic agreement that constituted the Columbia Medical Plan. The plan had a triangular structure. At the apex was the Columbia Hospital and Clinic Foundation, the umbrella group responsible for developing the hospital and offering the health and medical care. At another point were the insurance carriers (initially, only Connecticut General), responsible for financial support and marketing. Finally, an entity called the Johns Hopkins Medical Partnership was responsible for actually providing the medical care. Conspicuously absent was any direct consumer involvement, but plans called for the later establishment of a Members' Advisory Council.

Each group had a different power base. The insurance companies were the source of funds. The foundation negotiated the budget, receiving—and controlling—the funds. The physicians, in contrast, were salaried and had no discretionary funds. Although their power lay in their professional expertise, they lacked a strong, coordinated voice because they were inexperienced in budgetary negotiations. They were thus weak and unstructured administratively.[13]

The Columbia Medical Plan opened with two internists, two pediatricians, and one psychiatrist, receiving its first patients in temporary quarters in October 1969. The timing was unfortunate. The nation was involved in a recession, and the new community was growing at a slower rate than anticipated. Marketing of the plan during these early years also moved slowly, since HMOs were a new idea. Moreover, federal employees were initially not given the option of enrolling, and Blue Cross, the major carrier in that area, did not participate in marketing the program until 1972.[14]

Hospital construction began in March 1972,

and the hospital opened in the summer of 1973. The hospital was in financial trouble from the beginning, owing to substantial cost escalations over the 1968 estimates, the early need for more working capital, and lower-than-anticipated use. The hospital's financial problems, coupled with the continuing financial losses of the Columbia Medical Plan and the slower-than-anticipated membership growth, forced a major reorganization in 1974. The plan divested itself of the hospital, which became Howard County General, and added nongroup physicians to its staff. In response, the medical group moved out of the hospital, incorporated themselves as the Patuxent Medical Group, hired a business manager, and developed a new affiliation agreement with Johns Hopkins.

Under the new agreement, Hopkins no longer exerted any control over the group or the plan, but most plan physicians retained faculty appointments and continued to teach at Hopkins. The most generous assessment of this Hopkins venture was that it succeeded in part. Its teaching activities had to be considered a failure: medical students were not brought to Columbia for instruction. On the other hand, research in medical care flourished, largely through the work of Samuel Shapiro, who succeeded Peterson in 1973 as director of the Health Services Research and Development Center, and his staff.

The lack of enthusiasm from the clinical departments reflected the fact that Johns Hopkins in the 1960s was clearly not an institution oriented toward primary care. Perhaps more important, the Columbia Medical Plan was an idea ahead of its time. In the mid-1960s, few people had heard of prepaid health plans, and the idea had to be sold to consumers. Columbia's population base was simply not large enough to begin with and did not grow soon enough to allow for success in the short run. The early population and enrollment estimates were too optimistic, and revenues therefore lagged behind expenditures. When Hopkins relinquished control, the plan was not self-supporting, but it later became a financial success.

Hopkins learned many lessons from participating in the Columbia Medical Plan, and this was the real, if deferred, benefit of the experience for the medical institutions. For Johns Hopkins, an understanding of the potential value of an HMO to an academic medical center was only on the horizon in the 1960s. For the hospital, a new population can provide a new source of inpatient hospitalizations and specialty referrals. For the medical school, an HMO can provide a unique ambulatory practice for both teaching and research, especially in primary care, and an additional source of professional fee income. As one participant in the Columbia plan said, "The whole debate and those times loosened Hopkins from its kind of hidebound traditionality. And we started slowly along a path of opening it up."[15] When opportunities arrived two decades later to establish a Hopkins HMO, many of the key participants in the Columbia plan were still on the scene, able to use what they had learned from their previous experience.[16]

The East Baltimore Medical Plan

The ambivalence that marks most town-gown relationships was exacerbated during the 1960s as the economic disparity grew between the hospital and the surrounding black community. The fence around the hospital mandated by Johns Hopkins' will became a symbol of this disparity.[17]

As Clarence "Du" Burns, the first black mayor of Baltimore, commented,

> I was born right here [at the Johns Hopkins Hospital] and have lived in East Baltimore all my life. We always took pride in saying we were "Hopkins babies." This institution was reputed to be the greatest in the world and everybody wants to be tied to the greatest.
>
> But I will tell you this, we hated this place, even though I used to come up here with a little yellow card that my mother would give me. They would take care of our whole family; all we needed was the card.
>
> . . . This place had a black ward and a white ward. That stuck in our craw. There were such things as black and white toilets. So I learned to dis-

like this institution, yet took pride in saying I was a Hopkins baby.[18]

At the same time that the Columbia Medical Plan was under discussion, Hopkins faculty and administration were considering establishing a companion HMO closer to home. Faculty members were far more eager to establish such a facility in East Baltimore than in Columbia. The proposed East Baltimore HMO was closer to home and thus more manageable. It also satisfied the hospital founder's mandate to serve the "indigent sick" and "poor" of the area. The black community surrounding Johns Hopkins had similar ideas: "You're going out to Columbia, where folks can pay for their care," some said, "but what about health services for us?" The community was dissatisfied with the existing hospital clinics—the treatment, the long waits, the color barrier. After the riots of 1968, community leaders came forward with a demand for better health services. The main problem with existing services, they said, was access to medical care—and their solution was a community health center.[19]

In planning the health center, the major point of contention was control, i.e., ownership and decision making. The community insisted that it hold the reins, and Hopkins acceded. The governing board as finally constituted thus consisted of twenty members of the community and two representatives of Johns Hopkins. Board members included several community leaders who have since been important in the political life of East Baltimore, the city, and the state—including Clarence "Du" Burns. At Hopkins, the program was directed by the Office of Health Care Programs.[20]

By 1969, Hopkins and the community had reached a general agreement about the formation of an HMO and a health center. The objectives of the East Baltimore Medical Plan reflected the interests of both parties. The plan would provide a health care system more responsive to the needs of the inner-city population that was the traditional responsibility of the Johns Hopkins Medical Institutions. It would also develop a realistic model of health care delivery for the inner city in which physicians and other health personnel could be trained. To demonstrate that ambulatory care services could be improved in the inner city without additional *per capita* expenditures, it would substitute primary medical care for more expensive inpatient, emergency room, and multi-specialty outpatient care. Finally, it would demonstrate that prepaid group practices could be developed in the inner city with a minimum of new federal financing, by merging all the existing available local, state, and federal funds into one prepayment pool.[21]

These objectives required a single set of medical care benefits for all enrolled, one that was compatible with those provided by the state Medicaid program. The plan would also need a single administrative structure that would funnel local, state, and federal funds into one prepayment account for the common use of the plan. The crucial issue was to negotiate an acceptable contract with all major third-party financing agencies, particularly the state Medicaid program, to obtain prepayment capitation grants for eligible individuals.

All these conditions were met when the first phase of the plan began on March 1, 1971. Five thousand residents of four low-income housing developments were enrolled, and the plan was intended to accommodate 20,000 more. Funding was abundant, including public health service grants and special provisions by Medicare, and the accumulated funds were channeled through Hopkins to an organization known as the East Baltimore Community Corporation. In 1972, the East Baltimore Community Health Center opened in a church basement, and in 1979 it moved to a newly constructed ambulatory facility nearby.

Persistent problems concerned marketing and third-party payments, particularly Medicaid. Marketing was slow and difficult; almost ten years elapsed before employees of the City of Baltimore were finally included in the plan. The fragmented structure of governmental medical support for the needy created a lack of standardized benefit levels, a complexity of eligibility criteria, a multiplicity of administrative procedures, and a paucity of funds for new programs.

For patients, however, the establishment of the East Baltimore Medical Center resulted in accessible high-quality medical care. The East Baltimore facility was not quite like the private medical model, but it has been judged more satisfactory than the traditional hospital emergency room or outpatient department, and the community felt that it had the opportunity to change things if it was dissatisfied. The facility has been a source of jobs for members of the community, and its link with the local high school has provided opportunities for students interested in health care careers.

For Johns Hopkins, the importance of working with the community far outweighed the facility's shortcomings. Although some students from the School of Hygiene and Public Health were involved in a variety of programs, the center was not an important training facility for medical students, partly because of the low priority assigned by the community to the center's academic goals. The East Baltimore Medical Plan has, however, led to improved relations with the neighborhood, often at times when political and general community support has been crucial to the success of other activities of the medical institutions.[22]

To run a community-based HMO, "you must learn patience and flexibility as an institution, and that your way may not necessarily be the only way," said Torrey C. Brown, an associate professor of medicine who was instrumental in developing the center.[23] An institution cannot let frustration deter such a project, and it must be willing to recognize that the community's expectations are not necessarily those of the university.

The Johns Hopkins Health System

By the 1980s, it was evident that systems for the care of patients were becoming diversified. Across the country, for-profit organizations were increasingly taking control of facilities for medical care, and increasing numbers of patients were enrolling in HMOs and their variants. It was therefore essential that Hopkins' "market share" of medical care be not only protected but also enlarged—regionally, nationally, and internationally. The means for doing so was a vertically integrated system of medical care that would emphasize primary care (with special attention to chronic care facilities and home health care services), develop a Hopkins HMO, and increase the referral practice. To carry out this plan, Hopkins would have to affiliate with or acquire other hospitals.[24]

Coincidentally, the Baltimore City Hospitals had become an intolerable burden on the City of Baltimore, which decided in 1983 to put the institution up for contract management or to sell it. Hopkins was not interested in purchasing the hospital but did arrange to manage it in order to assess the situation. Within the first year, the hospitals' deficit was reduced from $7 million to just over $1 million, but Hopkins had concluded that, for the long term, the hospitals were not manageable under city ownership. Necessary capital replacement had been—and would continue to be—neglected, and a contract to manage the city-owned facility could not provide the fiscal and administrative freedom that Hopkins required to produce high-quality results.

The city then tried to find an investor-owned chain willing to buy the institution. Hopkins became aware that at least two such companies were interested. "We were simply unwilling to see a base of 11,000 inpatients and a burn unit go the way of investor-owned hospitals—to lose that market share," recalls Robert Heyssel.[25] Moreover, most of the institution's staff were Hopkins faculty members, and it was an important teaching resource for the Hopkins medical school—located at Hopkins' back door. "It had a very natural market area which looked good, as well as 103 acres of land strategically located in southeast Baltimore." It also included a 240-bed chronic disease hospital and the National Gerontological Research Institute. Moreover, the National Institute of Drug Abuse was in the process of moving to that site from Kentucky.

After lengthy negotiations with the city, Hopkins assumed the ownership and responsibility for the Baltimore City Hospitals in 1984, changing the name to the Francis Scott Key Medical Center. Admissions increased, and the operation became profitable.

Caring for patients at Francis Scott Key is an independent medical group, Chesapeake Physicians, formed in the early 1970s by the city-employed physicians at the Baltimore City Hospitals. By 1980, it had approximately 150 members. One requirement for membership is a faculty appointment at the Johns Hopkins University School of Medicine. Salaries are in line with those of full-time Hopkins-based faculty, and the dean and department heads control the salaries jointly. The appropriate chief of service at Hopkins helps to recruit these physicians, all of whom teach and many of whom engage in research activities. Medical students rotate through Francis Scott Key, and many of its residency programs are conducted jointly with Johns Hopkins. Several Hopkins divisions—geographic medicine and the burn unit, for example—actually have their primary base at Francis Scott Key.

The Chesapeake Physicians' clinical programs include three HMOs. The first is the labor-organized "Care First" HMO, which has contracted with the Chesapeake Physicians for physicians' services. The second is a small community health center in a blue-collar neighborhood near the hospital, which pays both capitation fees and fees for service. The third is a hospital-based HMO that originally served foster children and was later extended to their families and others.

At about the same time as arrangements were concluded for buying the Baltimore City Hospitals, the East Baltimore Health Plan went bankrupt, with only 7,000 persons enrolled. Hopkins took over that HMO as well. As at the Francis Scott Key Medical Center, medical care was provided by contract physicians.

The Johns Hopkins Health System was created as an umbrella organization, a holding company with several components, including the Johns Hopkins Health Plan. By the time final arrangements for the Johns Hopkins Health System were approved in June 1985 by the Board of Trustees of the Johns Hopkins Hospital, two of its parts were already in operation—a model for a broad regional association of independent physicians who contracted with Hopkins to provide care at Francis Scott Key, and the group practice model already in place as the East Baltimore Health Plan. The Johns Hopkins Health Plan also went into operation, helped by the acquisition of two other institutions: North Charles General Hospital, a smaller community hospital with a new facility and minimal debt; and the Wyman Park Health System, an outgrowth of the old United States Public Health Service Hospital. This institution had important contacts with the Department of Defense; its staff comprised approximately seventy physicians, many of whom already held Hopkins appointments. Both facilities are near Hopkins' Homewood campus and are therefore convenient to university faculty, staff, and students.

By March 1987, the Hopkins HMO had 26,000 members. Two-thirds were enrolled through employers; the remainder were Medicaid enrollees. Five ambulatory care clinics had already been built in East Baltimore and at fourteen other sites throughout the region.[26]

The early success of the Johns Hopkins Health System reflected the lessons learned in Columbia:[27]

1. A prepaid group practice will reach the break-even point only with a sizeable and guaranteed population base and a favorable economic climate. This base was not present in Columbia, and Columbia's potential depended on a continuation of the nation's economic growth of 1968—which was halted by the recession of 1970 and the gasoline crisis of 1973. The easiest place to start a prepayment group may be in the midst of a large city, in which substantial segments of the population are employed in a few major industries.

2. Saddling a plan with considerable initial debt will cause major difficulties. The benefit package and the co-payments must be carefully assessed. At Columbia, the former was probably too broad and too expensive, and the latter too low. Capital expenditures must be kept as low as possible.

3. The participating medical group must be given sufficient independence. In Columbia, the physicians' need to negotiate for every penny seriously weakened their governance.

4. A new group practice must be able to pay the standard fees for physicians, but fee-for-service for specialty care can cause a group considerable financial difficulty. One of the advantages of locating an HMO close to an academic medical center is the ready availability of specialty care, and charges can be negotiated to mutual benefit. Salaries for participating physicians must also be competitive. The HMO physicians cannot be second-class citizens in a setting where they have some relation to the academic community. One of the greatest challenges facing the academic medical center became clear with the Columbia venture—the problem of balancing service, research, and education against financial and academic rewards.

5. The existing faculty of an academic medical center will not be a good source of practitioners for a prepaid medical plan, since physicians who have made their careers in academic medicine will be less cost-conscious than is necessary for the effective management of the practice.

6. Before teaching can be introduced into an HMO, the plan must have a strong base of patients and money must be set aside to pay for the instruction.

7. Administrators should anticipate time- and energy-consuming struggles with the regional planning process, and the possibility of antagonistic county and state medical societies.

8. Attracting the consumer is crucial to the success of any HMO. The public did not initially understand the product at Columbia, and Connecticut General's mechanism for marketing the plan turned out to be more complex than anticipated. The initial neglect of the patient as a formal participant in the decision-making process also limited the extent to which satisfied patients would act as "marketers" of the program.

The corporate offices of the Johns Hopkins Health System are lean, primarily involved with marketing, planning, and group activities such as purchasing, information systems, and financial controls. The presidents of each of the other components are intended to have wide latitude in day-to-day operations and considerable discretion in selling their own services within an overall plan agreed to by all the institutions and the parent system.

The development of this new health system in a relatively brief time was accompanied by considerable stress within the institutions. Negotiations to acquire the various components necessitated rapid decision making, carried out without the usual open debate that characterizes the more leisurely committee-oriented academic process. It was difficult to arrange the movement of patients into these managed-care programs, and many community patients were displaced into other facilities. Another problem was the need to acquire a group of physicians to give private care, many of whom did not have the type of training traditionally associated with Hopkins physicians. The chiefs of service in the Johns Hopkins Hospital, called upon to provide specialty services, were faced with the necessity of assuring high-quality care and were startled by the promotion of the new system by advertising.

A serious problem concerns the availability of patients for instruction. The HMO model drains patients from the Hopkins outpatient clinics, as they tend to use the more conveniently located satellite clinics for medical care. Acceleration of this trend will result in a serious shortage of patients for teaching. The shift of patients into an HMO also creates difficulties on the inpatient services, because those admitted are coming into the hospital as patients of the HMO physician rather than of the house staff (see chapter 5). As one solution, the Department of Medicine put residents into the HMO, assigning third-year residents to train with a regular health-plan physician. The residents are satisfied with the experience because the patients are younger than those in the hospital and often have illnesses more amenable to medical treatment than patients seen in the hospital clinics. The physicians, for their part, enjoy teaching the residents, whose assistance permits the physicians to use their time more effectively.

The introduction of medical students into this ambulatory care setting is more difficult. Unlike residents, medical students cannot be contributing members of the HMO staff. Students still in the early learning stage of clinical medicine must be added in "dilute solution" to any highly efficient care-giving setting, such as an HMO. The resulting pattern placed one or two residents or students in many different sites around the city. This has made it difficult to ensure consistency in students' educational experiences.

Advertising the HMO is the source of another problem. When the Hopkins name is used to market the HMO, the public assumes that these physicians are equal to the ones on which the reputation of Hopkins was built. This is a difficult problem, and one that generates considerable emotion-laden discussion. One solution is a system of appointments that would distinguish between several types of physicians within the Hopkins family. The traditional one-track system would thus be replaced by a two- or even a three-track system.

Proponents of the Hopkins HMO believe these problems to be inevitable. They argue that the Johns Hopkins Hospital and School of Medicine need a firm, dependable patient base if they are to continue to educate physicians and carry out research as in the past. In 1985, less than 2 percent of the population of Baltimore was enrolled in an HMO; by 1987, the figure was 15 percent.[28] If Hopkins does not offer an HMO, they say, many of its patients will go elsewhere. As for the problem of physicians' credentials, Johns Hopkins, like all other academic medical centers beginning to compete for dollars in the marketplace, must develop new arrangements to prevent erosion of the traditional quality of teaching and research. A different type of physician with a different background is needed to staff an HMO, and members of the traditional academic faculty should not be required to participate in a type of practice in which they have neither interest nor training. The day of the renaissance physician is over, in any case, and proponents believe that the division of the faculty into clinicians and basic science investigators should now be echoed by the division of clinicians into primary care practitioners and those who instruct and perform research.

Less enthusiastic faculty and administrators

recognize that HMOs will surely grow as a system for providing health care, but believe that dissatisfaction with HMOs will probably lead many in the nation's expanding upper socioeconomic group to seek their health care in other ways. They see the possibility that a system of national health insurance will be instituted if the cost of medical care continues to escalate, but believe that the British experience teaches us that there will always be room for the private practice of medicine, and that Americans are used to seeking out quality to satisfy important needs. They also recognize that the demands of patient care activities tend to displace research and teaching, and if academic medical centers, including Hopkins, allow this tendency to prevail, they will soon be little-different from the ordinary community hospital.[29]

The history of Hopkins' ventures into the community is a series of experiments, efforts to develop models of medical practice and to carry out Hopkins' historic commitment to care for the indigent according to its founder's letter of intent. Medicine's growing complexity has rendered the traditional system of providing medical care ever more inadequate. It has become more difficult for faculty to give individual patients optimal care, more difficult for them to teach and conduct re-

search. The ghosts and shadows of earlier attempts at solutions remain—from the City of Baltimore's straightforward provision of capitation money to help local practitioners, to elaborate health maintenance programs developed first in Columbia and in East Baltimore.

With each experiment, it has become increasingly evident that the Johns Hopkins Medical Institutions' involvement in the delivery of medical care is closely connected to its responsibilities in medical education and medical research. How to balance these three activities—teaching, research, and patient care—has become a fundamental issue for the medical institutions. They must be organized so that the burden of medical care will not destroy the quality of medical education and the productivity of the academic program in medical research. The volume of medical care—and the resulting income—has grown logarithmically in the past decade. As Hopkins becomes increasingly dependent on income from this source, patient care threatens to overwhelm research and teaching. This potential conflict requires the wisest counsel, men and women who will interpret the structure of the medical institutions to permit the effective discharge of all three of these important responsibilities.

CHAPTER 11

THE NATURE OF DISCOVERY

Greater even than the greatest discovery is to keep open the way to future discoveries. This can only be done when the investigator freely dares, moved as by an inner propulsion, to attack problems not because they give promise of immediate value to the human race, but because they make an irresistible appeal by reason of an inner beauty. . . . From this point of view, the investigator is a man whose inner life is free in the best sense of the word. In short, there should be in research work a cultural character, an artistic quality, elements that give to painting, music, and poetry their high place in the life of man.

—John Jacob Abel

At the core of Johns Hopkins' heritage of excellence are its accomplishments in research. The impetus to discovery was a crucial part of Hopkins at its founding: an emphasis on the discovery of new information set Hopkins apart as the first graduate university in the United States. In the medical school, this keen sense of inquiry took the form of a drive to advance the potential for alleviating and preventing illness in human beings.

Alfred Blalock, professor of surgery at Johns Hopkins, explored what he called "the nature of discovery" in his presidential address before the American Surgical Association in 1956.[1] One type of discovery, he said, is the act of finding out something unknown, such as Harvey's discovery of the circulation of the blood. Another is the invention of something that did not exist before, such as the machinery necessary to use steam for locomotion. "The *idea* is the seed," said Blalock, quoting Claude Bernard. "The method is the earth furnishing the conditions in which it may develop, flourish and give the best fruit according

to its nature. But as only what has been sown in the ground will ever grow, so nothing will be developed by the experimental method except the ideas submitted to it."[2]

Blalock divided the "how" of discovery into four categories. Some discoveries are made by chance or accident, some by intention or design, some by intuition or imagination or hunch, and some by combinations of all of the above methods. Boundaries between categories are blurred, moreover, because the mode of discovery is often not clear-cut, and investigators cannot always recall exactly how they identified the clue that led to the solution of the problem under study.

The research performed at Johns Hopkins over the last century reflects all the diversity of Blalock's categories. Indeed, the contributions

Note: Some material in this chapter has appeared in A. McGehee Harvey's collections of essays, *Adventures in Medical Research* and *Research and Discovery in Medicine,* both published by the Johns Hopkins University Press. These essays were written with a future centennial volume in mind.

made at Hopkins over the last century are too numerous to document in anything but a catalogue. Some creative, productive investigators and some important discoveries are not mentioned in this chapter. They have been omitted not because they have been judged less important, but simply in response to the constraints of space. Each of the stories in this chapter is an example of a different facet of research at Hopkins—a different aspect of the nature of discovery.

The stories in this chapter were chosen for their interest, their variety, and their reflection of the Hopkins ideal: the way in which an institution can stimulate individuals training and working in a research-oriented environment to develop new knowledge. It is notable that many of the path-breaking articles cited, particularly those published in the early years, appeared in the *Bulletin of The Johns Hopkins Hospital*. The accounts that follow show that important discoveries were made not by professors alone, but also by fellows, residents, interns, students, and technicians—all a vital part of the Hopkins community. The diversity of the investigators is matched by the panorama of their discoveries, which span all fields of preclinical and clinical medicine.

A Genealogy of Research

Franklin P. Mall, one of Welch's first fellows, became the Johns Hopkins medical school's first professor of anatomy, and thus the head of the Department of Anatomy, at the age of thirty-one. His influence spanned all of medical education at the time, but his main interest was medical research.

After graduating from the University of Michigan Medical School, Mall went to Germany to study clinical medicine, and there his contacts with Wilhelm His and later with Carl Ludwig opened his eyes to the sciences of anatomy and physiology. Under Ludwig's tutelage, Mall investigated the blood vessels of the intestine, showing that as the vasculature develops, every segment of the organ has an equal supply of blood, and that the pattern of these vessels can be expressed as a

simple branching of one artery in five different orders. Mall subsequently showed that this simple concept—five different orders of arteries—was applicable to all organs.[3]

Returning to the United States in 1886, Mall spent the next three years in Welch's Pathological Laboratory. Mall's investigations of the stomach there displayed the same thoroughness as his study in Ludwig's laboratory of the blood and lymphatic supply of the intestine.

Welch's laboratory was also the site of Mall's notable collaboration with Halsted on intestinal contractions and their influence on blood flow. It was Mall who suggested what became Halsted's famous intestinal suture, and in a classic example of collaborative research, Halsted worked out his methods of intestinal anastomosis while Mall assisted with the operations and studied the structural results. The histological findings later published by Mall revealed that the best results were obtained when the sutures entered but did not penetrate the submucosa, whose predominance of white fibrous tissue was the only layer strong enough to hold the sutures.[4]

Mall's independent laboratory investigations in Baltimore concentrated on three subjects: embryology, the structure of organs in the adult as related to their function, and the beginnings of anthropological research. His embryologic studies included investigations of the development of the human diaphragm, ventral abdominal walls, body cavities, and loops of the intestines. In his various projects, he used three-dimensional wax models as well as human embryos. Wilhelm His wrote that Mall's work was a "signal advance," the first time that the development of any organ had been traced from its early stages through its transition forms to its condition in the adult.[5]

Mall's work on the spleen established its open circulation. His investigations of the structure of the liver produced one of the fundamental generalizations to emerge from his laboratory: that the anlage of the vascular system is the capillary. Artery and vein are thus secondary and are differentiated from capillaries by the flow of blood set in motion by the heart. Mall believed that throughout the vascular system, including the lymphatics, endothelium is the essential tissue. Muscle coats and connective tissue coats are accessories or, as their name suggests, adventitial. In this work, Mall brought to its fruition the concept he had first formulated in the study of the intestinal villus in Ludwig's laboratory: each organ contains a structural unit that is also a unit of function.[6]

Franklin P. Mall's Pupils

A slaughterhouse near Mall's laboratory provided an abundant supply of fresh embryo pigs in every stage of development, with hearts still beating. Mall turned the embryos over to his research fellows, to whom he assigned the problem of investigating the development of the blood vessels. To John B. MacCallum, Herbert M. Evans, George L. Streeter, and Florence R. Sabin, Mall suggested the problem of the origin of the lymphatic system, while to Eliot R. and Eleanor L. Clark, he suggested the study of the growth of the lymphatics in amphibian forms. The work of the first group led to the fundamental discovery that blood vessels come from a particular type of cell, the angioblast, and that endothelium is the primary tissue of the vascular system; the work on the lymphatic system likewise revealed the fundamental nature of the endothelial cell.[7]

Florence Rena Sabin   Florence R. Sabin, professor of histology, was the first woman to be appointed full professor at Hopkins and the first woman elected to membership in the National Academy of Sciences.

As a first-year medical student in 1896, Sabin soon came under Mall's influence. In her biography of Mall, she recognized him as her mentor: "The writer worked for twenty years under Mall; four years as a student, one as a fellow, and fifteen years on his staff. Her start in research as a medical student and her opportunity for a career in scientific medicine she owes wholly to him."[8]

Studying the development of the lymphatic channels in pig embryos, Sabin injected colored material into vessels in embryos as small as twenty-three millimeters in length. She demonstrated that lymphatics arise as buds from veins and grow outward as continuous channels by a process of further budding. Sabin established that lymphatics arise from veins by sprouts of endothelium, so that the entire system is derived from preexisting vessels. Furthermore, she showed that the peripheral ends of the lymphatics are closed, so that they neither open into the tissue spaces nor are they derived from these spaces.[9]

Sabin also studied the origin of endothelium. Using living tissue and the method of cell culture devised by another of Mall's students, Ross G. Harrison, she watched cellular growth in the hanging drop preparations and described the development of the earliest blood cells in explanted bits of blastoderm from chick embryo. On the second day of incubation of such cultures, she noted, only erythrocytes could be seen coming from the endothelial walls of the blood vessels. By the third day white cells appeared, arising partly from new cells that differentiated from mesenchyme without becoming part of the vessel's lining.[10]

Sabin later developed a technique to study preparations of living cells by staining them with dye. Her methods of supravital staining became useful research tools and were eventually employed by laboratory workers throughout the world. The characteristic differences in the intracellular distribution of the dyes enabled workers to identify many cell types and to study their functions under normal conditions and in disease. Among the cells Sabin studied were certain mononuclear units termed "monocytes." Her experiments indicated that these cells were involved in tissue reactions against infectious agents, particularly the tubercle bacillus.[11]

John Bruce MacCallum   Like Sabin, John B. MacCallum also came under Mall's influence while a medical student at Hopkins. MacCallum quickly learned the methods of cutting and staining microscopic sections and soon made impressive observations on the histology and histogenesis of the heart muscle cell. His investigations singled him out as a brilliant anatomist and embryologist. At twenty-one years of age, when his fellow students

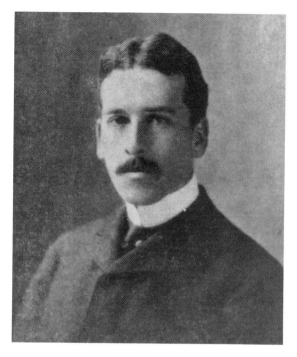

John Bruce MacCallum. (*Source*: A. Malloch, *Short Years: The Life and Letters of John Bruce MacCallum, 1876–1906* [Chicago: Normandie House, 1938].)

were still struggling with learning the anatomical names and the origins and insertions of muscles, MacCallum was carrying out original work on the structure of the heart.

In his first article, MacCallum concluded:

> It is to be emphasized, then, that in the protoplasm of the adult heart muscle cell, there are columns of fibrils, which run longitudinally surrounded by sarcoplasm, in a way that each bundle is surrounded by a varying number of small sarcoplasmic discs, the horizontal, separating partitions of which are continuous with Krause's line [the narrow striation across the fibril] on the fibril bundles.[12]

This article illustrates MacCallum's notable ability to think in three-dimensional terms. His schematic drawings, beautifully executed in pen and ink, show sarcoplasmic discs piled in columns like counters used in games, one on top of the other with the sides of the columns touching.[13]

MacCallum described what may be his most important anatomical work in an article in *Contributions to the Science of Medicine,* a volume dedi-

cated to Welch by his pupils. This article reported his discoveries concerning the arrangement and course of the muscle fibers of the heart—a subject very difficult for the student to grasp, as MacCallum points out. "The heart is a muscular pump," he wrote, "and when the heart muscle (or myocardium) contracts, blood is squeezed out of its chambers. That much the student knows; he can see that the heart muscle has several layers and that in each layer the fibers run in the same direction. He can see little order, however, as he attempts to trace their course. Each muscle has an origin (one place of attachment) and at the other end an insertion (the site of attachment), but in the case of the heart muscle, the fibers seem to run in almost every direction."[14] MacCallum's rapid unraveling of these complex arrangements is an example of his unusual creativity.

Ross Granville Harrison   Attempts to culture tissue *in vitro* were made as early as 1885, but more than twenty years elapsed before Ross G. Harrison, a pupil of Henry Newell Martin, became the first to devise a simple technique for growing tissue fragments outside the body. In his early studies of the embryonic development of the nervous system, he confronted a basic question: how does the embryonic animal body construct the fibers of the nerves that connect its various parts? Some embryologists supported the view that each fiber grows out from its cell, even to great lengths; others were equally certain that fibers are formed from short lengths built by local cells that somehow join end to end. No experimental proof existed for either mechanism.[15]

Harrison found the answer by actually watching nerve fibers as they grew. By removing a tiny portion of spinal cord from a frog embryo and placing it in a clear drop of coagulated lymph on a hollowed-out slide, Harrison prepared the first successful cultures of animal tissues. He observed the living fiber as it developed from a nerve cell at the periphery of the explant and grew out as far as the clot allowed it to spread. His experiment proved that these fibers, whether long or short, developed from one particular nerve cell in the brain, spinal cord, or outlying ganglia.[16]

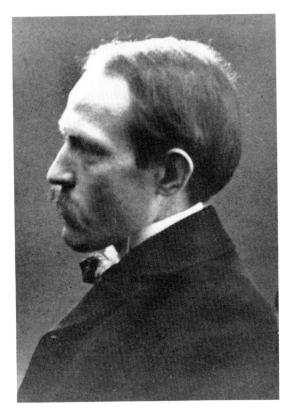

Ross G. Harrison. (*Source:* Alan M. Chesney Medical Archives, The Johns Hopkins Medical Institutions.)

professors who was not head of a department.

In 1910, Lewis married Margaret Reed, a student of Thomas Hunt Morgan. Reed had also worked in Berlin, with Rhoda Erdmann, cultivating amebae on nutrient agar made with physiological salt solution. In a later experiment, which involved explanting a small piece of bone marrow from a guinea pig into this medium, Reed demonstrated that bone marrow cells formed a membranelike growth on the surface of the agar and observed cells undergoing mitosis. This was probably the first *in vitro* culture of mammalian cells.

Working as a team, the Lewises began to cultivate bone marrow cells from guinea pig embryos. Modifying Harrison's method by using mammalian blood plasma instead of frog lymph, they succeeded in growing cells of many organs, but they recognized that most of the proliferating cells originated in connective tissue or endothelium.

To observe the fine structure of individual cells, the Lewises needed very clear media, so they devised a mixture of Locke's solution, agar, and bouillon. With this preparation, they found that

Thus, by a simple experiment, Harrison not only invented a research tool that was to revolutionize biology, he clarified one of the fundamental problems of the neuron theory. His demonstration of the nerve origins of the axon was vitally important in changing the direction of the entire field of neurology.[17]

Warren Harmon Lewis and Margaret Reed Lewis

Warren H. Lewis, whose studies of the embryology of the eye laid the groundwork for the modern theory of embryonic induction, was an active investigator for more than fifty years. Collaborating with his wife, Margaret R. Lewis, in an entirely different area, he also used techniques of tissue culture to investigate the nature of cells.[18]

Lewis became Mall's senior associate in 1907, and in 1914 the university recognized his stature by appointing him professor of physiological anatomy. He thus became one of the few full

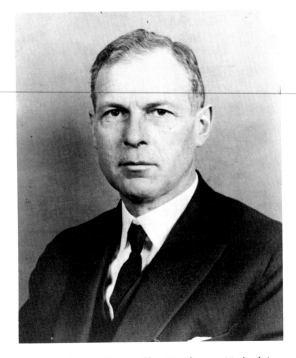

Warren H. Lewis. (*Source:* Alan M. Chesney Medical Archives, The Johns Hopkins Medical Institutions.)

connective tissue cells, endothelial cells, and nerve fibers would spread out into the fluid from the explanted tissue. This study represented the first attempt to grow cells in a solution containing only known constituents. In this respect, they were well ahead of their competitors, as little was known at the time about the factors—such as vitamins and trace elements—important in regulating growth.[19]

The Lewises steadily accumulated a comprehensive description of the living cell, including its nucleus, cytoplasm, and mitochondria, and the segregation vacuoles that the cells formed around phagocytosed particles. Then they shifted their objective to observations of the physiologic activities of cells, described the transformation of connective tissue cells into flattened mesothelial layers resembling those lining the peritoneal cavity, and observed the development of macrophages, epithelioid cells, and giant cells from mononuclear cells. They extended the work of their colleague Florence R. Sabin by demonstrating that monocytes and macrophages are not distinctive cell types but different developmental stages of the same cell. The last stage of Warren Lewis's career was devoted to the study of the cytologic features distinguishing the living malignant cell of connective-tissue origin from its normal counterpart, the fibroblast.[20]

Warren Lewis was also well known for his pioneering use of motion pictures to record microscopic observations. He began to employ time-lapse cinematography in 1929 and soon discovered that he could observe cellular activity in more detail by speeding up, on the screen, activities too slow in real time to be understood by direct observation. In 1931, Lewis observed a type of cell activity that he called "pinocytosis" (drinking by cells), and he recorded cells actively enfolding and engulfing drops of fluid from the surrounding medium. His time-lapse photographs of the physiologic activity of living cells—particularly his photographs of mammalian and zebrafish ova dividing—attracted widespread attention. Through the wide dissemination of his films, thousands of students around the world gained a vivid impression of the structure of the living nor-

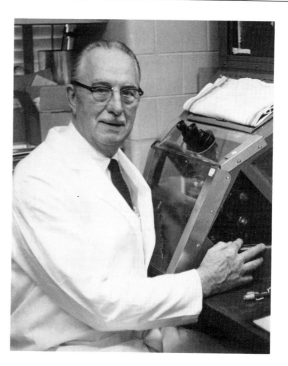

George O. Gey. (*Source:* Alan M. Chesney Medical Archives, The Johns Hopkins Medical Institutions.)

mal and malignant cells of the blood and connective tissues, and of processes such as cell division and phagocytosis.[21]

George Otto Gey   George O. Gey was a student of the Lewises, a distinguished pupil who worked at Johns Hopkins with tissue culture techniques for over forty-seven years. His association with the Lewises began in 1922, when he spent a year as a fellow in their laboratory. After six years as a cancer-research fellow in Wisconsin, Gey returned to Hopkins as director of the tissue culture laboratory in the Department of Surgery.

Gey was independently responsible for many new developments related to organoid and cell culture, intracellular and membrane cytology, and *in vitro* investigations in endocrinology, oncology, and virology. So numerous are the innovations that emerged from Gey's laboratory that one can list only some of them:[22] (1) the maintenance *in vitro* of organoid and hormonal tissues (thyroid, parathyroid, placenta, choriocarcinoma); (2) the "roller-tube" technique (used by Enders and his group in their Nobel Prize–winning cultivation of poliomyelitis virus in non–nervous system cells); (3) the continuous maintenance of normal and malignant human and rat cell lines; (4) flat-sided tubes and "flying cover slips" for cytologic studies; (5) collagen as a natural, often crucially important, substrate for fastidious cells and organoids; (6) the nutrition of cells in tissue extracts and body fluids and identification of their specific requirements for trace metals, amino acids, proteins, lipids, and carbohydrates.

Gey also advanced the field of virology by establishing the susceptibilities of normal and malignant cells as hosts for eastern equine encephalomyelitis virus; propagating cells and viruses simultaneously over long periods of time; and investigating the presence of viral particles in normal chick embryo cells.[23]

In the field of cancer research, Gey discovered many of the differences between a variety of malignant cells and their normal counterparts; established causes for the emergence and loss of malignancy in cell lines *in vitro*; and derived cell lines that have served as international workhorses in studies on cell nutrition, virology, and malignancy.[24]

Although Gey did not report his finding at the time, he was one of the first to prove that normal cells could become malignant while in culture. In 1939, the normal rat fibroblasts that Gey was growing took on the appearance and behavior of cancer cells; by injecting the cells into the same strain of rats from which they were derived, Gey confirmed their malignancy.[25]

George Gey's best-known contribution was the HeLa cell culture, the first established human cell line.[26] HeLa cell cultures have been used for studies of the nutritional requirements of cells in culture, of viral growth, of protein synthesis, of drug effects, and of somatic cell genetics, including genetic control mechanisms and mutations at the cellular level. The usefulness of this cell line to molecular and cell biology can hardly be overestimated.

Gey developed the HeLa cell when Richard TeLinde, the director of the Department of Gynecology, interested him in using his roller tube technique to grow cells from patients with carcinoma-*in-situ* of the cervix. Such cells would provide information about the growth characteristics of normal cervical epithelium, intraepithelial carcinoma, and invasive cancer. Gey was unsuccessful until he obtained cells from a thirty-one-year-old woman with intermenstrual spotting, whose biopsy revealed a carcinomatous lesion. Gey grew these cells readily and named the cell line after the patient, Henrietta Lacks.[27]

Gey also extended Warren Lewis's work with photography, synthesizing mechanical and optical means to investigate the living behavior of normal, malignant, and infected cells. His time-lapse, phase-motion photographs, supplemented with interference and electron microscopy, revealed the activity of the plasma-gel layer in producing membranous pseudopods, microfibrils, and spicules that contribute extracellular matrix; the continuous role of streaming hyaloplasm in intracellular nutrition and communication; the ways in which pinocytic and inclusion droplets become associated with mitochondria and the cytocentrum; the bizarre mitoses and the increased pinocytoses, feeding habits, and metastatic potential of malignant cells; and the degenerative damage caused by polio and eastern equine encephalomyelitis viruses. Gey's photographic records remain a tangible monument to his scientific work.[28]

Mall thus set a fine example for his students, and his was the classic "congenial atmosphere" for research. Not only did his younger colleagues become as productive as he was, but even the medical students were keenly stimulated to pursue their own independent investigations.

Discoveries by Medical Students

The fifteen students in the first class of the Johns Hopkins University School of Medicine were plunged into an atmosphere of intellectual excitement and inspiration. They were exposed to the great teachers—Welch, Osler, Halsted, Kelly—in whose laboratories and clinics they attempted to extend Billings' commitment to the pursuit of new knowledge.

Not surprisingly, the members of the Class of 1897 were a creative group. They were selected for their sound background in science as well as their intelligence. What is remarkable is that while they were still in medical school, three members of the first class made research discoveries whose importance endures to this day.

Thomas R. Brown and the Eosinophilia of Trichinosis

Thomas R. Brown was a fourth-year student taking Osler's clinical clerkship, when he was introduced to a twenty-three-year-old hobo who complained of generalized muscle pains. Brown found that his patient had an elevated number of white blood cells, 68 percent of which were eosinophils. The extreme tenderness of the patient's muscles, together with a fever, suggested myositis. Brown entertained a diagnosis of trichinosis when he discovered that the patient had repeatedly eaten incompletely cooked pork six or seven weeks earlier. Microscopic examination of muscle showed the presence of trichinae, confirming Brown's diagnosis. Although the disease was well known, it was Brown who related the elevated eosinophil count to the diagnosis.

Brown studied other similar cases and eventually published a comprehensive article about the increase of eosinophilic cells in the blood and muscle, the origin of these cells, and their diagnostic importance in trichinosis.[29]

Brown's interest in eosinophilia also led him to review the various situations associated with

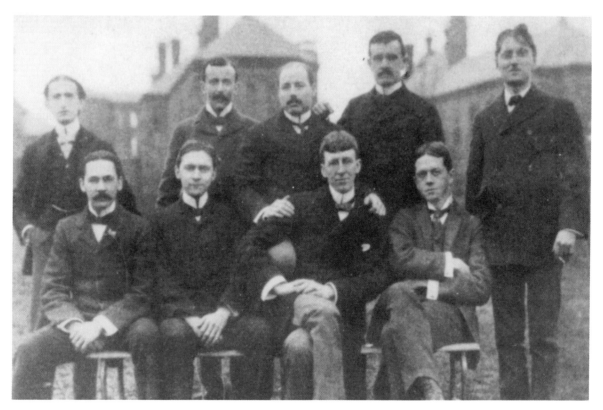

Original members of the Pithotomy Club, Class of 1897. *Standing, left to right,* Louis P. Hamburger, Joseph L. Nichols, Richard P. Strong, L. W. Day, Charles R. Bardeen; *seated, left to right,* James F. Mitchell, Eugene L. Opie, Thomas R. Brown, William G. MacCallum. (*Source:* J. A. Brown, *Dr. Tom Brown, Memories* [New York: Richard R. Smith, 1949].)

this hematologic disorder, and he was among the first to note the eosinophilia seen in adrenal insufficiency. His discovery of the eosinophilia of trichinosis was particularly valuable in identifying the cause of an epidemic of anemia ravaging Puerto Rico at the time. After reading Brown's article, Colonel Bailey Ashford concluded that his patients' eosinophilia, and consequent anemia was due to hookworm infestation.[30]

William G. MacCallum and Eugene L. Opie: Discoveries Related to Malaria, the Parathyroids, and Diabetes Mellitus

William G. MacCallum, the elder brother of John B. MacCallum and Welch's successor as director of the Department of Pathology, developed an interest in hematozoan infections during the third-year course in clinical microscopy directed by William S. Thayer. Baltimore was the site of widespread malarial infection in those days, and the disease was the subject of intensive study by Osler[31] and Thayer.[32] Laveran had discovered the malarial parasite in 1880; five years later, it was recognized that birds harbored a similar parasite, a hematozoan—a finding that stimulated the studies at Johns Hopkins.

MacCallum's fellow medical student Eugene L. Opie had identified two forms of the parasite in crows with malaria: a hyaline, nonstaining form and a granular form.[33] Opie suggested that the hyaline form alone might become flagellated. This distinction was confirmed by MacCallum, who also found that the granular forms were extruded as spheres recognizable among the nuclei of the red corpuscles that had contained them. As MacCallum described it, he observed the extrusion of the two adult forms from the corpuscle and saw that the flagellae tore themselves free and acted as fertilizing agents or spermatozoa. Only one flagellum gained admission to each granular sphere. It plunged itself into the sphere, which after some agitation of the pigment became quiet for fifteen or twenty minutes. The final result was a fusiform body with a small pigmented appendage and a refractive, nucleuslike body. MacCallum recog-

nized that this sequence of events was a sexual process.[34]

A few weeks later, MacCallum examined a fresh preparation from the blood of a woman with aestivo-autumnal malaria and found a large number of crescent forms. He was able to demonstrate the same sexual process in this preparation that he had seen in the bird malaria.

MacCallum later concentrated on the parathyroid glands, studying the influence of various factors, including diet, on experimentally produced tetany. He corroborated the findings of others that the subcutaneous or intravenous injection of an extract of the parathyroid gland would cause symptoms of tetany to disappear. When a patient who developed tetany after subtotal thyroidectomy was given an injection of a preparation made from four or five bovine parathyroid glands, symptoms disappeared within several hours.

In collaboration with Carl Voegtlin, MacCallum demonstrated that tetany was due to nervous system rather than muscle dysfunction. One series of experiments evaluated the effects of various mineral salts, particularly calcium, on patients with frank tetany produced by parathyroidectomy. In a second group of experiments on animals dying of tetany, MacCallum and Voegtlin studied changes in metabolism and alterations in the chemical composition of tissues.

MacCallum and Voegtlin had also shown that transfusion of a sufficiently large amount of blood from a normal dog would suppress symptoms in a dog with tetany. Their later experiments conclusively demonstrated the immediate and specific curative effect of a soluble calcium salt upon the tetany that followed parathyroidectomy.[35]

MacCallum's classmate Eugene L. Opie also began his career in scientific investigation during medical school. As Opie described his first venture into research:

During the laboratory course in pathology I found in a section of the pancreas a strange body which I showed to Dr. Welch when he made his unhurried rounds of the class. He told me it was a structure described by Langerhans in 1869. "Find out all you can about those islets of Langerhans," Welch said to me.[36]

This early interest in the pancreas would persist throughout Opie's life. It is plain from Opie's early papers, said Peyton Rous, that he started to discover things by questioning the meaning of everything that came under his eye:

> When examining postmortem material, he was no recorder of final states; the changes met in the dead had for him the liveliest of implications. He was an inquirer into riddles who sought after the meaning of diseased organs much as one might seek for the answers to charades.[37]

Studying postmortem sections from the pancreas of a diabetic patient, Opie observed the complete destruction of the islets of Langerhans by hyaline changes. While still a medical student, he disproved the current assumption that the islets were modified or underdeveloped acinar cells and went on to demonstrate by the perceptive collection of cases that severe injury to the islets is followed by diabetes mellitus.[38]

MacCallum read with interest Opie's article on the relation of the islets of Langerhans to the development of glycosuria. MacCallum knew that ligating the ducts of the pancreas to divert its secretion from the intestine caused digestive disturbances and injury to the gland—but not glycosuria. Although such obstruction results in atrophy of the secreting acini, the absence of glycosuria was generally ascribed to the gap between islets and ducts, which permitted the islets to remain intact. MacCallum also knew of the experiments by Mering and Minkowski in the 1880s showing that total extirpation of the pancreas in dogs resulted in a severe and total diabetes; they attributed this result to the lack of some substance secreted by the pancreas into the bloodstream.

MacCallum concluded that further investigation of the development of glycosuria depended on isolating the islets so that he could study them in their pure state. He would somehow have to keep the islets intact while ensuring

that the secreting tissue of the pancreas atrophied completely. Ligating the duct and separating it from the intestines had already been done, but it was difficult to keep the experimental animal alive long enough to allow the acini to atrophy. Instead of isolating the entire organ, MacCallum separated a portion of the pancreas from the remainder of the organ and ligated its duct. The dog remained alive until this portion of the pancreas had undergone extensive atrophy, at which point MacCallum removed the remaining normal portion of pancreatic tissue. The atrophied remnant was shown to be capable of warding off glycosuria, even when large amounts of dextrose were ingested. When the remnant itself was removed, glycosuria appeared at once.

This experiment clearly proved the specific control of carbohydrate metabolism by the islets of Langerhans. The procedure (duct ligation) employed by MacCallum to destroy the acinar tissue while leaving the islets intact was later adopted in 1921 by Banting and Best in their successful attempt to extract from the islets the antidiabetic hormone (insulin), which MacCallum's experiments had shown to be secreted by these cells.[39]

Discovery of an Abnormality of Hemoglobin in Sickle Cell Anemia: The First Molecular Disease

Johns Hopkins has been closely tied to the study of sickle cell anemia, particularly to the discovery that the disease is due to the genetically determined replacement of a single amino acid in a complex molecule. Sickle cell anemia was first described in 1910 by James B. Herrick, but the term was coined a decade later by a medical resident at Hopkins, Verne R. Mason.[40] Mason had graduated from the Hopkins medical school and remained on the staff as intern, resident, and instructor in medicine. In 1930, he became professor of clinical medicine at the new University of Southern California School of Medicine. Mason was Howard Hughes' personal physician and was instrumental in the founding of the Howard Hughes Medical Institute in 1953.

Mason's report, published in the *Journal of the American Medical Association,* was apparently the fourth description of a case of this disease. In his discussion, he advanced the idea that sickle cell anemia was a congenital anomaly. A year later, John Huck, another member of the Hopkins staff, presented strong evidence that the sickling phenomenon is a property of the red blood cell itself, subject to the laws of mendelian inheritance.[41] Huck, a 1918 graduate of Johns Hopkins, did the first genetic study of sickling. In the family of a patient with newly discovered sickle cell anemia, he and C. G. Guthrie noted that the red cells of both parents and of a number of the relatives were found to sickle.

Hopkins graduates who migrated elsewhere also made notable contributions to the field. Virgil Sydenstricker, Mason's classmate, was professor of medicine at the Medical College of Georgia for thirty-seven years. He maintained a lifelong interest in sickle cell anemia and made several important observations concerning the disorder. Another Johns Hopkins graduate, Lemuel Whitley Diggs (Class of 1926), studied sickle cell anemia over five decades of his career in Memphis. C. Lockard Conley states that Diggs was "the uncontested leader" in describing the pathologic features of sickle cell anemia and the mechanical factors responsible for the clogging of small arteries and the infarctions that underlie the clinical manifestations of this disorder.[42]

Although twenty-five years elapsed between Mason's article and Linus Pauling's epoch-making studies of sickle cell disease, the two events are linked through Johns Hopkins. In the mid-1930s, a Hopkins undergraduate, Irving J. Sherman, became interested in sickle cell anemia. As part of an advanced genetics course, he undertook a study of the hereditary pattern in sickle cell anemia and sickle cell trait. When Sherman entered the Hopkins medical school the following year, he approached Maxwell M. Wintrobe, a renowned hematologist and a member of the Department of Medicine, for permission to study sickle cells in his laboratory. While studying the sickling phenomenon, Sherman demonstrated that reduction

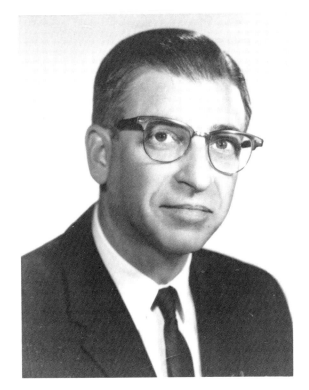

Irving J. Sherman

of oxygen tension enhanced its appearance.[43] Furthermore, he found that the oxygen tension at which sickling occurred was higher in patients with sickle cell anemia than in individuals with sickle cell trait. This discovery led to the demonstration that the venous blood of patients with sickle cell anemia contained a high percentage of sickled cell forms, whereas the venous blood of patients with sickle cell trait normally did not.

Later, Sherman did not recall the exact circumstances that led to his use of polarized light to examine the sickle cells, but he was excited by the birefringent effect, which he saw only in the sickled red blood cells. He believed that this effect indicated a change in the physical state of the hemoglobin. Because this physical change occurred only with reduced oxygen tension, and not in normal blood cells, he concluded that the hemoglobin molecule itself was different in sickle cells.

He was still working on the problem when he finished medical school in July 1940. He included his incomplete observations on the birefringence of sickled red cells in his final article on sickle cell hemoglobin in the hope that someone else would pursue the problem.

That "someone" turned out to be Linus Pauling, who learned about Sherman's results from William B. Castle, on a train ride back from a meeting. Pauling and his colleagues demonstrated the presence of an electrophoretically abnormal hemoglobin in sickle cell disease, and in 1949, their epoch-making article, "Sickle Cell Anemia: A Molecular Disease" appeared in *Science*.[44]

A Technologic Advance Spurs the Study of the Hemoglobinopathies

The delineation of hemoglobinopathies continued at Johns Hopkins under the leadership of C. Lockard Conley. Linus Pauling's laboratory had used an electrophoretic method that represented a modification of the Tiselius apparatus, technology not available in clinical research units. In 1953, Ernest W. Smith and C. Lockard Conley made a logarithmic advance in the study of abnormal hemoglobin when they used inexpensive, homemade equipment to demonstrate that hemoglobin components were separable by electrophoresis on filter paper. Smith and Conley's innovation is a striking illustration of the idea that important advances in research may depend upon the availability of a new laboratory technique.[45]

Smith and J. V. Torbert described a family with two different hemoglobin variants, sickle hemoglobin and a new form they named "hemoglobin Hopkins-2."[46] The pedigree indicated that the mutations were in different genes, leading to the conclusion that two different genes code for the molecule of hemoglobin present in adults. Smith and Torbert's conclusion antedated the discovery that the hemoglobin molecule is composed of two different types of subunits, alpha and beta.

The Conley group defined the characteristic clinical picture when sickle hemoglobin is combined with hemoglobin C or hemoglobin D. Samuel Charache described the first example of an abnormal hemoglobin that was accompanied by

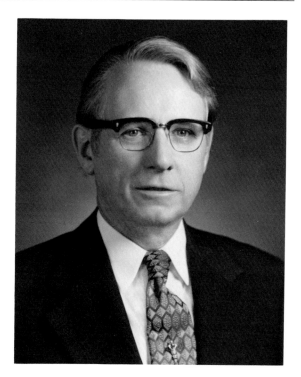

C. Lockard Conley

erythremia rather than anemia; this "hemoglobin Chesapeake" impeded the release of oxygen in the tissues. Subsequently, at least forty other hemoglobin variants causing plethora were described, including hemoglobin Osler, which was also discovered by Charache.

With David Weatherall (then a fellow, now Sir David, Nuffield Professor of Medicine at Oxford) and others, Conley found the first example of so-called hereditary persistence of fetal hemoglobin (HPFH) in homozygous form.[47] Normally, in the first months of life, an infant shows a progressive shift from production of fetal hemoglobin (Hb F), which predominates during most of the intrauterine period, to production of adult hemoglobin (Hb A). Some individuals have a genetic makeup that eliminates the "switch" from Hb F to Hb A. Persons with a single dose of the HPFH gene, i.e., heterozygotes, have part Hb A and part Hb F. Homozygotes, with a double dose of the HPFH gene, have 100 percent hemoglobin F. Conley recognized that the combination of high Hb F with the sickle cell gene had an ameliorating effect: the red cells did not sickle. Furthermore, the homozygous patient with only Hb F seemed to be a normally healthy adolescent.

These observations were the basis for the efforts by Samuel H. Boyer IV, Charache, George Dover, and others to switch hemoglobin production back from the sickling adult form to the nonsickling fetal form.[48]

Studies of the Thalassemias

The discovery of thalassemia minor at Hopkins emphasizes the importance of an alert technician on the clinical team. Thalassemia major (Cooley anemia), although very prevalent in Mediterranean countries, was first definitively described in Detroit, Michigan, by Thomas B. Cooley. The first cases of thalassemia minor, the heterozygous or single-dose form of thalassemia, were described in this country by Maxwell M. Wintrobe and colleagues at Johns Hopkins.[49]

What led to this discovery was the persistence of Regina Weistock, a laboratory technician. More than two years earlier, Weistock had noticed many stippled cells in the blood smear of a patient sent for study. The stippled cells suggested the possibility of lead poisoning, and because the patient was slightly jaundiced, Weistock decided on her own initiative to perform an osmotic fragility test on the blood sample. She expected it to show decreased resistance to hemolysis, but surprisingly, the result was the opposite. The cells were more resistant than normal, and a test for the presence of lead in the blood proved to be normal as well.

One month later, Weistock observed similar changes—and a normal lead level—in the blood of another patient. Wintrobe's only explanation at the time was human error: he suggested that Weistock had made a mistake in the fragility test.

But Weistock had confidence in her results. Two years later, a patient with subacute Cooley anemia was admitted to the hospital, and Wintrobe brought other members of the family to Hopkins to study their blood. When Weistock ex-

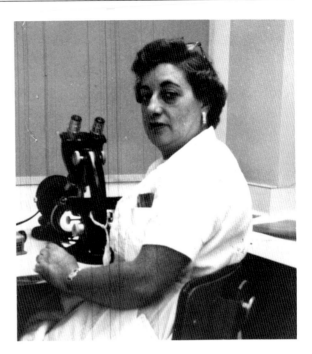

Regina Weistock

amined their blood smears, she immediately remembered the two earlier patients with similar findings. Reexamination of these patients revealed that all three had the same abnormalities, including increased resistance to hemolysis. Wintrobe promptly recognized that they were dealing with the hematologic abnormality associated with the thalassemia trait. Thus, carefully recorded observations by a competent technician and the prepared mind of a skillful hematologist were responsible for solving the enigma of this heritable disorder of hemoglobin synthesis.

At the same time, Wintrobe and his colleagues described consistent and typical blood changes in forty members of three Italian families in Baltimore, several of whom had enlarged spleens and mild jaundice. They realized that this was a mild form of thalassemia (thalassemia minor) and, in a footnote to their famous paper, they pointed out that they had seen the condition in both parents of a child with Cooley anemia. Thus was the heterozygous state defined.

At Hopkins, the investigation of thalassemia was extended by David Weatherall. As a fellow at

Johns Hopkins (from 1960 to 1965), he developed, with John Clegg and Michael Naughton, a technique that permitted the definition of the thalassemias in terms of defects either in alpha-globin synthesis or in beta-globin synthesis—the alpha-thalassemias or beta-thalassemias, respectively. Weatherall's discovery was based on the work of Vernon Ingram, who in 1956 demonstrated the single amino acid change that is responsible for sickle hemoglobin and three years later published with A. O. W. Strefton a classic paper on the genetic basis of the thalassemias.[50] Ingram and Strefton postulated the existence of the two basic types of thalassemia, which differ in their deficiency of alpha- or beta-globin.

The notion that unbalanced synthesis of one of the globin chains would result in deleterious accumulations of unpaired chains was originally developed by several workers, but the methods available in the early 1960s were too crude to allow researchers to effectively separate the two hemoglobin chains. Thus no one could provide a rigorously quantitative demonstration of unequal synthesis of alpha- and beta-globin in young red cells (reticulocytes). In the mid-1960s, Weatherall, Clegg, and Naughton evolved a simple method for separating the chains with almost 100 percent yield of the starting material.[51] Using reticulocytes incubated with radioactive amino acids *in vitro,* they could measure the total amounts of alpha and beta chains synthesized during the period of incubation.

Over the next few years, several groups applied these methods to the definition of the thalassemias. The work of Haig Kazazian was particularly valuable. By using combinations of DNA markers, called restriction fragment-length polymorphisms (RFLPs) to constitute a so-called haplotype, Kazazian and Stuart Orkin of Harvard found that the mutations in the beta subunit of hemoglobin that give rise to the frequent forms of thalassemia in the Mediterranean basin, in India, in Southeast Asia, and in Africa, tended to exist on the background of a particular haplotype. They demonstrated the usefulness of these haplotypes, as determined in the DNA of the fetus, for

the prenatal diagnosis of the thalassemias. Although most of the cases of thalassemia in persons from a particular geographic area tend to be of the same type, Kazazian identified over forty different forms of beta-thalassemia. He applied the polymerase chain reaction method to the diagnosis; the method involves amplifying the beta-globin gene or a relevant part of it and, with DNA clones, testing it for the various changes characteristic of beta-thalassemia.

Renaissance Investigators

Many Hopkins scientists made contributions of first-rank importance in more than a single area of research. Often their work spanned preclinical and clinical fields. These investigators thus not only augmented the fund of scientific knowledge—they also improved the scientific basis for the practice of medicine.

John Jacob Abel

John Jacob Abel, a pupil of Henry Newell Martin, became not only the first professor of pharmacology at Johns Hopkins but also the first full-time professor of pharmacology in the United States. His interest in pharmacology undoubtedly began during his fellowship in Martin's laboratory in 1884, where he participated in Martin's studies of the actions of drugs on the heart.

Abel's work on the isolation of hormones began in 1895, after his return to Baltimore from the University of Michigan. His first article, written with Albert C. Crawford in 1897, reported the isolation of epinephrine, a benzoyl derivative of the active principle of the adrenal medulla. Although pure epinephrine was later isolated by Jokichi Takamine, it was Abel who laid the foundation for this discovery.[52]

Much of Abel's research at Johns Hopkins was of a practical nature, and three of his discoveries yielded important clinical applications. In 1909, Abel and Leonard G. Rowntree, another member of the Hopkins Department of Pharma-

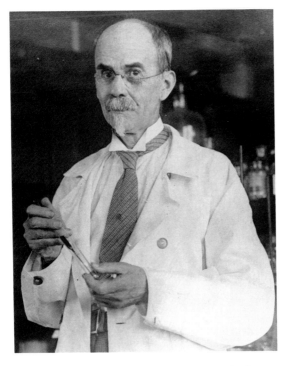

John Jacob Abel. (*Source*: Alan M. Chesney Medical Archives, The Johns Hopkins Medical Institutions.)

cology, who later joined Janeway's full-time staff in the Department of Medicine, reported the pharmacologic action of phthalein derivatives. This work was based on a description of phenolsulfonphthalein, a new chemical discovered by Ira Remsen, president of the Johns Hopkins University, when he was professor of chemistry. Geraghty and Rowntree studied the influence of substitutions in various parts of the molecule upon the compound's pharmacologic action, finding that phenolsulfonphthalein was excreted rapidly and completely by the normal kidney.[53] From this important observation came a classic test of renal function, which was used clinically for many years.

In 1913, Abel and his associates Rowntree and Benjamin B. Turner conceived a method of removing diffusible substances from the circulating blood of living animals by dialysis. Their basic idea became known as "vividiffusion," and their primary article on the subject discussed the rationale and implications of their studies:

There are numerous toxic states in which the eliminating organs of the body, more especially the kidneys, are incapable of removing from the body, at an adequate rate, the natural or unnatural substances whose accumulation is detrimental to life. In the hope of providing a substitute in such emergencies, which might tide over a dangerous crisis, as well as for the important information which it might be expected to provide, concerning the substances normally present in the blood, and also for the light that might thus be thrown on intermediary stages of metabolism, a method has been devised by which the blood of a living animal may be submitted to dialysis outside the body, and again returned to the natural circulation without exposure to air, infection by microorganisms, or any alteration which would necessarily be prejudicial to life.[54]

The method permitted the isolation of various diffusible substances in the blood. By identifying the amino acids alanine and valine and establishing the presence of histidine and creatinine, Abel provided the first incontestable evidence of their occurrence in normal blood, a fact of fundamental importance in the study of protein metabolism.

While engaged in their work on vividiffusion, Abel and his colleagues also carried out experiments in plasmapheresis. Their underlying idea was to devise a more scientific method for venesection. They demonstrated in dogs that large quantities of blood could be withdrawn repeatedly without apparent injury if the corpuscles separated by centrifugation from the plasma were suspended in Locke's solution and reinjected. Their 1914 article contains a prophetic sentence: "In view of the fact that mammalian corpuscles retain their stability for three or four days when kept on ice a supply of human corpuscles might possibly be kept in this manner in operating rooms for rapid injection in emergencies that would otherwise prove fatal."[55] Here again, Abel's interest in establishing fundamental principles did not blind him to the practical application of his work.

Later Research on Plasmapheresis: Its Benefits in Guillain-Barré Syndrome

Abel's work on plasmapheresis was extended by John W. Griffin and Guy M. McKhann, who between 1980 and 1984 directed a multicenter cooperative trial of this therapy for acute Guillain-Barré syndrome (GBS). With the marked decline in poliomyelitis, GBS has become the major cause of acute flaccid paralysis in healthy persons in the United States. Although most patients recover spontaneously, up to one-fourth require mechanical ventilation, many are left with some disability, and 2 to 5 percent die.

Griffin and McKhann suspected that the disease had an immunologic basis, and anecdotal reports suggested that patients could benefit from plasmapheresis. Their randomized trial of plasmapheresis versus conventional care in 245 patients severely ill with GBS involved exchanging 200 to 250 cc of plasma per kilogram of body weight over a period of seven to fourteen days.

Their results showed that plasmapheresis was particularly effective early in the course of the disease and in patients who required mechanical ventilation after entry into the study. Griffin, McKhann, and their large team of collaborators concluded that plasmapheresis is beneficial in patients with GBS of recent onset.[56]

Eli Kennerly Marshall, Jr.

Abel remained in the directorship of pharmacology until 1932, when he was succeeded by Eli Kennerly Marshall, Jr. One of the most versatile scientists at Johns Hopkins. Marshall held the directorships of two basic science departments, physiology and pharmacology.

Marshall began his career at Hopkins as an instructor in physiological chemistry under Walter Jones. Marshall's development of the technique for determining the presence of urea in biologic fluids was the first in a long series of major scientific contributions with important consequences for clinical medicine.[57]

Marshall's investigation of urease brought

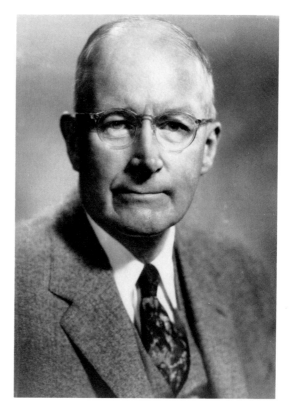

Eli Kennerly Marshall, Jr. (*Source:* Alan M. Chesney Medical Archives, The Johns Hopkins Medical Institutions.)

him to the attention of John J. Abel, who invited him to join the Department of Pharmacology. Marshall's rapid progress was partly due to the tutelage he received from Abel and from the conversations around the famous lunch table, that "exclusive and unofficial faculty club of the medical school" frequented by distinguished members of the faculty as well as visitors. It was the intellectual center of the medical school in those days, even though the amenities consisted solely of tea, bread, and cold cuts served on an old wooden table with its feet in kerosene to ward off the cockroaches.[58]

After two years with Abel, Marshall became head of pharmacology at Washington University in Saint Louis. He returned to Hopkins permanently in 1921, succeeding Howell as director of the Department of Physiology.

Marshall's greatest research contributions may have been made during this directorship.

One discovery led to a scientific confrontation that was eventually resolved in Marshall's favor. The controversial area was the mechanism of elimination of phenolsulfonphthalein, a process that Marshall believed was derived from secretion by the "convoluted" renal tubules.[59] Although Marshall's ideas about renal tubular secretion were strongly opposed by such leaders in the field as Arthur Cushny and A. Newton Richards, he amassed an enormous amount of supporting information, and his views were later substantiated by other investigators.[60]

Marshall also made the first measurements of cardiac output in unanesthetized dogs, using the Fick principle, with analysis of the arteriovenous oxygen difference. The method he developed for use in human beings employed nitrous oxide and ethylene, and it remained standard until the advent of cardiac catheterization.[61]

Marshall succeeded Abel as professor and director of the Department of Pharmacology and Experimental Therapeutics in 1932. He began his research there by investigating drug-induced respiratory depression. Marshall demonstrated that carbon dioxide alone is inadequate to drive the respiratory center and that anoxia plays a significant role in drug-induced respiratory depression. The clinical message was that administering oxygen under such circumstances is hazardous. Although his findings were not immediately appreciated in the clinic, physicians are now familiar with the danger of carbon dioxide narcosis when oxygen is administered to patients with severe obstructive pulmonary disease and respiratory acidosis.[62]

Marshall reoriented his research completely when the sulfonamides were first used in Baltimore by Perrin Long and Eleanor Bliss (see p. 278). After 1936, chemotherapy became his principal investigative interest. Within a year, he had published a quantitative method for mapping the absorption, distribution, and excretion of sulfonamides in animal and human subjects. He established rational dose schedules for the agent, and he soon met the need for a sulfonamide that could be administered intravenously, by introducing sodium sulfapyridine.[63]

Marshall also developed sulfaguanidine, a compound that, administered orally, was poorly absorbed and remained in the intestinal tract. This drug allowed the Allies to repulse the Japanese attack on Port Moresby during World War II. In 1942, every Australian and American soldier who could be mustered was mobilized for service in Port Moresby to withstand the arrival of the Japanese. When the Japanese reached the outskirts of the city, however, a severe outbreak of dysentery occurred among the Allies. Fortunately, a sizable amount of sulfaguanidine was found in the United States Army's medical supplies and was flown to Port Moresby in time for the Allied forces to recover and repel the Japanese attack.[64]

During World War II, Marshall abandoned his work on sulfanilamide to develop a better treatment for malaria. He and his colleagues at Hopkins studied malaria in birds and, with data obtained from the laboratory and from human volunteers, succeeded in defining the role of the four-amino and eight-amino quinolines in human malaria. The optimal dosage for the quinolines was controversial: some maintained that the drugs should be given to malarial patients in a regimen calculated to maintain a constant level of the agent in the blood. Marshall, who had introduced the concept of blood levels for the sulfonamides, demonstrated that this principle did not apply to the quinolines, whose pattern of distribution and mechanism of action were totally different from those of the sulfonamides.[65]

Marshall had the difficult task of succeeding not one but two of the remarkable and colorful members of the original faculty. He was nevertheless a distinguished example of the second generation of professors at Johns Hopkins, and his accomplishments placed him in the same rank with such giants as Abel and Howell. Marshall's work was original in theory and practice, and he stands in bold relief as a principal architect of the scientific age of chemotherapy.

Curt P. Richter

One of the most versatile investigators to grace the research laboratories at Johns Hopkins was Curt

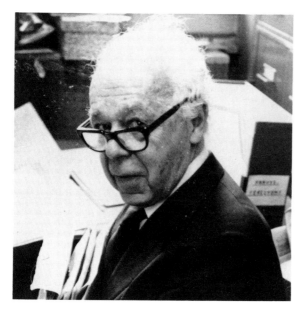

Curt P. Richter

ness, kindled his interest in "biologic clocks." Throughout his professional life, these two facets of animal activity remained his primary research concerns.[66]

When Watson left Hopkins, only eighteen months after Richter's arrival, Richter became a protégé of Adolf Meyer, director of the Department of Psychiatry. Thus was established the first experimental laboratory for psychobiology in the world. Richter identified Meyer as the most important influence at the time on his professional and personal development, and the two men became close friends. Meyer shared Watson's attitude toward formal course work. He invited Richter to attend his staff rounds and to lecture. He also allowed Richter to work with patients. Richter said of these years:

> My education from that point on was largely through conversations. I saw a great deal of Professor William H. Howell, who helped me with my experiments, and I had many long talks with him. It was the same way with Dr. Herbert Spencer Jennings at the University. These were all chance encounters when we would meet in the library and talk for an hour or two. This did more for me than all the courses I could take. The same way with Professor John J. Abel; I spent many hours with him. He followed my experiments and was very helpful, as was Professor Andrews in the biology department at Homewood. Later on, influence of that kind came particularly from Elmer McCollum of the School of Hygiene and Public Health. He took a great interest when I started my dietary self-selection studies. . . . I saw quite a good deal of W. G. MacCallum, mainly on an informal basis at the Maryland Club. Then there was Raymond Pearl, who was a close friend, and Dr. E. A. Park, who had a great influence on my work.[67]

P. Richter, whose career spanned almost seventy years. Richter arrived in Baltimore in 1919 to work with John B. Watson, the behavioral psychologist, who was a member of the Department of Psychiatry.

During Richter's first morning on the job, Watson told him, "I don't care what courses you take. As a matter of fact, you don't have to take any courses at all. All I care about is a good piece of research." To Richter, who was a poor classroom student, that seemed like a wonderful idea. He did, however, audit courses in anatomy and physiology, and he studied neurology with Henry Thomas, the first neurologist at Hopkins.

Watson assigned Richter a problem involving the study of learning in rats. Richter recalled that watching rats learn interested him far less than observing their bursts of activity. The fact that they were active—and the reasons for their activity—excited his curiosity, and he built cages containing devices that monitored the rats' slightest movement. Richter's discovery that the rats' activity occurred in clear-cut, regular ninety-minute cycles marked the beginning of his lifelong interest in periodic phenomena. His finding that the rats remained inactive during the day and active at night, even when kept in constant dark-

Some of Richter's early studies of activity in rats concerned the role of the endocrine glands. He determined the effects of removing the various glands, and the results of replacement therapy, on spontaneous running activity. He found that, although all the endocrine glands influence the control of activity, the most influential was the hypophysis. The role of specific glands differed among species, he found: in wild Norway rats, which have large adrenals, the adrenal gland was most important; in domestic rats, whose sex glands develop sooner, the gonads play the most important part.

When Richter extended his studies of activity to monkeys, he found that the prefrontal cortex of the brain, the tip of the striatum, and particularly cortical area 9 are important to the control of activity. In collaboration with Marion Hines, a member of the department of anatomy, he found that unilateral or bilateral removal of area 9 produced dramatic activity in monkeys. Working with C. Douglas Hawkes and Orthello Langworthy, neurologists at Hopkins, Richter produced the same type of activity by removing the frontal lobes in rats and cats.

Over the years, Richter compiled an extensive collection of case histories of both normal individuals and psychiatric patients with various periodic disturbances. He also produced a great variety of periodic phenomena in animals, by altering their endocrine glands, changing their diets, or treating them with drugs. His main objective in these experiments was to reproduce in animals the cyclic changes found in human beings. The cyclical behavior produced by interfering with the thyroid gland in rats, for example, closely resembled the behavior of catatonic schizophrenics.

The broadest implications of this work emerged from his finding that the twenty-four-hour and yearly cycles found in animals are non-homeostatic. These two cycles are independent of all external and internal disturbances, a factor that makes them such reliable timing devices.

Joel Elkes, chairman of the Department of Psychiatry from 1963 to 1975, referred to the "aesthetic beauty" of Richter's charts,

which recorded the precise, regular, and mysteriously stable shift of the biologic clocks from day to day. He described various kinds of clocks—homeostatic, central, and peripheral—and their accuracy is uncanny. This work presaged much of our present-day preoccupation with the rhythms that pervade daily life, including sleep and sleep disorders and the periodic somatic illnesses, which today

appear, at least in part, to be under hormonal control. The kinship between this approach to internal regulation and the concepts of self-regulation is apparent and, in view of present-day advances in biomonitoring and chemical assay techniques, offers a largely untilled field for research that is just now being cultivated.[68]

Richter's investigation of the electrical resistance of the skin inaugurated a new field of research, encompassing almost all functions of the body and personality. Through the study of more than three hundred patients at the Phipps Clinic and one hundred controls, he found that electrical skin resistance in the patients extended beyond both the lowest and highest limits of normal. Furthermore, the skin resistance levels varied with the type of psychiatric illness.

Richter then undertook a decade-long series of studies to determine the physiologic, neurologic, and physical factors on which electrical skin resistance depended. New instruments, electrodes, and techniques were designed to measure resistance on the skin from all parts of the body. The patients participating in these studies were gathered from most departments of the hospital, but mainly from medicine and surgery. Richter found that areas of skin denervated by sympathectomy, peripheral nerve lesions, or spinal cord transections could be mapped to the sharpest borders; various types of peripheral vascular disease gave characteristic patterns; and areas of abdominal sweating could be accurately defined. Characteristic patterns were also found in essential hypertension and other specific clinical conditions.

Of greatest interest was Richter's demonstration that the electrical skin resistance patterns on the surface of the body reflected pain that resulted from pressure on nerves, as well as pain referred from internal organs. He found that the skin resistance test could be used to detect the presence of lung tumors, particularly of the Pancoast type, and with John Bordley and George Hardy, of the Department of Otolaryngology, he demonstrated that by a simple conditioning process, the galvanic skin response could be used to test hearing in infants and children.

Richter's studies of nutrition stemmed from Raymond Pearl's early work on the effects of alcohol. Richter found that when rats are given solutions containing varying amounts of alcohol, they will reduce their intake of food by exactly the number of calories they are obtaining from the alcohol. This finding gave Richter the idea that animals have an inherent mechanism for regulating their dietary needs.

When he learned about the control of the adrenals over salt metabolism, he decided to investigate the effect of adrenalectomy on appetite for salt. Soon after adrenalectomy, his experimental animals began drinking large amounts of salt solution to keep themselves alive. Richter extended these observations to many other instances of homeostasis, including the role of parathyroid gland secretions in the metabolism of calcium.

When Richter began his studies of nutrition, he noted that in most other studies, subjects were given whole diets or diets comprising a variety of foodstuffs. It seemed to him that these earlier studies did not offer any conclusions about the nutritive value of any one foodstuff. With Emmett Holt, Jr., a member of the Department of Pediatrics, Richter devised diets consisting of a single foodstuff—a fat, a protein, or a carbohydrate—to learn how long a rat of a standard age could live on a single food, how active it would be, and how much it would eat. Then a single mineral or vitamin was added for choice. For example, on dextrose alone, rats survived for an average of thirty-six days, but when given access to a vitamin B_1 solution, they lived twice as long.

Foods found to have the best nutritive value were ultimately used in experiments in which rats were offered access to a variety of substances in separate containers. In one experiment, Richter and Holt offered the rats a choice of twenty purified foodstuffs in separate containers, including one fat, one protein, one carbohydrate, five mineral solutions, and six vitamin solutions. The rats made good choices from this selection of purified foodstuffs: they not only survived, but thrived, mated, and reproduced. It was obvious that their selection still lacked at least one nutritive sub-

stance, however, because none of the mothers succeeded in nursing their babies.

These brief descriptions of some of Curt Richter's research do not begin to encompass all his discoveries. His experiments have been characterized as "simple, ingenious, and elegant," of signal importance to psychology and biology.[69]

Arnold Rice Rich

MacCallum's successor as director of the Department of Pathology was Arnold R. Rich, many of whose important investigations were related to the problems of clinical medicine. One of his now-classic articles, an investigation of seven patients receiving sulfonamide therapy, established the role of hypersensitivity in the development of periarteritis nodosa.[70] None of these patients had any symptoms of periarteritis nodosa before the onset of the terminal, acute illness for which they were receiving serum or sulfonamides—their vascular lesions were all fresh. Rich concluded that these lesions could be a manifestation of the anaphylactic type of hypersensitivity.

In collaboration with John E. Gregory, Rich produced typical periarteritis in dogs by injecting a single large dose of foreign serum into the vein of a normal animal.[71] This procedure allowed for protracted circulation of antigen, which led to a hypersensitivity reaction.

A few years later, two independent groups of investigators—Frederick G. Germuth, Jr., and his group of pathologists at Johns Hopkins, and Frank J. Dixon and his colleagues at the University of Pittsburgh—found that they could produce serum sickness in rabbits by injecting combinations of foreign protein and antibody prepared in the test tube. Their studies showed that these injected "complexes" became trapped in the capillaries of the kidneys and led to changes resembling the human disease known as glomerulonephritis.[72]

The disease that Rich had produced was shown to be caused by an antigen-antibody complex. Given the name "immune complex disease," it could readily be produced in animals in the laboratory, but the discovery that it could also occur in response to viral infections in human beings (the so-called Australia antigen) had to await new techniques that would allow for the recognition of virus-antibody complexes.[73]

Rich's experimental work in the Department of Pathology spanned more than forty years and covered a wide range of subjects. His studies of jaundice and bile pigment metabolism were particularly important at a time when little was known about the mechanism and sites of hemoglobin breakdown. Rich and his co-workers showed that the pigment formed from hemoglobin in hemorrhages, known as hematoidin, was in fact bilirubin, and that it was formed not by extracellular enzymes or bacteria, but within the cells of the reticuloendothelial system. Rich conclusively demonstrated this phenomenon in tissue culture. He allowed reticuloendothelial phagocytes to engulf red cells, after which bilirubin would appear within the cells as the hemoglobin disappeared.[74] In further studies, Rich clarified the role of the liver in jaundice and was able to classify jaundice into two main types: retention and regurgitation.[75]

Another of Rich's interests, dating from the late 1920s, was the relation between bacterial allergy and immunity.[76] In those days, the hypersensitivity response was considered protective, even though it might result in tissue necrosis. The resulting exaggerated inflammation was believed necessary to wall off the noxious agent. In tuberculosis, for example, the dictum of the day was "the individual is as resistant as the shell of his tubercle." Rich and his collaborators disproved this theory, showing first in tuberculosis, next in syphilis, and then in other infections that although hypersensitivity and immunity might develop at the same time, they were independent phenomena.

Rich's group showed that hypersensitivity was dissociated from immunity in a variety of ways. Hypersensitivity might decrease while resistance remained, and cellular barriers were easily penetrated when resistance was low.[77] Furthermore, they found that antibodies rather than cell walls were responsible for checking the spread of bacteria.[78]

Rich expanded his studies of tuberculosis to investigate the general nature of resistance to this disease. One of his most fundamental contributions was the observation that bacterial allergy was a cellular phenomenon. He found that the cells themselves remained sensitized when grown in tissue culture. This property contrasted sharply with the behavior of cells in anaphylactic hypersensitivity, in which the ability to respond could be transferred with the serum.[79]

"For the pleasures of the cross-fertilization of thought between colleagues in different fields, I have been fortunately situated," Rich wrote,

> for pathology, concerned as it is with everything relating to all disease states from their beginnings to recovery or death, occupies a focal point for the interests of all special fields. Through the years, the day to day close association with my colleagues from all departments, as well as in our own, has been one of the happiest and most enriching advantages of my life, and I owe more than I could ever express to their stimulating thought and to their friendship.[80]

It was the academic life at Hopkins that made this cross-fertilization possible, that sustained and nourished these "renaissance physicians" for which Hopkins was known. This academic life was the realization of Gilman's vision:

> There is here an atmosphere of study, exhilarating and strengthening. It is a place where many men of diverse pursuits, coming from every part of the country and from many different colleges, are engaged in advanced intellectual work. The best of books and journals and instruments are procured as required, and are freely accessible. Diligence, perseverance and earnestness are expected from all. There are examples among the teachers of those who have already won distinction, and yet are laboring as industriously as the youngest scholar. There are lectures and conferences and discussions on questions of literary and scientific importance, by which the mind is quickened and the intellectual scope extended beyond the limits of a craft or technicality. There is an abundance of encouragement for laboratory research.[81]

Halsted and His School of Scientific Surgery

Foremost among those responsible for advancing the science of surgery was William S. Halsted, professor of surgery at Johns Hopkins from 1890 to 1922. While a young surgeon in New York, Halsted was described by one of his favorite residents, George J. Heuer, as

a bold, daring and original surgeon; a prodigious worker . . . a gay, cheerful soul, intimate with his students, holding open house for his friends, giving concerts at his home, enjoying people, and apparently one of them in their sports and pleasures.[82]

This picture of bonhomie is the obverse of the Baltimore Halsted:

thoughtful, careful, meticulous and preeminently a safe surgeon; a teacher as far removed from the quiz master as one could conceive possible; a worker indeed, but one who avoided hospital appointments, who limited his operative work, who sought leisure for study and reflection and became a profound thinker and surgical philosopher; and a man in relation with others, shy, retiring and remote, avoiding the crowd and its plaudits and preferring a seclusion which only a few choice friends were permitted to invade.[83]

This striking change in Halsted's personality resulted from his addiction to cocaine, which began in 1885. The previous year, a German investigator had discovered that cocaine would anesthetize the conjunctiva and cornea. Halsted recognized the importance of this agent, and with his associates Richard Hall and Frank Hartly began to study its potential value in surgical practice. They performed thousands of operations using cocaine as an anesthetic, but first they performed experiments upon themselves. It was only years later that the addictive effects of cocaine became known, and by that time Halsted and some of his associates had become dependent.

Although Halsted gained control over his addiction to cocaine, he continued to use morphine. During this period, he adopted a newly meticulous and methodical approach to surgery. His friend Welch had recommended him for the directorship of surgery at the new Johns Hopkins

Hospital, but the trustees were leery of taking him on. As Osler recalled:

With a morphia record, and an uncertainty as to the cure, the Trustees could not do more than put him on trial. He proved an immediate success, and his early work on methods of technique, the healing of wounds, on hernia and on breast cancer, brought much reputation to the Hospital. . . . His stand-offishness was much in the way of his popularity, but once beneath the crust people learned his true worth.[84]

When Osler and his colleagues recommended Halsted as full surgeon to the hospital in 1890, they were under the impression that he was no longer addicted. "He had worked so well and so energetically," Osler wrote, "that it did not seem possible that he could take the drug and do so much." But six months later, Osler saw him shaking as if from a severe chill, and this was Osler's first intimation that Halsted was still drug-dependent. Osler learned that Halsted could do his work comfortably and remain physically vigorous on a daily regimen of 3 grains of morphine. Halsted was later able to reduce the amount to 1-1/2 grains, and he may eventually have done without it entirely. Osler believed that no one else—even Welch—suspected that Halsted remained addicted through most of his life.[85]

Without a background for comparison, it is difficult to appreciate the importance of Halsted's contributions to the development of surgery. As Halsted's student Heuer has pointed out, the fundamental principles of surgery, such as the prevention of infection, the control of hemorrhage, the careful handling of tissues, and the promotion of drainage and wound healing were just beginning to be appreciated. The cranial and thoracic cavities were not entered on an elective basis, and brain surgery and thoracic surgery still awaited the future. Surgery of the thyroid was in its infancy, and no satisfactory operation for cancer of the breast, or for the successful treatment of hernia, had yet been developed. Gastric resection had not yet been accomplished, nor had intestinal resection. Surgery of the gallbladder and biliary tract was almost never attempted. So, as Heuer has said, surgery was a special, limited therapeutic field when Halsted came to Johns Hopkins.

On his arrival, Halsted set about identifying and extending the fundamental principles of surgery, one of which was the prevention of infection. He knew that neither the antiseptic nor the aseptic method alone could consistently prevent infection. Moreover, although instruments, dressings, and suture materials could be completely sterilized, neither the skin of the patient nor the hands of the surgeon and assistants could be sterilized by washing and antiseptic solutions. There was no way to avoid introducing organisms into a surgical wound, so Halsted turned to evaluating other aspects of preventing infection.

Halsted's studies revealed that normal tissues have a natural resistance to infection, but they lose this inherent resistance if they are crushed or if their blood supply is otherwise impaired. Halsted thus concluded that the soundest approach was to conduct surgical procedures with the minimum of injury to the tissues. He invented a clamp with a sharp point, now known as the Halsted artery forceps, whose purpose was to control hemorrhage with the least possible tissue damage. He employed the finest silk to tie the vessels, as silk can be securely sterilized and causes less reaction in the tissues than catgut. He was careful to transfix each bleeding point so that no blood would collect in tissue spaces, and to handle the tissues gently. He devised a subcutaneous suture that approximates skin without involving the outer layers, where pathogenic organisms are found. He did not drain clean wounds for fear of introducing infection along the drain. If drainage was required, if a wound needed packing, or an open wound needed frequent dressing, he avoided injury to the granulation tissue of healing by using a filmlike guttapercha tissue that did not adhere to wound surfaces.[86]

Halsted's contributions to surgical technique spanned the entire range of surgical practice. His keen interest in surgery of the thyroid gland led to signal advances in diagnosis as well as operative procedures. For this work, Halsted turned to experimental animals, transplanting the thyroid gland in dogs. He thus discovered the striking histologic changes indicative of hyperplasia and noted their similarity to the changes found in hyperthyroidism and exophthalmic goiter. Halsted devised an operation on the thyroid that reduced the danger of hemorrhage; he also recognized that the parathyroid glands protected against tetany, and he was careful to try not to excise them along with the thyroid. For intestinal anastomosis, he devised a special suture, called the Halsted mattress suture, which united the opposing peritoneal surfaces of the intestine, providing ideal conditions for healing. His contributions to the surgical treatment of breast cancer and the therapy of inguinal hernias changed the practice of surgery.[87]

Halsted's meticulously defined principles of surgical technique were all based upon scientific evidence. They had a far-reaching effect upon surgery, making it a much safer form of medical practice. The control of hemorrhage, the gentle handling of tissues, the use of the finest suture material, and the avoidance of tension on the tissues made it possible to spend the time necessary to do careful surgery without shock and without wound complications.

In his laboratory approach to surgical problems, in his residency program for training surgeons, and in his own meticulous surgical technique, Halsted guided American surgery along a new path. Many visitors who came to see him operate did not have the patience to watch him until the end of a procedure. His gentle and careful handling of tissues opened the way for radical surgery—operative procedures as decisively curative therapy. Before Halsted and his "school of safety," as Leriche called it, this approach made no sense; but with this methodical approach, Halsted and other surgeons of the time were able to give surgery true therapeutic power.[88]

Harvey Cushing and Walter Dandy: The Birth of Neurosurgery

"No greater change has come over the face of science," said Welch in 1907, "than the many subdivisions which have arisen. . . . We may regret the loss of many charming features which have been erased from the landscape of science by all of this minute specialization, of which no one can foresee the end, but such a sentiment is much the same and as unavailing as that for the return of the days of the stagecoach."[89]

Welch was referring to the natural sciences as a whole; specialization in the particular science of medicine did not occur until the early twentieth century. In the field of surgery, it was Halsted who was responsible for encouraging this "minute specialization," identifying students who could concentrate on the anatomy and physiology of one area of the body.

One such student was Harvey Cushing. Few realize that much of Cushing's important research was carried out during his sixteen years in Baltimore, from 1896 to 1912. Although he specialized in neurosurgery, Cushing's research spanned general medicine and surgery and included studies of blood pressure as well as investigations that extended Ringer and Locke's studies of "physiological" saline to the surgical clinic.

As a medical student in Boston, Cushing and Amory Codman had introduced "ether charts" on which the anesthetist would record the patient's pulse and respiration at regular intervals during an operation. Later, a year abroad took Cushing to the great laboratories of Europe. His interest in blood pressure was stimulated by Hugo Kronecker in Berne, where he studied the regulation of blood pressure, particularly in relation to pressure within the skull. Here Cushing learned that the level of blood pressure reflects an animal's physiologic condition: a significant drop during a surgical procedure indicates that the animal's condition is poor. Cushing revised the ether charts of his medical school days after a visit to Italy, where he first saw the Riva-Rocci sphygmomanometer. He quickly recognized it as an essential tool, and as soon as he returned to Baltimore, he insisted that blood pressure readings be taken during all operations.[90]

Cushing also was one of the first to draw attention to Ringer's discovery that so-called physiological salt solution, sodium chloride added to water, was inadequate for preserving excised tissues—a finding vitally important to clinical

medicine. Cushing perfused the hind leg vessels of a frog with solutions of differing ionic content, demonstrating that pure sodium chloride vitiated the capacity of the muscle to respond to stimulation of its nerves. If potassium chloride and calcium chloride were added, the irritability of the muscle was restored. The classic article that resulted from this work was published in 1901.[91]

The year 1900 marked the beginning of Cushing's concentration on disorders of the nervous system. His work in this field began with an interest in the surgical relief of trigeminal neuralgia, and the resulting article was a landmark in the development of neurosurgery.[92] His interest in the Gasserian ganglion led him to study the sensory distribution of the trigeminal nerve and of the nerves supplying the skin in other parts of the body. The resulting analysis of the areas of the skin supplied by the various branches of the trigeminal nerve is a classic neuroanatomic study, which shows that basic research can stem from the treatment of a clinical condition.[93]

From 1905 to 1912, Cushing was at the peak of his research career—a time he devoted to the study of the pituitary gland and the surgical treatment of its tumors. This interest came about through a tragic misdiagnosis. Cushing had operated on a young woman complaining of headaches and failure of vision. As he described the patient, "the face was fat and although 14 years of age she had failed to mature sexually." After he decompressed the brain first on one side and then on the other, her headaches improved, but her vision continued to deteriorate. His first diagnosis was obviously incorrect, but Cushing then concluded that his patient had a tumor in the occipital area. He exposed the cerebellum, after which the patient died. Autopsy revealed a large pituitary cyst. Soon afterwards, the surgeon Alfred Fröhlich sent Cushing a reprint of an article describing a similar patient—the first description of Fröhlich syndrome. Cushing's pride was hurt by his erroneous diagnosis, and from then on the pituitary became an obsessive interest.[94]

Cushing's studies of this gland coincided with the revelations of E. A. Schaefer, who in 1908 described his discovery of the active principle of the posterior pituitary. Cushing's important advantage was his command of the surgical techniques essential for approaching the pituitary gland of higher animals. It was this skill that enabled Cushing to connect hypophyseal adiposity with Fröhlich syndrome, a deduction that erased much confusion concerning sexual and asexual adiposity, and made Cushing a leader in the field.

The work that led to this discovery was performed by Cushing and L. L. Reford. They were replicating the 1907 experiments of Paulesco, who had devised an operation that permitted complete removal of the canine pituitary (hypophysectomy). Paulesco's animals invariably succumbed in a state of cachexia, as did most of Cushing's. Occasionally, however, Cushing and Reford's animals did not die but merely became fat. John Homans, the son of Cushing's teacher at Harvard, joined their pituitary study in 1908 and described Cushing's moment of insight:

> Some animals survived for many months. These animals were carefully looked after, but, on the whole, were passed by for the time being as freaks in which something had marred the completeness of the hypophysectomy. Finally, I remembered that one of these animals died; an extraordinarily fat, loggy [sic], sexless creature. I made the autopsy, merely noting the fact of the asexual adiposity which made no impression upon me whatever. One day Cushing caught sight of another of these animals while it was still alive, I am quite certain, and said at once: "Here is Fröhlich's asexual adiposity."[95]

The near or total absence of hypophysis in the animal led Cushing to conclude that the adiposity was the result of hypophyseal deficiency—in contrast to acromegaly, which represented an overfunction of the gland. Physicians were beginning to understand acromegaly, but until Cushing's discovery, they had also attributed asexual adiposity to an enlargement of the hypophysis. Cushing's work, performed in collaboration with Samuel J. Crowe and John Homans, resulted in an important monograph published in 1910.[96]

In further work on the pituitary, Cushing and his colleagues demonstrated in experimental animals that the gland normally exerts an important influence on the metabolic processes of the body. Extending their laboratory work to observations in human subjects, they described the disturbances that follow partial and complete removal of the gland and correlated them with the symptoms of pituitary disease.

Cushing introduced the terms "hypo-" and "hyperpituitarism" in a milestone paper in 1909. At the time, he was unaware that Marburg had devised the same terms the previous year. Marburg's deduction, however, was based entirely on clinical material, without experimental verification. Cushing, in contrast, used his research in the laboratory to show that absence of the anterior hypophysis was incompatible with life, and that its partial removal led to symptoms characteristic of lessened secretion (hypopituitarism) in human beings. He continued:

> A tumor of the gland, itself, or one arising in its neighborhood and implicating the gland by pressure, is naturally the lesion to which one or the other of these conditions has heretofore been attributed, though it is probable that over-secretion from simple hypertrophy, or under-secretion from atrophy, will be found to occur irrespective of tumor growth when examination of the pituitary body becomes a routine measure in the postmortem examination of all cases in which the conditions suggest one or the other of the symptom-complexes described.
>
> When due to tumor, surgery is the treatment that these conditions demand, and at present there are reasonably satisfactory ways of approaching the gland; but clinicians and surgeons must clearly distinguish between the local manifestations of the neoplasm due to involvement of structures in its neighborhood other than hypophysis, and those of a general character from disturbances of metabolism due to alterations of the hypophysis itself.[97]

Cushing's sixteen years in Baltimore ended with the publication of his classic monograph, "The Pituitary Body and Its Disorders." This was a landmark in the history of endocrinology, for it introduced a clinical concept of endocrine function that synthesized the growing body of knowledge in this field. In cases of acromegaly, Cushing found a preponderance of cells that stained with eosin, leading him to conclude that these cells produce the growth hormone and that the basophilic cells probably elaborate some other essential secretion—a prediction that illustrates his extraordinary clinical acumen.

Cushing's work on the pituitary gland continued even after his "retirement" in 1929 to the professorship of the history of medicine at Yale. Not until 1932 did Cushing's ideas crystallize. In that year, he presented his summary of basophil adenomas of the pituitary, and the syndrome that has taken his name, at a meeting of the Johns Hopkins Medical Society in the newly opened Hurd Hall.[98]

Cushing's move to Boston in 1912 left neurosurgical research at Hopkins under the direction of Walter E. Dandy, who had begun his training under Cushing. Dandy's discovery of ventriculography illustrates Louis Pasteur's oft-quoted statement, "In the field of observation, chance favors the prepared mind."

Dandy, then a surgical resident, was preparing to explore the abdomen of a patient with repeated intestinal hemorrhage. The hospital radiologist, Frederick Henry Baetjer, included the upper abdomen in a preoperative chest x-ray, which showed free air under the diaphragm. At operation, Dandy confirmed the presence of in-

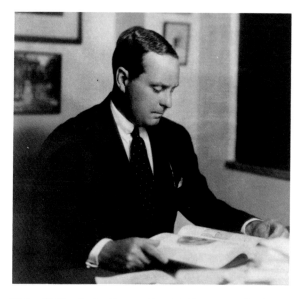

Walter E. Dandy, Jr. (*Source:* Alan M. Chesney Medical Archives, The Johns Hopkins Medical Institutions.)

traperitoneal air as well as the perforated typhoid ulcer through which it had escaped. Seeing this patient, Dandy must have ruminated on Halsted's frequent comments concerning the remarkable power of intestinal gases to perforate bone. It was not long before Dandy applied this characteristic of gases to his work on the brain.[99]

From this case and other clinical demonstrations of the radiographic properties of air, as well as his earlier laboratory studies of hydrocephalus, it was but a step for Dandy to conceive the idea of injecting a gas into the cerebral ventricles. The result revolutionized the diagnosis of brain tumors and, consequently, the field of neurosurgery.

Dandy needed to remove a little more cerebrospinal fluid than the contents of one ventricle and to replace this fluid with an equal quantity of air. Before the fontanelles closed, he could readily make a ventricular puncture through the interosseous defect. After the sutures were united, he had to make a small opening in the bone.[100]

The discovery of ventriculography was the logical result of Dandy's experimental and clinical studies of the ventricles and the circulation of the cerebrospinal fluid in hydrocephalus. It was not altogether a spontaneous and sudden inspiration, as Samuel J. Crowe recalled:

> In 1917 when Doctor Dandy was a house officer, he was very outspoken to his friends and associates about palliative brain surgery. A decompression, he said, relieves symptoms for a time, but when the cause is a growing tumor, the relief is not permanent. Early diagnosis, accurate localization and surgical removal are just as essential for the cure of a brain tumor as they are for a new growth in other parts of the body.[101]

In the laboratory, Dandy tested the possibility of filling the cerebral ventricles with several substances. By ventricular puncture, he removed a part of the cerebrospinal fluid, replacing it with an equal amount of a solution. The ventricles were then clearly outlined on x-ray. He repeated this procedure on animals with a simulated space-occupying tumor, and as he had predicted, the radiographs showed displacement of the ventricles. The substances he used, however, were far too irritating to inject into the central nervous system of patients. Ventriculography was possible only if a gas was substituted for the cerebrospinal fluid withdrawn. It was in this series of experiments that the idea of using air finally emerged.

At age twenty-seven, Dandy published the first of a series of ten classic articles on the nature of hydrocephalus and the circulation of the cerebrospinal fluid. Dandy and Blackfan produced dilatation of the lateral and third ventricles in dogs by obstructing the aqueduct of Sylvius; they also produced distention of one lateral ventricle by obstructing its foramen of Monroe. This distention could be prevented by removing the choroid plexus. Dandy demonstrated that hydrocephalus did not result from separating the Pacchionian granulations from the great veins. Thus, Dandy disproved the common belief that cerebrospinal fluid absorption occurs through these veins; instead, the fluid is absorbed directly into the blood vessels in the subarachnoid space. His theory was borne out in the autopsy room, as in every case of "idiopathic" hydrocephalus, an obstruction was demonstrated at the aqueduct of Sylvius, at the foramina of Luschka and Magendie, or along the basilar cisterns. Dandy's solid anatomic and physiologic studies, coupled with his clinical observations, allowed him to reclassify this disorder into communicating and noncommunicating types. The operations of choroid plexectomy and ventriculostomy were the logical outgrowth of his discoveries.[102]

Dandy's other pioneering advances included an operation for glossopharyngeal neuralgia, a surgical approach to the treatment of Ménière disease, and the recognition of protruded discs as one of the most frequent causes of back pain and sciatica.[103]

Dandy possessed a marvelous combination of qualities: a clear-thinking mind, enthusiasm, drive, a lively imagination, independence of thought and action, manual dexterity, and a colorful personality. He had the genius to conceive of new and startling operative techniques, the courage to try them, and the skill to make them succeed.

The Advent of Modern Cardiac Surgery

The past forty-five years have witnessed dramatic developments in cardiac surgery. Before 1944, surgeons believed that operating on the heart was impracticable. The British physician Stephen Paget wrote in 1896, "Surgery of the heart has probably reached the limit set by nature to all surgery. No new method and no new discovery can overcome the natural difficulties that attend a wound of the heart." Yet in a relatively short time, these difficulties were overcome, and operations on the heart became commonplace.

The event that triggered these advances in cardiovascular surgery was the famous "blue-baby" operation pioneered by Helen B. Taussig and Alfred Blalock of Johns Hopkins. The operation involved the creation of an artificial channel between the arteries of the lung and a branch of the aorta. The abnormality that they attempted to relieve was a curious combination of deformities of the heart known as the "tetralogy of Fallot."[104]

Blalock had succeeded Dean D. Lewis as director of surgery in 1941. Blalock's collaborator, Helen B. Taussig, had been appointed pediatrician in charge of the Cardiac Clinic at the Harriet Lane Home in 1930, at the age of twenty-nine. Taussig's particular interest was the study of rheumatic fever. Her new heart clinic acquired a fluoroscope, and her mentor Edwards A. Park suggested that if she matched her observations of each patient in different positions under the fluoroscope with information from x-rays and electrocardiograms, she might be able to discern the early changes of the heart in rheumatic fever.

Park also insisted that she study congenital heart disease—an assignment that she accepted with little enthusiasm. Taussig nevertheless observed in meticulous detail every child referred to the cardiac clinic.

House officers tended to ignore the embryonic cardiac clinic until an event in 1933 focused attention on Taussig and her studies. Fluoroscopy of one cyanotic infant revealed the absence of a right ventricular shadow. Taussig had made the diagnosis of absent right ventricle. A child admitted to the hospital a few weeks later had a similar radiograph, and when this second patient was presented at ward rounds, the resident, John Washington, thought he had put up the wrong film. Taussig demurred, pointing out that the film on display was of another child with the same malformation. The similarity of the cardiac findings in these two patients crystallized her impression that specific malformations caused specific changes in the size and shape of the heart.

Word of this incident spread, and house officers referred an increasing number of puzzling patients to her. Taussig perceived that some cyanotic patients did reasonably well as long as the ductus arteriosus was open, but when the ductus closed, they became more cyanotic. She soon reasoned that the basic problem was to re-establish the flow of blood to the lungs.

Trying to think of ways to keep the ductus open, Taussig searched the literature and considered such methods as nitrogen inhalation. Robert Gross in Boston was tying off the ductus in some patients, and it occurred to her that if one could close a ductus off, one could certainly put one in. Gross gave her no encouragement, but she did not abandon the idea. When Blalock performed the first closure of the ductus arteriosus at Hopkins in 1942, she praised his surgical skill but added that the really great day would come when he could build a ductus for a child who was dying of anoxemia, not when he tied off a ductus for a child who had a little too much blood going to the lungs.

Park later asked Blalock about the possibility of correcting narrowing (coarctation) of the aorta; although Blalock was noncommittal at the time, some months later, Park found on his desk an article by Blalock in which he had been named as coauthor, describing the use of the subclavian artery to bypass constricted aortas in dogs. Blalock was hesitant to use the operation in human beings, he told Park, because many of the dogs had become paraplegic when the aorta was cross-clamped. When Blalock discussed the procedure at a Harriet Lane conference, Taussig asked whether a similar operation could be devised to improve the pulmonary circulation in children with pulmonary stenosis. Blalock had the opera-

tive remedy at hand: the subclavian pulmonary anastomosis that he had performed in Nashville some years earlier in an attempt to produce pulmonary hypertension in the dog.

Opinions diverge about the origin of the Blalock-Taussig operation. Taussig remembered participating in a conversation with Blalock and Park in 1943 about the difficulties of cross-clamping the descending aorta. Park suggested using the carotid artery as a bypass, turning the carotid artery down and anastomosing it to the aorta below the coarctation. Taussig recalled speaking up: "If you put the carotid artery into the descending aorta, couldn't you put the subclavian artery into the pulmonary artery?" Park remembered the conversation differently, telling Mark Ravitch some twenty years later, "In my presence Taussig asked Blalock if he could not do something by operation to give patients with the tetralogy of Fallot adequate pulmonary circulation, on the grounds that such was what they required, but without suggesting how this could be done." Blalock's version was expressed in a letter in 1945: "I must say that if I made the statement to you that you could improve the condition of patients with aortic stenosis if you could find a means to allow more blood to reach the body, that I would still be far from solving the practical problems."[105]

However the idea developed, Blalock invited Taussig to work on the problem with him on the dogs in his laboratory. At first, laboratory experiments were directed toward the production of pulmonary stenosis, but the ligatures around the pulmonary artery cut through the arterial wall, removing the obstruction. Even when stenosis was produced, it alone did not result in oxygen unsaturation of the arterial blood. Taussig remembered suggesting to Vivien Thomas, Blalock's technician, that he put a branch of the right pulmonary artery into the left atrium, thereby causing venous blood to be directed to the aorta. After the dogs had developed polycythemia, the proximal end of the subclavian artery could be anastomosed to the pulmonary artery to determine whether a reduction in polycythemia would occur. That procedure alone did not alter the red blood cell count, so Thomas also removed part of the right lung. These two procedures resulted in some polycythemia, which appeared to be lessened by increasing the circulation to the other lung. Between 1943 and the end of 1944, operations were performed on more than 200 dogs, but the results of these experiments were not entirely clear.

On November 29, 1944, Blalock and Taussig decided to proceed with the anastomosis of the subclavian artery to the pulmonary artery in a cyanotic child. Taussig was convinced that the operation would help the patient, and despite the technical problems of operating on a very small and very ill child, Blalock's skill was equal to the task. The "blue-baby" operation was successful and brought deserved fame to both Alfred Blalock and Helen Taussig.[106]

The full potential of Blalock and Taussig's operation would not have been realized without the assistance of Richard J. Bing, who came to Johns Hopkins in 1943 to set up a laboratory that would extend the newly developed technique of cardiac catheterization. Bing developed this procedure as a diagnostic tool in the preoperative study of patients with heart disease; he also used it to make quantitative physiologic and biochemical measurements in patients with cardiovascular disease. His pathophysiologic studies of congenital malformations of the heart were published in a series of classic articles. Bing was one of the first to recognize the value of the catheter in investigating fundamental cardiac mechanisms in human beings, and he initiated some of the earliest studies of myocardial blood flow and myocardial oxygen consumption.[107]

The Discovery of Cardiopulmonary Resuscitation

William B. Kouwenhoven received the Albert and Mary Lasker Foundation Award in 1973 for three contributions: he and his colleagues confirmed that an electric shock could reverse ventricular fibrillation, developed the devices for both open- and closed-chest defibrillation, and devised the technique of "external cardiac massage."

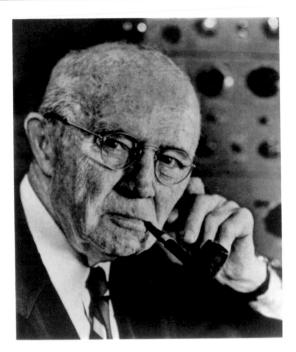

William B. Kouwenhoven. (*Source: Modern Medicine,* copyright © 1967 by the New York Times Media Company, Inc. Reproduced with permission.)

An electrical engineer by training, Kouwenhoven retired as professor of electrical engineering and dean of the Whiting School of Engineering at Hopkins in 1956 to become a lecturer in surgery. In 1969 he received the first honorary degree of doctor of medicine ever awarded by the Johns Hopkins University. Kouwenhoven's career illustrates the rewards of interdisciplinary cooperative research and displays a dedicated, creative scientist who continued to make important contributions long after he had attained emeritus status.[108]

Work on cardiopulmonary resuscitation began in the 1920s, supported by the electric utility companies, which were concerned about the increasing number of linemen killed by electric shock. Supervising the work at Johns Hopkins were Kouwenhoven and Orthello R. Langworthy, who studied the damage caused by electric shock. Using rats as experimental animals, they noted the effects of DC and AC shock of high and low voltages. Analysis of the problem in human subjects revealed that ventricular fibrillation occurred mainly from low-voltage shocks, while paralysis of respiration resulted from higher voltages.

Others working on the problem included Donald Hooker, then associate professor of physiology in the School of Hygiene and Public Health. Hooker was successful in defibrillating a dog's heart but was unable to start it beating again. Carl J. Wiggers of Case Western Reserve University in Cleveland attempted open-chest defibrillation in patients developing the arrhythmia during a surgical procedure. In 1947, Claude Beck, a 1921 graduate of the Johns Hopkins University School of Medicine, and one of the surgeons working with Wiggers, reported the first open-chest defibrillation in a human patient by applying electrodes directly to the surface of the heart. He also found that squeezing the exposed heart manually could provide circulation of the blood. At Hopkins, Howell called his group's attention to the work of Prevost and Batelly, who in 1889 used an electric countershock to arrest ventricular fibrillation in the animal heart. Howell asked the simple question: "Is this true?" The answer quietly came back to him: "Yes."

After World War II, Kouwenhoven moved to the Department of Surgery. His group's work was complemented in the early postwar years by the investigations of James Elam and Peter Safir of the Division of Anesthesiology, who perfected the mouth-to-mouth method of lung ventilation by expired air—an excellent method for oxygenating the blood, but one that does not produce any circulation.

Kouwenhoven and William Milnor began to develop a closed-chest defibrillator in 1950. They first used capacitor discharges with electrodes on opposite sides of the chest, but soon discovered that a brief AC current of twenty amperes would defibrillate the heart successfully.

Samuel Talbot, who was also investigating heart arrhythmias, asked Kouwenhoven and Milnor to demonstrate their method of defibrillating the canine heart: ventricular fibrillation was induced under anesthesia, and normal rhythm restored by a shock applied through electrodes attached to the sides of the dog's chest. Because Talbot's experiments required strapping a vest stud-

ded with contact electrodes around the chest, however, no space was available for the defibrillating electrodes. Forced to adapt their method to Talbot's requirements, Kouwenhoven and Milnor found that their procedure was just as effective when one electrode was placed over the suprasternal notch and the other over the apex of the heart. In fact, these placements were superior to the original ones, since the current then flowed longitudinally through the heart, allowing the intensity of the shock to be reduced by 50 percent. After hundreds of tests in the laboratory, the Hopkins AC defibrillator was used on a human subject for the first time in March 1957.[109]

Tests with the defibrillator had shown a rise in blood pressure when a countershock was applied to the heart. G. Guy Knickerbocker, a member of Kouwenhoven's staff, also noticed a slight rise in blood pressure when the electrodes were pressed on an animal's chest, even before the countershock was applied. Knickerbocker wondered whether manual compression of the thorax might be effective in producing circulation of the blood. In experiments in which pressure was applied to the sides of the chest as well as to the sternum, a number of animals suffered broken costal junctions and ribs, but their blood pressure rose to 40 percent of normal. Hopkins surgeons were excited by this result—particularly Henry T. Bahnson, who had recently joined Kouwenhoven's group. Further studies showed that a dog could be kept alive for ten minutes by applying rhythmic pressure over the lower third of the sternum with a force of 80 to 100 pounds at a rate of one application per second. In February 1958, Bahnson finally had the opportunity to try this technique on a patient, successfully resuscitating a two-year-old child whose heart was in ventricular fibrillation. In the same year, James Jude, a resident surgeon working with Kouwenhoven, successfully applied external cardiac massage to an obese woman in her forties who had developed ventricular fibrillation while undergoing anesthesia.

The portable defibrillator was also developed by Kouwenhoven and his group. To avoid accidental condenser discharges, the electrodes do not connect to the charged condensers unless both electrodes are applied to the chest with a force of at least twelve pounds. This defibrillator has saved many lives and has become part of the equipment of all modern hospitals.

Both of Kouwenhoven's innovations, the defibrillator and closed-chest cardiac massage, were developed further during the 1970s by Myron Weisfeldt's group at Johns Hopkins. They showed that a prolonged phase of chest compression is important for most effective movement of blood during closed chest cardiac massage.[110] The circulation of blood in the current method of cardiopulmonary resuscitation (CPR) was shown to be more the result of rise in intrathoracic pressure, propelling blood out of the thoracic cavity (with a drawing in of blood from the venous system with the elastic recoil) than it is compression of ventricles between sternum and vertebral column.[111] This mechanism of the circulation in CPR had been suggested by J. Michael Criley, an Osler resident who also trained in cardiology at Johns Hopkins. Criley discovered that a patient who was conscious at the onset of ventricular fibrillation could maintain consciousness by coughing every two or three seconds.[112]

Working at Sinai Hospital, Mieczyslaw Mirowski of the Hopkins Department of Medicine developed an implantable automatic defibrillator, an extension of Kouwenhoven's devices.[113] The first was installed in 1980 at Johns Hopkins in a patient with repeated life-threatening episodes of ventricular fibrillation.

Advances in Preventive Medicine

The ultimate objective of medical research is the prevention of disease, and the prevention of disease through basic research is the most promising approach to reducing the enormous cost of medical care. Lewis Thomas has referred to "decisive" technology for prevention of disease, including immunization against disease caused by bacteria and viruses, the treatment and prevention of infectious diseases with antibiotics and chemicals, and the prevention of nutritional disorders through a balanced diet with adequate vitamin intake.[114]

Johns Hopkins has been the site of many discoveries leading to such "decisive" advances, five of which will be recounted here.

The Conquest of Rickets

The key to the problem of rickets was to discover what prevented the deposition of calcium salts into the bone and bone-forming cartilage. In 1914 W. McKim Marriott and John Howland developed better biochemical methods for the determination of calcium and phosphorus in the serum—a necessary step, since only a limited amount of blood could be obtained from infants. They showed that in the active phase of the so-called idiopathic tetany of infancy, the serum calcium was substantially less than normal. Later, they found that the serum concentration in cases of rickets without tetany was normal or only slightly reduced.

Meanwhile, Elmer V. McCollum had joined the group working on this problem. McCollum had come to Hopkins with a fine background in nutrition research. He and Marguerite Davis had demonstrated the existence of vitamin A, the first fat-soluble vitamin to be described. McCollum had set up his rat colony in Hopkins' newly founded School of Hygiene and Public Health. In the autumn of 1918, Howland asked McCollum whether anyone had ever produced experimental rickets in animals; McCollum invited Howland to inspect his rats, some of which appeared to be rachitic. Howland saw that the gross appearance of the thorax in these rats was similar to the thorax in children with severe rickets. These animals had the typical "pigeon breast" (Harrison's groove) and the characteristically wide costochondral junctions of the ribs.

McCollum had not yet been able to identify the dietary factors involved. His laboratory notes, however, included careful records of the composition and source of the rats' diets. It was time to bring in an expert in bone histology and pathology, McCollum and Howland believed, to discover the nature of the various dietary defects that would produce abnormalities in growing bones. Howland cabled Edwards A. Park to return to Baltimore; in the meantime, Paul G. Shipley was assigned to supervise the histologic studies.

The group's studies benefited from clues provided in 1918 by Sir Edward Mellanby, who demonstrated that certain fats (butterfat and, notably, cod-liver oil) prevented the bone lesions caused by his experimental diets. When the Hopkins group published their first results, in 1921, they had completed studies of the effects of about 300 experimental diets on hundreds of rats. They found that, although the bones of young rats were highly responsive to dietary defects, the most significant factors for safeguarding normal bone growth were the ratio between the calcium and the phosphorus in the food and the kind of fats supplied. Low calcium and high phosphorus, or low phosphorus and high calcium, were disturbing to bone growth; the former relationship caused rickets complicated by tetany. Despite unfavorable ratios between calcium and phosphorus, rickets could be avoided if the diet contained a little cod-liver oil or a large amount of butterfat.

The following year, Howland included Hopkins pediatrician Benjamin Kramer in the studies. Kramer was one of the pediatricians with formal training in chemistry attracted to Howland's interest in using chemical techniques for the investigation of disease. Using more elegant micromethods that Kramer had devised for analyzing inorganic ions in serum, Howland and Kramer confirmed that calcium concentrations remain essentially normal or only slightly reduced in children with the disease; equally important, the concentration of serum phosphorus in uncomplicated rickets was always much lower than normal. Kramer's determinations showed that blood phosphate levels were low in the animals with rachitic lesions.

The group also demonstrated that vitamin A was not the controlling substance in rickets, thus identifying a second fat-soluble vitamin, an antirachitic substance that they named vitamin D.

Their experiments involved placing young rats on a rickets-producing diet and exposing some of them to five hours of Baltimore summer sunshine each day. These rats were completely protected against rickets. The rats who received the same deficient diet but were kept out of the sunlight, on the other hand, developed severe, acute rickets within three weeks.

The Hopkins group then developed a quantitative test for vitamin D, based upon the extent of deposition of calcium salts in the line of provisional calcification in the long bones of small rats rendered rachitic by a deficient diet. This procedure was adopted in 1922 as the pharmacopoeial method for standardizing vitamin D.[115]

William Henry Howell, Jay McLean, and the Discovery of Heparin

In 1915, William H. Howell assigned a second-year medical student, Jay McLean, the problem of isolating from heart and liver certain "phosphatides" that were believed to induce clotting. In the

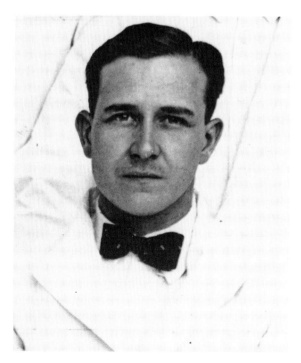

Jay McLean. (*Source:* Alan M. Chesney Medical Archives, The Johns Hopkins Medical Institutions.)

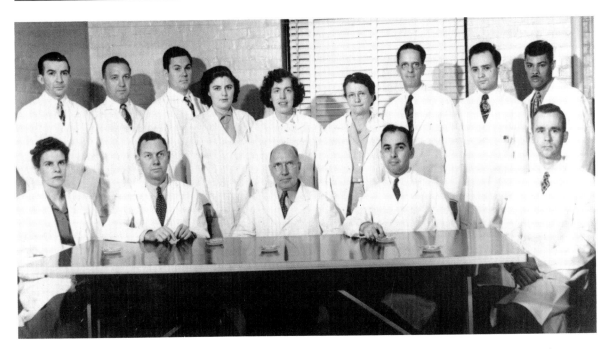

Members of the Polio Research Group. *Seated, left to right,* Isabel Morgan, Howard A. Howe, Kenneth Maxcy, David Bodian. (*Source:* Alan M. Chesney Medical Archives, The Johns Hopkins Medical Institutions.)

process of working on the problem, McLean obtained a product that was presumed to be a phosphatide—but that instead of inducing clotting, actually retarded it. From this point on, Howell continued the investigation of this "anticoagulant," which he named "heparin" because it was derived from the liver.[116]

McLean's article on the thromboplastic action of cephalin, published in the *American Journal of Physiology,* illustrates the then-primitive state of knowledge about coagulation of blood. In it, he concluded:

> The heparphosphatid on the other hand when purified by many precipitations in alcohol at 60° has no thromboplastic action and in fact shows a marked power to inhibit the coagulation. The anticoagulating action of this phosphatid is being studied and will be reported upon later. Cuorin and heparphosphatid when dry have no odor, but when moist with warm alcohol have a characteristic odor common to both. It is possible that on further purification the heparphosphatid may be shown to be identical with cuorin.[117]

McLean later attributed his discovery to his strength of will, saying, "The discovery of heparin came as a result of my determination to accomplish something by my own ability. It was this determination to become a physiologically based surgeon, rather than an anatomy-based surgeon, that led to the discovery of heparin."[118] His discovery also showed the influence of serendipity on scientific progress (see p. 281).

Howard A. Howe and David Bodian: Pioneers in Poliomyelitis Research

Research on the cause and prevention of poliomyelitis began at Johns Hopkins in 1936, when Howard A. Howe and his associates in the Department of Anatomy, Robert Ecke and Talmadge Peel, demonstrated in rhesus monkeys that the polio virus could spread along known nerve fiber pathways in the brain. In 1938, David Bodian joined Howe's group as a research fellow—a momentous event for the future of poliomyelitis research.

Within two years, Bodian and his co-workers had established themselves as one of the nation's outstanding poliomyelitis research teams. Their early studies of monkeys revealed the interaction of the polio virus with the nervous system, the way in which it spread through the nerve fibers, its route of entry into the nervous system, and factors that might affect the resistance of nerve cells to infection with the virus. In 1939, they demonstrated the preferential nerve fiber pathways of polio virus in the brain and the existence of susceptible and refractory centers of viral multiplication. Two years later, they found evidence for intraneuronal multiplication of polio virus and its spread within axons.[119] They also determined the rate at which the polio virus spread in peripheral nerve axons in a retrograde direction, and they were the first, independent of Sabin, to demonstrate that chimpanzees could be infected with polio virus by feeding, without the involvement of the olfactory bulbs. The results of their studies called into question the belief that the olfactory bulb was the major route of the virus's entry in human beings.

The team also discovered that the degree of pathologic involvement in nonparalytic cases of polio could be as severe as in paralytic cases. In nonparalytic cases, the destroyed neurons in the spinal cord were too widely separated to inactivate a single functional group; consequently, patients experienced no demonstrable loss of motor power.[120]

Meanwhile, Kenneth Maxcy, a faculty member at the Johns Hopkins School of Hygiene and Public Health, was considering the problem of poliomyelitis from another perspective. He believed that the logical approach to its solution lay in a broad program, whose staff would study the spread of the virus in a community along with its spread in the human body. Maxcy set out to establish a research center at the school of hygiene for the study of polio and other viruses. He intended to start with a nucleus of scientists in pathology, anatomy, virology, and epidemiology, and then to add investigators from biochemistry and biophysics.[121]

Maxcy knew that he would need funds not only to establish the center, but to give its staff at least five years of security. In 1941, he applied to the National Foundation for Infantile Paralysis for a long-term grant—an unusual request for the

time, as research grants were usually awarded yearly and for modest amounts.

After several months of negotiations, the foundation agreed to Maxcy's proposal. In return for a five-year grant of $300,000 a year, the Johns Hopkins University would establish a research center in the School of Hygiene and Public Health devoted solely to the study of poliomyelitis. For its part, the foundation would also give the director of the center and his associates full authority for determining the direction of the center's research.

Maxcy's plan was strengthened when Howe and Bodian agreed to join the research center. Howe moved from the medical school to the school of hygiene. Bodian, who had left Hopkins in 1942 to become assistant professor of anatomy at Western Reserve, returned later that year to join Maxcy's group. Substantial laboratory space was made available for the group in the new Hunterian Building (Hunterian II).

Also joining the group in 1942 was Isabel Morgan, daughter of the first American-born Nobel laureate, Thomas Hunt Morgan. Isabel Morgan came to Hopkins from the Rockefeller Institute, where she had begun immunologic studies of encephalitis viruses with Peter Olitsky. With her arrival, Maxcy's team began their comprehensive studies of the epidemiologic, immunologic, and pathologic aspects of poliomyelitis.

Morgan's first task was to discover whether she could induce resistance to an intracerebral inoculation of live polio virus. A next step was to look for a correlation between antibody and resistance.[122]

Morgan finally demonstrated the hoped-for resistance by giving monkeys several intramuscular injections of a strain of polio virus inactivated with formalin. As anticipated, she found a correlation between resistance to infection and level of antibody.

Bodian, Howe, and Morgan next made the important observation that there were only three major immunologic types of polio virus and that in contrast to influenza virus, they were genetically stable. Since development of an effective vaccine depended on the inclusion of all existing virus types, the National Foundation for Infantile

Paralysis established a large typing program in four laboratories.[123]

Howe extended Morgan's original observations by immunizing chimpanzees and monkeys against all three types of polio virus with both formalin-inactivated and live-virus vaccines. Most virologists still believed that a formalin-inactivated virus could not be used for immunization against poliomyelitis, but Howe soon provided evidence that, although animals that received formalin-inactivated vaccine developed an alimentary infection and shed virus in their stools, they nevertheless resisted paralysis upon intracerebral and oral challenge. Most important, he found satisfactory antibody responses to all three polio virus types and noted that adjuvants could stimulate antibody responses to small amounts of formalin-treated material.

About a year later, Howe inoculated a few mentally impaired children in a Maryland home with formalin-inactivated vaccine. All of them developed antibodies against all three polio types. By 1951, Morgan had convincingly demonstrated that rhesus monkeys could be immunized with formalin-inactivated viruses of all three basic immunologic types—so successfully that the animals were resistant to polio virus given by any route.

Bodian also discovered the polyvalent characteristics of polio virus antibody in human gamma globulin, demonstrating that it contained antibody in equal titer to all three types. William Hammon then set up a field trial of the effectiveness of pooled gamma globulin in preventing poliomyelitis.

The pathway of the virus to the central nervous system was, however, still undetermined. The hope was that the polio virus was transmitted through the bloodstream, as in this case a smaller antibody titer would be required to provide immunity than if the portal of entry was the peripheral nerves. Hammon's field trial showed that even a small amount of antibody protected against paralytic poliomyelitis.

Bodian, and Dorothy Horstmann at Yale, appreciated the importance of this observation, which indicated that polio virus travels from its portal of entry to the central nervous system by way of the bloodstream. Both began the search for evidence of viremia: they hoped to find the presence of virus in blood samples from monkeys and chimpanzees several days after they were fed the polio virus. Other investigators had taken blood specimens after paralysis had set in—too late in the course of the disease. By sampling blood between the time of feeding and the development of paralysis, however, Bodian and Horstmann were independently able to establish the presence of virus in the blood.[124]

After demonstrating viremia in animals, Bodian and Horstmann found that they could establish its presence early in the course of the disease in patients. The result was their demonstration of viremia in abortive cases of poliomyelitis. Further studies with chimpanzees pointed to a correlation between the occurrence of viremia and subsequent paralytic infection.

These key discoveries created a sound foun-

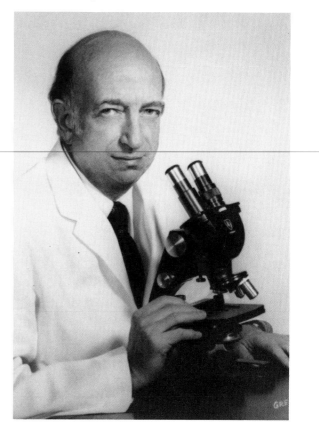

Arnall Patz. (*Source:* Leonard L. Greif, Jr.)

dation for development of polio vaccines, beginning with the Salk vaccine in 1954, and Hopkins' contributions to the conquest of polio continued through the 1950s. In 1956, the Hopkins group determined the sites of polio virus multiplication in tissue of chimpanzees after virus feeding. In 1960, they demonstrated that low levels of passive serum antibody are capable of limiting polio virus excretion from the throat, but much higher antibody levels are required before fecal shedding of virus is affected.[125]

The Pathogenesis of Retrolental Fibroplasia

For his controlled study of oxygen in the nursery that demonstrated the role of excessive oxygenation in the pathogenesis of retrolental fibroplasia of premature infants, Arnall Patz won the Albert Lasker Award in 1956. Patz, who became professor of ophthalmology and director of the department, was first associated with Johns Hopkins during his internship at Sinai Hospital in 1945. In 1955, he became a part-time member of the Wilmer Institute, and in 1970, a full-time member of the Hopkins faculty.

The retinopathy of prematurity (formerly called retrolental fibroplasia) was first identified in 1942. Within a decade, it had become the largest cause of blindness in children in the United States and a major cause of childhood blindness throughout the developed countries. Patz's experimental production of a close counterpart to the human disease in young mice and kittens supported his findings that implicated oxygen as the cause.

His work on retrolental fibroplasia led him to concentrate on a disease with similar features, diabetic retinopathy. The new blood vessels that had formed in the eyes of the experimental animals in his previous study were similar in many ways to the abnormal new vessels that occur in this disease. Working with scientists from the Applied Physics Laboratory at Hopkins, Patz developed the first argon lasers to be used in ophthalmology. He also was one of those who developed laser treatment for retinal disorders, and he conducted the first controlled clinical study to demonstrate the benefits of laser treatment for diabetic macular edema, the fluid leakage into the central macula that is the main cause of visual impairment in diabetic patients.[126]

Sulfonamide in the Prevention of Chronic Rheumatic Heart Disease

In 1957, Caroline Bedell Thomas received the James D. Bruce Memorial Award in Preventive Medicine of the American College of Physicians—an award commemorating her use of sulfanilamide for prophylaxis of hemolytic streptococcal infections to prevent recurrence of acute rheumatic fever. After receiving her medical degree from Johns Hopkins in 1929, Thomas completed residency training in medicine and spent two years as a National Research Council Fellow in physiology. She then returned to the Department of Medicine at Hopkins, at a time when no woman had a full-time appointment on the faculty. She was not to be an exception to this unwritten rule, but Edward P. Carter, who was in charge of the Cardiovascular Division in the Department of Medicine, suggested that Thomas organize a cardiac clinic for adult patients, and department director Warfield T. Longcope approved.

With her associate Richard France, Thomas began to treat patients in September 1935, on the second floor of the Carnegie outpatient building. The large number of young adults who came to the clinic with recurrent rheumatic fever led Thomas and France to ponder what they could do to interrupt the rheumatic cycle. The next year, Perrin H. Long returned from London having seen the miraculous effects of sulfanilamide on streptococcal infections. Long reported on his discovery one day at the lunch table in the Doctor's Dining Room, and added the startling statement that when small doses of this drug were injected into the peritoneum of a mouse before it was inoculated with a beta hemolytic *Streptococcus,* no infection ensued. While all of his listeners were excited over the prospect of treating and curing fatal streptococcal infections such as meningitis, Thomas's thoughts were on her young rheumatic patients.

She conceived the idea of preventing the beta hemolytic streptococcal infections that preceded the onset of the rheumatic state by giving patients one gram of sulfanilamide every day. The prophylactic use of this agent in patients susceptible to rheumatic fever was indeed highly successful. Not only did it prevent acute beta hemolytic streptococcal infections, but not a single major attack of acute rheumatic fever occurred in the treated groups. In contrast, in the untreated groups, a number of major episodes of acute rheumatic fever were observed.[127]

The Advent of Successful Chemotherapy: Sulfanilamide

When Calvin Coolidge, Jr., son of the thirtieth president of the United States, died of blood poisoning in 1924, all the medical expertise of the country was brought to bear on the problem, but nothing could stem the relentless progress of the disease. Some twelve years later, Franklin D. Roosevelt, Jr., developed septicemia—but this time the result was very different. Perrin H. Long, of the Department of Preventive Medicine, had been engaged in clinical studies with the drug sulfanilamide and was receiving calls from all over the world, asking him for advice about its use. He was also receiving a full quota of good-natured ribbing from his colleagues, who would call, announce themselves as some famous individual, and give Dr. Long a dramatic but fictitious story about their problem. A. McGehee Harvey remembers one such occasion: "I was sitting with Long late one evening on Osler 7, the communicable disease floor, when his phone rang; I answered it and a woman's voice asked for Dr. Long. I heard him say, 'You can't fool me this time. I know you're not Eleanor Roosevelt,' and he hung up the phone. Within seconds it rang again. This time, he said meekly, 'Yes, Mrs. Roosevelt, this is Dr. Long.' " The next day, the newspaper headlines announced that the president's son was ill; later headlines signaled the news that he had been cured by sulfanilamide, a drug supplied by Perrin H. Long and Eleanor A. Bliss of Johns Hopkins.

Early work on sulfonamide compounds had been performed in Germany by Gerhard Domagk, who in 1935 had successfully treated streptococcal infections in mice with prontosil. The next six years witnessed a substantial advance in the treatment of infectious diseases.

In the United States, Long and Bliss had been developing specific antisera for the treatment of streptococcal infections. Their work was at an advanced stage when, early in 1936, they read reports about prontosil in the German literature. Their interest in the sulfonamide compounds grew when that summer, they met the British investigator Leonard Colebrook, who was studying the effects of these drugs in human infections, at a medical meeting in London. They also had the opportunity to talk with Colebrook's associate, who had developed septicemia by accidentally infecting himself with streptococci and was treated successfully with prontosil. This story convinced Long and Bliss of the value of the drug, and they immediately made arrangements to bring some of it back to Baltimore. Supplies were limited, but fortunately the Jackson Laboratory of the DuPont Company was able to provide them with the drug. They confirmed that para-aminobenzene sulfonamide (sulfanilamide) is the effective portion of the prontosil molecule and proposed that it acts by a bacteriostatic rather than a bactericidal effect.

Their immediate results in treating experimental hemolytic streptococcal infections with sulfanilamide seemed miraculous. Eight of the first ten mice treated survived, while all of the untreated controls died within twenty-four hours. When they found that large doses of sulfanilamide were not too toxic for mice, the decision was made to try the drug on patients. An opportunity soon arrived when a seven-year-old child, severely ill with erysipelas, was admitted to the Johns Hopkins Hospital. Antitoxin had been given repeatedly without any improvement, but within twelve hours after the administration of sulfanilamide, the child's temperature was normal. The next patient treated was a woman dangerously ill with "childbed fever." Within twenty-four hours after sulfanilamide administration had begun, her temperature was normal. Any skepticism about the drug was soon erased as, in patient after patient, streptococcal tonsillitis and pharyngitis, erysipelas, acute otitis media, and streptococcal bacteremia were promptly cured by its administration. By November 1936, Long and Bliss had accumulated enough experimental and clinical observations to warrant a report at the meeting of the Southern Medical Association held in Baltimore—a report that heralded the development of a series of new sulfonamide derivatives.[128]

Long and Bliss's clinical investigations of the later additions to the sulfonamide family were similar to their early studies. Pharmacologic studies were added when W. Harry Feinstone joined their group late in 1937, but most of the pharmacologic work on the sulfonamides was done at Johns Hopkins by E. Kennerly Marshall, Jr., (see p. 258).[129]

The Clinical Application of Biochemical Research in Pediatrics

The foundation of biochemical investigation in pediatrics was laid by L. Emmett Holt, who under the aegis of the Rockefeller Institute established well-equipped laboratories at the Babies Hospital in New York in 1910 and 1911. One of Holt's associates in these laboratories, John Howland, came to Baltimore in 1912 as the full-time head of the Department of Pediatrics at Johns Hopkins. The next fifteen years saw the flowering of pediatric biochemistry. Much of the basic work in pediatric research during this time was done by Howland and the remarkable group of young men associated with him in the Harriet Lane Home.

When Howland came to Baltimore, Hopkins had no functioning pediatrics department. Clemens von Pirquet, the nominal head of the department, had returned to Germany, and pediatrics had neither a hospital nor a staff. In selecting his initial staff, Howland demonstrated almost unerring judgment, a quality whose importance cannot be overvalued in a department head. Most of the faculty he appointed later became directors of medical school departments of pediatrics.

Edwards A. Park described the stimulating environment that Howland created in the Harriet Lane Home:

It must be remembered that this pediatric oasis was set in the larger oasis of Johns Hopkins, then still in its early glory, filled with interesting and distinguished men, engaged in important work and having wide outlooks. . . . Dr. Holt established pediatrics in this country as a special branch of medicine, defining it, putting it in order and assigning it the welfare of the child in health as well as in disease. John Howland, on the other hand, modernized pediatrics. He changed the course of pediatrics by substituting for bedside observation and conjecture, the study of disease through laboratory methods and experiments. He caused pediatrics to become a rapidly expanding subject. He did this by example—by the development of a model clinic; model from the point of view of administration, medical care, teaching, research and spirit. . . . He created and sent out missionaries, his pupils, filled with ideas and his spirit. A new era in medicine founded on the application of scientific methods to the study of clinical problems was coming anyway . . . but Howland started the move in pediatrics and the Harriet Lane Home under his guidance was the first full-time university clinic to win complete success.[130]

The Acidosis of Infantile Diarrhea

Howland perceived clearly the importance of chemistry for the investigation of disease in children, and his first success was the demonstration that acidosis existed in children with diarrhea.[131] Howland selected the problem; his collaborator W. McKim Marriott's expertise in developing new methods made the problem solvable. Their study offered a new explanation for the symptoms of what was called "alimentary intoxication"—marked dyspnea without signs of respiratory obstruction, accompanied by restlessness, stupor, and coma.

Howland and Marriott showed that these manifestations were the result of loss of base, which resulted in acidosis. The evidence was clear and convincing: they demonstrated a marked increase of urinary ammonia, a severe reduction of carbon dioxide tension in the alveolar air, an increase in the hydrogen ion concentration of the blood, and an increase by a factor of three to five in the amount of sodium bicarbonate required to alkalinize the urine. They were able to correct the acidosis in part or wholly by administration of sodium bicarbonate.

The Rebirth of Parenteral Therapy

When W. McKim Marriott and K. Utheim discovered that blood volume was the critical dimension in the treatment of infant diarrhea, they were reviving a topic that had been abandoned for a century. The long-forgotten report of William B. O'Shaughnessy in 1832 established the loss of water, neutral salts, and free alkali in the blood of cholera patients, accounting for these losses in the diarrheal stool. Thomas Latta, a physician who lived near Edinburgh, applied these findings by injecting intravenously a solution containing sodium chloride and sodium bicarbonate in a woman severely ill with cholera. Despite her dramatic improvement, investigation of replacement therapy languished for the next 100 years.

The spur to further research at Hopkins came from Kenneth Blackfan, Howland's resident from 1912 to 1923, whose observations demonstrate the importance of physicians at the bedside to advances in medical science. Blackfan was convinced that infants dehydrated by diarrheal disease needed more salt solution than could be provided by subcutaneous infusions. He showed that adequate replacement of fluid was followed by a dramatic reduction in mortality.[132]

James L. Gamble and "Gamblegrams"

When James L. Gamble joined Howland's department in 1914, he had decided to abandon a career in clinical medicine and dedicate his life "to the study of disease by means of chemistry." A graduate of the Harvard Medical School, Gamble had worked in several laboratories in the United States

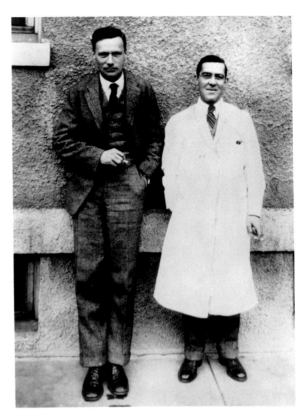

Left, James L. Gamble, and *right,* Kenneth D. Blackfan. (*Source:* Alan M. Chesney Medical Archives, The Johns Hopkins Medical Institutions.)

and in Europe. His close contact with Lawrence J. Henderson, from whom he received further training in biologic chemistry, stimulated his interest in problems of electrolyte physiology—an interest that Gamble carried with him to Baltimore.[133]

At Howland's suggestion, Gamble began work with two Canadians, Graham Ross and F. F. Tisdall, investigating the treatment of epilepsy by the ketosis of starvation. Since there was no food intake or feces, the balance studies could be carried out using only measurements on the daily urine collections and blood plasma. The execution of the experiment was laborious and extended over nearly two years. The analytical determinations were also tedious, but in Robert F. Loeb's words, "rarely have data been subjected to more original deductive reasoning."[134] The results are best summarized in Gamble's own words:

One, the data display in operation the two adjustable components of the acid-base construction of urine (titrable acidity and ammonia production) which Henderson and Palmer described and which permit the removal of anion excess within the prescribed limits for urine acidity without expenditure of fixed base beyond the quantity which properly presents for removal.

Two, they show the determining role of fixed base in sustaining the osmolar value of the body fluids because of the adjustability of the total anion value by change in bicarbonate ion so as to produce total cation-anion equality.

They show further, the relation of the volume of the body fluids to fixed base content on the premise of preservation of the normal osmolar value with corollary that, so long as the kidney is operating accurately, loss (or gain) of water and electrolytes will be parallel. On this basis the data was used to allocate losses of water from the body fluid compartments from measurements of outgo of intracellular and of extracellular base.[135]

Gamble's elucidation of these data in simple graphic form came to be widely known as "Gamblegrams." Perhaps even more significant than the contribution of these experiments to the knowledge of electrolyte physiology was their influence on clinical research. Most clinical investigation at the time consisted of a recording of endless observations made with some new method. Gamble, in contrast, applied chemical means in one crucial experiment. In Loeb's words, "These experiments constituted a pioneer approach to the interpretation of quantitative description in terms of the mechanisms involved. Meaning received the primary emphasis."[136]

Serendipity and the Process of Discovery

"As their highnesses traveled," wrote Horace Walpole to his friend Horace Mann in 1754, "they were always making discoveries, by *accident* or *sagacity,* of things which they were not in quest of." Walpole was recounting a fairy tale entitled

"The Three Princes of Serendip" (the ancient name for Sri Lanka), and in his letter he coined the word "serendipity" to denote this type of discovery.

Serendipity can play an important part in research. While some results emerge from the meticulous, methodical trudge from point *A* to point *B*, a few have an element of whimsy—as Walter Cannon wrote, "the happy faculty, or luck, of finding unforeseen evidence of one's ideas or, with surprise, coming upon new objects or relations which were not being sought."[137]

As important as the serendipitous event is the investigator's ability to recognize it. In research, this ability can translate into clinical acumen—as in the case of John Eager Howard, one of whose discoveries was based on his recognition of the similarity between two patients examined fifteen years apart. In other cases, "serendipity" can mean being in the right place at the right time: had goitrous dogs not been roaming about the train station in Cleveland as David Marine arrived for his internship, he might have gone on to an entirely different career.

The stories that follow illustrate examples of serendipity in research discoveries made at Johns Hopkins. All are characterized by the investigator's powers of observation: the ability to capture the fortunate moment, recognize the value of the information, and pursue it productively.

John Eager Howard: The Recognition of Unilateral Renal Hypertension

A leading figure in medicine at Johns Hopkins for more than fifty years was John Eager Howard III. He was a keen clinical observer, and it was his clinical acumen, coupled with a fortunate coincidence, that led to his most notable discovery.

A member of one of the most prominent families in Maryland history and a great-great-grandson of the first John Eager Howard, the Revolutionary War hero, JEH (as he was known) graduated from the Johns Hopkins medical school in 1928. After two years of training at the Massachusetts General Hospital, he returned to

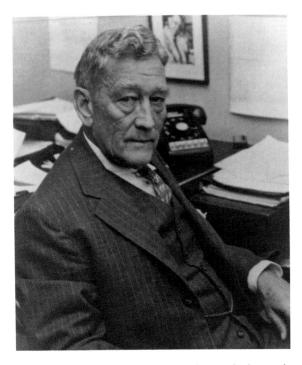

John Eager Howard. (*Source: Johns Hopkins Medical Journal* 131[1972]:79.)

Johns Hopkins and was continuously associated with this institution until his death in 1985.

One of his early forays into clinical investigation was conducted in collaboration with Reed Ellsworth, a member of the Department of Medicine and a man of remarkable talent, who died of tuberculosis early in a promising career. Together they devised the Ellsworth-Howard test, an early method for testing responsiveness to parathyroid hormone. This work focused Howard's attention on calcium metabolism and renal stone formation, the subject of his later important contributions.

In the 1930s, Howard turned to the study of pheochromocytoma; with Halsey Barker, he reviewed the literature in search of clinical features that would be identifiable at the bedside. Because of this interest, Howard was asked to see a patient with sudden right-sided abdominal pain. The tentative diagnosis was appendicitis, but surgical exploration of the abdomen revealed a normal appendix. Soon after operation, the patient suddenly developed severe hypertension, leading to a

tentative diagnosis of pheochromocytoma. Indeed, perirenal air injection suggested a mass above the right kidney. When the abdomen was explored a second time, however, the surgeon, Hugh Young, removed not a pheochromocytoma but a renal mass he believed was malignant. The report of the pathologist, Morgan Berthrong, revealed the mass to be an infarct (damaged tissue from impeded blood supply to the area). The patient's hypertension soon disappeared.

Some fifteen years later, another patient was admitted to the hospital with sudden right lower abdominal pain. Abdominal exploration revealed nothing abnormal, but two weeks later the patient returned with florid hypertension. He was thought to have acute nephritis, and over the next two weeks, his condition worsened. When Howard examined this patient, he immediately recalled the earlier patient with a renal mass. Howard recommended a nephrectomy even though the intravenous pyelogram was normal. As he had suspected, the kidney that was removed contained a grayish yellow area exactly like that in the first patient. As in the first patient, this patient's hypertension disappeared within a week.

Morgan Berthrong was again the pathologist, and he again found a localized infarction. In contrast to the many kidneys seen each year with similar-appearing lesions but in patients without high blood pressure, Berthrong identified in these two kidneys a perimeter of incomplete infarction surrounding the completely dead renal tissue. Thus was born Howard's interest in high blood pressure associated with areas in the kidney partially deprived of blood.

Howard's next goal was to find a way to detect the deprived tissue clinically. Edmund Yendt, a fellow in Howard's group, called attention to published experiments in which one renal artery was gradually narrowed and urine from the left and right kidneys was collected simultaneously but independently. A striking reduction was found in the volume of urine coming from the side with restricted arterial flow, along with a decreased sodium concentration. Howard and Yendt proceeded to demonstrate the same findings in patients with unilateral renal ischemia. Although the procedure, which became known as the Howard test, required expert urologic technique and meticulous care in the collection of urine, it proved useful in identifying those cases in which stenosis of major renal arteries was responsible for hypertension.[138]

The Thyroid and Its Diseases: The Discoveries of David Marine, Alan M. Chesney, and the Team of Julia and Cosmo Mackenzie

As a medical student at Hopkins, David Marine was inspired by Halsted to seek a career in research; his field of study, however, was chosen by happenstance. After graduation in 1905, Marine went to Cleveland for an internship in pathology. On his way from the train station, he noticed that many of the dogs roaming the streets had large thyroid glands. His interest in the thyroid had been awakened by Halsted's experimental studies of the gland. Arriving at the hospital, he was asked by his new chief what area of investigation he was interested in. Marine recalled the dogs he had just seen and replied, "the thyroid."

Marine thought that the canine goiters might be due to a lack of iodine in the dogs' food and water supply. Testing his hypothesis in the laboratory, he produced goiters in dogs by depriving them of dietary iodine. Marine believed that endemic goiter could be produced solely by a lack of iodine. Goiter prophylaxis by the addition of iodine to the diet had been tried as early as 1860, but the method had fallen into disuse. In 1916, Marine and Allyn Kimball revived this method to prevent goiter in school children in Akron, Ohio. Marine urged that iodine be added to drinking water and table salt, but his proposals drew as much opposition as did later proposals to add fluoride to the water supply. It took another ten years to convince the public that Marine's simple measure would prevent endemic goiter.

By 1924, Marine had worked out the theory now known as the "Marine cycle." It stated that at a time of increased demand, thyrotropic hormone from the pituitary stimulates the cells lining the follicles. As a result, the individual cells increase in size (hypertrophy). Further action of thyrotropic hormone causes the individual cells to multiply by cell division, so that the size and volume of the individual follicles are increased (hyperplasia). If an excess of iodine is made available, the enlarged follicles fill up with colloid. This excessive secretion ceases after a time, but the follicles remain permanently enlarged in their resting state (involution). A continuation of this state leads to degeneration of the gland substance and production of a simple colloid goiter.[139]

Three years after Marine first advanced his important theory of goiter production, a chance observation by Alan M. Chesney led to the proof of another mechanism for the production of goiter—the presence of an active "goitrogen." The colony of rabbits in Chesney's experimental studies of syphilis was developing large goiters, and Chesney was quick to recognize the potential importance of this unexpected finding.

Bruce Webster was assigned to search for the cause of the thyroid enlargement. A Jacques Loeb fellow in medicine, Webster had arrived in Baltimore only a few months before to work in the division of metabolism with George A. Harrop. After a trip to New York to confer with Marine, then director of the laboratories at Montefiore Hospital, Webster began an intensive study of Chesney's rabbit colony.

The result was a series of articles on endemic goiter in rabbits. The first article, published in 1928 in the *Bulletin of The Johns Hopkins Hospital*, established that although most of the rabbits in the colony developed goiter, the event had no relationship to the syphilitic infection.[140] Grossly and microscopically, the thyroid appeared to be a hyperplastic gland. The second paper, published simultaneously, demonstrated that heat production in the goitrous animals was 16.6 percent lower than in the normal ones, and that the rabbits with the largest goiters showed the greatest depression in metabolic rate.[141] The third of the series reported that when iodine was administered to these goitrous rabbits, the metabolic rate increased, they rapidly became emaciated, and in most cases, they died.[142]

The severity of the reaction was directly related to the extent of the preexisting hyperplasia. Webster found that iodine tended to bring about involution of the hyperplastic thyroid gland, with a lowering of the alveolar epithelium. He observed areas of involution resembling colloid adenomata and both diffuse and localized areas of persistent hyperplasia.

Webster and Chesney's subsequent articles on the subject showed that the rabbits' diet, which consisted almost exclusively of cabbage, appeared to be the major etiologic factor, and that iodine administered orally protected the animal completely against the goiter-producing factor.[143] This important discovery was substantiated by Marine. Since then, small outbreaks of goiter have been reported in human populations, in communities compelled by circumstances to exist mainly on cabbage.

Webster and Marine refined their observations by investigating seasonal variations in endemic goiter in rabbits. They found that cabbage maturing in the spring and summer months has little goiter-producing potential, while cabbage maturing in late autumn has much greater goiter-producing power. Other plants of the genus *Brassica* were also found to be goitrogens. Since these plants contain mustard oils, Marine and his co-workers were prompted to investigate thyroidal actions of the isothiocyanates and their cyanide precursors. In 1932, they demonstrated that acetonitrile and related compounds can produce thyroid hyperplasia and that the effect can be antagonized by iodine.

The discoveries of Cosmo G. Mackenzie and his wife Julia concerning the goitrogenic activity of several well-defined compounds emerged serendipitously, not from direct study of the thyroid gland but from an effort to explain the perplexing contradictions in the symptoms produced by vitamin E deficiency in the rabbit and in the rat. Within only a few months, the Mackenzies uncovered the goitrogenic activity of the sulfonamides, para-aminobenzoic acid, and the thioureas.

The Mackenzies were based in the School of Hygiene and Public Health at Hopkins, but their work related to the research of faculty members in

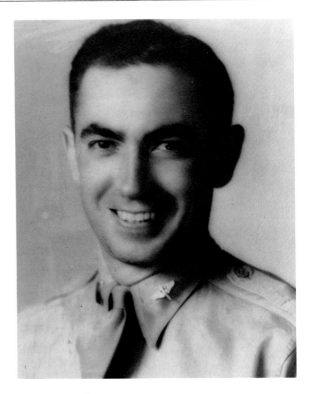

Cosmo G. Mackenzie

the School of Medicine as well. Their investigations of vitamin E deficiency built on Goetsch and Pappenheimer's description in 1931 of a dietary deficiency disease in rabbits and guinea pigs characterized by dystrophy of striated muscles. Goetsch and Pappenheimer had destroyed the vitamin E in the diet of these animals by treating their food with an ethereal solution of ferric chloride. Yet potent samples of wheat-germ oil, which had been shown to cure vitamin E deficiency in female rats, failed to cure the acute degeneration of the voluntary muscles in these animals.

Elmer V. McCollum, professor of biochemistry in the school of hygiene, suggested that the Mackenzies pursue this exciting development by investigating the nutritional factors responsible for this lethal disease. The Mackenzies thought that the response to vitamin E deficiency might reflect a difference between species, a variation due to the synthesis of small amounts of vitamin E by the intestinal flora of the rat. They tested this hypothesis by administering a sulfaguanidine-containing mash to their animals. This sul-

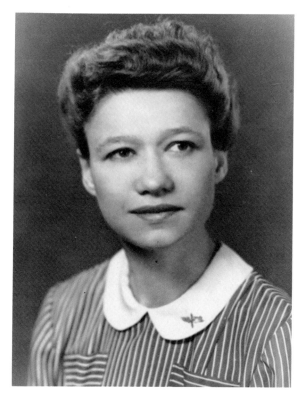

Julia B. Mackenzie

fonamide derivative, which had been synthesized in 1940 by Eli Kennerly Marshall, Jr., professor of pharmacology in the medical school, was poorly absorbed in the intestinal tract and had been shown to reduce the concentration of coliform bacteria in the feces of mice. The Mackenzies tested the effect of the mash on weanling rats fed a purified diet containing all of the then-known vitamins except vitamin E. The control animals grew normally and were healthy in appearance, but the animals fed sulfaguanidine grew at a slower rate for the first few weeks, then stopped growing and began to bleed from the eyes. Autopsies of both control and experimental animals showed that the organs and tissues were grossly normal with one exception: in the animals fed sulfaguanidine, both lobes of the thyroid were greatly enlarged and hyperemic.

The experiments were repeated on weanling rats, but now 10 percent yeast was added to the sulfaguanidine-containing diet. The results were startling. Although the yeast-supplemented ani-

mals grew at a normal rate and did not bleed from the eyes, their thyroid glands were just as large and hyperemic as the glands of those that had received sulfaguanidine alone. The Mackenzies concluded that sulfaguanidine produced a nutritional deficiency of unknown nature and, most important, an independent enlargement of the thyroid gland. Histological examination of the gland revealed changes resembling Graves disease. The flat epithelial cells that normally line the follicles had been transformed into columnar cells of such height as to practically obliterate the lumen, which was essentially devoid of colloid. The results were a spectacular display of completely hyperplastic thyroid glands.

The Mackenzies had now come to a fork in the road. They could pursue the nutritional aspects of the problem, attempting to isolate and identify the factor in yeast that prevented the nutritional deficiency caused by sulfaguanidine, or they could investigate the mechanism of sulfaguanidine's action on the thyroid. Their decision to pursue the latter path was based on several factors. In her years as a nurse, Julia Mackenzie had seen the devastating effects of toxic goiter and of myxedema. Her husband recalled the winter of 1912, when his mother's sister, who was suffering from Graves disease, had come to stay with them; he had been scolded for calling attention to her loss of weight, and his family had "whispered" about her erratic behavior. Her cure by subtotal thyroidectomy left an indelible impression on him. As students at Hopkins, both of the Mackenzies had taken Arnold Rich's special course in pathology for students in the school of hygiene— a memorable series of lectures that stimulated their interest in the causes and mechanisms of human disease.

An additional aspect of their decision was even simpler and perhaps more scientific. They appreciated that their observation of goitrogenic activity in a stable compound of known chemical structure represented a substantial step toward solving the problem that had frustrated Marine and Chesney: the isolation of the active goitrogenic factor.

Further experiments with sulfaguanidine revealed that additional sodium iodide (administered either subcutaneously or in the rats' diet) furnished no protection against the sulfaguanidine-induced goiter. Thus the Mackenzies' compound, sulfaguanidine, was unique among goitrogens in producing an enlargement of the thyroid that could not be prevented by iodine. Indeed, iodine actually increased the size of the thyroid in the sulfaguanidine-treated rats.

They next added para-aminobenzoic acid to the experimental diet, as a study of D. D. Woods in 1940 had shown that this compound inhibited the bacteriostatic action of sulfonamides. It not only failed to prevent the action of sulfaguanidine on the thyroid but also, when fed alone, it exhibited goitrogenic activity in its own right, although to a lesser extent than sulfaguanidine. The Mackenzies now had two goitrogenic organic compounds of known chemical structure.

The Mackenzies then turned to the study of goitrogenic properties of other sulfa drugs. Thousands of experiments with these compounds had not yielded any mention of an effect on the thyroid, and the Mackenzies therefore assumed that their compound was unique among the sulfa drugs and that its goitrogenic activity was related to the guanidine moiety of the molecules. They found that guanidine and sulfanilic acid, administered both separately and together, did not produce any effect on the thyroid. Large doses of urea also provided negative results.

Could the spatial relations between the sulfur and guanidine molecules make sulfur derivatives, and analogs of guanidine and urea, worth investigating? The first compound they tested was thiourea. Its effect on the thyroid was dramatic, exceeding that of sulfaguanidine. They then proceeded to test sulfanilamide, sulfathiazole, sulfapyridine, and sulfamethyldiazine on rats, and without exception each of them produced thyroid enlargement. Similar responses were obtained in mice and dogs. At the same time, the Mackenzies tried a variety of thiourea derivatives, and all except acetylthiourea elicited the typical thyroid response.

Arnold Rich examined these glands histologically, concluding that the rats were hyper-

thyroid. He recalled having seen similar sections of thyroid glands from rats fed phenylthiourea by Curt Richter and Katherine Clisby, members of the Department of Psychiatry at Johns Hopkins. This compound is tasteless to some humans but bitter-tasting to others, a difference that is genetically determined. Richter and Clisby were studying this compound in rats to see if they exhibited similar taste discrimination. They found that the compound produced severe edema and, in those animals that survived, an enlargement of the thyroid. Thus, as Rich recognized, these workers had independently observed the effect of the thioureas on the thyroid. Rich pointed out that these rat glands, like those of the Mackenzies, showed an increase in the height of the epithelium and a depletion of colloid. Rich and Richter thought this was a compensatory response to the drug's propensity to lower the body temperature.

The Mackenzies, however, tried unsuccessfully during the next few weeks to demonstrate a fall in body temperature in young rats fed thiourea and sulfaguanidine. They believed the question could be settled only by measuring the basal metabolic rate. World War II had begun, however, there was already a shortage of metal, and the machine shop was so busy that no suitable measuring instrument could be constructed. Enthusiastic about the study, E. V. McCollum called the Carnegie Institution and asked if the Mackenzies might borrow the metabolic chamber originally used on rats by Francis G. Benedict in his classic studies on basal metabolism. The Carnegie officials graciously agreed to remove the apparatus from their museum. It was, therefore, with Benedict's copper chamber, with its water-sealed bellows, that the Mackenzies conclusively demonstrated that young rats fed sulfaguanidine or thiourea exhibited, after two weeks of goitrogen administration, a decline in oxygen consumption of 20 percent. Of a variety of compounds tested, only desiccated thyroid and thyroxine restored the basal metabolic rate to normal and completely abolished the hyperplastic appearance of the gland.

The next question was the mode of action. The Mackenzies showed that in thyroidectomized rats, the drug did not inhibit the action of thyroxin on the target tissues. Furthermore, minute doses of the hormone restored the basal metabolic rate to normal. They concluded that these drugs must block the synthesis of the thyroid hormone. Next, they demonstrated that in hypophysectomized animals the antithyroid drugs exerted no hyperplastic effect on the thyroid. Finally, in normal animals, the drugs produced histologic changes in the pituitary that were typical of thyroidectomy. Their conclusions were that the sulfanilamides and thiourea inhibited the synthesis of thyroxine and that this in turn lowered the basal metabolic rate. The normal feedback mechanism stimulated release of thyrotropic hormone, which in turn produced the spectacular hyperplasia without resulting in the synthesis of thyroxine.[144]

William S. Tillett's Discovery of Streptokinase

An unexpected laboratory result also provided the basis for William S. Tillett's discovery of streptokinase and the application of the agent to clinical medicine.

A graduate of the Johns Hopkins University School of Medicine in 1917, Tillett took an internship and assistant residency in medicine at Hopkins as well. From 1922 to 1930, he was a member of the resident staff at the Hospital of the Rockefeller Institute, where he was assigned to work with Thomas Rivers, another Hopkins graduate, on viral diseases. Tillett was subsequently transferred to Rufus Cole's pneumonia service; he then joined Oswald T. Avery's research group, where he remained until 1930.

Tillett returned to Baltimore as associate professor of medicine and director of the department's Biological Division. During investigations with hemolytic streptococci, he noted that normal human plasma was capable of "agglutinating" these organisms, while serum was not. He suspected that fibrinogen, was, in some way, responsible for this agglutination. If his assumption was correct, he reasoned that the addition of a fresh broth culture of hemolytic streptococci to a specimen of oxalated human plasma would, after a

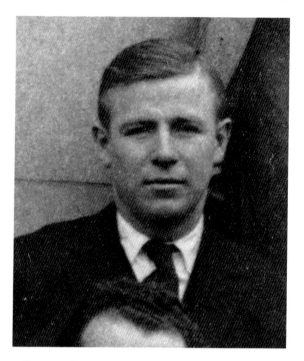

William S. Tillett. (*Source:* Alan M. Chesney Medical Archives, The Johns Hopkins Medical Institutions.)

short period of incubation, tie up all the fibrinogen; subsequent recalcification of the plasma should no longer lead to clotting. When he did the experiment, he was disappointed to find that clotting occurred just as rapidly as in the control. Later, to his surprise, he found that the previously clotted test sample was now liquid. He repeated the experiment several times and soon established that hemolytic streptococci elaborated a fibrinolytic principle that became known as streptokinase. Tillett quickly envisioned the value of this principle in dissolving the thick fibrinous exudates that frequently complicate empyemas and meningitis.

The exploitation of this finding, however, came not at Hopkins, but at the New York University School of Medicine, where he moved in 1937 to become head of the Department of Bacteriology and later, head of the Department of Medicine. His observations on streptokinase proved to be the key for unraveling the hitherto little-recognized human fibrinolytic enzyme system, and several of his associates then laid the foundation for the biochemical characterization of this important system.

Tillett personally pursued the clinical applications of streptokinase, which led to the discovery of streptodornase, the concept of enzymatic debridement, and the first practical application of injected enzymes for therapeutic purposes. Tillett's ultimate goal, however, was the dissolution of intravascular thrombi with streptokinase, and he and his associates provided the experimental evidence and basic framework for development of the field of therapeutic thrombolysis.[145]

Subsequent Clinical Applications of Streptokinase

The clinical application of streptokinase was assisted by Henry Wagner's development of diagnostic techniques for the detection of pulmonary embolism. Wagner was the first director of the Division of Nuclear Medicine, a joint effort between

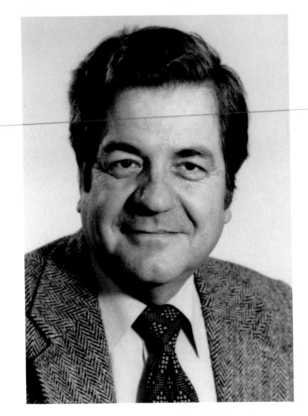

Henry N. Wagner, Jr. (*Source:* Tadder/Baltimore.)

the Departments of Radiology and Medicine. Cardiopulmonary bypass was coming into use in the early 1960s, and David Sabiston of the Department of Surgery was among the first to apply it in the treatment of patients with massive pulmonary embolism. Pulmonary embolectomy, using cardiopulmonary bypass, was an advance over previous surgical procedures but required a readily available test in order to select patients for operation. In 1963, Wagner's group became the first to use radioactive tracers for the rapid diagnosis of pulmonary embolism.

George Taplin had developed radioactively labeled albumin aggregates to study the reticuloendothelial system.[146] With an average diameter of ten millimicrons, these particles were larger than the pulmonary capillaries. Wagner and his group found that by injecting these large albumin particles intravenously, one could view the distribution of pulmonary arterial blood flow. In experiments in dogs, Sabiston and Wagner inserted a balloon filled with contrast medium through the superior vena cava and right ventricle until it lodged in a branch of the pulmonary artery. Nuclear imaging delineated the effect of the experimental clot on regional pulmonary arterial flow.

These experiments were followed by use of the technique in human beings by sending radiolabeled microemboli to detect thromboemboli.[147] By the mid-1960s, both lung scanning and pulmonary arteriography became widely used.

Just as pulmonary embolectomy in critically ill patients led to the development of lung scanning, a series of experiments with urokinase stimulated the concurrent use of arteriography and lung scanning to monitor the effect of thrombolytic therapy. The question was whether urokinase was valuable in the treatment of patients with pulmonary embolism. The same question was subsequently asked of Tillett's streptokinase. Like streptokinase, urokinase is an enzyme that activates plasmin, but urokinase is produced by kidney cells, not bacteria. The trial of urokinase in pulmonary embolism during the early 1970s was one of the first large-scale collaborative clinical efforts in this country. William R. Bell of Johns Hopkins was a major clinical participant and chaired the editorial committee that assembled the report.[148]

Similar studies of streptokinase and urokinase in acute myocardial infarction opened the way for the trial of intravenous tissue plasminogen activator (t-PA), produced in bacteria by methods of recombinant DNA, in the same disorder. Alan D. Guerci and others in Myron L. Weisfeldt's cardiology group at Hopkins demonstrated the usefulness of early intravenous administration of t-PA, permitting deferral of cardiac catheterization and coronary angioplasty.[149]

A Remedy for Motion Sickness: The Story of Leslie N. Gay

The history of Johns Hopkins is filled with stories of department directors who selected an able but inexperienced person to advance an unexplored field. Leslie Gay was one such individual. A graduate of the Johns Hopkins medical school in 1917, Gay returned to Baltimore in 1922 after residency training in Boston. His return coincided with a growing interest in allergy among physicians. As Gay recalled the conversation that would change his career, he was stopped in the hall by G. Canby Robinson, interim chairman of the Department of Medicine. Robinson said, "Gay, I want you to start an allergy clinic." Gay's prompt answer was, "I don't know anything about allergy." Robinson replied, "Nobody else does either."[150]

The Allergy Clinic opened in 1923, in a small room in the old dispensary building. At the time, it was only the third allergy clinic in the United States. At first, the only other worker was Nathan Herman, but Gay and Herman were soon joined by other young staff members. From their experience in the clinic came the first extensive clinical trial of ephedrine, a study of one hundred patients with asthma that Gay and Herman published in the Bulletin of The Johns Hopkins Hospital.[151] In 1929, they also began systematic surveys of pollen in the atmosphere in conjunction with the Department of Botany at the university. At the time, these surveys were pioneering investigations. The first studies of the effect of an air-conditioned environment on patients with hay fever

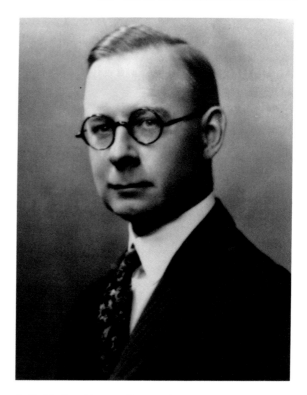

Leslie N. Gay. (*Source:* Alan M. Chesney Medical Archives, The Johns Hopkins Medical Institutions.)

and asthma were also carried out in the mid-1930s by Gay and his associates.[152]

In association with Edmund Keeney, a 1935 graduate of the Hopkins School of Medicine, Gay and Herman developed long-acting epinephrine for use in the patient suffering from chronic asthma.[153] Like long-acting protamine zinc insulin, long-acting epinephrine saved patients from having to take multiple doses of regular epinephrine.

The most exciting work in the Allergy Clinic after World War II was a study of drugs with antihistaminic action. In 1948 one of these drugs, compound 1694 (later known as Dramamine), was found by accident to have a remarkable effect in preventing motion sickness. A woman being treated for hives with this compound told Gay that every time she rode a trolley car, she had been incapacited by severe motion sickness. Since taking the new drug, however, she had experienced no further difficulty. Gay perceived the importance of this observation and pursued it experimentally: he gave the patient placebo capsules, made of sugar. She came back within two or three days, greatly disappointed that her motion sickness had returned.[154]

The search was next made for a means of testing this effect on a large scale. Gay met with General Omar Bradley, chief of staff of the United States Army, in October 1948. On the twenty-seventh of November, Gay and his associates began a twelve-day voyage from New York to Bremerhaven on a troop ship. On board were 1500 young, healthy soldiers, who were divided into subject and control groups. The voyage was beset by severe North Atlantic storms, and seasickness became a serious problem. The results of Gay's experiment were dramatic, in that Dramamine appeared to be successful not only in preventing seasickness but also in relieving seasickness after it had developed. A man taking the placebo, with resulting severe seasickness of several days' duration, would be given Dramamine by rectum. Within fifteen minutes he would be feeling well enough to ask for food and drink. On this ship's previous voyage, between 50 and 100 soldiers had been so incapacitated as to require intravenous fluids during the twelve-day passage, but on this voyage not a single man required such fluid replacement. The subsequent development of many other drugs capable of preventing motion sickness is a well-known story, but many do not realize that these discoveries began as an example of serendipity in research in the Allergy Clinic at the Johns Hopkins Hospital.[155]

Louis Hamman: The Influence of a Research Environment on Clinical Practice

The career of Louis Hamman illustrates not only the force of serendipity but also the influence of an exciting research environment on a physician's later clinical practice. Hamman's talent as a diagnostician lay in his uncanny ability to gather clinical facts, organize them effectively, arrive at the correct diagnosis, and thus establish the best basis for the management of the patient's problem. The seventy-five articles he published in the course of his career contained important new information, presented in a delightfully literate manner.

The best of his work emphasized prognosis—in Hamman's view, the highest accomplishment of medical practice. The foundation of prognosis, Hamman said, is correct diagnosis, and the function of diagnosis is to direct and guide treatment.[156]

Hamman performed all his investigative work on normal volunteer subjects or on patients. He never worked with experimental animals, although he followed the work of others and used their information effectively in his teaching and practice.[157] The opening of the Phipps Tuberculosis Clinic in 1905 provided Hamman with the opportunity to study the diagnosis and treatment of that disease. With Samuel Wolman, member of the Department of Medicine (and older brother of Abel Wolman, another noted member of the Hopkins faculty), he conducted a series of pioneering investigations of the clinical use of tuberculin and, in 1912, published the results in a comprehensive book, *Tuberculin in Diagnosis and Treatment.*

The following year, Hamman turned to the study of blood glucose. A 1913 report on the hyperglycemia following a normal person's ingestion of starchy foods suggested to Hamman the possibility of applying a similar approach to the study of carbohydrate tolerance in various diseases. He hoped that information about carbohydrate tolerance would be helpful in making the differential diagnosis, and the resulting estimation of a patient's ability to dispose promptly of a certain amount of glucose taken at one time into the stomach became known as the "glucose tolerance test."

Hamman and his co-worker, I. I. Hirschman, did not receive proper credit for their pioneering observations. Although Janney and Isaacson are credited with the present-day concept of the glucose tolerance test, and Staub and Traugott with the description of the blood sugar response to a second dose of orally administered glucose, it was Hamman who first delineated both principles. He presented his results at the May 1916 meeting of the Association of American Physicians, and his full report appeared in the *Archives of Internal Medicine* in November 1917. Janney and Isaacson's work was reported in February 1917 and published in April 1918, a year after Hamman's paper appeared. Staub and Traugott reported the so-called Staub-Traugott effect even later—several years after Hamman's description of the phenomenon.[158]

The story of Hamman's recognition of spontaneous mediastinal emphysema is illuminated by his keen clinical perception and his ability to reason logically from the clinical information available. In February 1933, Hamman was called to Washington to see a robust, vigorous, fifty-one-year-old physician who had suddenly developed an intense pain in the chest. The electrocardiogram was normal and the patient felt well, but auscultation of the heart revealed that each contraction was accompanied by an extraordinary crunching, bubbling sound, the likes of which Hamman had never heard before. The peculiar sound disappeared after a few days.

Hamman did not connect this patient's problem with an episode he had discussed years before with his colleague Benjamin Baker. As Baker recalled:

As far as I know, I was probably the first case of spontaneous mediastinal emphysema with anything close to recognition of the underlying process. The event occurred when I was an assistant resident working in the heart station. While bending over the desk making routine electrocardiographic measurements, I suddenly noticed a vague discomfort in my chest which did not disturb me greatly. However, I was surprised and preplexed to hear a strange noise within my own thorax. I found that by leaning back in my chair the noise would disappear and on leaning forward it would return. This occurred over and over. I then called my colleague, Dr. Donald MacEachern [who later became professor of neurology at the Neurological Institute in Montreal], who leaned over the desk with me and agreed that he could also hear the noise in certain positions. We listened with a stethoscope and heard a strange crunching sound over the precordium which disappeared when I leaned back in my chair. I was in the midst of a

minor respiratory infection with a little tracheitis and cough at the time this happened. Our explanation was that there was an emphysematous bleb against which the heart beat in certain positions and made the strange noise. Drs. Longcope, Thayer, and Carter took this strange situation under advisement for several days without arriving at any definitive diagnosis. Subsequently, when I went into practice with Dr. Hamman, we frequently discussed various clinical experiences, and I remember telling him about this. We speculated about its mechanism.[159]

In June 1933, about four months later, Hamman examined a young boy whose heart produced the same sound under circumstances that left no doubt about its origin and cause. There was also subcutaneous crepitation over the front of the neck, a clear indication of mediastinal emphysema, although the patient had not undergone any trauma. Thus Hamman coined the term "spontaneous mediastinal emphysema." He subsequently saw additional cases of this disorder and concluded that the cause of pain in the disorder was the rupture of pulmonary alveoli, which allows air to escape into the interstitial tissues of the lung. If only a small amount of air escapes, the patient may experience no symptoms at all, or only localized pain. If a larger amount of air escapes, however, it may travel along the interstitial bands to the pleura and form a vesicle there. The resulting pleural membrane stretches and often ruptures. "This seems to me," Hamman wrote, "the most reasonable explanation for the recurrence of spontaneous mediastinal emphysema. The symptoms produced may be severe and may closely simulate those of coronary occlusion or pericarditis."[160]

John Eager Howard modestly defined *serendipity* as "*some fellows have all the luck.*"[161] In discussing his discovery of the factor that inhibits calcification in urine, however, he also recognized the responsibility that serendipity places upon its beneficiaries:

as with every new finding, greater challenges lie ahead. It now behooves us to find out what tissues in the body give rise to this or these substances with so amazing a potential to prevent crystallization. It may be as exciting to the concrete industry as to medicine. Also we must discern whether these substances are natural by-products of normal metabolism, what factors stimulate or retard their production and release into the circulation, and whether the urine of stone formers contains less of them or has a substance which inhibits the inhibitor, or indeed, whether these inhibitory substances have anything to do with formation of kidney stones. Perhaps the observation of their presence in urine was purely serendipitous to the discovery of their far greater potential importance in tissue metabolism, to biology in general, and to medical physiology and practice.[162]

"Thus, as always," Howard concluded, "successful outcome of one investigation inevitably points the way to many more experiments."

Clinical Investigation of Chronic Disease in an Outpatient Setting

During the first decade of the twentieth century, great discoveries were made in relation to syphilis—its transmission to animals, the identification of the spirochete, the Wassermann test, and Ehrlich's introduction of Salvarsan. In 1915, Johns Hopkins established a clinic devoted entirely to the clinical and experimental study of this disease. The later discovery that penicillin was treponemicidal led to such a dramatic decline in the number of new cases that the Syphilis Clinic was reorganized. The clinical and epidemiologic techniques and the facilities that had been created to study and manage this single disease were used to investigate other chronic diseases and, finally, to form the base for a pioneering program in medical genetics.

From its inception, the Syphilis Clinic was a subdivision of the Medical Clinic. In 1915 the word syphilis was taboo, so the new clinic had to be camouflaged under a name that meant nothing to laymen in order to help protect the confidentiality of patients. The designation chosen was "Department L," derived from *lues venerea,* an old name for the disease.

George Walker was the clinic's first director; his principal assistant was Albert Keidel, who was the first to administer Salvarsan in Maryland. The clinic grew rapidly, and in 1921 Keidel officially succeeded Walker as director. Perhaps the most important of their early clinical studies were those dealing with the effects of various forms of treatment in selected groups of patients. It was in this clinic that the continuous treatment for early syphilis was introduced in America. Keidel and Joseph Earle Moore, another faculty member of the Department of Medicine, pointed out that full curative treatment was particularly important in early syphilis, whereas in late syphilis the objective was to control the presenting lesions. They described a definitive plan of management consisting of seventy weeks of continuous treatment with alternating courses of arsphenamine and bismuth. Although their system of continuous treatment was instituted in 1916, Keidel and Moore did not describe it in the medical literature until 1926. Priority in publication, therefore, belongs to Almkvist, whose first paper on the subject appeared in 1920.

Upon Keidel's retirement in 1929, Joseph Earle Moore was placed in charge of the clinic. Among his valuable contributions were his elucidation of the natural history of neurosyphilis and the recognition of the occurrence of false-positive serologic tests for syphilis in certain acute and chronic diseases. A major accomplishment was Moore's demonstration that an outpatient clinic could be used as a productive clinical research facility.

Before World War I, funds were not available to organize an experimental laboratory. After the war, however, venereal disease was receiving more attention, and funds were attracted to the clinic from a number of sources. In 1921, a full-time member of the Department of Medicine, Alan M. Chesney, was put in charge of research and teaching in syphilis. Chesney approached the problems of syphilis through the study of both patients and experimental animals. These two lines of research overlapped in so many phases that no sharp distinction could be drawn between them.

Chesney's classic experiments on immunity

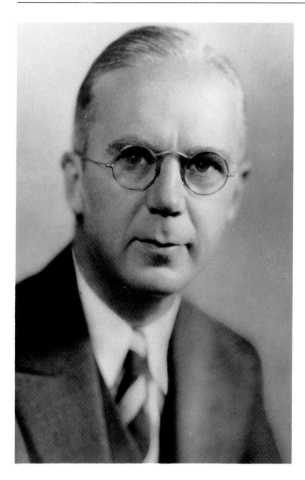

Joseph Earle Moore. (*Source:* Alan M. Chesney Medical Archives, The Johns Hopkins Medical Institutions.)

in syphilis were well described in his monograph on the subject, published in 1926.[163] At the time, experimentalists were divided regarding the existence of acquired immunity. Chesney's experiments indicated that a true acquired immunity developed during the course of experimental syphilis. Summarizing his own experiments and the earlier experiments of others, he concluded that the determining factor in the development of such immunity was the duration of the primary or immunizing infection before its termination by treatment. If the immunizing infection lasted less than three months, reinoculation of the homologous strain by the same route as the original inoculation was usually followed by clinical reinfection. If the immunizing infection was terminated by treatment after three months, similar re-

inoculation with the homologous strain usually did not result in symptomatic infection. Investigators agreed on these observations but differed as to whether this failure to react to the second infection represented a true immunity or whether it represented an altered reactivity of the animal due to the persistence of the original infection. Numerous studies substantiating Chesney's conclusions appeared after his review.

When the discovery of penicillin suddenly changed the character of the Syphilis Clinic, Moore realized that the organization and the methods he had developed for long-term follow-up and study of syphilis could be applied to other chronic diseases. He reoriented the Syphilis Clinic to the study and treatment of chronic diseases. In particular, he began to study the natural history of three classes of patients whose records he had accumulated in the long years of his attention to syphilis.

First, Moore developed the idea that since patients with systemic lupus erythematosus were known to have a false-positive serologic test for syphilis, the myriad of patients who had come to the Syphilis Clinic with this serologic abnormality could form the base of a long-term prospective study of the pathogenesis of the connective tissue diseases. This study was made possible by the development of the specific treponemal immobilization test by Robert Nelson and Manfred Mayer in the Department of Microbiology at Hopkins, and the subject proved to be a fertile field for clinical investigation.

Second, Moore proposed to study the natural history of hypertensive vascular disease. For this project, he had available a mass of clinical data gathered over many years in the clinic, including the serial recording of patients' blood pressure.

Finally, he saw the opportunity to make observations on the natural history of serum hepatitis. Many such cases had accumulated in the clinic's files because intravenous arsenicals often used in the treatment of syphilis resulted in exposure to contaminated serum and consequent hepatitis.

Moore's assistant in running this multi-

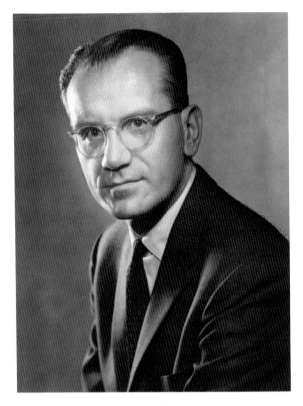

Victor A. McKusick. (*Source:* Udel Bros.)

It was as a cardiologist in the early 1950s that McKusick first came in contact with the genetic disorder known as the Marfan syndrome, largely because its most serious symptoms were cardiovascular in nature. Knowing that animal studies had shown that a defect in a single gene could produce a wide variety of effects throughout the body, McKusick was the first to suggest that a single gene defect in connective tissue could be responsible for the great variety of manifestations seen in patients with the Marfan syndrome. He soon extended this idea to a number of other genetic diseases that had defective connective tissue as a common denominator. These early interests culminated in publication in 1956 of his monograph entitled, "Heritable Disorders of Connective Tissue," a conceptual and clinical landmark in medical genetics. The directorship of the Joseph Earle Moore Clinic in 1957 was a turning point in his career, for it was at that time that he also organized the Medical Genetics Division, one of the first in the country, within the Department of Medicine.

McKusick's studies of the Amish, which began in the 1960s, demonstrated the importance of inbred populations for identifying previously unrecognized recessive diseases as well as for further delineating known disorders. His research demonstrated the dynamics of genes in such populations as well as the so-called "founder effect": the distribution and often disproportionate impact of the founding ancestors' genes over the course of generations in a population that was relatively closed genetically. These observations in the Amish laid the foundation for explaining the higher frequency of certain disorders in other ethnic groups, including Tay-Sachs disease, a neurodegenerative disorder, in Ashkenazic Jews.

In 1973, McKusick joined forces with Frank Ruddle of Yale University and other geneticists around the world to organize the international human gene mapping workshops. Their objective was to map the genes on all twenty-two chromosome pairs, plus the X and Y chromosomes. By June 1976, at least one gene had been located on every chromosome. McKusick maintains a hu-

faceted chronic disease clinic was Ernest W. Smith, who succeeded Moore as head of the clinic from 1954 to 1957. Other participants conducted follow-up clinics: Albert H. Owens in oncology, Lawrence E. Shulman in connective tissue disease, and W. Gordon Walker in renal disease.[164]

When Victor A. McKusick became head of the clinic in 1957, its name was changed to the Joseph Earle Moore Clinic, and its direction was altered to include the expanding field of genetic diseases.

McKusick was a 1946 graduate of the Johns Hopkins medical school. His first clinical investigation identified the hereditary syndrome of intestinal polyps and melanin spots on the lips, which later became known as the Peutz-Jeghers syndrome. This work, published in 1949, brought him in contact with Bentley Glass of Hopkins' Department of Biology, who was to be his mentor in genetics during the next fifteen years.

man gene map at Hopkins in an easily accessible format. The chromosomal location of most genes is discovered by various combinations of techniques: by family studies of linkage that match a defective gene with a marker, by somatic cell hybridization, by high-resolution microscopy, or by recombinant DNA techniques.

McKusick regards the orientation of genes on a chromosome as the modern anatomy. The location of genes has proved useful in a variety of ways, including prenatal diagnosis and carrier identification for diseases such as Huntington disease, the thalassemias, sickle cell anemia, and muscular dystrophy. Application of the techniques for studying DNA directly has also made it possible to detect many mendelian disorders.

The first gene to be assigned to a specific chromosome in human beings was the color-blindness gene. In 1911, Edmund B. Wilson, noted cytologist and an 1881 recipient of the Ph.D. degree from Johns Hopkins, concluded that this gene must be located on the X chromosome because of the characteristic pedigree pattern of this trait, and because of the apparent presence of XX chromosomes in human females and XY chromosomes in males. By similar deductions, over sixty other genes had been assigned to the X chromosome by 1968, when the first gene—coding for the Duffy blood type—was mapped to a specific autosome, or non–sex chromosome, by Roger Donahue, a doctoral candidate in human genetics at Hopkins. Other Hopkins faculty members who have mapped genes include Barbara Migeon, who located the thymidine kinase gene on chromosome 17, and Haig Kazazian, who studied the fine structure of hemoglobin genes.

The facilities that Hopkins offers, those of a large general hospital, gave McKusick the opportunity to search the specialty clinics for patients with the variety of manifestations that characterize heritable entities. At the same time, Hopkins' special resources for follow-up of patients and study of family members enabled him to generate new information on these disorders. Thus, from its beginnings as an effort to manage a single, sexually transmitted disease, the Syphilis Clinic developed into a major center for the study of the genetic diseases of human beings.[165]

Pathways in Neuroscience

Adolf Meyer and the Development of Psychobiology

As the first head of the Phipps Clinics at Johns Hopkins, and a leader in psychiatric treatment, education, and research, Adolf Meyer redefined the relation between mind and brain. At the same time, according to his successor, John C. Whitehorn, his most important contribution to psychiatry was the formulation of clinical psychiatric conditions as reaction types, rather than as mere impersonal disease processes.[166]

Meyer stressed the importance of a sense of professional responsibility in carrying out his formulation, which required in the study of each case a full biography and medical history, "to justify one in a pertinent statement of the life situation to which the person is reacting." Without such a detailed biographical study of the patient as an individual, Meyer's reaction types would be merely a new set of synonyms for the older clinical entities. In Whitehorn's words, Meyer abhorred mere verbal fluency and plausibility in psychiatric discussion. He carefully avoided dramatic or spectacular gestures in his professional work and in his teaching. Because of the austerity of his thought and the thoroughness of his psychiatric formulations, Meyer's lectures and teaching clinics presented difficulties to those who would have preferred some simpler approach. Those who trained under Meyer were uniformly impressed, however, by the simplicity and style of his communications with patients.[167]

Meyer began his scientific career at a time when traditional concepts of neurology were undergoing enormous change. Two key events colored his professional development. The first was a sharp challenge to the traditional views concerning the basic structure of the nervous system. A newly formulated view of the neuron theory, supported by the work of Ross G. Harrison, contradicted previous beliefs. Harrison and others showed that nerve cells and nerve fibers are not separate and independent but are both elements of each neuron. They maintained that each nerve fiber is an outgrowth from a cell body and that it is the cell, with all its processes, that forms the morphologic and functional unit within the nervous system. Recent developments in neurohistopathology were also of great immediate interest. New techniques permitted visualization of the cellular components of the central nervous system with a clarity previously unattainable.

Meyer took an active interest in both of these advances. He published numerous, varied neuropathologic case reports. These reports, in addition to their histopathologic data, contained occasionally significant deductions regarding normal anatomic arrangement and function. Among Meyer's best-known discoveries were his observation concerning the course of the optic fibers in what Jerzy Rose referred to as the "endbrain" (cortex), his study of central neuritis, and his analysis of aphasia.[168]

Meyer's early training took place in Europe, where he studied with many of the outstanding neurologists and psychiatrists in Paris, Edinburgh, Berlin, Vienna, and London. He arrived in the United States in 1892 and held positions in pathology and psychiatry at an asylum in Kankakee, at the University of Chicago, and at the Worcester (Massachusetts) State Hospital, which was affiliated with Clark University. Guided by G. Stanley Hall, a psychologist who had trained at the Johns Hopkins University, Clark University was one of the active centers of experimental psychology in the United States.

As a pathologist, Meyer believed that the study of disease, in its full scientific context, demanded thorough clinical study and review of the life experience of each person whose body and brain came to the autopsy table and to microscopic examination. He emphasized that such information was essential for the understanding of what he termed an "experiment of nature," in which a psychotic reaction formed part of the life experience. Meyer's devotion to this concept led him to strive forcefully against the great inertia and conservatism in state hospital systems, which inevitably brought about a heightened interest in the genetic dynamic study of patients' lives. His most important contribution at this time was his study of central neuritis as a complication of alcoholism.

Meyer came to Johns Hopkins in 1910, after eight years in the New York State Hospital Service. The Phipps Clinic became Meyer's clinical and experimental laboratory in psychiatry and neurology for the remainder of his active years. Here he assembled a brilliant program, which was carried out over the years by some of the world's most distinguished scholars in the fields of psychiatry and neurology. A residency in this clinic became a cherished prize for psychiatrists from all parts of the world, who then returned home to establish new facilities for the extension of Meyer's novel concepts.[169]

Meyer's research built on the acceptance of the neuron theory as a fundamental truth. Using comparative embryologic data, he proposed an approach to the central nervous system that replaced the traditional topographic divisions of the brain with systems composed of combinations of neurons with interrelated activities. Meyer thus arrived at his segmental and suprasegmental mechanisms of cerebellum, midbrain, and forebrain.

Meyer's idea was radical at the time. It was not unusual to consider the fiber and its cell of origin as a unit, but to consider the afferent neurons, the intermediate neural chain, and the efferent neurons as an anatomic grouping was a daring extension of current concepts. The principle underlying Meyer's assumption was that every recognized anatomic level must be capable itself of integrated action. Not until much later were such concepts accepted.[170]

Meyer retained his interest in neuroanatomy throughout his life, despite his later preoccupation with psychiatric problems. To him, psychiatry, neurology, and neuroanatomy were all part of the total picture.

Like his approach to neuroanatomy, Meyer's interest in psychiatry focused on the broad, difficult problems in the field. His 1906 publication on schizophrenia is regarded as a classic contribution. In contrast to Kraepelin, who espoused the concept of the impersonal disease entity based on hypothetical metabolic factors, Meyer viewed schizophrenic patients as the victims of faulty training and faulty use of potential resources. Meyer's contribution was to elevate the mental hygiene of the preschizophrenic state to a level of importance equal to that of the treatment of the disease itself.[171]

Similar clinical acuity and incisiveness were evident in Meyer's article on the treatment of paranoia, part of a textbook published in 1913. Based on Meyer's own experience, this work is a practical approach to getting along with, and influencing, paranoid patients. As one of his colleagues at Johns Hopkins, Wendell S. Muncie, wrote, "It is clearly documented that Meyer had to his credit one of the few authentic cures in an authentic paranoid condition."[172]

He taught his students to take the broadest possible view of psychiatric problems, in order to prevent the premature creation of theories that eventually would only hinder progress in the field. Each investigator in his department was encouraged to pursue his own special interest, and Meyer's only request was that the results be made available to all.[173]

Meyer showed that the varied manifestations of mental disease could be studied with precision. Through his own investigations, he was convinced that much mental disease was preventable. To this end, Meyer coined the term "mental hygiene" and participated in the mental hygiene movement founded by Clifford Beers in 1907. This movement's publications were responsible for the wide dissemination of the ideas of the psychobiologic school. Meyer's contributions thus became a living part of the community and of the great reservoir of common knowledge.[174]

The opening of the Henry Phipps Psychiatric Clinic in 1913 marked the dawn of a new era in psychiatric education. The high standards set in teaching, practice, and research soon spread to other cities, as Meyer's disciples joined the faculties of other schools. Meyer adapted Osler's resi-

dency system to train psychiatrists in his new approach to the patient. By stressing direct observation of the patient, another instance of "learning by doing," he insisted that residents and students collect all their information by observation before preparing their own formulation of the case and their plan of treatment.

A former student, Franklin P. Ebaugh, recalled Meyer's approach:

It was at the daily ward rounds that Dr. Meyer was seen at his best. With the touch of the master clinician and teacher, he imparted a spark to the meeting which makes the spirit of medicine a vital, living force. . . . In the staff conferences one noted his willingness to spend time in detailed inquiry about the essential facts in each case and to discuss, formulate and reformulate facts in the light of new information and additional opinions of staff members. The sensitive management of the patient's conflicts, the tact and the understanding of human nature shown in his relations to the patient were the highest expression of the physician's art.[175]

In discussing his dynamic theory, Meyer emphasized that he concerned himself not with symptoms but with reactions that required understanding and readjustment in one way or another. He constantly emphasized the importance of information gathering—determining the conditions under which behavior occurs and the factors that affect it and, finally, determining the range of results to be analyzed.

At least 60 percent of all the residents and fellows trained by Meyer at the Phipps Clinic pursued careers in academic psychiatry. At the time of his retirement, this group of physicians constituted approximately 10 percent of the teachers of psychiatry in this country. Joel Elkes, who was director of the Department of Psychiatry and Behavioral Sciences and of the Henry Phipps Psychiatric Clinic from 1963 to 1975, summarized Meyer's attitudes:

Meyer believed there was a deep connection between psychiatry and the life sciences, and he regarded *symbolic life* and *behavior* as fundamental parts of general biology. His views emphasized environment as a tool and an opportunity and viewed the reciprocal relationships between organism and environment as a system. The affinities with contemporary views on self-regulation, developmental and social ecology, social biology, and modern systems theory are apparent. Such concepts as consistency, coping, and competence were no strangers to Adolf Meyer. His "attention to life habits" echoes the mental-hygiene movement of his native Europe of the time.[176]

The Development of Neurophysiology: Philip Bard and Vernon Mountcastle

The first three professors of physiology appointed to the medical school—Martin, Howell, and Marshall—were giants in their field. The next department head, Philip Bard, seemed unlikely to attain equal stature when he arrived in Baltimore at the age of thirty-four, for he had published only three articles based on his own independent investigations. Over the ensuing thirty-one years, however, Bard lived up to the high standards set by his predecessors in physiology.

An important influence on Bard's future career was the great physiologist E. Newton Harvey, with whom Bard spent a graduate year at Princeton. Bard's studies with Walter Cannon in Boston turned him toward the area of research that would form the continuing theme of his scientific career: the physiology of the nervous system.[177]

When Bard arrived in Baltimore, he had become adept at performing intracranial surgical procedures in cats, dogs, and monkeys. There were so many problems that seemed approachable by these techniques, Bard said, that he failed to learn the elements of electrophysiology, which became the technique most responsible for advancing knowledge of the nervous system. Bard and fellow department member Clinton Woolsey were using the technique of cortical ablation on monkeys to determine the control of the placing and hopping reactions by the precentral and postcentral gyri of the cortex. By 1936, they had realized the limitations of cortical ablation, and they turned to electrophysiologic methods to continue their investigations. Wade Marshall, another member of the department, set up a cathode-ray

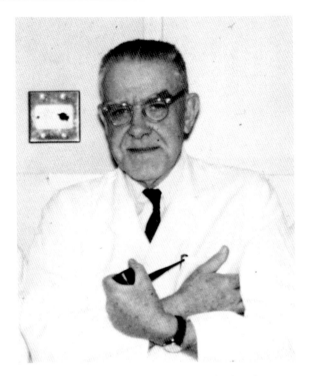

Philip Bard. (*Source:* Alan M. Chesney Medical Archives, The Johns Hopkins Medical Institutions.)

oscillograph with amplifiers, and the three investigators began to study the question of whether evoked potentials would throw further light on the cortical representation of somatic sensibility. The use of the oscillograph in this context was a pioneering technique, and their study resulted in the first systematic mapping of the primate postcentral gyrus. Woolsey applied the method widely, and many of Bard's pupils who subsequently entered the laboratory learned to use it to analyze central sensory systems. Bard himself, while he encouraged work in these directions, returned to his old-fashioned ablation technique for further experiments.[178]

With Woolsey and Chandler Brooks, a physiologist in the department with a particular interest in neurophysiology, Bard carried out an extensive comparative study of the cortical control of the postural reactions, showing their increasing corticalization in phylogeny and their loss following discrete local lesions of the somatotopically related portions of the sensory and motor cortices. As Bard's successor Vernon Mountcastle has pointed out, these studies represent the limit to which the methods of surgical ablation and clinical examination could be pushed in the elucidation of cortical function, and they culminated in Bard's Harvey Lecture of 1938.[179] Bard subsequently studied hypothalamic function in regulating sexual behavior and the reproductive cycle, in governing the pituitary gland and its target organs, in regulating body temperature, and in producing fever.[180]

Bard's vision of the Department of Physiology was far ahead of its time. Bard and Chandler Brooks were both physiologists and neurophysiologists; Woolsey was a comparative neuroanatomist who used physiological methods; Jerzy Rose was a neuroanatomist; Reginald B. Bromley was an experimental psychologist; and Evelyn Howard was an endocrinologist and neuroendocrinologist. By 1946, Bard had created what was essentially a department of neuroscience.

Bard's successor when he retired in 1964 was Vernon B. Mountcastle, then forty-four years of

age. During his forty-year career, Mountcastle has concentrated on four main aspects of the nervous system: the organization of sensory systems and the cortex; the neural mechanisms of information processing in sensory systems; the causal relation between neural events in sensory systems of primates and their sensory capacities; and the cortical mechanisms of perception. He found that the cortex is organized in vertical columns of related cells, each column making up a single processing unit. For example, a given area of skin—a sensory field—is served by three different types of sensory fibers, each of which detects a different sensory stimulus. This discovery, made in 1957, is the basis of the current understanding of cortical function. As Mountcastle pointed out, there is nothing specifically "motor" about the motor cortex or "sensory" about the sensory cortex. It is the input each receives and the ongoing connections it makes to other brain areas that gives it the characteristics we label as "motor" or "sensory." In his view, if one could understand the functioning of a single cortical column, it would provide the basic means of understanding the function of all other areas and contribute greatly to knowledge of the workings of the brain.[181]

Mountcastle's interest in submodality perception—the many kinds of touch—had been stimulated in 1948 by Philip Bard's observations. Mountcastle realized that the use of newly available cellular techniques might reveal a more understandable map of the somatic sensory system, but major technical innovations (including new microelectrodes) and quantifiable stimuli were still required. Mountcastle was instrumental in developing these new tools, which were responsible for the advance of modern cortical physiology.

Mountcastle discovered that at the cellular level, all areas of the somatic sensory system contain a segregation of submodalities that could not be recognized using less sophisticated techniques. His studies showed that single nerve cells respond either to superficial touch stimuli or to pressure stimuli, but not to both. Cells responding to one type of stimulus were grouped together.

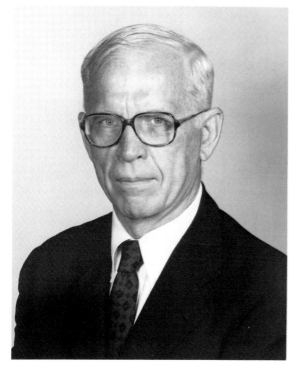

Vernon B. Mountcastle.

In a classic article published in 1957, Mountcastle described his basic observation that submodalities are located in the cortex as vertical columns running from the surface of the brain to the white matter beneath. All cells in a given column received information from a specific point on the skin and from a certain type of receptor, either superficial or deep. Thus, each region of the skin projected its signals to a specific area of the cortex, and other types of receptor stimuli were routed to adjacent columns. The organization of neurons in vertical columns was, therefore, the unique mechanism that allowed the cortex to handle the various functions related to the same region of the body. Each column was an integrating unit, made up of a myriad of neurons, that represented the initial level in the cortex for translating sensory experience into conscious awareness.[182]

Mountcastle's work extended the contributions of Santiago Ramon y Cajal, who, almost a century earlier, had used morphologic techniques to describe for the first time the network of interconnections between populations of nerve cells. Using techniques of modern cell physiology, Mountcastle helped to reveal the functional significance for perception of these interconnections. He showed that the connections sort out and transform sensory information on the way to and within the cortex, that the cortex is organized into functional modules, and that this organization can be altered by experience.[183]

For his numerous significant discoveries, Mountcastle was awarded the National Medal of Science in 1986.[184]

Myasthenia Gravis and the Thymus Gland

Studies of myasthenia gravis at Johns Hopkins have spanned the past fifty years, and investigators from the early years have had the satisfaction of seeing their questions answered by current investigators with new tools and new approaches.

In 1935, while interns on the Osler Service, Richard Whitehill and A. McGehee Harvey demonstrated the value of neostigmine as a specific diagnostic test in patients with myasthenia gravis.[185] They also confirmed that quinine produced an increase in the muscular weakness in patients with this disease.

Just two years later, Sir Henry Dale's Herter Lecture in Baltimore outlined his Nobel Prize–winning work in demonstrating the relation of acetylcholine to transmission of the nerve impulse across the neuromuscular junction. Harvey obtained a fellowship to work in Dale's laboratory, where he used Dale's novel techniques to study the mechanism of action of quinine on neuromuscular function. These studies revealed several effects of the drug on skeletal muscle, including its propensity to abolish the response of normal mammalian muscle to injected acetylcholine. This phenomenon proved to be largely due to the curariform action of quinine, which was demonstrated for the first time in these experiments.[186]

Many years earlier, F. Jolly had pointed out the analogy between curare poisoning and the fatigability of the muscles in patients with myasthenia gravis. Curare, the generic name for a variety of South American arrow poisons, has a long and exotic history, having been employed for centuries by Indians along the Amazon River to kill wild animals for food. It produces death from muscle paralysis, the key feature of which is the type of fatigability seen in myasthenia gravis.

To determine the nature of myasthenia gravis, Harvey's next step was to study normal and partially curarized animals. He would need to develop quantitative methods that would enable him to relate the results in animals to similar neuromuscular defects in human beings. Several key findings in the experimental animals were successfully reproduced in later experiments in human subjects: (1) the response to acetylcholine excitation and the late depression of neuromuscular function produced by acetylcholine; (2) the conversion of the single response of the muscle to nerve stimulation of an evanescent tetanus by neostigmine; (3) the phenomenon of facilitation and depression of neuromuscular transmission in the partially curarized animal; and (4) the post-tetanic facilitation seen in the partially curarized animal.

Not long afterwards, while working in collaboration with Richard L. Masland, Harvey successfully overcame previous difficulties in obtaining satisfactory electromyographic recording of maximal nerve stimulation in human subjects.[187] Electrodes for recording the muscle action potential were fixed to the skin over the muscle. The stimulating electrode was pressed firmly over the ulnar nerve, just below the elbow. With the action potential observed on the cathode-ray oscillograph, the strength of the nerve stimulus was gradually increased until the action potential reached its maximum size. Subjects were then partially curarized, and the investigators recorded the time course of the response to paired nerve stimuli given at varying intervals. The results made it clear that the method was entirely suitable for studying the physiology and pharmacology of neuromuscular transmission in human beings.

The next step taken by Masland and Harvey was to study the electromyogram in patients with myasthenia gravis. They quickly discovered that the response of the myasthenic muscle to a single maximum motor nerve stimulus excited a reduced number of muscle fibers, indicating a partial block in neuromuscular transmission.[188] The response to a second nerve impulse was further reduced, as in the partially curarized individual. When the nerve was stimulated with a series of electrical impulses—in other words, a tetany—the resulting muscle action potentials showed a progressive decline in voltage. The abnormalities in the electromyogram in myasthenia gravis were abolished by neostigmine but increased by a very small dose of quinine.

Harvey continued his studies as a medical resident at Johns Hopkins, in collaboration with fellow resident Joseph L. Lilienthal, Jr. In 1941, they showed that when neostigmine was injected into the brachial artery, it produced a prolonged paresis of the injected extremity, during which a muscle action potential evoked by supramaximal stimulation of the ulnar nerve was followed by repetitive activity. This result was undoubtedly due to the persistence of acetylcholine released from the nerve ending. The initial response to a single stimulus remained normal, showing that the block in neuromuscular transmission caused by neostigmine was different from that produced by partial curarization.[189] These experiments furnished clear evidence that one could observe the state of neuromuscular transmission in human beings as accurately as one could determine the status of a patient with diabetes mellitus by estimating the blood glucose. They indicated a striking similarity between the neuromuscular block in the patient with myasthenia gravis and that produced by curare in the experimental animal.

The studies carried out between 1939 and 1941 strongly suggested that a curarelike action was responsible for the neuromuscular block. Later work done by Harvey and Lilienthal, and then by David Grob, Richard J. Johns, and Harvey, provided convincing evidence that the abnormality in neuromuscular function in myasthenia gravis was an inadequate response of the motor endplates (now referred to as the acetylcholine receptors) to the transmitter substance acetylcholine, which is released from the nerve endings with each nerve impulse.[190]

To Harvey and Lilienthal in 1940, it seemed logical that there might be a curarelike substance present in serum which was responsible for the dysfunction. They therefore turned their attention to the thymus gland as the possible source of such a substance. Many patients with myasthenia gravis were known to have abnormal thymus glands, in some cases tumor of the thymus. The possibility that there might be a curarelike substance in serum released from the thymus was also enhanced by the occasional observation of neonatal myasthenia. Infants born of a myasthenic mother may have a characteristic difficulty in feeding due to weakness of the circumoral and other facial muscles—a weakness that is relieved by administration of neostigmine. This neonatal myasthenia persists for only a few weeks, then spontaneously disappears and has no tendency to return at a later age. The explanation suggested by these two investigators was that a curarelike substance capable of crossing the placental membrane was present in the mother's serum.

When Alfred Blalock became professor of

surgery at Hopkins in 1941, Lilienthal and Harvey approached him with the proposition that the effect of total removal of the thymus be determined in a series of well-studied patients with myasthenia gravis. The literature at that time contained several reports of surgical removal of a thymic tumor with what appeared to be a beneficial influence on the course of the disease. In none of these cases was an effort made to search for and remove all thymic tissue. The fifth such operation had been carried out in 1939 by Blalock, who removed a cystic tumor from the thymic region. He saw no other thymic tissue, although his search of the anterior mediastinum was not a thorough one.

Experimental evidence was thus incomplete, and Lilienthal and Harvey felt justified in proposing to Blalock that he systematically remove all of the thymic tissue from a series of patients with myasthenia. Frank Ford, who had followed their work carefully, agreed with the proposal, and his stature and influence were helpful in persuading Blalock to undertake this approach. Three principal methods were employed in estimating the effect of thymectomy in these patients: (1) the degree of clinical fatigability without medication was compared with that following a given dose of neostigmine; (2) quantitative studies of the response to nerve stimulation of the type described were carried out, and the effect of neostigmine on this response to nerve stimulation was also determined; and (3) the general course of the disease and the total need of the patient for neostigmine were recorded.[191]

For the first few months after the operation, several of the patients showed progressive improvement in strength and no longer required neostigmine therapy. Five months after the operative procedure, electromyographic studies demonstrated that a larger number of muscle fibers were responding to maximal motor nerve stimulus and that there was greater efficiency in the transmission of pairs and trains (tetani) of maximal motor nerve stimuli across the neuromuscular junction. In addition, the intra-arterial injection of neostigmine now produced repetitive responses to a single stimulus, whereas before

thymectomy, these responses had been absent. Finally, two patients showed normal local paresis and depression of neuromuscular function.[192]

These studies indicated that in some patients, the thymus played an important role in the pathogenesis of myasthenia gravis. Although there was no absolute proof that improvement was related to thymectomy, subsequent experience indicates that this was the case. For the first time, objective evidence of the thymus's function had been obtained in human beings.[193]

Harvey and his co-workers had correctly deduced that the abnormality resided in the acetylcholine receptors, that a circulating substance was involved in the process, and that the thymus gland was involved in the pathogenesis of myasthenia gravis. The concepts of autoimmune disease and the new immunology, however, had not yet been introduced when their work was performed. An exciting new phase of investigation soon began, in which Daniel Drachman played a key role.

Drachman's work made use of the investigations of C. C. Chang and C. Y. Lee, Taiwanese pharmacologists whose 1966 article discussed their electrophysiological study of the neuromuscular blocking action of cobra neurotoxin, which paralyzed the victims of the many-banded krait (*Bungarus multicintus*).[194] Because this alpha-bungarotoxin (alpha-BuTx) bound specifically, quantitatively, and irreversibly to the acetylcholine receptor (AChR), it seemed to Drachman an ideal tool for studying the defect in myasthenia gravis.

Douglas Fambrough, then in his first year as a staff member of the Carnegie Institution, had obtained some of the material and was using radiolabeled alpha-BuTx to study neuromuscular junctions in experimental animals. At Drachman's suggestion, he and his group measured the junctional receptors in myasthenic patients. When Drachman learned to localize the "motor points" (i.e., neuromuscular junction—containing regions) in muscle biopsies, he obtained biopsies from a series of myasthenic and nonmyasthenic individuals, quickly placed the biopsied material in a holding medium, and drove it over to the Carnegie Institution, where Fambrough incubated it with radiolabeled bungarotoxin, teased the muscle fibers, and calculated the radioactivity.

Scintillation counting and autoradiograms showed a striking decrease in the number of acetylcholine receptors per neuromuscular junction in myasthenic patients as compared to controls.[195] This observation clearly substantiated the evidence obtained by Harvey and his co-workers that the defect in myasthenia gravis was in the acetylcholine receptors at the postsynaptic membrane.

To determine whether a decrease in the number of receptors could in fact reproduce all of the features of myasthenia gravis, Drachman, Satyamurti, a fellow, and Fred Slone, a premedical student, used cobra venom to block a portion of the AChRs at neuromuscular junctions in rats. These functionally blocked junctions in rats showed precisely the same decremental responses demonstrated more than thirty years previously by Harvey and Masland in human patients with myasthenia. This result was compatible with the belief that the AChR was the site of the defect.[196]

At about the same time, it was reported elsewhere that animals immunized with AChR purified from the electric organ of electric rays developed a disorder similar to human myasthenia gravis. Other investigators recognized that this was attributable to an autoimmune process directed against AChRs, but the nature of the autoimmune process was unclear. Antibodies were present, but the neuromuscular junctions in these animals with experimental myasthenia gravis were heavily infiltrated with lymphocytes and macrophages. Myasthenia gravis was therefore widely believed to be a cell-mediated autoimmune disorder, despite the fact that antibodies against AChRs were also present in the sera of both human myasthenic patients and animals with experimental autoimmune myasthenia gravis. Drachman remembered earlier observations on neonatal myasthenia, which suggested the importance of the antibody response. The role of antibodies had been more or less discredited by numerous experiments showing that the injection of serum from myasthenic patients into a variety of animals failed to reproduce the features of my-

asthenia gravis in the recipients. Drachman reasoned that the reaction to exposure to serum antibodies might take longer than the duration of the exposure in previous experiments. Accordingly, he and his co-workers transferred human serum antibodies repeatedly, for periods ranging from days to weeks. By measuring both the number of AChRs at neuromuscular junctions and also the electrical potentials generated by neurotransmission (miniature endplate potentials as well as endplate potentials), they showed that passive transfer of serum from myasthenic human beings to mice faithfully reproduced the features of myasthenia gravis; and in a follow-up study, they demonstrated that immunoglobulin G (IgG) was responsible.[197]

To reveal how the antibodies exerted their effect at the neuromuscular junction, they used a system of *in vitro* tissue culture. Skeletal muscle cells from fetal rats were cultured in Petri dishes. These cells had large numbers of AChRs, and their turnover could be followed by labeling them with ^{125}I-alpha-BuTx. Drachman and his colleagues demonstrated that the degradation rate of AChRs was greatly accelerated by adding serum IgG from myasthenic patients to the culture medium.[198] It has been shown that sera from over 90 percent of patients with myasthenia cause accelerated degradation of AChRs. This provided the first evidence that antibodies to a cell membrane receptor could induce the accelerated loss of the receptor. This principle has now proven to be generally true in a wide variety of autoimmune disorders.

Drachman's group also carried out a series of studies on the mechanisms by which antibodies directed against AChR cause accelerated degradation of the receptors. They first showed that the receptors must be cross-linked by the divalent antibodies in order for degradation to be accelerated. Monovalent antibody fragments (Fab′ fragments) bind to the AChRs but fail to cause accelerated degradation. When "piggyback" antibodies directed against the Fab′ fragments are added, however, this cross-linkage induces accelerated degradation. Only the AChRs that have antibodies bound to them are degraded at an accelerated rate. They demonstrated by freeze-fracture electron microscopy that the cross-linked AChRs are first clustered together in patches, prior to their accelerated loss. The rate-limiting step in this process is endocytosis. Once endocytosed, the AChRs are readily degraded by lysosomes within the muscle cells.[199]

In addition to the effect on receptor turnover, circulating antibodies in myasthenia gravis can result in blockade of the ligand-binding site of the AChR. Again, using the rat skeletal muscle tissue culture system, Drachman and his group showed that under optimal conditions, sera from over 85 percent of myasthenic patients interfere with binding of alpha-BuTx to the receptors.

It was known that the antibody titer in myasthenic patients does not correlate with the severity of the clinical disorder. Drachman and his co-workers suspected that the functional activity of the antibodies, resulting in blockade and/or accelerated degradation of the AChRs, might correspond more closely with the patient's clinical status. Accordingly, they measured in vitro blockade and accelerated degradation, using sera from fifty myasthenic patients with varying degrees of clinical involvement. Their findings revealed that the functional ability of the antibodies to cause loss of AChRs through blockade and accelerated degradation corresponded more closely with the clinical severity of the disorder than did the antibody titers.

Most of their studies of accelerated degradation were demonstrations in tissue culture. This experimental system differs from the situation at the normal neuromuscular junction, since AChRs in cultured muscles are distributed over the entire surface of the muscle cell and are normally degraded at a rapid rate. In contrast, AChRs in normally innervated muscle fibers are located only at the neuromuscular junctions and are relatively stable, with a half-life of ten to twelve days. It was, therefore, important to determine whether junctional AChRs are degraded at an accelerated rate in the presence of anti-AChR antibodies. Drachman and his colleagues tested this question both in vivo and in vitro and found that anti-AChR antibodies from myasthenic patients caused accelerated degradation of junctional AChRs.[200]

A key question is the origin of myasthenia gravis. Clearly the thymus gland plays an important role. It was known that the thymus gland contains peculiar muscle-like or "myoid" cells, which Drachman thought might bear AChRs. If so, their presence in thymus might lead to the autoimmune response. Drachman's group cultured thymus glands from normal rats and from human myasthenic patients who underwent thymectomy, and found in both instances that muscle cells grew out. These cells behaved like normal muscle cells in all respects; most important, the researchers demonstrated that these cells had surface AChRs that bound ^{125}I-alpha-BuTx. The presence of AChR-bearing muscle cells in apposition to immunocompetent cells within the thymus may well set the stage for the initiation of the autoimmune reaction, but the factor that triggers myasthenia gravis has yet to be determined.[201]

The Department of Neuroscience: Transmitters and Receptors

Although the study of transmitters and receptors is central to the work of the Department of Neuroscience, the research described above antedated the creation of a separate department in 1980, and transmitters and receptors continue to interest investigators throughout the School of Medicine. Solomon H. Snyder, the first director of the Department of Neuroscience, was directly influenced by the work of one of these other investigators.

Early work at Johns Hopkins was performed by William H. Howell, who studied the vagus inhibition of the heart and its relation to inorganic salts in the blood. It was well known that an increase in the percentage of neutral potassium salts, especially potassium chloride, present in the blood or other circulating media, caused the heart to beat at a slower rate and eventually to come to rest in a condition of diastole, with loss of tone, just as with vagus inhibition. Later, Howell and W. W. Duke demonstrated that when the vagus nerve is stimulated, potassium is released into the perfusion fluid. Thus, in an era when acetylcholine was unknown, Howell came close to establishing the concept of chemical transmission at nerve endings.[202]

Some years later, in the Department of Medicine, A. McGehee Harvey and his colleagues David Grob, Richard J. Johns, and Joseph L. Lilienthal, Jr., studied the effect of a lipid-soluble anticholinesterase compound, di-isopropyl-fluorophosphate (DFP). Their administration of DFP to human subjects resulted in peculiar central nervous system symptoms as well as electro-encephalographic changes indicating increased neural activity. The EEG changes consisted of an increase in the frequency and irregularity of the rhythm, and the intermittent appearance of abnormal waves similar to those seen in patients with grand mal epilepsy. These effects of DFP on the central nervous system and their inhibition by atropine led these investigators to believe that the acetylcholine cycle played a role in central neural function. The techniques were not available at the time to pursue these observations further in human subjects, but Harvey and his colleagues were among the first to suggest that acetylcholine could act as a transmitter in the central nervous system as well as at peripheral neuromuscular junctions.[203]

The first to make significant contributions to the study of receptors at Johns Hopkins was Pedro Cuatrecasas, an associate professor of pharmacology and medicine. After residency training on the Osler Medical Service, Cuatrecasas had worked at the NIH with Christian Anfinson, studying the structure and catalytic mechanisms of a crystalline staphylococcal nuclease. His work attracted widespread attention when he popularized the method known as affinity chromatography. The possibility of isolating enzymes and proteins by binding them to a specific substrate analogue, which was itself covalently bound to a polymer, had been considered for many years, but it was Cuatrecasas who first developed this technique for widespread use. By preparing inhibitory substrate analogues or other suitable ligands covalently linked to Sepharose, he was able to purify in a single step staphylococcal nuclease, alpha-chymotrypsin, carboxypeptidase A, and avidin from egg white.

Cuatrecasas returned to Johns Hopkins in

1970 to head the Division of Clinical Pharmacology. Continuing the use of his chromatographic techniques, he found that the "receptors" for insulin are located on the surface rather than in the interior of fat and liver cells. When he extracted the cell membrane–bound insulin receptors and partially purified them in a water-soluble form, he discovered that several important cell functions are regulated by processes that occurred in the thin structure called the plasma membrane, on the surface of the cell.

Not only insulin but also other peptide hormones appeared to exert their effect by interacting with specific molecules in cell membranes. He found that other processes, such as the regulation of ion and sugar transport and the triggering of immune reactions by specific antigens, are also controlled by events mediated at a receptor on the cell surface.[204]

Cuatrecasas was continuing his studies on the nature of membrane receptors for a variety of hormones, growth-promoting substances, and drugs when he began a collaboration with Solomon H. Snyder. Their laboratories were on the same floor, and Snyder was intrigued by Cuatrecasas' work on insulin receptor binding. Snyder became interested in a collaborative effort when he saw an article on the amino acid sequence of proinsulin and noted its many similarities to nerve growth factor. Because of its importance for neuroscience, Snyder had targeted nerve growth factor as an interesting subject for research. He thought that it might interact with receptors in a manner similar to insulin, which Cuatrecasas had described. With Cuatrecasas' continuing advice, Snyder and Shailesh Banerjee quickly succeeded in identifying the receptors for nerve growth factor. Studying them in the soluble state, they identified their unique regulation by calcium ions.

In 1972, as the recipient of an NIH Drug Abuse Research grant, Snyder was searching for an exciting approach to research on the subject. Avram Goldstein of Stanford had attempted to identify opiate receptors, but with little success. Yet Snyder felt that specific receptors for opiates should exist. With his experience in nerve growth factor receptors, Snyder improved on Goldstein's strategy. Candace Pert, a graduate student at Hopkins, was finishing work on the uptake of choline into acetylcholine nerves. Snyder and Pert successfully applied the techniques used in studies of nerve growth factor to their search for opiate receptors.

It is now well established that information processing in the brain largely involves communication among neurons through release of neurotransmitters at synapses. In most instances, neurotransmitters were first identified as endogenous substances, and only then were their receptors characterized. In contrast, after Pert and Snyder found the receptors for the enkephalins, they used the receptors to identify and isolate the opiatelike peptides. The enkephalins (or natural opiates) function in the same way as the addictive opiate narcotics, regulating the body functions that are also strongly influenced by opiate drugs. Pert and Snyder knew that understanding the actions of these substances was the key to understanding brain function, and could lead the way to the synthesis of nonaddictive pain relievers.

In his studies with Cuatrecasas on nerve growth factor, Snyder had mastered the important technical skills needed for this work. Snyder and his co-workers used an intensely radioactive form of an opiate, which allowed them to measure very low concentrations of the drug. In addition, they were able to wash away the nonspecific binding while preserving the specific attachments to opiate receptors. They discovered that opiate receptors are localized to the synaptic membrane, evidence that they are receptors for a natural neurotransmitter.[205]

In other studies with Michael Kuhar, Pert and Snyder found that the medial portion of the thalamus contains a large number of opiate receptors, while the lateral thalamus has few. The lateral thalamus deals with stimuli such as light pressure and touch, which are not influenced by opiates. The medial thalamus, on the other hand, is involved with the type of pain that opiates are most successful in relieving.[206]

Kuhar developed techniques to visualize radioactive-labeled opiate molecules microsco-

pically and showed that opiate receptors were concentrated in a variety of small, discrete regions. In the spinal cord, these receptors occupied a narrow vertical band of gray matter known as the substantia gelatinosa. The presence of these receptors was convincing evidence that the opiate drugs act in both the brain and the spinal cord.

Another investigation built on the common knowledge that opiate drugs are psychologically addictive. In one component of the area of the brain that regulates emotions—the amygdala—Snyder and his group found the largest concentration of opiate receptors.

With Gavril Pasternak, Snyder showed that brain extracts contained a material that competed with radioactive-labeled opiate drugs in binding to opiate receptors. The quantity of this material in various regions of the brain paralleled the number of opiate receptors.[207]

Two years later, investigators in Scotland published an article delineating the chemical structure of the morphinelike material that they had isolated from the brain. Rabi Simantov and Snyder independently isolated the enkephalins, finding the same two peptide structures.

With Carol LaMotte, Pert and Snyder also demonstrated that the opiate receptors of the spinal cord are located on the nerve endings of the sensory nerves. They suggested that the enkephalins inhibit the release of the excitatory transmitter, which results in a decrease in pain.[208]

Snyder and his co-workers identified other transmitters and their receptors and established the importance of these neurochemicals in such disorders as schizophrenia and Parkinson's disease. Existence of receptors for dopamine, for example, had been predicted, but it was Snyder's group that provided evidence for their existence and later showed that antischizophrenic drugs act by blocking dopamine receptors. Snyder's group was also able to determine antischizophrenic drug concentrations in a patient's blood, thus making the clinical use of these drugs more controllable.[209]

One of the most exciting recent techniques for the study of the living chemistry of the brain is positron emission tomography (PET scanning), an application developed by Henry N. Wagner, Jr., and Michael Kuhar. Their research was a natural consequence of Kuhar's work with Snyder in mapping dopamine and opiate receptors by autoradiography. Wagner's objective was to label these substances, or related molecules, with carbon-11 or fluorine-18, both of which had to be prepared nearby using a cyclotron because of their short half-life. With funds from an NIH grant, Wagner and Kuhar obtained the cyclotron, putting it into operation in the hospital by January 1982. Using carbon-11 N-methyl spiperone, they carried out the first imaging of a neuroreceptor (the dopamine receptor) in the human brain on May 25, 1983.[210]

One year later, Wagner and Kuhar also became the first to image opiate receptors in the human brain. Wagner was his own experimental subject for both this study and for the mapping of the dopamine receptor. Later experiments showed that dopamine receptors are increased in the brain of schizophrenic patients and that an increased number of opiate receptors are present at the loci of epileptic seizures.[211]

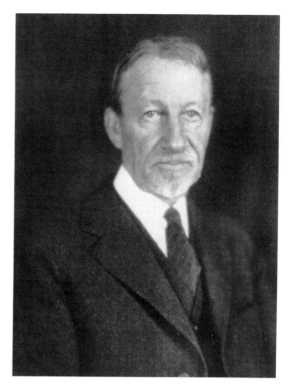

William H. Howell. (*Source: Bulletin of the Johns Hopkins Hospital* 68[1941]:291.)

Uniformity and Differentiation in Modern-Day Research

When the Johns Hopkins University School of Medicine opened its doors in 1893, the preclinical sciences were becoming differentiated and professionalized. Franklin P. Mall singlehandedly created a new school of anatomy, and his disciples spread his particular pedagogical approach and research interests across the country. As the first professor of pharmacology, John J. Abel imposed a characteristic stamp on his department. Out of pharmacology grew the Department of Physiological Chemistry, a discipline that had only recently taken root under Russell H. Chittenden at Yale. William H. Howell carried on the development of physiology in this country—a movement that owed much to his mentor, Henry Newell Martin.

Thus, a century ago, the basic science departments enjoyed strong leadership and increasingly demarcated boundaries. The provinces of anatomy, physiology, biochemistry, and pharmacology existed comfortably side by side, each with its own well-defined intellectual purview.

A portent of the dramatic changes that were occurring in medical science was the ease with which E. Kennerly Marshall, Jr., in 1932, shifted from a successful career as professor of physiology to an even more distinguished one as professor of pharmacology. His ability to be productive in more than one field was aided by his fundamental training as a chemist. Given his background in chemistry, he probably could have had a third distinguished career as professor of biochemistry.

More recently, advances in biochemical knowledge and the development of molecular biology and recombinant DNA technology have led to dramatic changes in the nature of the preclinical sciences. In Mall's day, each department member could investigate many areas of his field. Now, departments must house a large number of scientists, each of whom concentrates on a relatively small part of the discipline.

Moreover, the distinctions between these sciences basic to medicine have blurred, drawing them together. To accommodate to this new uniformity, the medical school curriculum has been restructured. In scientific investigation as well as in education, the preclinical sciences have become less distinctive, in their research tools and even in their areas of interest, not only from each other but from the clinical sciences as well.

"What we have now," said one senior staff member at Hopkins, "is seven departments of molecular biology." Indeed, in the past decade, many science departments have changed their names. Reports of departmental research by directors of three present-day departments (anatomy, biological chemistry, and pharmacology) illustrate these profound changes in the nature of scientific investigation.

The Department of Anatomy

David Bodian's successor as director of anatomy in 1977 was Thomas D. Pollard, who classified himself professionally as a cell biologist.[212] The changes that occurred in the Department of Anat-

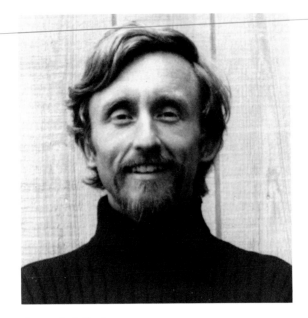

Thomas D. Pollard

omy over the next decade illustrated the response in one department to a growing trend across the entire medical school: the unification of the biomedical sciences.[213]

Pollard believed that the term "anatomy" was too narrow to encompass the faculty's current work on biological structure. The department was therefore renamed "the Department of Cell Biology and Anatomy," a name that reflected the department's broadened research and teaching interests. The members of the department recruited by Pollard were biochemically oriented cell biologists interested in the question of how macromolecular structure and dynamics can explain the major activities of cells. This new generation of scientists was drawn to specific biologic questions but was comfortable using methods from any of the traditional disciplines of anatomy, biochemistry, biophysics, immunology, and molecular biology. Thus, because it was difficult to classify this type of work in accordance with time-honored disciplines, those who studied the molecular basis of cell structure and function called themselves "cell biologists" rather than anatomists, physiologists, or biochemists.

Pollard was one of the pioneers who showed that contractile proteins, closely related to actin, myosin, and their associated proteins in muscle, were present in all eukaryotic cells. These proteins not only produce the movements of cells but also account for the gel-like consistency of cytoplasm. He and his students characterized in detail the molecular mechanisms of a variety of these cytoplasmic contractile proteins. Their focus on one biological question, the mechanism of cell motility, and their use of a wide range of methods including protein chemistry, biochemical kinetics, immunochemistry, light and electron microscopy, gene cloning, and x-ray crystallography epitomizes the approach of the cell biologists in the 1980s.

Other members of the department used a similar range of methods in other areas of cell biology. Ueli Aebi used electron microscopy and image processing to decipher the structure of the actin molecule, the actin filament and intermediate filaments. Vann Bennett discovered and characterized the molecular interactions that connect the plasma membranes of cells to the underlying framework of cytoplasmic structural proteins. William Earnshaw used immunochemical methods to identify the first protein to be localized at the centromere of chromosomes and used molecular biologic methods to clone and sequence DNA corresponding to this protein. He also discovered that the DNA-unwinding protein topoisomerase-II is a major component of the chromosome scaffold, where it may help to anchor loops of DNA. Larry Gerace discovered and characterized the lamins, structural proteins that stabilize the nuclear envelope and control its reversible disassembly during mitosis. He also identified the first protein associated with nuclear pores, the portals that control movements of macromolecules in and out of the nucleus. Ann Hubbard used quantitative biochemical and morphologic techniques to characterize the biosynthesis and incorporation of proteins into specific domains of the plasma membrane and to follow the movements of receptor proteins from the plasma membrane to various compartments inside the cell. Douglas Murphy discovered that microtubules, protein polymers forming part of the so-called cytoskeleton, can anneal end to end, and that specialized forms of the constituent tubulin molecules can sort from each other during polymerization.

Pollard also strengthened teaching and research in the department's traditional sphere of gross anatomy by appointing the noted physical anthropologist Alan Walker to extend the department's traditional interest in anthropology, begun by Franklin P. Mall and continued by Adolph Schultz and William L. Straus. Walker recruited an able group of junior faculty interested in vertebrate evolution and biomechanics. This group used both paleontological field work and, in the laboratory, new analytical techniques to study vertebrate evolution and function. Working with African colleagues, Walker and Mark Teaford from Hopkins have made three historic and widely publicized fossil discoveries: the most complete skeleton ever found of *Homo erectus*; the most complete collection of skeletons of *Proconsul,* an important link in the primate evolutionary

tree: and a striking skull of a hyperrobust early hominid. Walker and Teaford also pioneered the use of electron microscopy to analyze the wear on teeth for clues about the dietary habits of early man. Kenneth Rose did pioneering work on the earliest mammals, obtaining a number of important fossils from Wyoming, including some unusually complete records of gradual evolution at the species level. Christopher Ruff used methods from mechanical engineering to study evolutionary changes in human long bones and the process of osteoporosis. Patty Shipman used electron microscopy of scratches and cuts on bones to document the earliest uses of tools in butchery and more recent examples of cannibalism.

The Department of Pharmacology

Anchoring the history of the Department of Pharmacology at Johns Hopkins is the department's persistent strength in chemistry, which has contributed significantly to its success. Neither John Jacob Abel nor his successors were "trained pharmacologists." At a time when the practice of pharmacology was a trade rather than a profession and most medical school departments trained rather than educated their students, the department at Hopkins emphasized a chemical approach to the investigation of drugs. The wisdom of this concentration on biochemistry emerged with the development of molecular biology as the key to growth in pharmacology.[214]

E. Kennerly Marshall, Jr., was succeeded as head of the department in 1955 by Gilbert H. Mudge. Mudge's particular interest was the kidney, and as a faculty member at Columbia University, he made significant contributions to the understanding of its biochemical mechanisms. The mechanisms governing the regulatory functions of the kidney have also been a continuing research interest of the pharmacology department at Hopkins since its inception, and every department director has made important contributions in this field.

Mudge appointed two faculty members with particular expertise in the fields of renal function and electrolyte transport: Irwin M. Weiner and

Mackenzie Walser. Studying the renal excretion of drugs, most of which are weak organic acids or bases, Weiner and Mudge demonstrated that the renal tubule contains separate mechanisms for the secretion of these weak acids and bases, and that these mechanisms do not compete with each other.[215] They also investigated the mechanism of transport of charged organic compounds, determining that the secretion and reabsorption of organic acids and bases proceed independently across renal tubule membranes in both directions and that they occur in different parts of the renal tubule.[216] Their studies established for the first time the physicochemical requirements for these processes, including the important role of lipid solubility and ionization.

Weiner, Levy, and Mudge[217] also discovered that the potency of a series of mercurial diuretics (virtually the only effective diuretics then available) was correlated closely with the ease of cleavage of the carbon-mercury bond by sulfhydryl groups, suggesting that the effectiveness of these compounds depended upon the interactions of the mercuric ions with vital sulfhydryl groups involved in renal function. Complementing these discoveries were Walser's studies of renal ion transport and his development of methods for combating renal failure in human beings.

Urea had been universally regarded as the sole end product of nitrogen metabolism in human beings until 1959, when Walser and L. J. Bodenlos reported that about 25 percent of the urea synthesized by the liver was continuously degraded by ureases of the intestinal flora. This observation proved to be important in devising novel treatments for renal failure. It was already known that alpha-keto-analogues of five of the nutritionally essential amino acids could sustain growth in rats fed diets devoid of the corresponding amino acids. Other investigators coupled Walser's observation with this information and suggested that the administration of these keto acids to uremic patients might lower blood urea, promote nitrogen reutilization, and reduce the requirements for dietary proteins.

Walser and his colleagues made it possible to test these predictions by developing large-scale methods for synthesizing the keto-analogues of valine, leucine, isoleucine, methionine, and phenylalanine, and by designing techniques to measure their levels in body fluids. They demonstrated that the keto-analogues are converted to their respective amino acids by normal animal tissues and established safe upper limits of keto-acid dosage. On the basis of animal studies, they developed a mixture of keto acids for testing in uremic patients. It quickly became apparent that the mixture exerted a protein-sparing effect and that its administration appeared to slow the progress of chronic renal failure.

A reliable method of assessing the progression of chronic renal failure on a long-term basis was fundamental to these studies. With William E. Mitch, a member of the Department of Medicine, Walser developed an empirical method for evaluating renal function based on a reciprocal plot of the creatinine value with respect to time.

When Mudge left Johns Hopkins in 1962 to become dean of the Dartmouth Medical School, he was succeeded by Paul Talalay. Talalay's appointment coincided with major changes in the methods of discovery, evaluation, and testing of drugs for potential human use. With the discovery of the teratogenicity of thalidomide, entirely new and formalized procedures for the ethical clinical evaluation of both safety and toxicity in human beings were mandated. At the same time, important advances in the basic biomedical sciences inevitably pointed to new biochemical and molecular approaches to pharmacology and drug development. These approaches were amenable to formal and informal arrangements with other departments, through collaborative projects and joint appointment of faculty members, and Talalay intensified these collaborative efforts. Some departments work very successfully in isolation, said Paul Talalay, "but what I am proudest of is to see the influence of this department diffused throughout the institution."[218]

Under Talalay's leadership, the Division of Clinical Pharmacology, a joint venture begun by A. McGehee Harvey and Marshall, became more closely integrated into its two parent departments, medicine and pharmacology. Harvey obtained funds to build new quarters for the division on Osler 5, near the NIH-supported clinical research ward. The faculty of the division was expanded and became more involved in the teaching of pharmacology through the preclinical and the clinical years of medical school. These developments emerged from the pioneering work of Louis Lasagna during his years as head of clinical pharmacology, and continued under Lasagna's successors, Pedro Cuatrecasas and Paul S. Lietman.

Talalay also established a unique association with the Department of Urology through the Brady Laboratory for Reproductive Biology, which opened in 1965 under the direction of H. Guy Williams-Ashman. Since Ashman's departure in 1969, the laboratory has been directed by Donald S. Coffey. Similar collaborative ventures were established in pediatric and developmental pharmacology under the direction of Paul S. Lietman; in psychopharmacology under Solomon H. Snyder; in pharmacology in relation to obstetrics and gynecology under David A. Blake; and in parasitology under Ernest Bueding, professor of pathobiology in the School of Hygiene and Public Health.

Talalay also recognized the utility for modern pharmacology of physical instrumentation, particularly the mass spectrometer and nuclear magnetic resonance. Enthusiasm for the most modern equipment was also a departmental tradition. In the early 1920s, Abel had become intrigued by the possibilities of characterizing organic molecules by means of their infrared absorption spectra. He reputedly spent more than half of one year's departmental budget to buy rock salt crystals and other accessories for construction of an infrared spectrophotometer.

Talalay's efforts soon led to the development of a mass spectrometry center, which served not only his department but the university at large. Catherine Fenselau, an expert mass spectrometrist, joined the department in 1967 with a particular interest in new methods of obtaining useful fragments of organic molecules. As an example of her collaborative work, Fenselau and O. Michael Colvin of the Oncology Center developed a number of the new metabolites of cyclophospha-

mide, which led to the introduction of new and modified analogues with favorable chemotherapeutic activities.

At Hopkins, Talalay continued his work begun at the University of Chicago on the enzymatic mechanisms underlying the transformations of steroid hormones. He and his group made the important discovery of the hydroxysteroid dehydrogenases, a family of nicotinamide nucleotide–linked alcohol dehydrogenases that promote the reversible interconversions of hydroxy and carbonyl functions on the steroid nucleus and side chain with a high degree of steric and positional specificity. Working with H. Guy Williams-Ashman, Talalay showed that hydroxysteroid dehydrogenases with dual nicotinamide nucleotide specificity present in animal tissues could promote the reversible steroid-dependent transport of hydrogen between reduced and oxidized nicotinamide nucleotides. The mechanisms of these reactions were found to be a general property of the hydroxysteroid dehydrogenases and to involve reversible steroid oxidation-reduction reactions. Talalay and Williams-Ashman proposed an entirely novel theory for the mechanism of action of steroid hormones, based on their ability to function as coenzymes of hydrogen transport between nicotinamide nucleotides through the participation of hydroxysteroid dehydrogenases with dual nucleotide specificity.

With the use of purified hydroxysteroid dehydrogenases, Talalay was the first to propose and implement a system for the quantitative microanalysis of steroid hormones.[219] He demonstrated the versatility of these enzymatic methods for measuring and resolving specific groups of steroids, assigning steric configurations, determining purity and stereospecific synthesis of steroids. The utility of these analytical tools was dramatically enhanced by the technique of nicotinamide nucleotide cycling, which made it possible to measure subpicomole quantities of steroids. These methods can be used to analyze not only the steroid content of body fluids but also the much lower levels of steroids present in many tissues.

The most extensive studies of enzymatic

mechanisms have been carried out on the keto-steroid isomerase reaction, first described by Talalay in both microbial and animal systems.[220] His laboratory has also been responsible for recent advances in delineating the catalytic mechanism of the reaction. Beginning in 1977, however, these research interests of Talalay's laboratory were overshadowed by the development of an inter-disciplinary program of research on chemical protection against cancer.

Although sporadic experiments since the 1920s had demonstrated that one chemical agent can block the carcinogenicity of another, the potential importance of this phenomenon was not widely appreciated. Efforts to develop chemoprotective measures against carcinogens and mutagens were initiated by Talalay and Ernest Bueding in the late 1970s. Bueding had shown that a number of chemotherapeutic agents, including those used for the treatment of parasitic diseases, were mutagenic and carcinogenic, but it was not clear whether chemotherapeutic properties and toxicities could be dissociated.

Studies with the common food antioxidant butylated hydroxyanisole (BHA) demonstrated that these properties could indeed be dissociated. Talalay and Bueding confirmed that BHA and related antioxidants provided substantial protection against carcinogenicity as well as reducing mutagenic effects of carcinogens administered in vivo. A research program was then initiated to devise practical strategies for the chemoprotection of human beings by analyzing the molecular mechanisms of BHA and related compounds.

The first studies with BHA in rodents demonstrated elevations in the levels of detoxification enzymes including glutathione-S transferases, epoxide hydrolase, and glucuronosyltransferase in the livers and many extrahepatic tissues of mice and rats. These findings led Talalay to suggest that chemoprotection could be accounted for largely by elevations of detoxification enzymes. Previous studies had attributed chemoprotection to alterations in phase I (activational) enzyme patterns. Because BHA caused only small or inconsistent changes in these phase I enzymes, however, Talalay and his colleagues concluded that the ele-

vation of phase II enzymes was sufficient for chemoprotection. Many synthetic and natural anticarcinogenic agents, comprising a wide variety of chemical structures, were found to induce enzymes that inactivate the ultimate reactive forms of various carcinogens.

Talalay and his colleagues also developed in vitro cell culture systems to analyze anticarcinogenic agents. Their simple assay system for one chemoprotective enzyme (quinone reductase) allowed rapid and efficient screening of natural products and components of the human diet for anticarcinogenic activity.

Talalay and associates also identified the specific functional groups responsible for enzyme induction by analyzing the molecular events involved. Although the structures of compounds capable of eliciting chemoprotective enzyme induction are diverse, all either contain, or are converted to, agents with specific positively charged electrophilic centers that signal the induction of chemoprotective enzymes. This work enhanced the exciting prospect of predicting and designing new chemoprotectors against cancer.

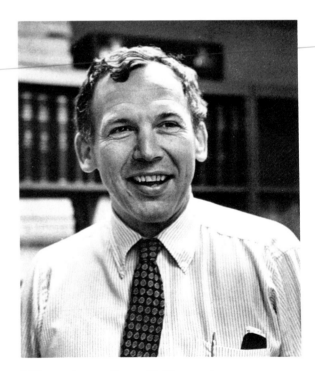

J. Thomas August. (*Source:* Ted Burrows.)

J. Thomas August became director of the pharmacology department in 1975, at a time when rapid advances in molecular science had highlighted the need to expand various aspects of pharmacologic research. August identified three areas essential to the department's growth: molecular virology, immunopharmacology, and molecular biology of cell membranes. He acquired additional faculty members in each of these areas and, as a formal demonstration of the department's commitment to molecular research, changed its name to "the Department of Pharmacology and Molecular Sciences."[221]

Molecular Virology During the past two decades, studies of the clinically important herpesviruses and retroviruses (including the virus for the acquired immune deficiency syndrome) have benefited enormously from the application of the powerful approaches of molecular biochemistry, recombinant DNA technology, and molecular genetics. Gary Hayward and Wade Gibson, whom August recruited in 1976, shared his long-standing interest and expertise in the molecular biology of retroviruses.

Hayward's research was instrumental in elucidating the structure of the genomes of cytomegalovirus (CMV) and Epstein-Barr virus (EBV). His characterization and mapping of these genomes brought to light the unusual clusters of internal tandem repeats typical of the genomic organization of EBV, and the inverted repeats of CMV. In addition, he found extensive cross-homology between the herpesvirus (HSV) sequences and the repetitive elements of mammalian cell DNA. Hayward went on to construct complete libraries of DNA fragments for HSV, CMV, and EBV; the fragments were cloned in bacteria plasmids, making possible a new level of functional and sequence analysis of these complex viral genomes.

Through his pioneering functional studies of the herpesviruses, Hayward also developed a DNA transfection technique that made possible the functional analysis of specific elements controlling gene expression during both lytic infection and latency and reactivation.

Wade Gibson's interest in the synthesis, structure, and function of specific proteins of herpesviruses has complemented Hayward's research. Gibson chose to focus on CMV, a sexually transmitted agent associated not only with opportunistic infections but also with birth defects, neuromuscular disease (Charcot-Marie-Tooth syndrome) and malignancy (Kaposi sarcoma) as well. He identified and characterized four CMV proteins that play central roles in the life cycle of the virus, two with structural importance (matrix protein and assembly protein) and two with regulatory roles (an immediate-early protein, IE 94, and a DNA-binding protein).

Gibson also identified and characterized the molecular structure of CMV proteins (particularly enzymes) that might be appropriate targets for specific antiviral therapy and immunodiagnosis. In particular, he demonstrated that *D,L*-alpha-difluormethylornithine (DFMA) could block CMV replication in pretreated cells and was also effective against herpes simplex. Related work involved characterization of a virion-associated protein kinase and production of CMV-specific immunologic reagents for use in diagnosis and in studies of the expression of such proteins.

Immunopharmacology With the development of techniques for monoclonal antibody production, immunologic reagents have come to play a vital role in the diagnosis and treatment of infections and malignancy. A major contribution to the use of monoclonal antibodies for diagnosis and therapy of cancer was made by Mette Strand, who joined the pharmacology department in 1977. She developed techniques for conjugating derivatives of metal chelates (such as EDTA and DTPA) to immunoglobulins under conditions that preserved the antigen-binding capacity of the antibodies. Using these methods, she was able to obtain both positron and gamma camera images without subtraction or enhancement. She also demonstrated the applicability of these subjugation methods to radioimmunotherapy of tumors, using a murine erythroleukemia model system. Her approach employed short-range, highly potent alpha-emitting isotopes that could be targeted to malignant cells by chelation to tumor antigen-specific monoclonal antibodies; because of their short path lengths in tissue, these high-energy isotopes were much less damaging to the healthy tissue surrounding the tumor than were gamma emitters such as radioiodine.

Monoclonal antibodies have also been used by James Hildreth to characterize a number of specific surface antigens of human leukocytes. Hildreth, who was appointed to the faculty in 1987, brought with him a number of monoclonal antibodies he had prepared against human lymphoid cells and selected for their ability to inhibit specific immune functions *in vitro*. He obtained strong evidence to suggest that several of these antibodies could be useful clinically in the prevention of graft rejection. These include a series of antibodies that block Fc receptor function; several that identify CD44, a common human leukocyte antigen that appears to be involved in allograft rejection; and others that react with the leukocyte antigen LFA-1 and are highly immunosuppressive *in vitro*. These LFA-1-specific antibodies have already shown promise in clinical trials involving kidney transplant patients.

Molecular Biology of Cell Membranes   The essential functions carried out by cell membranes have only recently yielded to understanding at the molecular level. The pharmacology department has focused particularly on the involvement of membrane components in the essential processes of adhesion, ligand-specific binding, and immune recognition. The importance of cell adhesion in morphogenesis and the importance of differentiation in morphogenesis and immune function have been recognized for nearly a century. It is only in the past few decades, however, that the molecular events mediating these processes have begun to be identified. This information has immense importance for the control and treatment of malignancy, immune disorders, and developmental defects.

The department's progress in this area was significantly strengthened by the presence of Mette Strand and the recruitment of Ronald

Schnaar, who joined the faculty in 1979. An expert in the molecular dissection of carbohydrate-dependent cell adhesion, Schnaar developed "cell surface analogues," a major contribution to the study of cell-cell recognition. These analogues are plastic surfaces to which carbohydrates of defined composition are covalently attached in configurations that mimic their *in vivo* cell surface arrangement. Using these substrates, Schnaar demonstrated the ability of carbohydrates to elicit specific cell adhesion *in vitro*, finding that a number of cell types could selectively recognize and bind to specific carbohydrate-derivatized substrates and that the binding process resulted in altered cell behavior.

This system also allowed Schnaar to define the exquisite carbohydrate specificity underlying the adhesion process and to dissect the cell response into three steps. He then further refined his cell surface analogue by developing a new ligand-linker molecule for attaching the sugar ligand to the plastic surface by means of a cleavable disulfide bond. This permitted him to dissociate the cell-ligand complex from the plastic substrate and analyze the binding reaction at the molecular level.

Schnaar has applied his experimental system to the study of a number of mammalian cell types, including hepatocytes, macrophages, lymphocytes, and neural retinal cells. In nerve tissue, he has begun to identify the receptors involved in carbohydrate-based recognition and to examine the role of these recognition/binding processes in nerve cell development and differentiation.

The structure and function of cell surface molecules has also been a major interest of J. Thomas August, who uses monoclonal antibodies to isolate, purify, and characterize several molecules involved in the functional activities of mouse and human cells. These molecules include Pgp-1 (LY-24), a cell surface allodifferentiation antigen that is involved in adhesive interactions of cells and has the interesting property of acting as a specific marker of memory T cells; the alpha-2-macroglobulin receptor, a glycoprotein now implicated as the polyoma virus receptor and as a cell surface molecule involved in stimulating cell division; and lysosomal membrane glycoproteins (LAMPs), which are being used to study the biogenesis, structure, and function of lysosomes. LAMPs have amino acid sequences and biochemical properties highly similar to those of cell surface differentiation and oncogenesis markers detected on mouse and human tumor cell lines.

Mette Strand chose to examine surface membrane antigen expression and function in a very different system—in parasites of the genus *Schistosoma,* the causative organism in human schistosomiasis. This disease has represented a particular challenge for vaccine development because the organisms are able to survive and reproduce for decades within the infected individuals, despite their production of a measurable humoral and cellular immune response to the parasites. Strand addressed this problem by isolating the major surface antigens recognized by a panel of schistosome-specific monoclonal antibodies and identifying a series of "vaccine-specific" antigens that are particularly immunogenic in vaccinated mice. By use of recombinant DNA techniques, she isolated and cloned the gene encoding several of these surface antigens. She also sequenced a clone that appeared to encode schistosome myosin. This antigen was recognized by mouse sera that had been shown to be capable of passively transferring partial protection against challenge infection, a result that suggests that myosin expressed at the surface of the organism (an unprecedented occurrence) might serve as an important target of vaccine-induced immune attack. This discovery has direct significance for the development of a vaccine against schistosomiasis, a major goal in this field of research.

The research history of the Department of Pharmacology and Molecular Science provides a chronologic panorama of the rapid changes in the nature and substance of basic research over the past century. The advent of the new molecular biology has transformed the background and training of faculty members and altered the targets of scientific interest in this and other preclinical departments.

The Department of Physiological Chemistry

William M. Clark was succeeded as director of the Department of Physiological Chemistry in 1952 by Albert L. Lehninger. Lehninger's most important scientific contributions were his elucidation of oxidative phosphorylation and other energy-coupling mechanisms associated with the electron transport chain; his discovery of the importance of the mitochondrion in respiration and in the compartmentation of metabolism in the cell; and his findings concerning the role of mitochondria in regulating calcium distribution in cells and tissues, and in biologic calcification.[222]

Lehninger's success rested on his development in 1948 of the sucrose procedure for centrifugal recovery of cell organelles. Lehninger and his graduate student Eugene P. Kennedy (who later became professor of biological chemistry at Harvard) were able to find, only weeks after the sucrose method was described, that the mitochondrial function of liver cells contained virtually all the organized oxidative activity of the cell. This basic discovery started a new direction in biochemistry—an awareness of the metabolic role of intracellular structure and of highly organized enzyme complexes, at a time when the conventional goal of most enzymologists was to discard "cell debris" and to solubilize and purify enzymes as chemical entities.

Shortly after moving to Baltimore, Lehninger (with Sigurd Olaf Nielsen) demonstrated that one of the three respiratory chain phosphorylations occurs on electron transport from cytochrome C to oxygen. With another colleague, Bengt Borgstrom, Lehninger showed that two phosphorylations occur between NADH and cytochrome C. Lehninger's discovery in 1951 that NADH cannot pass through the membrane of intact mitochondria was a crucial element in his demonstration that oxidative phosphorylation occurs during electron transport. Lehninger emphasized that failure of NADH to pass through the membrane effectively compartmentalizes the nicotinamide adenine dinucleotide of the cell into cytosolic and mitochondrial pools. Moreover, he showed that NADH formed by glycolysis could not directly enter the mitochondria and indicated that some other pathway was required, one that would necessarily be crucially important to the integration and regulation of glycolysis and respiration. These findings began a new era in the understanding of cell metabolism.

Lehninger was one of the earliest students of respiratory energy coupling to consider ion transport as an important means of energy conservation by mitochondria. Studies with James Gamble on potassium ion transport revealed a rapid incorporation of potassium ion into respiring mitochondria and submitochondrial vesicles. Later, following the observations by his associate Frank Vasington that calcium ions are rapidly accumulated by a respiring mitochondrion, Lehninger and Carlo S. Rossi carried out a classic study of the stoichiometric relationship between the number of calcium ions transported into the mitochondrial matrix and the number of electrons flowing from substrate oxygen. They were the first to report stoichiometric coupling of ion transport to electron flow in mitochondria, finding that two calcium ions passed each of the three energy-conserving sites of the respiratory chain. Similarly, they showed that ATP hydrolysis led to calcium ion uptake. They also discovered that phosphate is accumulated together with the calcium ion and defined the quantitative relationship between the uptake of calcium ions, the uptake of phosphate, electron flow, and respiratory activation by calcium ions.

With his colleagues Rossi and John W. Greenawalt, Lehninger had observed that accumulation of calcium and phosphate by isolated mitochondria leads to formation of electron-dense insoluble deposits in the mitochondrial matrix, which could be visualized by electron microscopy. These deposits of calcium phosphate, which x-ray diffraction revealed to be amorphous, appeared to be involved in the biologic process of calcification. Lehninger assembled his evidence into a general hypothesis of biologic calcification.

As department director, Lehninger extended the accomplishments of his two predecessors. His

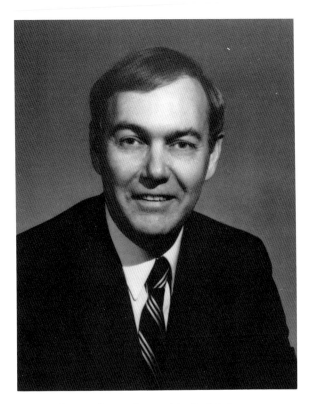

M. Daniel Lane. (*Source:* Leonard L. Greif, Jr.)

own accomplishments included sole authorship of a comprehensive textbook of general biochemistry. In an era of specialization, he may have been the last scientist to write such a volume singlehandedly.

Lehninger's successor as director was Malcolm Daniel Lane, who arrived in 1978. Lane intended to bring the department into the forefront of research in the rapidly developing areas of molecular biology and cell regulation, while maintaining a rigorous underpinning of basic biochemistry. Under his direction, "the Department of Physiological Chemistry" became "the Department of Biological Chemistry." He recruited six young assistant professors (Gerald Hart, Barbara Sollner-Webb, Leroy Liu, Peter Devreotes, Don Cleveland, and David Shortle), each of whom has achieved international prominence in his or her respective area of research.

Before moving to Hopkins, Lane was most widely known for his work on enzymatic CO_2 fixation, studies he continued well into the 1970s.

He made his most important contributions to the field of regulatory biochemistry, however, after he joined the faculty at Hopkins.

As is often the case in basic research, Lane was led into this area by questions raised in previous studies. In this instance, Lane's question was: Is the lipogenic process regulated in living cells as predicted by his *in vitro* studies with purified acetyl-CoA carboxylase? To test his hypothesis, Lane and his colleagues developed two model cell culture systems, the chick hepatocyte and the mouse preadipocyte. The wisdom of conducting these experiments in parallel with studies at the molecular level was borne out over the next decade.[223]

During the early and mid-1980s, Lane and his group made several significant discoveries. They found the precise mechanism whereby glucagon (acting via cyclic AMP) reciprocally regulated fatty acid biosynthesis and ketogenesis in the chick hepatocyte. The site of control of fatty acid synthesis was proved to be acetyl-CoA carboxylase, which oscillates between an inactive monomeric form, in the presence of glucagon, and active polymeric filaments in the absence of the hormone. Lane's laboratory simultaneously discovered that the set of enzymes that carry out the identical initial steps of ketogenesis and cholesterogenesis are not only independently regulated but are also located in different intracellular compartments.

Lane's group also described the pathway by which very low density lipoprotein (VLDL) is assembled as it traverses the secretory system of the hepatocyte. VLDL is the precursor of low-density lipoprotein (LDL) and major carrier of plasma triglyceride, the product of hepatic lipogenesis.

In another area, Lane and his colleagues made pioneering contributions in elucidating the role of the insulin receptor in mediating the cellular actions of insulin. They defined the mechanism by which cells control the level of their receptor and thereby regulate cellular responsiveness to insulin. In a now-classic series of articles, they defined the complicated posttranslational processing pathway the proreceptor must undergo during its long journey to the cell surface where it functions. More recently, they discovered a cellular protein target of the insulin receptor kinase, which appears to mediate the multiple actions of insulin—most important, the activation of glucose uptake.

Lane and his group also defined the differentiation program during which the mouse preadipocyte undergoes conversion (in cell culture) into cells possessing the biochemical and morphologic characteristics of adipocytes. Their systematic approach laid the groundwork for the subsequent isolation and sequencing of several genes that undergo differentiation-induced expression. Specific regulatory regions of these genes were identified and studied to define the precise mechanism or mechanisms responsible for the coordinate activation of their expression.

The recent contrasting trends of uniformity and differentiation in research have populated laboratories with investigators whose skills and perspective are at once narrower and broader than those of investigators of the past. In Welch's laboratory of a century ago, a relatively small number of scientists, all of whom shared a basically similar store of information, worked on comparatively general problems. In contrast, today's scientific investigation requires a large and specialized faculty, each of whom is expert in a particular, and comparatively restricted, area of knowledge.

At the same time, there has been a remarkable convergence of research in all departments of the medical school. The boundaries between biological chemistry, pharmacology, and molecular science, cell biology and anatomy, and physiology have become increasingly blurred. As a result, faculty members often hold appointments in more than one department, either simultaneously or sequentially. The separation between clinical and preclinical departments has become so indistinct that the director of pediatrics at Hopkins, John W. Littlefield, later became director of physiology.

These two trends, uniformity and differentiation, thrive in the traditional Hopkins atmosphere of professional camaraderie. Some miss

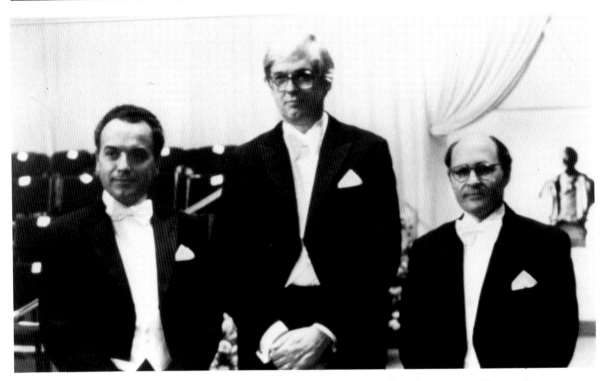

Nobel Laureates, 1978. *Left to right,* Werner Arber, Hamilton O. Smith, and Daniel Nathans. (*Source:* Alan M. Chesney Medical Archives, The Johns Hopkins Medical Institutions.)

the days when the faculty was small enough to allow you to greet by name all those you passed in the main hospital corridor. Despite growth and change, however, the "sweet spirit of the place," in Osler's words, remains to unify the hospital and medical school, as it has for one hundred years.

Daniel Nathans and Hamilton O. Smith: Recipients of the Nobel Prize for Physiology or Medicine

Daniel Nathans and Hamilton O. Smith of Johns Hopkins, and Werner Arber of Switzerland, won the Nobel Prize in 1978 for their discovery of restriction enzymes and the application of these enzymes in the study of molecular genetics. The use of recombinant DNA for cloning human genes depends on these site-specific restriction endonucleases, which cut the DNA into pieces of predictable size. These pieces can then be used to determine the sequence of genes on chromo-

somes and to analyze the chemical structure of genes and of regions of DNA that regulate their function. Restriction enzymes also provide the starting point for the creation of new combinations of genes. The discoveries of Nathans, Smith, and Arber opened up new avenues to the study of the organization and expression of genes and provided the opportunity to solve basic problems in developmental biology. Recombinant DNA techniques for cloning human genes, which are now in such widespread use, also stem from their work.[224]

Arber hypothesized that restriction enzymes bind to DNA at specific sites containing recurring structural elements composed of specific base-pair sequences. Smith discovered the first site-specific restriction enzyme in the late 1960s, while investigating the ability of bacterial cells to take up "naked" DNA from the surrounding medium. He showed that these cells produce a substance that cuts the double-stranded DNA molecule at specific sites, and recognized that he was dealing with the site-specific enzyme formulated earlier by Arber. Smith verified this idea by isolating a purified bacterial restriction enzyme and showing that it separated DNA in the middle of a specific symmetrical sequence.[225] Smith later found these restriction enzymes useful for studying the mechanisms by which proteins recognize and then interact with specific sequences in DNA.

Smith's finding was the basis of Nathans' work on the mapping of DNA. Nathans employed these site-specific restriction enzymes to isolate specific chromosome segments from the DNA of simian virus 40. He then mapped the genes of this tumor virus, which made it possible to identify the genes required for manufacture of the tumor-producing protein. Nathans' group also used site-specific restriction enzymes to create mutations in the chromosome of the simian virus in order to demonstrate how the viral genes are regulated.[226]

Concluding Comments

Probably no contribution for which the Nobel Prize has been awarded in recent years has had more influence on medical research than the work of Werner Arber, Daniel Nathans, and Hamilton O. Smith. Their discovery and application of restriction enzymes marked the beginning of a new era in medicine, the era of recombinant DNA. As the scalpel for dissecting the human genome, restriction enzymes are at the center of most research in molecular genetics. Cutting the DNA into fragments of manageable size is the first step in cloning a gene, and cloning itself can be the first step in delineating the changes that occur in disease. Cloning has permitted the preparation of DNA probes that can be used in prenatal diagnosis and the detection of carriers, and the synthesis of therapeutic agents in bacteria. Examples of such therapeutic agents are insulin, growth hormone, and tissue plasminogen activator.

This new era of molecular genetics is analogous to the bacteriologic era of almost precisely a century earlier. Discoveries in bacteriology not only produced technological innovations that led to an increased understanding of diagnosis and treatment but also utterly changed physicians' and the public's perceptions of health and disease. One hundred and fifty years ago, asthma, dropsy, jaundice, and anemia were thought of as diseases in their own right. As scientific knowledge advanced, physicians realized that these disorders had varied causes.

In his 1929 monograph *Nosography,* Knut Faber pointed out the influence of bacteriology and of mendelism on the perception of disease. The credit that Faber gave to Mendel was only the beginning of the influence of genetic knowledge on nosology, or the classification of diseases, for this knowledge of molecular genetics has fundamentally altered nosologic ideas. The clearest example of the recent clarification of nosologic thought may be the classification of cancer as somatic cell genetic disease. The ability to define specific lesions in DNA associated with specific types of neoplasia led to the conclusion that these changes, which often occur in multiple steps, in the aggregate represent the truly basic cause of the cancer.

Restriction enzymes are fundamental to efforts to map and sequence the entire human genome, providing the fragments for analysis and sequencing. Variation in cutting by these site-specific endonucleases results in variations from person to person in the length of fragments produced, simply because people vary, to some extent, in the nucleotides they have at specific sites. This form of variation, called "restriction fragment length polymorphism" (RFLP) has been a powerful tool: these polymorphisms have been used as linkage markers for mapping chromosomes and in making diagnoses by the linkage principle.

Huntington disease, for example, was the first of a considerable number of genetic disorders of unknown biochemical basis that were mapped to specific chromosome sites through discovery of linkage to one of these DNA markers. This linkage is the basis of the program of Susan and Marshall Folstein, faculty members in the Departments of Medicine, and Psychiatry and Behavioral Sciences at Johns Hopkins, who were able to diagnose Huntington disease before the person at risk developed the abnormality. In both white and black families with Huntington disease, and in those with somewhat atypical clinical presentations, the Folsteins were able to confirm the linkage of the disease to markers on the end of the short arm of chromosome 4. The Folsteins used the principle of linkage in both preclinical and prenatal diagnosis of Huntington disease.

In the study of the thalassemias, Haig Kazazian of the Department of Pediatrics used combinations of RFLPs to define the mutations that underlie the many different forms of thalassemia and to diagnose the disorder. Similarly, Bert Vogelstein and his colleagues at the Oncology Center used RFLPs to define specific DNA changes in colon cancer and other malignancies.

The use of DNA technology by these and other members of the clinical departments points up the pervasive applicability of molecular genetics to the study of disease during the last decade. In the study of development, for example, members of the Department of Physiology use molecular genetic methods, including transgenic mice, i.e., mice derived from fertilized eggs into which human or other genes have been injected. Although some scientists view this emphasis on molecular genetics as excessive—detrimental to consideration of the organism as a whole—it is

difficult to identify any department not touched by its influence.

The more one understands about the principles that govern life, the closer together the various disciplines of medical science are drawn. Not only have the boundaries between the preclinical sciences become less and less distinct, but the same is true of the boundaries between the preclinical and the clinical sciences as these fundamental approaches are applied to the study of disease. Nature's experiments, as exemplified by human disease processes, often provide insights that would not be appreciated in the study of the normal individual. Medical research today is approaching a unity that Pasteur appreciated long ago:

> There does not exist a category of science to which one can give the name applied science. There are science and the applications of science, bound together as the fruit to the tree which bears it.[227]

A century of discovery at Johns Hopkins represents the achievement of the goal set by John Shaw Billings in 1889—that the hospital and medical school produce investigators as well as practitioners, "to give the world men who can not only sail by the old charts but who can make new and better ones for the use of others."

EPILOGUE

President Gilman . . . I congratulate you, sir, on the prodigious advancement of medical teaching, which has resulted from the labors of the Johns Hopkins faculty of medicine. The twenty-five years just past are the most extraordinary twenty-five years in the whole history of our race. Nothing is done as it was done twenty-five years ago; the whole social and industrial organization of our country has changed; the whole university organization of our country has changed; but among all the changes there is none greater than that wrought in the development of medical teaching and research; and these men whom you, sir, summoned here have led the way.

—President Charles W. Eliot of Harvard, 1901

The Johns Hopkins Hospital and the Johns Hopkins University School of Medicine developed as models of their kind not because they produced a succession of medical, scientific, and educational "firsts," but because it was at Hopkins that several key ideas were first gathered together and implemented in one place.

Most important was the central academic theme of graduate training within a research-centered environment. This presupposed more stringent entrance requirements for students, as inadequately prepared students could not benefit from the advanced training offered. It also led to new approaches to teaching, as the principles of "self-education" and "learning by doing" removed students from the lecture halls and placed them in the laboratories and wards. The hospital was easily accessible to students because of the unique link between it and the medical school, the administrative structure that placed the same individual at the head of a clinical department in both institutions. To obtain the best professors for this research-centered environment, the ones who would attract the best graduate students, it was necessary to expand the arena of choice by eliminating the provincialism that characterized most medical faculties. Professors at Johns Hopkins were therefore brought from around the world. Once they arrived, it was important that they be able to devote their full time to carrying out their investigations, free from the need to augment their income by caring for patients. Ideally, the medical school and hospital would provide the faculty member's entire livelihood. Thus the system of so-called full-time professorships was inaugurated, first in the preclinical sciences and later in the clinical departments. Finally, to extend the growth of scientific investigation, Hopkins developed the principle of exporting its graduates as teachers, investigators, and administrators.

In the late nineteenth century, these were unorthodox approaches to the problems and responsibilities of American medicine. Their remarkableness was not diminished by the fact that isolated changes had been tried at other hospitals and medical schools. The crucial difference at Hopkins was their aggregate effect, the result of the modification of each idea by the others.

As important as the ideas to be implemented was the timing of their implementation. Historian Richard Shryock remarked that if Daniel C. Gilman, the first president of the Johns Hopkins University, had been given the opportunity to create the university fifty years earlier, he could not have been successful.[1] In the late 1800s, however, the time was right for the creation of the Johns Hopkins Hospital and the Johns Hopkins University School of Medicine: it was time for an explosion of progress.

It was George Rosen, professor of public health and a historian of medicine, who characterized the advance of medical science as a series of "explosion phenomena."[2] He borrowed a phrase applied by Walter W. Rostow to economic development, "take-off into sustained growth," to describe the crescendo from a period of relative inactivity to a "critical explosive level." Arnold R. Rich used a similar concept, the alternation of "quiescence" and "flux," to describe the history of medical education.[3] He later expanded this idea to include almost all human endeavor. The most important periods of flux, according to Rich, originate in a widespread, spontaneous feeling that the existing form of any enterprise is inadequate to permit the best expression of its purposes. This feeling intensifies; thought and energy are extensively applied to render the form of endeavor more suitable to current demands or expectations. As participants experiment, changes— often unduly radical or reactionary—are tested freely. Finally, a modified form comes to be regarded as enough of an improvement to permit a temporary relaxation of activity. Another period of quiescence ensues, during which the outward form of the activity remains relatively static. Inactivity at these times is only apparent, however, since imperceptible changes may be occurring that will lead a new generation to find the outlines, laws, or dimensions that will form the basis of a new period of flux.

The events surrounding the creation of the Johns Hopkins Hospital and the School of Medicine illustrate Rosen and Rich's models. The quiet growth of knowledge and interest in bacteriology reached a critical level in about 1880. It was followed by the explosive discovery, within little more than a decade, of the bacterial cause of many diseases. Coincidentally, in the last quarter of the nineteenth century, there was great dissatis-faction with the state of medical education and medical practice in the United States. A group of enthusiastic young medical scientists recognized the revolutionary changes in medical research under way in Germany and were determined to improve the situation by making it possible to provide for similar activities here. These events took place just as the Hopkins epic was unfolding.

The founding of the hospital and medical school also coincided with the growth of private wealth in the United States. Johns Hopkins' bequest was the largest endowment for medical purposes up to that time. It made several innovations possible: the medical school could pay professors, restrict class size, and establish clinical facilities under faculty control.

Johns Hopkins supplied more than merely the financial wherewithal, however. He also provided the philosophical structure. His decision to found both an educational and a medical enterprise—a university and a hospital—was crucial, as was his designation of the relationship between these two organizations, which were linked by overlapping boards of trustees. This is spelled out in his statement to the hospital trustees: "In all your arrangements in relation to this hospital, you will bear constantly in mind that it is my wish and purpose that the institutions should ultimately form part of the medical school of that university for which I have made ample provision in my will."

As early as 1885, a joint committee of trustees of the university and hospital devised the plan to give the directors of the clinical departments full responsibility for their department in both the hospital and the medical school. This plan was unusual for the time. Most hospitals were staffed by local practitioners, who controlled staff privileges and policies, and teaching was not generally considered a part of the hospital's responsibilities. At Johns Hopkins, in contrast, the unified organizational structure gave the hospital the professional services of the teachers in the medical school while providing the medical school with advantages for clinical training unexcelled at the time.

Many of the innovations that characterized

the hospital and medical school depended on the close connection specified by their founder, and educational programs impossible in medical schools without an affiliated hospital were carried out smoothly at Hopkins. In contrast, most medical schools lacked the authority to place students on wards as clinical clerks, and the permission of hospital boards was frequently difficult to obtain. Clinical research in such medical schools was hampered by the same difficulties. Hopkins became the first medical school to make "learning by doing" a matter of stated policy—and then carry that policy out—because of this link between hospital and medical school. Other schools offered bits and pieces of self-education for medical students; others recognized the importance of clinical experience but, lacking control of a teaching hospital, were unable to execute it.

In ensuring that the hospital would be linked to the medical school and the medical school to the university as a whole, Johns Hopkins created a powerful complex that would have a basic and enduring influence on medical care, medical education, and medical research in the United States. Along with the two boards of trustees, President Gilman and John Shaw Billings, his consultant, established the principles to realize the founder's intent. And the early faculty—particularly William H. Welch, Franklin P. Mall, and William Osler—devised the procedures that were the concrete representations of these principles.

The specific execution of Johns Hopkins' general idea thus reflected a unified vision, extending from the founder through the faculty, residents, and students. Those who implemented the plan were not simply following directives; their belief in the principles underlying the hospital and medical school unified all who worked and studied there. The resulting harmony, the sense of collegiality that remains to this day, was explored by Alan Gregg at the commemoration of Welch's 100th birthday:

I suggest that something extraordinarily precious comes out of the close but entirely free association of really superior people. To this emergent quality I give the name—the heritage of excellence, mostly because it lasts so long and because it never comes

from, nor appeals to, mediocrities. . . . By really superior people I mean persons so spirited and yet so balanced, so gifted and yet so incomplete, so mature and yet so eager that they can remain in close contact with but a few of their kind and yet experience no surfeit, boredom or friction.

The exact nature of the contacts between a few absolutely first-rate people is completely unpredictable except in point of its astonishing quality. All you can know about it in advance is that it will be memorable and that it will spread outward and afterward. This almost unearthly and certainly intangible product of the interchange between superior persons cannot be seen but it can be felt and truly like an atmosphere it can be breathed. Indeed, it is an inspiration. . . .

What Welch and his colleagues did and believed and wrote is not as important now—nor anywhere near as important—as the heritage of excellence their contacts with each other have left us.[4]

Most important to the development of the hospital and medical school was the success of their parent university. The Johns Hopkins University was the first modern university in this country, the first to adopt the European idea of university education. Gilman is credited with introducing this system into the United States—a system that recognized the importance of research and insisted that all its faculty be investigators. As he wrote:

When this university began, it was a common complaint, still uttered in many places, that the ablest teachers were absorbed in routine and were forced to spend their strength in the discipline of tyros, so that they had no time for carrying forward their studies or for adding to human knowledge. Here the position was taken at the outset that the chief professors should have ample time to carry on the higher work for which they have shown themselves qualified, and also that younger men, as they gave evidence of uncommon qualities, should likewise be encouraged to devote themselves to study. Even those who were candidates for degrees were taught what was meant by profitable investigation. They were shown how to discover the limits of the known; how to extend, even by minute accretions, the realm of knowledge; how to co-operate with other men in the prosecution of inquiry; and how to record in exact language, and on the printed page, the results attained. Investigation has thus been among us the duty of every leading professor, and he has been the guide and inspirer of fellows and pupils, whose work may not bear his name, but whose results are truly products of the inspiration and guidance which he has freely bestowed.[5]

Gilman's views were nevertheless controversial. The presidents of Harvard, Michigan, and Cornell Universities cautioned him against emphasizing graduate studies, believing that the United States was not ready for a school that went beyond college or technical education. Only Gilman envisioned graduate training and research as processes that could be undertaken here at once.

It was Gilman who emphasized "learning by doing," a particular method of education that required the student to acquire knowledge rather than receive it passively. "Learning by doing" was implemented through small classes and individualized laboratory work. The method was intended to teach students how to create new knowledge, not simply to inculcate them with a fixed body of accumulated information. It was better to teach students how to learn and how to continue the process of self-education after formal schooling was over.

Nor was the idea of education limited to those formally recognized as students. The faculty and students were linked by graduate assistants, and as "all one body," in Gilman's words, all were engaged in the pursuit of knowledge. By providing fellowships and assistantships to attract well-qualified applicants, Gilman created training opportunities that had previously been available only in Europe.

Gilman saw as one of the great opportunities of the new university the chance to disseminate critical scholarship in the United States by sending Hopkins' graduates to faculty positions in other institutions. Later, the export of Hopkins-trained physicians would become a notable feature of the hospital and medical school. Setting the pattern for the export of graduates was the biology laboratory of Henry Newell Martin, established in 1876 as the first medical science laboratory at Johns Hopkins and one of the two real centers of research in physiology at the time.

Many of Martin's fellows achieved eminence at medical schools across the country. Four joined the Johns Hopkins medical school's first faculty—William T. Councilman in pathology, William Henry Howell in physiology, John Jacob Abel in pharmacology, and Ross G. Harrison in anatomy.

The same emphasis upon research and advanced instruction that Gilman created at the Johns Hopkins University became the keystone of the program of medical education and medical research when the Johns Hopkins Hospital opened in 1889 and the Johns Hopkins University School of Medicine opened in 1893. As advisor to Gilman and the hospital and university trustees, John Shaw Billings was appointed to design the hospital buildings in 1876, the year the university opened. He could not begin, however, until he knew how the hospital buildings were to be used, and he helped to develop the educational policies that would underlie their construction. The hospital buildings were therefore planned with special reference to their utility for higher medical education and research. The hospital was also intended to represent the best in hospital construction of the day, particularly with regard to sanitary arrangements, heating, ventilation, and other facilities to encourage cleanliness and prevent the spread of disease.

When Billings began his formal consideration of plans for the medical school in 1877, the year after the university opened, he gave a series of lectures about medical education at the university. One talk asked the question, In view of the present condition of medical education in this country, how should the Johns Hopkins University organize its medical school? Billings' answer emphasized the desirability of establishing a medical course that would give students abundant opportunity to observe disease in the patient at the bedside. Because the hospital would be limited in its capacity to allow bedside instruction, the medical school should limit its classes to twenty-five students. Billings also stressed the idea that the medical school should educate students to add to medicine's store of knowledge, not simply to absorb what was already known.

Thirteen years elapsed between the start of

construction and the opening of the hospital. The delay was caused by the trustees' conservative financial approach. The best hospital, one that would meet all the requirements of the new program in medical education and research, was a costly proposition. In an example of Quaker prudence, however, the trustees would not touch the endowment's capital; they would spend only the annual income for hospital construction. Consequently, the building proceeded year by year, halting when each year's funds were exhausted.

Paradoxically, the delay was an example of the good fortune to which Abraham Flexner referred when he invoked the importance of chance in the creation of the Hopkins model. Although, at the time, the delay was a source of distress to all involved, in retrospect, the years that elapsed between the beginning of hospital construction and the admission of the first patient gave Gilman and Billings the time to establish the educational plan that would be put into effect when the medical school opened, and to begin to identify those individuals who would best fit their ideals as research professors.

Although the hospital opened in 1889, the medical school was not ready until four years later. The failure of the Baltimore and Ohio Railroad, whose stock represented almost half of Johns Hopkins' endowment, diminished the amount of money available to the university. It was only the substantial sum offered by the national Women's Fund Committee, led by M. Carey Thomas and Mary Garrett, that enabled the medical school to open in 1893. This bequest came with two important stipulations: women had to be admitted to the medical school on equal terms with men, and all entering medical students were required to have a bachelor's degree and a knowledge of French and German. This insistence on intellectual excellence affirmed the ideas of the medical school's founding faculty, set forth almost a decade earlier.

The founding faculty of the medical school, appointed in 1883, ten years before the school opened, consisted of Billings, Martin, and Ira Remsen (professor of chemistry at the university). In a series of three meetings the following year,

they drew up concrete plans for the medical school, which included several features that were novel for the time. Admissions requirements would include knowledge of French and German as well as knowledge of physics, chemistry, biology, physiology, and histology. The curriculum would encourage research, and laboratories would be established for the study of such subjects as physiology, pathological anatomy and histology, pharmacology, and public health. They also decided to establish a program of fellowships, based on the system already in place in the university. These awards would be given to graduate students, and their holders would not be permitted to engage in private medical practice. Instead, clinical fellows would be given room and board in the hospital so that they could devote themselves to the study of patients; and fellows in preclinical fields would work in the laboratories.

None of these first three men actually served on the faculty of the medical school. Nine years elapsed between their series of meetings and the opening of the medical school, and by then all three had assumed other positions.

The first active member of the medical school faculty was William H. Welch, who was appointed professor of pathology in 1884. In keeping with the idea that the hospital was part of the university, he established a laboratory in the hospital in 1886, even before the hospital was opened for patients. This Pathological Laboratory was the first site of research in the Johns Hopkins Hospital. Here were gathered a brilliant group of young scientists for advanced study. Welch's students included William S. Halsted, Franklin P. Mall, Lewellys F. Barker, and J. Whitridge Williams, all of whom became department heads at Hopkins, as well as many others who made notable contributions elsewhere. Among them were Walter Reed and James Carroll, who discovered the cause of yellow fever.

The heads of the clinical departments were brought from around the country. William Osler and Howard A. Kelly came from Philadelphia to head the Departments of Medicine and Gynecology, respectively; Halsted, who had come to Welch's laboratory from New York, remained to become head of the Department of Surgery. Hopkins' policy of obtaining its medical school faculty from outside its immediate environs was a novel idea in the 1880s. In other medical schools, faculty members were drawn from the pool of local physicians, who taught the preclinical sciences while continuing to practice medicine. Hospitals and medical schools were responsible for appointing their own staffs, and medical schools found it difficult at the time to appoint clinical professors from other communities because they would have no access to hospital beds for teaching and research. The decision at Hopkins to make appointments based on qualifications alone signaled the end of provincialism in the selection of faculty members.

Plans for the medical school were thus well under way long before the hospital was ready. Had the hospital been envisioned merely as a facility for the care of patients, this planning would have been premature. Furthermore, the trustees would have had the hospital constructed more cheaply and opened it sooner. Instead, the hospital was seen as a part of the medical school; with Billings' help, Gilman and the trustees organized the hospital as the clinical laboratory of the medical school. Welch later attributed the success of the Hopkins residency program to this educational partnership between the hospital and the medical school, saying, "The list of those who have been resident physicians, surgeons, gynecologists and obstetricians will help you to realize that this has been one of the distinctive features of our organization. Such provision for the higher grades was in large measure due to the fact that the Hospital was started before the Medical School opened. The Hospital was therefore an educational institution."[6]

Like the delay in the opening of the hospital, the delay in the opening of the medical school was, in retrospect, beneficial. It gave Welch's laboratory time to become established as a mecca for aspiring young scientists. Among them were future Hopkins faculty members, the next leaders of the two institutions. This four-year hiatus also gave the clinical chiefs time to organize their services in the hospital, to set the unique residency

training program in motion, and to gain experience in teaching with a limited number of postgraduate students. By the time the first class of medical students reached the clinical years, in 1895, the hospital was well prepared to integrate them into its organization.

Welch pointed out that the fate of the hospital and medical school might have been very different had both institutions opened simultaneously: "When I was appointed it was intended to proceed with the selection of other members of the medical faculty, so as to be ready to open the school at the same time that the hospital was opened, which it was thought then would be in two or three years. Then came the financial difficulties due to failure of the B. & O. to pay dividends on the stock, and I found myself somewhat stranded as regards medical teaching and human autopsies. If we had been able to proceed, say in 1885 or 1886, with the selection of other members of the Faculty we should probably have missed Mall, Abel, Halsted, Kelly and, above all, Osler."[7]

Even with the faculty in place, this second delay could have brought disaster—other institutions were courting Welch and Osler while they waited for the medical school to open—but it was a blessing in disguise. Vital tasks were completed that would have been more difficult to carry out with the first class of medical students in place. In sum, the two periods of waiting allowed the Hopkins innovations to crystallize.

The educational programs devised by both the preclinical and the clinical faculty reflected many of Gilman's precepts. Like Gilman, John Shaw Billings was a key proponent of "learning by doing." As Billings expressed the idea, "an important part of the higher education of modern times is the teaching how to increase knowledge; and the best way of teaching this, as of many other things, is by doing it and by causing pupils to do it."[8] In both the preclinical and the clinical sciences, "doing" required the use of all the senses, not just the ears.

Learning by doing was emphasized in the first two (preclinical) years of medical school by study in the laboratory. Elsewhere at the time, these subjects were taught mostly by textbooks and lectures, a system that Welch termed very defective. Welch believed that students could learn the fundamental importance of accurate observation and experiment only in the laboratory, and not through didactic lectures and recitations based on textbooks.

The medical school curriculum was a novel program that gave serious attention to all the preclinical sciences. Anatomy, which for centuries had been the only subject taught in the laboratory, was joined at Johns Hopkins by four preclinical sciences: physiology, pharmacology, pathology, and physiological chemistry.

The clinical departments also emphasized original work along with advancing the quality of practice and enhancing the educational process. Osler's approaches to instruction in medicine were unusual at the time. The importance of accurate history-taking and physical examination had been generally recognized, but Osler was also one of the first to introduce systematized courses of instruction in these skills. Osler established clinical laboratories next to the wards. In these laboratories, students in their final two (clinical) years were taught to apply the laboratory methods of chemistry, physics, and biology to the study of patients. Instruction in the principles of these methods was followed by drill in their application, and each student became skilled in all the important aspects of clinical examination of the blood and other body constituents. In this endeavor, Osler said, students began to regard the microscope as a clinical tool, not as a mere toy.[9]

Osler also devised the clinical clerkship, a form of "learning by doing" that Welch identified as one of Hopkins' most important contributions to medical education. The clinical clerkship extended the principle of preceptorships, which themselves had derived from the apprenticeships of medieval times. It was more than a teaching device: unlike ward classes, the clinical clerkship constituted part of the regular, orderly machinery of the hospital. The students' feeling of responsibility on realizing that the facts they had collected had contributed to the patient's diagnosis and treatment were important to their development as physicians. Moreover, the clinical clerkship also contributed to the welfare of patients: by performing necessary procedures, students assumed responsibility for part of the patients' care.

Other schools had created experiences for the students on the hospital wards, but it was not until Osler reached Hopkins that conditions were ideal for the establishment of the modern clinical clerkship. Here he could put in place, for the first time, a systematized clerkship. Because the same individuals were department heads in the hospital and the medical school, the hospital was open to students as a teaching facility. Class sizes were small, so that all students could participate in instruction at the bedside.

This emphasis on an equally excellent education for all students was also a novel idea at the time. Four paths were open to medical students in the United States who wished to supplement the generally mediocre education available at proprietary medical schools. One choice was an apprenticeship with a practicing physician. Not surprisingly, the educational quality of apprenticeships varied widely, depending on the preceptor's competence and willingness to teach and supervise. Another possibility was attendance at a non-degree-granting medical school (these operated during summer vacations, when degree-granting schools were not in session). A third alternative was service in a hospital as a "house pupil," either before or after receiving the medical degree. House pupils were usually the elite, selected by competitive examination, and they lived in the hospital and managed cases. The fourth choice was study abroad, usually after the student had completed the regular course of medical lectures. Here, too, the possibilities for an excellent education were limited. At the eminent British teaching hospitals, a student aristocracy held the positions that offered a close relationship to patients and the opportunity for laboratory research. In France, hospital residencies were reserved for a few, who were chosen by examination. In Germany, medical students were excluded from the laboratory, as opportunities for research were limited to advanced students. At Hopkins, however, every student could participate in laboratory work, and every student became an essential part of the hospital wards. The Hopkins system thus adapted European ideas to an egalitarian American setting, and it standardized medical education in the United States.[10]

Osler believed that the education of medical students was among the greatest achievements of the Johns Hopkins Hospital. "A type of medical school was to be created new to this country," he said, "in which teacher and student alike should be in the fighting line. That is lesson number one of our first quarter century, judged by which we stand or fall. And lesson number two was the demonstration that the student of medicine has his place in the hospital as part of its machinery just as much as in the anatomical laboratory, and that to combine successfully in his education practice with science, the academic freedom of the university must be transplanted to the hospital."[11]

After graduation, medical students often remained at Hopkins as fellows and residents, the medical school's counterparts to the university's graduate students. Before the opening of the Johns Hopkins Hospital, opportunities for in-hospital, post-internship training in medical or surgical specialties were unknown in the United States. As in the university, the unique clinical residencies established by Osler, Kelly, and Halsted bridged the gap between the faculty and the medical students, forming a continuum that united the care of patients, the advancement of medical knowledge, and the continuing education of all three groups. The average length of service and other features differed somewhat between the clinical services, but the total arrangement added up to a graduate school within the hospital. The value of the system was indicated by its eventual adoption in practically all teaching hospitals. The presence of these residents led to better patient care and also contributed to the high quality of the educational program for medical students. Both fellows and residents extended the spectrum of postgraduate education from pure "bench" science to specialized clinical training, and these programs contributed substantially to Johns Hopkins' preeminence as an institution dedicated to the advancement of scientific and clinical knowledge.

Both Welch and Billings were strong advocates of a new type of American medical school—a center of basic as well as applied science. Their object was to train investigators as well as practitioners, scientists who could relate the growing knowledge in the preclinical fields to the study of disease in the clinical departments. Welch agreed with the view that little research would be done if the preclinical sciences were taught by local practitioners, as was the case in most schools at that time. All the preclinical science professors at Hopkins were therefore appointed to so-called full-time positions. Their salaries were paid by the university, and they were thus able to devote all their time to research and teaching, without the need to care for patients.

Although a few full-time preclinical chairs existed in medical schools nationwide, Johns Hopkins was the first medical school in the United States to place all of its preclinical departments on a full-time basis. Like Osler's clinical clerkships, full-time professorships became a regular feature of the medical school. This decision professionalized the preclinical departments, first at Johns Hopkins and then nationwide as the system spread to other medical schools. The success of the research activities in Welch's Department of Pathology, Franklin P. Mall's Department of Anatomy, John Jacob Abel's Department of Pharmacology, William H. Howell's Department of Physiology, and Walter Jones' Department of Physiological Chemistry substantiated the wisdom of organizing these departments on a full-time basis.

By the turn of the century, a preclinical scientist could secure a position as a teacher and a director of a laboratory in his special branch of science, but the clinical sciences were still undeveloped. American hospitals in general did not offer similar opportunities for training in the clinical sciences, and even for those who were trained, the prospect of securing a stable position was poor.

Franklin P. Mall, the first professor of anatomy at Johns Hopkins, was a quiet crusader for the idea of extending the full-time system to the clinical departments. His enthusiasm was shared by Lewellys F. Barker, whose speech in 1902 on the subject of full-time clinical departments raised the issue across the nation. When he became director of medicine in 1905, Barker extended the full-time system by establishing three research divisions whose directors were paid wholly by the medical school: the Biological Division was devoted to the study of infectious diseases, the Physiological Division focused on cardiovascular problems, and the Chemical Division applied biochemical techniques to the study of disease. But sufficient funds were not available to transform the directorship of medicine into a full-time post.

It was Welch who was instrumental in obtaining the money necessary to place the Departments of Medicine, Surgery, and Pediatrics on a full-time basis. In 1911, the Rockefeller Foundation's General Education Board was ready to offer Johns Hopkins a substantial endowment for this purpose, but two years elapsed before Welch was able to persuade the faculty to accept.

The principle of full-time faculty in both the preclinical and the clinical sciences has been characterized as a turning point in medicine in this country, the innovation that has given rise to the nation's leadership in medicine. Most schools have adopted some variation of the full-time plan, but medical education and medical research have benefited from the full-time plan even in schools in which it was not formally or fully adopted. The very existence of the arrangement in certain research-oriented schools put pressure on professors in all clinical departments to give heed to research. It was an important step in cementing a sound relationship between medical school and university.

The application of the full-time system to the clinical departments was the last great medical innovation put in place at Johns Hopkins. The foundation for Hopkins' future growth was thus established by 1914, the hospital's twenty-fifth anniversary. "In many ways," wrote Alan M. Chesney, "those first twenty-five years constitute the most interesting and most important part of the story of the Hospital and of that of its partner, the School of Medicine, for it was during those years that the two institutions had the oppor-

tunity to initiate and to carry out pioneering work in the supremely important field of medical education."[12]

By its twenty-fifth anniversary, the hospital's vitality was apparent: its endowment, the value of its physical plant, its bed capacity, and the number of outpatient visits had all increased substantially since its opening. Growth in the medical school could also be measured by the number of men and women it had sent out to populate other medical schools nationwide. Rather than retaining all of its well-trained graduates and young faculty, Billings and his colleagues intended that they bring the specific innovations developed at Johns Hopkins to other medical schools across the country. The export of graduates "fitted to make research" was the fulfillment of the wish that Billings had expressed at the opening of the hospital.

Hopkins graduates, residents, fellows, and young faculty members spread into varied fields of medicine, influencing practice, research, and education. The Flexner Report of 1910 added to the renown of the Hopkins model when Abraham Flexner cited the Johns Hopkins medical school as the outstanding institution of its kind in the United States. When the Rockefeller Foundation provided funds to establish new medical schools based on the Hopkins model, Hopkins graduates were brought to the new schools as deans and faculty members. At the University of Rochester and Duke University, for example, Hopkins-trained administrators influenced the entire pattern of medical education.

The success of the Hopkins migration helped to transform American medicine, and what was put forth as a model is now firmly entrenched. Today we accept as commonplace aspects of academic medicine the ideals promulgated by Gilman, Billings, Welch, Osler, and the rest of the Hopkins founders. That acceptance may be Hopkins' greatest contribution.

The spread of these ideals diffused the uniqueness of the Johns Hopkins medical school and hospital. As its graduates helped to create other strong schools, Johns Hopkins became one of many. By sending its graduates out to staff an increasing number of strong sister institutions with research-oriented faculties, Hopkins lost its unique position of unrivaled leadership. Shryock points out the paradox: the fact that Hopkins training is no longer as distinctive as it was one hundred years ago suggests the hospital and med-

ical school's greatest achievement. Viewed from this perspective, he writes, the loss of Hopkins' once unique position becomes a persuasive measure of its enormous success.[13]

NOTES

Introduction

1. Abraham Flexner to Henry Sigerist, November 29, 1943, Alan M. Chesney Medical Archives, the Johns Hopkins Medical Institutions.

2. Roger L. Geiger, *To Advance Knowledge: The Growth of American Research Universities, 1900–1940* (New York: Oxford University Press, 1986), pp. 7–8.

3. Kenneth M. Ludmerer, *Learning to Heal: The Development of American Medical Education* (New York: Basic Books, 1985), p. 57.

4. William H. Welch, "Address at the Twenty-Fifth Anniversary of the Johns Hopkins Hospital, 1889–1914," *Johns Hopkins Hosp. Bull.* 25 (1914): 364. The *Bulletin of The Johns Hopkins Hospital* was known as *The Johns Hopkins Hospital Bulletin* before 1924. Its name was changed again in 1967, to *The Johns Hopkins Medical Journal*.

5. William Osler, "Looking Back: Communication at the Twenty-Fifth Anniversary of the Johns Hopkins Hospital, 1889–1914," *Johns Hopkins Hosp. Bull.* 25 (1914): 354.

6. Ibid.

7. Welch, "Address at the Twenty-Fifth Anniversary," p. 364.

8. Ethel Johns and Blanche Pfefferkorn, *The Johns Hopkins Hospital School of Nursing, 1889–1949* (Baltimore, Johns Hopkins Press, 1954); Elizabeth Fee, *Disease and Discovery: A History of the Johns Hopkins School of Hygiene and Public Health, 1916–1939* (Baltimore: Johns Hopkins University Press, 1987).

Chapter 1   The Opening of the Hospital and Medical School

Epigraph: William Osler, cited in Harvey Cushing, *The Life of Sir William Osler,* 2 vols. (London: Oxford University Press, 1925), 1:303.

1. *Hospital Plans: Five Essays Relating to the Construction, Organization and Management of Hospitals* (New York: William Wood & Co., 1875), p. xvii.

2. Helen M. Thom, *Johns Hopkins: A Silhouette* (Baltimore: Johns Hopkins Press, 1929); John C. French, *A History of the University Founded by Johns Hopkins* (Baltimore: Johns Hopkins Press, 1946), pp. 10–17.

3. John C. French, "Mr. Johns Hopkins and Dr. Macaulay's 'Medical Improvement,' " *Bull. Hist. Med.* 27 (1953): 562–66.

4. *Hospital Plans,* pp. xv–xviii.

5. Henry M. Hurd, "History of the Johns Hopkins Hospital," unpublished manscript, Alan M. Chesney Medical Archives, the Johns Hopkins Medical Institutions. This manuscript was written soon after Hurd's retirement in 1911.

6. French, *A History of the University,* pp. 17–22.

7. Alan M. Chesney, *The Johns Hopkins Hospital and the Johns Hopkins University School of Medicine,* 3 vols. (Baltimore: Johns Hopkins Press, 1943) 1:5–7.

8. French, *A History of the University,* pp. 17–22; Chesney, *The Johns Hopkins Hospital* 1:7–10; Hugh Hawkins, *Pioneer: A History of The Johns Hopkins University, 1874–1889* (Ithaca, N.Y.: Cornell University Press, 1960), pp. 4–5.

9. Hugh Hawkins, "Three University Presidents Testify," *American Quarterly* 11 (1959): 99–119.

10. Gert H. Brieger, "The California Origins of the Johns Hopkins Medical School," *Bull. Hist. Med.* 51 (1977): 339–52.

11. Daniel C. Gilman, "The Johns Hopkins University in Its Beginning," inaugural address at the opening of the Johns Hopkins University, 1876, in Daniel C. Gilman, *University Problems in the United States* (New York: Century Co., 1897), pp. 22–23.

12. Fabian Franklin, *The Life of Daniel Coit Gilman* (New

York: Dodd, Mead & Co., 1910); Abraham Flexner, *Daniel Coit Gilman* (New York: Harcourt, Brace & Co., 1946); Kenneth M. Ludmerer, *Learning to Heal: The Development of American Medical Education* (New York: Basic Books, 1985), p. 58.

13. Hawkins, *Pioneer*, pp. 22–23.

14. Ibid., pp. 57–62.

15. Daniel C. Gilman, "Hopkins," *Cosmopolitan* 11 (1891): 466.

16. Hawkins, *Pioneer*, chap. 5; Francesco Cordasco, *The Shaping of American Graduate Education: Daniel Coit Gilman and the Protean Ph.D.* (Totowa, N.J.: Rowman & Littlefield, 1973); Laurence R. Veysey, *The Emergence of the American University* (Chicago: University of Chicago Press, 1965).

17. French, *A History of the University*, pp. 40–41.

18. Richard Shryock, *The Unique Influence of the Johns Hopkins University in American Medicine* (Copenhagen: Ejnar Munksgaard, 1953), pp. 7–10.

19. Hawkins, *Pioneer*, pp. 9–14.

20. Ludmerer, *Learning to Heal*, chap. 3.

21. Shyrock, *Influence of The Johns Hopkins University*, p. 9.

22. Daniel C. Gilman, "Charity and Knowledge: Address at the opening of the Johns Hopkins Hospital, 1889," reprinted in Chesney, *The Johns Hopkins Hospital* 1:261.

23. Daniel C. Gilman, *The Launching of a University and Other Papers* (New York: Dodd, Mead & Co., 1906), p. 41.

24. *Hospital Plans*; Gert H. Brieger, "The Original Plans for the Johns Hopkins Hospital and Their Historical Significance," *Bull. Hist. Med.* 39 (1965): 518–28.

25. Ibid., p. 4.

26. Fielding H. Garrison, *John Shaw Billings: A Memoir* (New York: G. P. Putnam's Sons, 1915); John Shaw Billings, "The Surgical Treatment of Epilepsy," *Cincinnati Lancet and Observer* 4 (1861): 334–41; John D. French, and Louise Darling, "The Surgical Treatment of Epilepsy in 1861," *J. Int. Coll. Surg.* 34 (1960): 685–91.

27. John Shaw Billings, *A Report on Barracks and Hospitals; with Descriptions of Military Posts* (Washington, D.C.: Surgeon General's Office, United States War Department, 1870).

28. Dorothy Schullian, "Alfred Alexander Woodhull, John Shaw Billings, and the Johns Hopkins Hospital, 8 June 1871," *J. Hist. Med.* 13 (1958): 531–37.

29. John Shaw Billings, *Johns Hopkins Hospital: Reports and Papers Relating to Construction and Organization*, no. 1, 1876, Privately printed.

30. Donald Fleming, *William H. Welch and the Rise of Modern Medicine* (Boston: Little, Brown & Co., 1954), p. 84.

31. Billings to Gilman, November 11, 1876, Gilman Papers, Ferdinand Hamburger, Jr., Archives, the Johns Hopkins University, cited in W. Bruce Fye, "Daniel Gilman, John Shaw Billings and the Foundation of Johns Hopkins," unpublished manuscript, 1977. Used by permission.

32. Garrison, *John Shaw Billings*, p. 198.

33. John Shaw Billings to John Warren, September 13, 1878, Billings Papers, New York Public Library.

34. Ibid.

35. *Hospital Plans*.

36. John Shaw Billings, address at the opening of the Johns Hopkins Hospital, 1889, reprinted in Chesney, *The Johns Hopkins Hospital* 1:241–55.

37. John Shaw Billings, "Suggestions on Medical Education," ed. Alan M. Chesney, *Bull. Hist. Med.* 6 (1938): 318.

38. Chesney, *The Johns Hopkins Hospital* 1:95.

39. William H. Wilson, *Medical and Dental Register of the City of Baltimore, with Medical Directory of Maryland*, 1884.

40. Ibid.

41. Chesney, *The Johns Hopkins Hospital* 1:95–96; W. Bruce Fye, *The Development of American Physiology* (Baltimore: Johns Hopkins University Press, 1987), chap. 4.

42. A. McGehee Harvey, *Adventures in Medical Research* (Baltimore: Johns Hopkins University Press, 1974), pp. 84–96.

43. Daniel C. Gilman, report of January 1, 1876, cited in French, *A History of the University*, pp. 33–34; see also Fye, *Development of American Physiology*; Carl P. Swanson, "A History of Biology at the Johns Hopkins University," *Bios* 22 (1951): 223–62.

44. Harvey, *Adventures in Medical Research*, pp. 84–96.

45. Gilman, "The Johns Hopkins University," p. 23.

46. Gert H. Brieger, "Fit to Study Medicine: Notes for a History of Pre-Medical Education in America," *Bull. Hist. Med.* 57 (1983): 1–21.

47. Swanson, "Biology at the Johns Hopkins University," pp. 223–62.

48. Fye, *Development of American Physiology*.

49. Henry N. Martin, cited in Harvey, *Adventures in Medical Research*, p. 90.

50. Henry N. Martin, "A New Method of Studying the Mammalian Heart," in *Studies from the Biological Laboratory of the Johns Hopkins University*, vol. 2 (Baltimore: Johns Hopkins University, 1881), p. 119.

51. Gilman, *Launching of a University*, p. 52.

52. J. George Adami, "Address at Opening of New Medical Building," *The Art of Healing and the Science of Medicine* (Ann Arbor: University of Michigan, 1901), p. 47.

53. Chesney, *The Johns Hopkins Hospital* 1:79–82.

54. Ibid., 1:82.

55. *Development of American Physiology*, p. 166.

56. Simon Flexner and James T. Flexner, *William Henry Welch and the Heroic Age of American Medicine* (New York: Viking Press, 1941), pp. 128–34; Fleming, *William H. Welch*, pp. 65–70.

57. Flexner and Flexner, *William Henry Welch*, chap. 6 and 7; Fleming, *William H. Welch*, pp. 34–54.

58. Fleming, *William H. Welch*, p. 80.

59. Ibid., p. 81.

60. Chesney, *The Johns Hopkins Hospital* 1:91–92; see also Flexner and Flexner, *William Henry Welch*, p. 152.

61. Flexner and Flexner, *William Henry Welch*, pp. 160–70; Harvey, *Adventures in Medical Research*, pp. 39–40.

62. Harvey, *Adventures in Medical Research*, pp. 39–40; Fleming, *William H. Welch*, p. 128.

63. Fleming, *William H. Welch*, p. 126.

64. A. McGehee Harvey, "Johns Hopkins and Yellow Fever: A Story of Tragedy and Triumph," *Johns Hopkins Med. J.* 149 (1981): 25.

65. Fleming, *William H. Welch*, p. 82.

66. Harvey, *Adventures in Medical Research*, pp. 39–40.

67. Fleming, *William H. Welch*, p. 86; Harvey, *Adventures in Medical Research*, pp. 69–73.

68. Cushing, *Sir William Osler*, vol. 1.

69. Chesney, *The Johns Hopkins Hospital* 1:114–17; Audrey Davis, *Dr. Kelly of Hopkins* (Baltimore: Johns Hopkins Press, 1959); Harvey, *Adventures in Medical Research*, pp. 10–15.

70. Hawkins, *Pioneer*, pp. 322–23; Chesney, *The Johns Hopkins Hospital* 1:100–102.

71. Chesney, *The Johns Hopkins Hospital* 1:100–102; Henry M. Hurd, "History of the Johns Hopkins Hospital," unpublished manuscript, Alan M. Chesney Medical Archives.

72. Chesney, *The Johns Hopkins Hospital* 1:145–46.

73. Henri A. LaFleur, "Early Days at the Johns Hopkins Hospital with Dr. Osler," *Can. Med. Assoc. J.*, memorial no. (May 1920): 42.

74. Margaret Janeway Billings, "Recollection of the Dedication of the Johns Hopkins Hospital," in Dorothy Schullian, typewritten notes, John Shaw Billings Papers, National Library of Medicine, Bethesda, Maryland.

75. Admissions and discharge book, 1889, Alan M. Chesney Medical Archives, the Johns Hopkins Medical Institutions; A. M. Carr, "The Early History of the Hospital and the Training School," *Johns Hopkins Nurses Alumnae Magazine*, June 1909, pp. 61–62.

76. Henry M. Hurd, *First Report of the Superintendent of the Johns Hopkins Hospital* (Baltimore: Johns Hopkins Press, 1890).

77. Thomas S. Cullen, *Henry Mills Hurd: The First Superintendent of the Johns Hopkins Hospital* (Baltimore: Johns Hopkins Press, 1920); A. McGehee Harvey, Henry Mills Hurd: The First Superintendent of the Johns Hopkins Hospital and the First Professor of Psychiatry," *Johns Hopkins Med. J.* 148 (1981): 135.

78. Henry M. Hurd, *The Institutional Care of the Insane in the United States and Canada*, 4 vols. (Baltimore: Johns Hopkins Press, 1916); Henry M. Hurd, "A History of Institutional Care of the Insane in the United States and Canada," *Am. J. Insanity* 67 (1910–11): 587.

79. French, *A History of the University*, pp. 219–27.

80. Thomas B. Turner, *Heritage of Excellence* (Baltimore: Johns Hopkins University Press, 1974), pp. 251, 253.

81. Ethel Johns and Blanche Pfefferkorn, *The Johns Hopkins Hospital School of Nursing, 1889–1949* (Baltimore: Johns Hopkins Press, 1954); Janet W. James, "Isabel Hampton and the Professionalization of Nursing in the 1890's," in *The Therapeutic Revolution*, ed. Morris J. Vogel and Charles E. Rosenberg (Philadelphia: University of Pennsylvania Press, 1979), pp. 201–44.

82. Chesney, *The Johns Hopkins Hospital* 1:193–221, 1:291–94.

83. Cushing, *Sir William Osler* 1:373.

84. William H. Welch, "Address at the Twenty-Fifth Anniversary of the Johns Hopkins Hospital, 1889–1914," *Johns Hopkins Hosp. Bull.* 25 (1914): 365.

85. Florence R. Sabin, *Franklin P. Mall, The Story of a Mind* (Baltimore: Johns Hopkins Press, 1934); George W. Corner, "Franklin Paine Mall," in *Dictionary of Scientific Biography*, ed. Charles C. Gillispie, 16 vols. (New York: Charles Scribner's Sons, 1970–80), 9:55–58; Harvey, *Adventures in Medical Research*, pp. 97–102.

86. Harvey, *Adventures in Medical Research*, pp. 97–102.

87. Anne C. Rodman, "William Henry Howell," in *Dictionary of Scientific Biography*, ed. Gillispie, 6:525–27.

88. Charles E. Rosenberg, "John Jacob Abel," in *Dictionary of Scientific Biography*, ed. Gillispie, 1:9–12; Harvey, *Adventures in Medical Research*, pp. 49–58.

89. Harvey, *Adventures in Medical Research*, pp. 49–58.

90. Chesney, *The Johns Hopkins Hospital* 2:1–10; Jeannie A. Brown, *Dr. Tom Brown, Memories* (New York: Richard R. Smith, 1949).

91. Chesney, *The Johns Hopkins Hospital* 1:86–88.

Chapter 2   The Early Days, 1893–1905

Epigraph: William Osler, "Looking Back: Communication at the Twenty-Fifth Anniversary of the Johns Hopkins Hospital, 1889–1914," *Johns Hopkins Hosp. Bull.* 25 (1914): 354.

1. Alan M. Chesney, *The Johns Hopkins Hospital and the Johns Hopkins University School of Medicine*, 3 vols. (Baltimore: Johns Hopkins Press, 1943–63), 2:22.

2. A. McGehee Harvey, *Adventures in Medical Research* (Baltimore: Johns Hopkins University Press, 1974),

pp. 188–94; Howard A. Kelly, "John Whitridge Williams (1866–1931)," *Am J. Surg.* 15 (1932): 169; Lawrence D. Longo, "John Whitridge Williams and Academic Obstetrics in America," *Trans. Stud. Coll. Phys. Phila.* 3 (1981): 221–54.

3. Harvey, *Adventures in Medical Research,* pp. 114–18; J. S. Nicholas, "Ross G. Harrison," in *Biographical Memoirs of the National Academy of Sciences,* vol. 35 (New York: Columbia University Press, 1961), p. 132.

4. Hugh Young, *A Surgeon's Autobiography* (New York: Harcourt, Brace & Co., 1940), p. 76.

5. John F. Fulton, *Harvey Cushing: A Biography* (Springfield, Ill.: Charles C Thomas, 1946); Elizabeth L. Thomson, *Harvey Cushing: Surgeon, Author, Artist* (1950; New York: Neale Watson Academic Publications, 1981).

6. Harvey Cushing, "Instruction in Operative Medicine," *Johns Hopkins Hosp. Bull.* 17 (1906): 123–24. (See Part 2 of this book's companion volume.)

7. Rollin T. Woodyatt "President's Address," *Trans. Assoc. Am. Phys.* 51 (1936): 1.

8. Chesney, *The Johns Hopkins Hospital* 2:43–47.

9. Ibid., 2:234.

10. Harvey Cushing, *The Life of Sir William Osler,* 2 vols. (London: Oxford University Press, 1925), 1:314.

11. Chesney, *The Johns Hopkins Hospital* 2:117.

12. G. Canby Robinson, *Adventures in Medical Education* (Cambridge: Harvard University Press, 1957), p. 40.

13. Ibid., p. 43.

14. Ibid., p. 44.

15. Cited in Chesney, *The Johns Hopkins Hospital* 2:37.

16. Cited in Chesney, *The Johns Hopkins Hospital* 2:127; see also Joseph Pratt, *A Year with Osler: 1896–1897* (Baltimore: Johns Hopkins Press, 1949).

17. George W. Heuer, "Dr. Halsted," *Bull. Johns Hopkins Hosp.* 90, suppl., (February 1952): 27.

18. Kenneth M. Ludmerer, *Learning to Heal: The Development of American Medical Education* (New York: Basic Books, 1985), pp. 68–69.

19. William Osler, "The Natural Method of Teaching the Subject of Medicine," *JAMA* 36 (1901): 1673.

20. William Osler, *The Principles and Practice of Medicine* (New York: D. Appleton & Co., 1892).

21. Ludmerer, *Learning to Heal,* p. 69.

22. Rufus I. Cole, "Perfectionism in Medicine," *Bull. Johns Hopkins Hosp.* 79 (1946): 196.

23. Chesney, *The Johns Hopkins Hospital* 2:159–61.

24. The approximate date was arrived at by comparing the listing of house medical officers in the annual reports of the hospital superintendent with the names of the medical school graduates in the same year.

25. Chesney, *The Johns Hopkins Hospital* 1:131.

26. Ibid., 2:137.

27. Ibid., 2:292–93.

28. Ibid., 2:372.

29. J. M. T. Finney, *A Surgeon's Life* (New York: G. P. Putnam's Sons, 1940); Chesney, *The Johns Hopkins Hospital* 2:156–58.

30. Harvey, *Adventures in Medical Research,* pp. 71–74; Samuel J. Crowe, *Halsted of Johns Hopkins: The Man and His Men* (Springfield, Ill.: Charles C Thomas, 1957), pp. 61–64.

31. A. McGehee Harvey, "Johns Hopkins's Pioneer Venture into International Medicine: The Commission to the Philippine Islands," *Johns Hopkins Med. J.* 147 (1980): 13.

32. Fifteenth Report of the Superintendent of the Johns Hopkins Hospital (Baltimore: The Johns Hopkins Press, 1903).

33. Chesney, *The Johns Hopkins Hospital* 2:422.

34. Jacques Kelly, *Bygone Baltimore* (Norfolk: Donning Co., 1982), Chap. 3; Harold A. Williams, *Baltimore Afire* (1954; Baltimore: Schneidereith, 1979); Chesney, *The Johns Hopkins Hospital* 2:376.

35. Chesney, *The Johns Hopkins Hospital* 2:376–96.

36. Young, *A Surgeon's Autobiography,* p. 66.

37. William H. Welch, address delivered at memorial exercises at the Johns Hopkins University for William Osler, March 22, 1920, cited in Chesney, *The Johns Hopkins Hospital* 2:405–6.

38. William Osler, "The Fixed Period," in William Osler, *Aequanimitas with Other Addresses* (Philadelphia: P. Blakiston's Son & Co., 1932), p. 393.

39. Thomas McCrae, *The Influence of Pathology upon the Clinical Medicine of William Osler,* Bulletin no. 9, Sir William Osler memorial no. (Montreal: International Association of Medical Museums, 1926).

40. This account of Barker's recruitment is taken from Lewellys F. Barker, *Time and the Physician* (New York: G. P. Putnam's Sons, 1942), chap. 10.

41. Lewellys F. Barker, "The Laboratories of the Medical Clinic," *Johns Hopkins Hosp. Bull.* 18 (1907): 193.

42. Harvey, *Adventures in Medical Research,* pp. 127–32.

43. Ibid., pp. 132–38.

44. Ibid., pp. 133–34; Donald Fleming, *William H. Welch and the Rise of Modern Medicine* (Boston: Little, Brown & Co., 1954), pp. 127–28.

45. William Osler, "The Fixed Period," pp. 388–89.

46. William Henry Welch, "Address at Commencement of the Johns Hopkins University," *Johns Hopkins Hosp. Bull.* 9 (1898): 151. See also Ludmerer, *Learning to Heal,* p. 70.

47. Evarts Graham, "Report of the Surgical Service 1928–29 to the Director of Barnes Hospital," Archives, Washington University School of Medicine, cited in A. McGehee

Harvey, *Science at the Bedside* (Baltimore: Johns Hopkins University Press, 1981), p. 438.

Chapter 3   Consolidation and Growth, 1905–1942

Epigraph: William Osler, "Looking Back: Communication at the Twenty-Fifth Anniversary of the Johns Hopkins Hospital, 1889–1914," *Johns Hopkins Hosp. Bull.* 25 (1914): 354.

1. Kenneth M. Ludmerer, *Learning to Heal: The Development of American Medical Education* (New York: Basic Books, 1985), pp. 87–93.

2. Abraham Flexner, *Medical Education in the United States and Canada,* Bull. no. 4 (New York: The Carnegie Foundation for the Advancement of Teaching, 1910); Gert H. Brieger, "The Flexner Report: Revised or Revisited?" *Medical Heritage,* 1, no. 1 (1985): 25–34.

3. Ludmerer, *Learning to Heal,* chap. 9.

4. Flexner, *Medical Education in the United States and Canada,* p. 53; Ludmerer, *Learning to Heal,* p. 174.

5. Ludmerer, *Learning to Heal,* pp. 177–90.

6. Abraham Flexner, *The General Education Board: An Account of its Activities, 1902–1914* (New York: General Education Board, 1915), p. 162; Ludmerer, *Learning to Heal,* p. 177.

7. Abraham Flexner, *I Remember* (New York: Simon & Schuster, 1940), pp. 176–77.

8. William Osler to President Remsen of the Johns Hopkins University, "Whole-Time Clinical Professors," September 1, 1911, Alan M. Chesney Medical Archives, the Johns Hopkins Medical Institutions; see also Donald Fleming, "The Full-Time Controversy," *J. Med. Educ.* 30, no. 7 (1955): 398–406.

9. Richard Shryock, *The Unique Influence of the Johns Hopkins University in American Medicine* (Copenhagen: Ejnar Munksgaard, 1953), p. 40.

10. Alan M. Chesney, *The Johns Hopkins Hospital and the Johns Hopkins University School of Medicine,* 3 vols. (Baltimore: Johns Hopkins Press, 1943–63), 3:260–62.

11. Ludmerer, *Learning to Heal,* pp. 207–13.

12. Abraham Flexner, anecdote of Dr. Welch, March 26, 1935, File "William Welch," Abraham Flexner Papers, Library of Congress; see also Ludmerer, *Learning to Heal,* p. 213.

13. Lewellys Barker, *Time and the Physician* (New York: G. P. Putnam's Sons, 1942), chap. 9.

14. A. McGehee Harvey, *Science at the Bedside* (Baltimore: Johns Hopkins University Press, 1981), pp. 153–59; Theodore C. Janeway, "Important Contributions to Clinical Medicine during the Past Thirty Years from the Study of Human Blood Pressure," *Johns Hopkins Hosp. Bull.* 266 (1915): 341; Lewellys F. Barker, "Theodore Caldwell Janeway," *Science* 447 (1918): 273.

15. Theodore C. Janeway, *The Clinical Study of Blood Pressure, Etc.* (New York: D. Appleton & Co., 1904); Nathan Flaxman, "Janeway on Hypertension: Theodore Caldwell Janeway (1872–1917)," *Bull. Hist. Med.* 9 (1941): 505; Robert Kaiser, "Thinking About High Blood Pressure: Theodore C. Janeway and the Clinical Investigation of Hypertension," (Master's essay, Institute of the History of Medicine, the Johns Hopkins Medical Institutions, 1985).

16. Knud Faber, *Nosography in Modern Internal Medicine* (New York: Paul B. Hoeber, 1923), chap. 5; Barker, "Theodore Caldwell Janeway," p. 273.

17. Barker, "Theodore Caldwell Janeway," p. 273.

18. Harvey, *Science at the Bedside,* pp. 166–68; Edward P. Carter, "William Sydney Thayer (June 23, 1864–December 10, 1932)," *Bull. Johns Hopkins Hosp.* 52 (1933): 1; Edith G. Reid, *The Life and Convictions of William Sydney Thayer—Physician* (London: Oxford University Press, 1936); William S. Thayer and John Hewetson, *Lectures of Malarial Fever* (New York: D. Appleton, 1897).

19. Richard Wagner, *Clemens von Pirquet: His Life and Work* (Baltimore: Johns Hopkins Press, 1968).

20. Chesney, *The Johns Hopkins Hospital,* vol. 3.

21. Emmett Holt, "The Children's Hospital, the Medical School and the Public," *Johns Hopkins Hosp. Bull.* 24 (1913): 89–92.

22. Edwards A. Park, "John Howland," *Science* 64 (1926): 80.

23. Stanley Cobb, "Acceptance of the Kober Medal," *Trans. Assoc. Am. Phys.* 69 (1956): 41.

24. Thomas B. Turner, *Heritage of Excellence* (Baltimore: Johns Hopkins University Press, 1974), pp. 104–5, 539.

25. A. McGehee Harvey, *Adventures in Medical Research* (Baltimore: Johns Hopkins University Press, 1974), pp. 22–31; Simon Flexner, "William George MacCallum" *Science* 99 (1944): 290; Wiley D. Forbus, "William George MacCallum (1874–1944)," *J. Pathol.* 56 (1944): 603.

26. Harvey, *Adventures in Medical Research,* pp. 396–99; Thomas H. Marin, "Eli Kennerly Marshall, Jr. (1889–1966)," *Bull. Johns Hopkins Hosp.* 119 (1966): 247.

27. A. McGehee Harvey, "The Department of Physiological Chemistry: Its Historical Evolution," *Johns Hopkins Med. J.* 139 (1976): 257.

28. Harvey, *Adventures in Medical Research,* pp. 158–61; A. McGehee Harvey, *The Interurban Clinical Club (1905–1976)* (Philadelphia: Interurban Clinical Club, 1976), p. 42.

29. A. McGehee Harvey, *The Association of American Physicians, 1886–1986* (Baltimore: Association of American Physicians, 1986), pp. 277–78.

30. Harvey, *Adventures in Medical Research,* pp. 215–17;

Harold E. Harrison, "Edwards A. Park: An Appreciation of the Man," *Johns Hopkins Med. J.* 132 (1973): 361.

31. J. M. T. Finney, *A Surgeon's Life* (New York: G. P. Putnam's Sons, 1940).

32. Turner, *Heritage of Excellence,* pp. 408–409; Gert H. Brieger, "Dean DeWitt Lewis," in *Dictionary of American Biography,* suppl. 3. ed. Edward T. James (New York: Charles Scribner's Sons, 1973), pp. 457–58.

33. Harvey, *Adventures in Medical Research,* pp. 188–94; Howard A. Kelly, "John Whitridge Williams (1866–1931)," *Am. J. Surg.* 15 (1932): 169.

34. Harvey, *Adventures in Medical Research,* pp. 173–75.

35. Margaret Brogden, "The Johns Hopkins Hospital Department of Social Service, 1907–1931," *Soc. Sci. Review* 38 (1964): 88–98; Turner, *Heritage of Excellence,* pp. 324–28.

36. Harvey, *Adventures in Medical Research,* pp. 175–83; Thomas S. Cullen, "Max Broedel, 1870–1941: Director of the First Department of Art as Applied to Medicine," *Bull. Med. Libr. Assoc.* 33 (1945): 5; Max Broedel, "The Origin, Growth, and Future of Medical Illustration at Johns Hopkins Hospital and Medical School," *Johns Hopkins Hosp. Bull.* 26 (1915): 185.

37. Thomas S. Cullen, *Henry Mills Hurd* (Baltimore: Johns Hopkins Press, 1920); Henry M. Hurd, "History of the Johns Hopkins Hospital," unpublished manuscript, Alan M. Chesney Medical Archives, the Johns Hopkins Medical Institutions; Shryock, *Unique Influence of The Johns Hopkins University;* Chesney, *The Johns Hopkins Hospital* 3:64–74.

38. Franklin P. Ebaugh, "Adolf Meyer's Contribution to Psychiatric Education," *Bull. Johns Hopkins Hosp.* 89, suppl. (1951): 65.

39. Frederick F. Russell, to Simon Flexner, August 7, 1939, in Simon Flexner and James T. Flexner, *William Henry Welch and the Heroic Age of American Medicine* (New York: Viking Press, 1941), p. 363.

40. William H. Welch, *Public Health in Theory and Practice* (New Haven: Yale University Press, 1925).

41. Ludmerer, *Learning to Heal,* pp. 29–38.

42. Elizabeth Fee, *Disease and Discovery: A History of the Johns Hopkins School of Hygiene and Public Health, 1916–1939* (Baltimore: Johns Hopkins University Press, 1987).

43. Turner, *Heritage of Excellence,* p. 382.

44. Gert H. Brieger, "Fielding H. Garrison: The Man and His Book," *Trans. Stud. Coll. Phys. Phila.* 3, no. 1 (1981): 1–21.

45. Turner, *Heritage of Excellence,* pp. 381–83; Harvey, *Adventures in Medical Research,* pp. 378–89.

46. Harvey, *Adventures in Medical Research,* pp. 383–89; Owsei Temkin et al., "In Memory of Henry E. Sigerist," *Bull. Hist. Med.* 31 (1957): 295.

47. Turner, *Heritage of Excellence,* pp. 426–31.

48. M. Elliott Randolph and Robert B. Welch, *The Wilmer Ophthalmological Institute: The First Fifty Years, 1925–1975* (Baltimore: Williams & Wilkins, 1976).

49. Material about the building boom of the 1920s is derived mainly from Turner, *Heritage of Excellence,* chap. 7.

50. Turner, *Heritage of Excellence,* pp. 134–36.

51. Ibid., chap. 13; James Bordley III and A. McGehee Harvey, *Two Centuries of American Medicine* (Philadelphia: W. B. Saunders, 1976); A. M. Harvey and James Bordley III, *Differential Diagnosis* (Philadelphia: W. B. Saunders, 1970).

52. Turner, *Heritage of Excellence,* pp. 267–68.

53. Augusta Tucker, *Miss Susie Slagle's* (1939; Baltimore: Johns Hopkins University Press, 1987).

54. Survey report, 1931, in Turner, *Heritage of Excellence,* p. 286.

55. Turner, *Heritage of Excellence,* p. 436; R. Austrian, "Perrin Hamilton Long (1899–1965)," *Trans. Assoc. Am. Phys.* 79 (1966): 59.

56. Turner, *Heritage of Excellence,* p. 299.

57. Ibid., pp. 501–505.

58. Turner, *Heritage of Excellence,* pp. 279–86.

Chapter 4 The War Years and the Postwar Expansion, 1942–1968

Epigraph: John Z. Bowers and Elizabeth F. Purcell, *Advances in American Medicine: Essays at the Bicentennial,* 2 vols. (New York: Josiah C. Macy, Jr., Foundation, 1976), 2:843.

1. Bowers and Purcell, *Advances in American Medicine* 2:843; James Bordley III and A. McGehee Harvey, *Two Centuries of American Medicine* (Philadelphia: W. B. Saunders Co., 1976), p. 358.

2. Stephen P. Strickland, *Politics, Science, and Dread Disease,* (Cambridge: Harvard University Press, 1972), p. 16.

3. Thomas B. Turner, *Heritage of Excellence* (Baltimore: Johns Hopkins University Press, 1974), pp. 476–77.

4. Robert H. Ebert, "Medical Education at the Peak of the Era of Experimental Medicine," *Daedalus* 115, no. 2 (1986): 58.

5. Ibid., p. 19; Vannevar Bush, *Science: The Endless Frontier* (Washington, D.C.: U.S. Govt. Printing Office, 1945).

6. Strickland, *Politics, Science, and Dread Disease,* pp. 23–31; Paul Starr, *The Social Transformation of American Medicine* (New York: Basic Books, 1982), pp. 340–43.

7. Paul B. Beeson, "The Changing Role Model, and the Shift in Power," in *Daedalus* 115, no. 2 (1986): 90.

8. Joseph B. Murtaugh, "Biomedical Sciences," in *Science and the Evolution of Public Policy,* ed. James A. Shannon, (New York: Rockefeller University Press, 1973), p. 157;

Bordley and Harvey, *Two Centuries of American Medicine,* pp. 388–90.

9. Strickland, *Politics, Science, and Dread Disease,* chap. 4, p. 259.

10. Ibid., p. 252.

11. Starr, *Social Transformation of American Medicine,* p. 354; Kenneth M. Ludmerer, *Learning to Heal: The Development of American Medical Education* (New York: Basic Books, 1985), pp. 262–63.

12. Strickland, *Politics, Science, and Dread Disease,* chap. 3.

13. Bordley and Harvey, *Two Centuries of American Medicine,* p. 424.

14. Strickland, *Politics, Science, and Dread Disease,* chap. 5.

15. Bowers and Purcell, *Advances in American Medicine* 2: 544.

16. Murtaugh, "Biomedical Research," p. 165.

17. James A. Shannon, "Federal Support of Biomedical Sciences: Development and Academic Impact," *J. Med. Educ.* 51, suppl. (1976): 1–98.

18. Robert Ebert, "Biomedical Research Policy: A Reevaluation," *Trans. Assoc. Am. Phys.* 86 (1973): 1–7.

19. Bordley and Harvey, *Two Centuries of American Medicine,* p. 431.

20. Robert H. Ebert, "Medical Education," pp. 55–81.

21. Ebert, "Biomedical Research Policy," pp. 1–7.

22. Ebert, "Medical Education," pp. 62–63.

23. Starr, *Social Transformation of American Medicine,* p. 360.

24. Thomas B. Turner, *Accounting of a Stewardship* (Baltimore: Johns Hopkins University School of Medicine, 1969), p. 37.

25. Ludmerer, *Learning to Heal,* p. 215; Ebert, "Medical Education," pp. 62–63; Starr, *Social Transformation of American Medicine,* pp. 352–53.

26. Ebert, "Medical Education," pp. 55–81.

27. Murtaugh, "Biomedical Sciences," p. 175.

28. James A. Shannon, "The University Medical Center and Medical Education," *Trans. Assoc. Am. Phys.* 81 (1968): 31–39; see also Vernon Lippard, *A Half-Century of American Medical Education* (New York: Josiah Macy, Jr., Foundation, 1974).

29. David E. Rogers, "Where have we been? Where are we going?" *Daedalus* 115, no. 2 (1986): 210.

30. Turner, *Accounting of a Stewardship,* p. 6.

31. Ibid., pp. 5, 33.

32. Ibid., pp. 6, 34.

33. Turner, *Accounting of a Stewardship,* p. 34.

34. Thomas B. Turner, *Part of Medicine, Part of Me* (Baltimore: Johns Hopkins University School of Medicine, 1981), p. 122.

35. Turner, *Accounting of a Stewardship,* p. 20.

36. Ibid., p. 34.

37. Turner, *Part of Medicine,* p. 131.

38. In the pages that follow, information about members of the faculty and administration was obtained from the biographical files of the Alan M. Chesney Medical Archives and from the minutes of the Advisory Board, the Johns Hopkins Medical Institutions.

39. Turner, *Heritage of Excellence,* pp. 506–508.

40. Ibid., pp. 508–9.

41. Ibid., pp. 501–5.

42. Ibid., p. 518.

43. Ibid., p. 516.

44. Richard J. Johns, "About the Author," A. McGehee Harvey, *Adventures in Medical Research* (Baltimore: Johns Hopkins Press, 1972), pp. 461–64.

45. Turner, *Heritage of Excellence,* p. 527.

46. Harold E. Harrison to A. McGehee Harvey, personal communication, 1987.

47. M. Elliott Randolph and Robert B. Welch, *The Wilmer Ophthalmological Institute: The First Fifty Years, 1925–1975* (Baltimore: Williams & Wilkins, 1976).

48. Turner, *Heritage of Excellence,* p. 521.

49. Arnold R. Rich, "Acceptance of the Kober Medal," *Trans. Assoc. Am. Phys.* 71 (1958): 46–49.

50. Paul Talalay to A. McGehee Harvey, personal communication, 1987.

51. A. McGehee Harvey, "The Department of Physiological Chemistry: Its Historical Evolution," *Johns Hopkins Med. J.* 139 (1976): 257.

52. Turner, *Heritage of Excellence,* pp. 376–80.

53. Vivien Thomas, *Pioneering Research in Surgical Shock and Cardiovascular Surgery: Vivien Thomas and His Work with Alfred Blalock: An Autobiography.* (Philadelphia: University of Pennsylvania Press, 1985).

54. J. Alex Haller, introduction at the 75th anniversary symposium for the Harriet Lane Home, November 20, 1987.

55. George D. Zuidema, oral history of Department of Surgery 1964–1984, recorded 1988, Alan M. Chesney Medical Archives, the Johns Hopkins Medical Institutions.

56. George D. Zuidema to A. McGehee Harvey, personal communication, 1987.

57. Howard W. Jones, Georgeanna S. Jones, and William E. Ticknor, *Richard Wesley TeLinde* (Baltimore: Williams & Wilkins, 1986).

58. Allan C. Barnes, introductory remarks, Johns Hopkins Medical Institutions' 75th Anniversary Symposium on Social Responsibility of Gynecology and Obstetrics, 1964.

59. Guy M. McKhann to A. McGehee Harvey, personal communication, 1987.

60. Ibid.

61. Harvey, *Adventures in Medical Research,* pp. 340–47; untitled article, *Hopkins Medical News* 1, no. 5 (November 1976): 1; "W. Horsley Gantt—A legend in his own time," *Johns Hopkins Med. J.* 139 (1976): 121; Joel Elkes, "Self-Regulation and Behavioral Medicine: The Early Beginnings," *Psych. Annals* 11, no. 2 (February 1981): 15.

62. H. Hanford Hopkins IV to A. McGehee Harvey, personal communication, 1980.

63. Turner, *Accounting of a Stewardship,* pp. 39–40.

64. Ibid., p. 40; "Biomedical Engineering," *Hopkins Medical News* 5, no. 6 (January 1981): 1.

65. Turner, *Accounting of a Stewardship,* p. 41; "Laboratory Medicine," *Hopkins Medical News* 6, no. 5 (November 1981): 1.

66. Turner, *Accounting of a Stewardship,* p. 40.

67. Albert H. Owens, Jr., to A. McGehee Harvey, personal communication, 1987.

68. Turner, *Heritage of Excellence,* pp. 9–11.

69. Turner, *Accounting of a Stewardship,* p. 11.

70. Turner, *Accounting of a Stewardship,* p. 6.

71. Ibid., p. 6.

72. Minutes of the Medical Planning and Development Committee, Alan M. Chesney Medical Archives, the Johns Hopkins Medical Institutions.

73. Robert H. Ebert, "Presidential Address," *Trans. Assoc. Am. Phys.* 86 (1973): 5; Turner, *Accounting of a Stewardship,* pp. 33–37.

Chapter 5 Renewal and Redirection, 1968–1989

Epigraph: James A. Shannon, "Acceptance of the George M. Kober Medal for 1982," *Trans. Assoc. Am. Phys.* 95 (1982): cxlviii–cxlix.

1. Walsh D. McDermott, "Acceptance of the Kober Medal," *Trans. Assoc. Am. Phys.* 88 (1975): 40–43.

2. Ibid.

3. A. McGehee Harvey, *The Interurban Clinical Club (1905–1976)* (Philadelphia: Interurban Clinical Club, 1976), pp. 513–14. Unless otherwise noted, the information about members of the faculty and administration in this chapter has been drawn from the biographical files of the Alan M. Chesney Medical Archives and the minutes of the Advisory Board, the Johns Hopkins Medical Institutions.

4. Franklin C. McLean, "University of Chicago: Medicine in the Division of Biological Sciences," in *Methods and Problems in Medical Education,* ed. Franklin C. McLean and Nellie Gorgas, 19th ser. (New York: Rockefeller Foundation, 1931).

5. A. McGehee Harvey and Susan L. Abrams, *"For the Welfare of Mankind": The Commonwealth Fund and American Medicine* (Baltimore: Johns Hopkins University Press, 1986).

6. Victor A. McKusick to A. McGehee Harvey, personal communication, 1988.

7. Ibid.

8. George D. Zuidema, oral history of the Department of Surgery, 1964 to 1984, recorded 1988, Alan M. Chesney Medical Archives, the Johns Hopkins Medical Institutions.

9. Ibid.

10. John Shaw Billings, *Description of the Johns Hopkins Hospital* (Baltimore: Johns Hopkins Hospital, 1890).

11. "New Center for Emergency Medicine Completed," *Hopkins Medical News* 6, no. 1 (March 1981): 2–4.

12. "New Department Links Brain Chemistry with Behavior, Drugs, and Disease," *Hopkins Medical News* 5, no. 4 (September 1980): 2–5; "Johns Hopkins Psychiatry and Neurology," *Hopkins Medical News* 8, no. 5 (November/December 1982): 1; Solomon H. Snyder to A. McGehee Harvey, personal communication, 1988.

13. "New Department Links Brain Chemistry," pp. 2–5.

14. Solomon H. Snyder to A. McGehee Harvey, October 26, 1987.

15. Thomas B. Turner to A. McGehee Harvey, personal communication, 1988.

16. John Harvey to A. McGehee Harvey, personal communication, 1974; W. Gordon Walker to A. McGehee Harvey, personal communication, 1988; Philip A. Norman to A. McGehee Harvey, personal communication, 1988; "Good Samaritan Hospital," Files, Alan M. Chesney Medical Archives, the Johns Hopkins Medical Institutions.

17. "The Legacy of Howard Hughes," *Hopkins Medical News* 10, no. 3 (Winter 1987): 12–20.

18. Daniel Nathans to A. McGehee Harvey, personal communication, 1987.

19. Information furnished by Dean Richard S. Ross, 1988.

20. Mark L. Batshaw et al., "Academic Promotion at a Medical School," *N. Engl. J. Med.* 318 (1988): 741.

21. Thomas B. Turner, *Accounting of a Stewardship* (Baltimore: Johns Hopkins University School of Medicine, 1969), p. 37.

22. Thomas B. Turner to A. McGehee Harvey, personal communication, 1988; untitled article, *Hopkins Medical News* 4, no. 2 (May 1979): 1.

23. Vernon B. Mountcastle to A. McGehee Harvey, personal communication, 1988.

24. Report of the Mountcastle Committee, Alan M. Chesney Medical Archives, the Johns Hopkins Medical Institutions.

25. "A Curriculum for the Second Century of Johns Hop-

kins Medicine," report of the Curriculum Committee of the Johns Hopkins University School of Medicine, 1988.

26. "Physicians for the Twenty-First Century," report of the Panel on the General Professional Education of the Physician and College Preparation for Medicine, Association of American Medical Colleges, 1984.

27. Richard S. Ross to A. McGehee Harvey, personal communication, 1988.

28. Paul Talalay to Susan L. Abrams, personal communication, 1988.

29. Victor A. McKusick, "A Plan for Reorganization of the Osler Medical Service," *Johns Hopkins Med. J.* 136 (1975): 231.

30. Extensive use has been made of the article by Robert M. Heyssel et al., "Decentralized Management in a Teaching Hospital," *N. Engl. J. Med.* 310 (1984): 1477–80. See also David B. Starkweather, "The Rationale for Decentralization in Large Hospitals," *Hospital Administration* 15, no. 2 (1970): 27–45.

31. Robert Heyssel to A. McGehee Harvey, personal communication, April 26, 1988.

32. Richard S. Ross to A. McGehee, personal communication, 1988.

33. Robert Heyssel to A. McGehee Harvey, personal communication, April 26, 1988.

34. Robert Heyssel, "The Hopkins Experience: The Hospital Perspective," address delivered at Duke University Medical Center, March 9, 1987.

35. Robert Heyssel to A. McGehee Harvey, personal communication, April 26, 1988.

36. Thomas B. Turner, quoted in Richard S. Ross, "The Hopkins Experience: The Academic Perspective," address delivered at Duke University Medical Center, March 9, 1987.

37. Ross, "The Hopkins Experience."

38. Heyssel, "The Hopkins Experience."

39. "The Johns Hopkins Health System," *Hopkins Medical News* 11, no. 1 (Summer 1987): 6.

Chapter 6   Women at the Medical School

Epigraph: Minute adopted by the Board of Trustees, the Johns Hopkins University, October 28, 1890, Alan M. Chesney Medical Archives, the Johns Hopkins Medical Institutions.

1. Agnes C. Vietor, *A Woman's Quest: The Life of Marie E. Zakrzewska* (New York: D. Appleton & Co., 1924), p. 436.

2. Mary R. Walsh, *Doctors Wanted: No Women Need Apply: Sexual Barriers in the Medical Profession, 1835–1975* (New Haven: Yale University Press, 1977), pp. 169–70.

3. Cora B. Marrett, "On the Evolution of Women's Med-

ical Societies," *Bull. Hist. Med.* 53 (1979): 434–49.

4. Walsh, *Doctors Wanted*, p. 193.

5. Gert H. Brieger, "Looking Backward: The First Woman Medical Student," *University of California San Francisco Magazine,* June–September 1979, p. 42.

6. Harold J. Abrahams, *The Extinct Medical Schools of Baltimore, Maryland* (Baltimore: Maryland Historical Society, 1969).

7. Walsh, *Doctors Wanted*, p. 179.

8. Regina M. Morantz-Sanchez, *Sympathy and Science: Women Physicians in American Medicine* (New York: Oxford University Press, 1985), p. 81.

9. Lilian Welsh, *Reminiscences of Thirty Years in Baltimore* (Baltimore: Norman, Remington Co., 1925), p. 37.

10. Women's Fund Committee, general circular, 1890, Alan M. Chesney Medical Archives, the Johns Hopkins Medical Institutions.

11. Untitled article, *Maryland Medical Journal* 24, no. 2 (November 8, 1890): 29.

12. Ibid.

13. Harvey Cushing, *The Life of Sir William Osler,* 2 vols. (London: Oxford University Press, 1925), 1: 387–88.

14. Mary E. Garrett to George W. Dobbin, April 27, 1891, Alan M. Chesney Medical Archives, the Johns Hopkins Medical Institutions.

15. Mary Gwinn to Logan Pearsall Smith, copy, early 1938, Alan M. Chesney Medical Archives, the Johns Hopkins Medical Institutions.

16. James Cardinal Gibbons, "On the Opening of the Johns Hopkins Medical School to Women," letter, *Century,* February 1891, pp. 632–33.

17. "Women and Medicine," editorial, *Nation,* February 12, 1891, p. 131.

18. Editorial, *Republican* (Springfield, Mass.), November 3, 1890.

19. Editorial, *Rocky Mountain News* (Denver, Colo.), November 9, 1890.

20. "The Temptation of Johns Hopkins," editorial, *Medical Record,* November 15, 1890.

21. Emily Blackwell, "The Temptation of Johns Hopkins," letter, *Medical Record,* December 6, 1890, p. 650.

22. William Osler to President Remsen of the Johns Hopkins University, "Whole-Time Clinical Professors," September 1, 1911, Alan M. Chesney Medical Archives, the Johns Hopkins Medical Institutions.

23. William H. Welch to Emma W. Walcott, November 11, 1890, Alan M. Chesney Medical Archives, the Johns Hopkins Medical Institutions. See also Donald Fleming, *William H. Welch and the Rise of Modern Medicine* (Boston: Little, Brown & Co., 1954), p. 98.

24. William H. Welch to Daniel C. Gilman, July 6, 1897,

Alan M. Chesney Medical Archives, the Johns Hopkins Medical Institutions.

25. Simon Flexner and James T. Flexner, *William Henry Welch and the Heroic Age of American Medicine* (New York: Viking Press, 1941), p. 218.

26. William H. Welch to Franklin P. Mall, November 7, 1891, Mall Papers, Alan M. Chesney Medical Archives, the Johns Hopkins Medical Institutions.

27. Hugh Hawkins, *Pioneer: A History of The Johns Hopkins University, 1874–1889* (Ithaca: Cornell University Press, 1960), p. 323.

28. Cushing, *Sir William Osler* 1:398–99.

29. Dorothy R. Mendenhall, manuscript autobiography, 10, Smith College Archives, cited in Morantz-Sanchez, *Sympathy and Science,* pp. 114–15.

30. Morantz-Sanchez, *Sympathy and Science,* p. 142.

31. Mendenhall, manuscript autobiography, 8, cited in Morantz-Sanchez, *Sympathy and Science,* p. 115.

32. William H. Welch to Daniel C. Gilman, June 21, 1898, Alan M. Chesney Medical Archives, the Johns Hopkins Medical Institutions.

33. Flexner and Flexner, *William Henry Welch,* p. 230.

34. Ibid., pp. 230–31.

35. David L. Edsall to J. Whitridge Williams, October 28, 1918, Alan M. Chesney Medical Archives, the Johns Hopkins Medical Institutions; J. Whitridge Williams to David L. Edsall, October 31, 1918, Alan M. Chesney Medical Archives, the Johns Hopkins Medical Institutions.

36. Welsh, *Reminiscences,* p. 46.

37. Ibid., p. 44.

38. Morantz-Sanchez, *Sympathy and Science,* p. 100.

39. Welsh, *Reminiscences,* pp. 44, 166–67.

40. John F. Goucher to Daniel C. Gilman, March 13, 1893, Alan M. Chesney Medical Archives, the Johns Hopkins Medical Institutions.

41. John F. Goucher to Daniel C. Gilman, May 31, 1893, Alan M. Chesney Medical Archives, the Johns Hopkins Institutions; memorandum, n.d., folder of correspondence between Daniel C. Gilman and John F. Goucher, 1893, Alan M. Chesney Medical Archives, the Johns Hopkins Medical Institutions.

42. Flexner and Flexner, *William Henry Welch,* p. 230.

43. Henry M. Hurd to Howard A. Kelly, September 4, 1897, Alan M. Chesney Medical Archives, the Johns Hopkins Medical Instituions.

44. Mary S. Packard, autobiographical notes, Alan M. Chesney Medical Archives, the Johns Hopkins Medical Institutions.

45. "Statistics, 1919–1920," *JAMA* 75 (1920): 383; "Medical Education," *JAMA* 144 (1950): 119.

46. Walsh, *Doctors Wanted,* p. 239.

47. Walsh, *Doctors Wanted,* p. 240.

48. Ibid., p. 203.

49. Ibid., p. 261.

50. Ibid., pp. 178–206; Morantz-Sanchez, *Sympathy and Science,* p. 87; Regina M. Morantz, Cynthia S. Pomerleau, and Carol H. Fenichel, *In Her Own Words: Oral Histories of Women Physicians* (Westport, Conn.: Greenwood Press, 1982), p. 25; Kenneth M. Ludmerer, *Learning to Heal: The Development of American Medical Education* (New York: Basic Books, 1985), p. 60. See also Abrahams, *Extinct Medical Schools.*

51. "Medical Education," p. 119.

52. Ibid.

53. J. Whitridge Williams to David L. Edsall, October 31, 1918, Alan M. Chesney Medical Archives, the Johns Hopkins Medical Institutions.

54. Welsh, *Reminiscences,* p. 46.

55. Carol J. Johns, interview by Susan L. Abrams, Baltimore, July 21, 1986.

56. Bessie L. Moses to Elinor Bleumel, September 6, 1955, Sabin manuscripts, Box 30, Smith College Archives, cited in Morantz-Sanchez, *Sympathy and Science,* pp. 264–65.

57. Ada C. Notestein, "The Sixth President of Smith," *Smith Alumnae Quarterly,* Winter 1959.

58. Mendenhall, manuscript autobiography, 22, cited in Morantz-Sanchez, *Sympathy and Science,* p. 178.

59. Mendenhall, manuscript autobiography, 2–21, cited in Morantz-Sanchez, *Sympathy and Science,* p. 177.

60. Welsh, *Reminiscences,* p. 46.

61. Walsh, *Doctors Wanted,* p. 184; "Survey of Women Physicians Graduating from Medical School 1925–1940," *J. Med. Educ.* 32 (1957): 33; Caroline B. Thomas, "What Becomes of Medical Students: The Dark Side," *Johns Hopkins Med. J.* 138 (1976): 189.

62. Welsh, *Reminiscences,* p. 39.

63. Response to questionnaire, Goucher College Alumnae Office.

64. Ibid.

65. "Medical Education," p. 119.

66. Caroline B. Thomas, interview by Susan L. Abrams, Baltimore, June 23, 1986.

67. Caroline B. Thomas, "Fulfilling the Promise: Hopkins Women before World War II," presented at the Mary Elizabeth Garrett Symposium: Women Physicians in Contemporary Society, Johns Hopkins Medical Institutions, October 7, 1979.

68. Harriet G. Guild, interview by Susan L. Abrams, Baltimore, July 8, 1986.

69. "Medical Education," p. 587.

70. Carol J. Johns, interview by Susan L. Abrams, Baltimore, July 21, 1986.

71. "Medical Education," p. 587.

72. Letter to director of Goucher College Alumnae Office, March 31, 1956.

73. Carol Lopate, *Women in Medicine* (Baltimore: Johns Hopkins Press, 1968), p. 169.

74. Jacqueline Seaver, "Women Doctors in Spite of Everything," *New York Times Magazine,* March 26, 1961, p. 67.

75. "Medical Education," p. 853.

76. Franklin P. Mall to Mabel S. Glover, June 6, 1894, Alan M. Chesney Medical Archives, the Johns Hopkins Medical Institutions.

77. Morantz, Pomerleau, and Fenichel, *In Her Own Words,* p. 32; Alice S. Rossi, "Why So Few Women Become Engineers, Doctors, and Scientists," in *Women and the Scientific Professions,* ed. Jacquelyn A. Mattfeld and Carol G. Van Aken (Cambridge: MIT Press, 1965); Phoebe A. Williams, "Women in Medicine: Some Themes and Variations," *J. Med. Educ.* 46 (1971): 584–91.

78. Thomas, "What Becomes of Medical Students," p. 189.

79. Davis G. Johnson, and Edwin B. Hutchins, "Doctor or Dropout: A Study of Medical Student Attrition," *J. Med. Educ.* 41 (1966): 1099–1269.

80. Jeremiah A. Barondess, "Are Women Different? Some Trends in the Assimilation of Women in Medicine," *J. Am. Women's Assoc.* 36 (1981): 95–104.

81. A. McGehee Harvey, *Adventures in Medical Research* (Baltimore: Johns Hopkins University Press, 1974), pp. 228–29. Information about Gertrude Stein was kindly provided by Gene Nakajima, in correspondence and in his unpublished manuscript, "Gertrude Stein's Medical Education at Johns Hopkins," and is used by permission. See also Elinor Bleumel, *Florence Sabin: Colorado Woman of the Century* (Boulder: University of Colorado Press, 1959), p. 75.

82. Harvey, *Adventures in Medical Research,* pp. 228–29.

83. Nancy Morris Davis to the Trustees of the Johns Hopkins University, *Johns Hopkins University Circular* 83 (November 1890): 14, Alan M. Chesney Medical Archives, the Johns Hopkins Medical Institutions.

84. Minute of the Board of Trustees, the Johns Hopkins University, *Johns Hopkins University Circular* 83 (November 1890): 14. Alan M. Chesney Medical Archives, the Johns Hopkins Medical Institutions.

85. M. Carey Thomas, "Women at Johns Hopkins," letter, *Nation,* February 5, 1891.

86. Gibbons, "On the opening," pp. 632–33.

87. Helen MacMurchy, "Hospital Appointments: Are They Open to Women?" *N.Y. Med. J.,* April 27, 1901, pp. 712–15.

88. Ibid.

89. Welsh, *Reminiscences,* p. 41.

90. Mendenhall, manscript autobiography, n.p., cited in Morantz-Sanchez, *Sympathy and Science,* pp. 166–67.

91. Vivien Thomas, *Pioneering Research in Surgical Shock and Cardiovascular Surgery* (Philadelphia: University of Pennsylvania Press, 1985), p. 121.

92. Harriet G. Guild, interview by Susan L. Abrams, Baltimore, July 8, 1986.

93. Morantz-Sanchez, *Sympathy and Science,* p. 335.

94. Ibid., pp. 99, 148.

95. Carol S. Shapiro et al., "Careers of Women Physicians: A Survey of Women Graduates from Seven Medical Schools, 1945–1951," *J. Med. Educ.* 43 (1968): 1033–40; "Survey of Women Physicians," p. 34; Lee Powers, Rexford D. Parmelle, and Harry Wiesenfelder, "Practice Patterns of Women and Men Physicians," *J. Med. Educ.* 44 (1969): 481.

96. H. Westling-Wikstrand, M. A. Monk, and C. B. Thomas, "Some Characteristics Related to the Career Status of Women Physicians," *Johns Hopkins Med. J.* 127 (1970): 275–76.

97. Powers, Parmelle, and Wiesenfelder, "Practice Patterns," p. 481; Madelaine R. Brown to Caroline B. Thomas, March 18, 1952, Alan M. Chesney Medical Archives, the Johns Hopkins Medical Institutions.

98. Madelaine R. Brown to Caroline B. Thomas, March 18, 1952, Alan M. Chesney Medical Archives, the Johns Hopkins Medical Institutions.

99. Westling-Wikstrand, Monk, and Thomas, "Career Status of Women Physicians," *Johns Hopkins Med. J.,* p. 274.

100. George W. Corner, *The Seven Ages of a Medical Scientist* (Philadelphia: University of Pennsylvania Press, 1981), p. 147.

101. Bleumel, *Florence Sabin,* p. 218.

102. Ibid., pp. 217–18.

103. Lawrence S. Kubie to Alan M. Chesney, June 16, 1961, Alan M. Chesney Medical Archives, the Johns Hopkins Medical Institutions. See also Lawrence S. Kubie, "Florence Rena Sabin, 1871–1953," *Perspect. Biol. Med.* 4, no. 3 (1961): 306–15.

104. Lewis H. Weed to Florence R. Sabin, May 30, 1925, Alan M. Chesney Medical Archives, the Johns Hopkins Medical Institutions.

105. Harvey, *Adventures in Medical Research,* pp. 224–47.

106. Ibid., pp. 230–31.

107. A. McGehee Harvey, *Science at the Bedside* (Baltimore: Johns Hopkins University Press, 1981), p. 345.

108. Information from biographical folders in Alan M. Chesney Medical Archives, The Johns Hopkins Medical Institutions. See also Barbara Sicherman et al., *Notable American Women—The Modern Period* (Cambridge: Harvard University Press, Belknap Press, 1980); Jacques Cattell Press, ed., *American Men and Women of Science* (New York: R. R. Bowker Co., 1975).

109. "Quotations from the Will of M. Carey Thomas," Alan M. Chesney Medical Archives, the Johns Hopkins Medical Institutions.

110. John Price Jones to Lewis H. Weed, January 27, 1925, Alan M. Chesney Medical Archives, the Johns Hopkins Medical Institutions.

111. Alan M. Chesney, *The Johns Hopkins Hospital and The Johns Hopkins University School of Medicine*, 3 vols. (Baltimore: Johns Hopkins University Press, 1943–63), 2:47.

112. Caroline B. Thomas, "How Women Medical Students First Came to Hopkins: A Chronicle," Staff newsletter, the Johns Hopkins Hospital, 1, no. 4 (February 1975).

113. Pearl V. Konttas, president of the Women's Association of the Johns Hopkins Medical School, memorandum, 1922, Alan M. Chesney Medical Archives, the Johns Hopkins Medical Institutions.

114. Thomas, "How Women Medical Students."

115. Carol J. Johns, president, Johns Hopkins Women's Medical Alumnae Association, to members, April 15, 1958, Alan M. Chesney Medical Archives, the Johns Hopkins Medical Institutions.

116. Morantz-Sanchez, *Sympathy and Science*, p. 85.

117. Richard Shryock, "Women in American Medicine," *J. Am. Med. Women's Assoc.* 5 (September 1950): 375.

118. Ludmerer, *Learning to Heal*, p. 14.

119. Walsh, *Doctors Wanted*, p. 139; Morantz, Pomerleau, and Fenichel, *In Her Own Words*, p. 18.

120. Walsh, *Doctors Wanted*, pp. 140, 143.

121. Morantz, Pomerleau, and Fenichel, *In Her Own Words*, p. 270.

122. Mary E. Garrett to the trustees of the Johns Hopkins University, December 22, 1892, Alan M. Chesney Medical Archives, the Johns Hopkins Medical Institutions. Katharine P. Loring to C. Morton Stewart, trustee of the Johns Hopkins Hospital, February 10, 1893, Alan M. Chesney Medical Archives, the Johns Hopkins Medical Institutions.

123. Morantz-Sanchez, *Sympathy and Science*, p. 142.

124. Ibid., p. 328.

125. Betty Friedan, *The Feminine Mystique* (New York: W. W. Norton & Co., 1963), p. 100.

126. Florence R. Sabin to P. H. Long, January 13, 1933, American Philosophical Society Archives, Philadelphia.

127. Florence R. Sabin to Helen B. Taussig, April 16, 1936, American Philosophical Society Archives, Philadelphia.

128. Walsh, *Doctors Wanted*, p. 279.

129. Morantz-Sanchez, *Sympathy and Science*, p. 328.

Chapter 7 "Learning by Doing"

Epigraph: John Dewey, "Johns Hopkins University," *Michigan Argonaut* 3 (1885): 292.

1. This point has been made forcefully by Kenneth M. Ludmerer in his book *Learning to Heal: The Development of American Medical Education* (New York: Basic Books, 1985). Our purpose here is to elaborate on this theme in the context of medicine at Johns Hopkins.

2. Daniel C. Gilman, *University Problems in the United States* (New York: Century Co. 1898).

3. Daniel C. Gilman, "The Johns Hopkins University in Its Beginning," inaugural address at the opening of the Johns Hopkins University, 1876, in Gilman, *University Problems* (New York: Century Co., 1897), p. 35.

4. Daniel C. Gilman, "Hand-craft and Rede-craft—A Plea for the First-Named," in Daniel C. Gilman, *The Launching of a University and Other Papers* (New York: Dodd, Mead, 1906), pp. 287–88.

5. Oscar Handlin, *John Dewey's Challenge to Education* (New York: Harper & Brothers, 1959), pp. 18–19, 33.

6. Laurence R. Veysey, *The Emergence of the American University* (Chicago: University of Chicago Press, 1965).

7. Oscar Handlin and Mary F. Handlin, *The American College and American Culture* (New York: Carnegie Foundation for the Advancement of Teaching, 1970).

8. Lawrence A. Cremin, *The Transformation of the School* (New York: Alfred A. Knopf, 1961), pp. 100–102.

9. Hugh Hawkins, *Pioneer: A History of the Johns Hopkins University, 1874–1889* (Ithaca: Cornell University Press, 1960), pp. 300–303.

10. John Shaw Billings, "The National Board of Health," *Plumber and Sanitary Engineer*, 3 (1880): 47, cited in Ludmerer, *Learning to Heal*, p. 64.

11. Ibid.

12. Henry K. Beecher and Mark D. Altschule, *Medicine at Harvard: The First Three Hundred Years* (Hanover, N.H.: University Press of New England, 1977), p. 111.

13. William H. Welch, "The Material Needs of Medical Education (1899)," reprinted in *Papers and Addresses by William Henry Welch*, 3 vols. (Baltimore: Johns Hopkins Press, 1920), 3: 68.

14. William H. Welch, "Some of the Advantages of the Union of Medical School and University (1888)," reprinted in Welch, *Papers and Addresses*, 3:30.

15. Welch, "Material Needs of Medical Education," 3:68.

16. John H. Warner, "Physiology," *The Education of American Physicians*, ed. Ronald L. Numbers (Berkeley and Los Angeles: University of California Press, 1980). See also William T. Porter, "The Teaching of Physiology in Medical Schools," *Boston Med. Surg. J.* 139 (1898): 647–48; Martin Kaufman, *American Medical Education: The Formative Years, 1765–1910* (Westport, Conn.: Greenwood Press, 1976), p. 148.

17. William H. Welch, "The Medical Curriculum (1910)," reprinted in Welch, *Papers and Addresses* 3:104–8.

18. David L. Cowen, "Materia Medica and Pharmacology," *Education of American Physicians*, ed. Numbers, p. 105. See also *John Jacob Abel, M.D: A Collection of Papers by and about the Father of American Pharmacology* (Baltimore: Williams & Wilkins, 1957).

19. John J. Abel, "On the Teaching of Pharmacology, Materia Medica, and Therapeutics in Our Medical Schools," *Phila. Med. J.*, September 1, 1900, pp. 9–10.

20. William H. Welch, "Laboratory Methods of Teaching," in Welch, *Papers and Addresses* 3:71.

21. Abel, "On the Teaching of Pharmacology," p. 18.

22. G. Canby Robinson, *Adventures in Medical Education* (Cambridge: Harvard University Press, 1957), p. 45.

23. William H. Welch, address at commencement, June 1893, in Announcement, the Johns Hopkins Medical School, 1893, Alan M. Chesney Medical Archives, the Johns Hopkins Medical Institutions.

24. Abel, "On the Teaching of Pharmacology," pp. 7–8.

25. Franklin P. Mall, "The Anatomical Course and Laboratory of the Johns Hopkins University," *Johns Hopkins Hosp. Bull.* 7 (1896): 85–100. See also Florence R. Sabin, *Franklin Paine Mall, The Story of a Mind* (Baltimore: Johns Hopkins Press, 1934), chap. 6.

26. Mall, "Anatomical Course and Laboratory," p. 86.

27. John B. Blake, "Anatomy," in *Education of American Physicians*, ed. Numbers, pp. 29–47.

28. Mall, "Anatomical Course and Laboratory," p. 86.

29. Sabin, *Franklin Paine Mall*, p. 138. See also Lewellys F. Barker and Charles R. Bardeen, "An Outline of the Course in Normal Histology and Microscopic Anatomy," *Johns Hopkins Hosp. Bull.* 7 (1896): 100–109.

30. Sabin, *Franklin Paine Mall*, p. 139.

31. Saul Benison, "Alan Gregg, An Oral History Memoir," Columbia University Oral History Research Office, 1956, pp. 33–35, quoted in Saul Benison, *Tom Rivers, Reflections on a Life in Medicine and Science* (Cambridge: MIT Press, 1967), p. 9.

32. Franklin P. Mall, "Liberty in Medical Education," *Phila. Med. J.* 3 (1899): 720, reprinted in *Science and Education*, ed. J. McKeen Cattell (New York: Science Press, 1913), 2:211–22.

33. Ibid.

34. Ibid.

35. Sabin, *Franklin P. Mall*, pp. 189–90.

36. Ibid., p. 190.

37. Franklin P. Mall, "The Value of Research in the Medical School," *Mich. Alumnus* 8 (1904): 395, cited in Sabin, *Franklin Paine Mall*, pp. 202–3.

38. Welch, "Material Needs of Medical Education," 3:68.

39. Welch, "Laboratory Methods of Teaching," 3:72.

40. Howard A. Kelly, "Methods of Teaching Gynecology," *Phila. Med. J.*, September 1, 1900, p. 392.

41. Gert H. Brieger, "Surgery," in *Education of American Physicians*, ed. Numbers, pp. 175–204. See also Harvey Cushing, "Instruction in Operative Medicine," *Bull. Johns Hopkins Hosp.* 17 (1906): 123–24.

42. E. Scott Carmichael, "The Surgical Department and Teaching of Surgery in the Johns Hopkins Hospital," *Scottish Med. Surg. J.* 22 (1908): 513–17.

43. "Medical Schools and Hospitals," editorial, *JAMA*, 35 (1900): 501.

44. William H. Welch, "The Relation of the Hospital to Medical Education and Research (1907)," reprinted in Welch, *Papers and Addresses* 3:134. See also Edward C. Atwater, "Internal Medicine," in *Education of American Physicians*, ed. Numbers, pp. 143–74. See also Ludmerer, *Learning to Heal*, chap. 8.

45. Harvey Cushing, *The Life of Sir William Osler*, 2 vols. (London: Oxford University Press, 1925), 2:372 et seq., 2:543–54.

46. William Osler, "The Natural Method of Teaching the Subject of Medicine," *JAMA* 36 (1901): 1673. See also William Osler, "The Hospital as a College," in *Aequanimitas* (New York: McGraw-Hill, 1932), pp. 311–25.

47. Percy M. Dawson, cited in Alan M. Chesney, *The Johns Hopkins Hospital and the Johns Hopkins University School of Medicine*, 3 vols. (Baltimore: Johns Hopkins Press, 1943–63), 2:128–29.

48. Lewellys F. Barker, "Osler as Chief of a Medical Clinic," *Bull. Johns Hopkins Hosp.* 30 (1919): 189–93. See also Atwater, "Internal Medicine," pp. 143–74; Ludmerer, *Learning to Heal*, pp. 60–61, 68–69.

49. The July 1919 issue (vol. 30) of *The Johns Hopkins Hospital Bulletin* contains eighteen articles about William Osler as teacher and clinician.

50. Atwater, "Internal Medicine," pp. 156–57.

51. William Osler, "Influence of Louis on American Medicine," *Johns Hopkins Hosp. Bull.* 8 (1897): 161.

52. A. McGehee Harvey, *Science at the Bedside* (Baltimore: Johns Hopkins University Press, 1981), pp. 6–13.

53. Ludmerer, *Learning to Heal*, pp. 21, 61. See also John

Duffy, ed., *The Rudolph Matas History of Medicine in Louisiana*, 2 vols. (Baton Rouge: Louisiana State University Press, 1958–1962), vol. 2, chap. 8.

54. Atwater, "Internal Medicine," pp. 143–74; quotation on p. 166.

55. George W. Corner, *The Seven Ages of a Medical Scientist* (Philadelphia: University of Pennsylvania Press, 1981), p. 80.

56. E. Scott Carmichael, "The Surgical Department and Teaching of Surgery in the Johns Hopkins Hospital," *Scottish Med. Surg. J.* 22 (1908): 515.

57. Ibid., pp. 513–17.

58. Harvey Cushing to Jay McLean, January 24, 1920, reprinted in John F. Fulton, *Harvey Cushing: A Biography* (Springfield, Ill.: Charles C Thomas, 1946), pp. 217–22.

59. Brieger, "Surgery," pp. 175–204. See also Cushing, "Instruction in Operative Medicine," pp. 123–24.

60. John F. Fulton, *Harvey Cushing: A Biography* (Springfield, Ill.: Charles C Thomas, 1946). See also Elizabeth L. Thomson, *Harvey Cushing: Surgeon, Author, Artist* (New York: Neale Watson Academic Publications, 1981), chap. 14.

61. Bertram M. Bernheim, *The Story of The Johns Hopkins* (New York: Whittlesey House, 1948), pp. 88–89.

62. Harvey W. Cushing and J. R. B. Branch, "Experimental and Clinical Notes on Chronic Valvular Lesions in the Dog and Their Possible Relation to a Future Surgery of the Cardiac Valve," *J. Med. Res.* 17 (1908): 471.

63. Kelly, "Methods of Teaching Gynecology," p. 392. See also Audrey W. Davis, *Dr. Kelly of Hopkins* (Baltimore: Johns Hopkins Press, 1959); Lawrence D. Longo, "Obstetrics and Gynecology," in *Education of American Physicians*, ed. Numbers, pp. 205–25; and Lawrence D. Longo, "John Whitridge Williams and Academic Obstetrics in America," *Trans. Coll. Phys. Phila.* 3 (1981): 221–54.

64. J. Whitridge Williams, "Teaching Obstetrics," *Bull. Am. Acad. Med.* 3 (1897–98): 409.

65. Ibid., p. 411.

66. Corner, *Seven Ages of a Medical Scientist*, p. 62.

67. Williams, "Teaching Obstetrics," p. 412.

68. Edward C. Atwater, "Making Fewer Mistakes: A History of Students and Patients," *Bull. Hist. Med.* 57 (1983): 165–87.

69. William H. Welch, "The Relation of the Hospital to Medical Education and Research (1907)," reprinted in Welch, *Papers and Addresses* 3:135.

70. Ibid., 3:136–37.

71. Abraham Flexner, *Medical Education in the United States and Canada*, Bull. no. 4 (New York: Carnegie Foundation for the Advancement of Teaching, 1910). See also Ludmerer, *Learning to Heal*, pp. 171–73.

72. Ludmerer, *Learning to Heal*, pp. 176–77.

73. Flexner, *Medical Education in the United States*, pp. 68–69. See also Abraham Flexner, *I Remember* (New York: Simon & Schuster, 1940) and Abraham Flexner, *Medical Education: A Comparative Study* (New York: Macmillan, 1925).

74. Flexner, *I Remember*, p. 250.

75. Joseph Ratner, "Introduction to John Dewey's Philosophy," in Rollo Handy, Edward C. Harwood, John Dewey, and Joseph Ratner, *Useful Procedures of Inquiry, by Rollo Handy and E. C. Harwood: Including Knowing and the Known, by John Dewey and Arthur F. Bentley, and Introduction to John Dewey's Philosophy, by Joseph Ratner* (Great Barrington, Mass.: Behavioral Research Council, 1973).

76. Philip P. Wiener, *Evolution and the Founders of Pragmatism* (Cambridge: Harvard University Press, 1949), p. 20.

77. Flexner, *Medical Education in the United States*, p. 68; Abraham Flexner, *Medical Education in Europe* (New York: Carnegie Foundation for the Advancement of Teaching, 1912), p. 168.

78. Arthur G. Wirth, *John Dewey as Educator* (New York: John Wiley & Sons, 1966), p. 10. Wirth cites Frances Littlefield Davenport, "The Education of John Dewey" (Ed.D. thesis, University of California, Los Angeles, 1946), p. 22.

79. Neil Coughlan, *Young John Dewey* (Chicago: University of Chicago Press, 1975), p. 18.

80. Richard J. Bernstein, *John Dewey* (New York: Washington Square Press, 1966), p. 14. See also George Dykhuizen, *The Life and Mind of John Dewey* (Carbondale: Southern Illinois University Press, 1973), pp. 28–43.

81. John Dewey, *Experience and Education* (New York: Macmillan, 1938), p. 87.

82. Ibid., p. 88. See also John Dewey, *Democracy and Education* (New York: Macmillan, 1916), p. 150; John Dewey, *Dictionary of Education* (New York: Philosophical Library, 1959), p. 121.

83. Dewey, *Experience and Education*, pp. 19–20. See also Donald Fleming, *William Henry Welch and the Rise of Modern Medicine* (Boston: Little, Brown & Co., 1954), p. 103.

84. John Dewey and Evelyn Dewey, *Schools of To-Morrow* (New York: E. P. Dutton, 1915), p. 16.

85. Dewey, *Experience and Education*, chaps. 3, 6, 7. See also Reginald D. Archambault, ed., *Dewey on Education* (New York: Random House, 1966); Sidney Hook, *John Dewey, Philosopher of Science and Freedom: a Symposium* (New York: Dial Press, 1950).

86. Dewey, *Experience and Education*, pp. 96–104. See also Wirth, *John Dewey as Educator*, pp. 282–83.

87. Sidney Hook, "Dewey: His Philosophy of Education and Its Critics," in *Dewey on Education*, ed. Archambault, pp. 127–60; Oscar Handlin, *John Dewey's Challenge*, p. 46.

88. Dewey and Dewey, *Schools of To-Morrow*, p. 70.

89. Dewey, *Experience and Education*, pp. 25, 87.

90. Flexner, *Medical Education in the United States*, p.69.

91. Longo, "Obstetrics and Gynecology," pp. 205–24.

92. Abel, "On the Teaching of Pharmacology," p. 12.

93. Thomas B. Turner, *Heritage of Excellence* (Baltimore: Johns Hopkins University Press, 1974), pp. 173–75.

94. Report of Curriculum Committee of the Johns Hopkins University School of Medicine, 1921, Alan M. Chesney Medical Archives, the Johns Hopkins Medical Institutions.

95. *The Johns Hopkins University Circular: Catalog and Announcement for 1921–1922 of the Medical Department*, n.s., no. 5, whole no. 333, October, 1921, p. 58.

96. *The Johns Hopkins University Circular: Catalog and Announcement for 1922–1923 of the Medical Department*, n.s., no. 6, whole no. 340, October 1922, p. 52.

97. *The Johns Hopkins University Circular: Catalog and Announcement for 1923–1924 of the Medical Department*, n.s., no. 6, whole no. 347, October 1923, p. 54.

98. Report of Curriculum Committee of the Johns Hopkins University School of Medicine, 1927, Alan M. Chesney Medical Archives, the Johns Hopkins Medical Institutions. See also Turner, *Heritage of Excellence*, pp. 173–75.

99. Turner, *Heritage of Excellence*, pp. 173–75.

100. Ibid., p. 175.

101. Arnold R. Rich, "Reflections of the Relation of the Curriculum to Certain Problems in Medical Education," *Bull. Johns Hopkins Hosp.* 69 (1931): 121–69.

102. Ibid., p. 155.

103. Ibid., p. 128.

104. Ibid., pp. 141–42.

105. Ibid., pp. 128–36.

106. Ibid., pp. 139–41.

107. Greer Williams, *Western Reserve's Experiment in Medical Education and Its Outcome* (New York: Oxford University Press, 1980).

108. Report of Curriculum Committee of the Johns Hopkins University School of Medicine, 1955, Alan M. Chesney Medical Archives, the Johns Hopkins Medical Institutions.

109. Samuel Asper, "A Revised Program of Medical Education at Johns Hopkins," *J. Med. Educ.* 33 (1958): 225; A. McGehee Harvey and Susan L. Abrams, *"For the Wel-*

fare of Mankind": The Commonwealth Fund and American Medicine (Baltimore: Johns Hopkins University Press, 1986).

110. Daniel Funkenstein, *Medical Students, Medical Schools and Society During Five Eras: Factors Affecting the Career Choices of Physicians 1958–76* (Cambridge, Mass.: Ballinger Publishing Co., 1978). See also Robert Ebert, "Medical Education," *Daedalus* 115, no. 2 (1986): 55–81.

111. Vernon W. Lippard and Elizabeth F. Purcell, *The Changing Medical Curriculum: Report of a Conference* (New York: Josiah C. Macy Foundation, 1972).

112. Robert R. Wagner, "The Basic Medical Sciences, the Revolution in Biology and the Future of Medical Education," *Yale J. Biol. Med.* 35 (1962): 1–11. See also Paul B. Beeson, "The Changing Role Model, and the Shift in Power," *Daedalus* 115, no. 2 (1986): 83–97.

113. Ebert, "Medical Education," p. 65.

114. Lippard and Purcell, *Changing Medical Curriculum*, p. vii.

115. Ibid., p. 10.

116. Ebert, "Medical Education," p. 67.

117. Ibid., pp. 68–72. See also John S. Millis, *The Graduate Education of Physicians* (Chicago: American Medical Association, 1966); Stanley R. Truman, *The History of the Founding of the American Academy of General Practice* (St. Louis: Warren H. Green, 1969).

118. Ebert, "Medical Education," pp. 72–75.

119. Robert G. Petersdorf, "Medical Schools and Research: Is the Tail Wagging the Dog?" *Daedalus* 115, no. 2 (1986): 99–118.

120. Report of the Curriculum Committee of 1975, Vernon H. Mountcastle, chairperson.

121. Harvey and Abrams, *"For the Welfare of Mankind"*, pp. 267–68.

122. Association of American Medical Colleges, "Physicians for the Twenty-First Century," *J. Med. Educ.* 59, part 2 (1984): 1–200.

123. "A Curriculum for the Second Century of Johns Hopkins Medicine," report of the Curriculum Committee, 1987, Gert H. Brieger, chairperson.

124. Paul Talalay, remarks at Yale-Duke Conference in Medical Education, Durham, N.C., April 20–22, 1986.

125. Ibid.

126. Report of Educational Policy Committee of Johns Hopkins School of Medicine to the Advisory Board, November 27, 1961, Alan M. Chesney Medical Archives, the Johns Hopkins Medical Institutions.

127. James A. Shannon, "Federal Support of Biomedical Sciences: Development and Academic Impact," *J. Med. Educ.* 51, suppl. (1976): 1–98.

128. Ibid.

129. John C. French, *A History of the University Founded by Johns Hopkins* (Baltimore: Johns Hopkins Press, 1946), pp. 39–44.

130. Chesney, *The Johns Hopkins Hospital* 1:79.

131. John Shaw Billings, "Hospital Construction and Organization," in *Hospital Plans: Five Essays Relating to the Construction, Organization and Management of Hospitals,* (New York, William Wood & Co., 1875), p. 5.

132. John Shaw Billings, "Suggestions on Medical Education from a Course of Lectures by John Shaw Billings," ed. Alan M. Chesney, *Bull. Inst. Hist. Med.* 6 (1938): 326.

133. Lewellys F. Barker, "Organization of the Laboratory in the Medical Clinic of The Johns Hopkins Hospital," *Johns Hopkins Hosp. Bull.* 18 (1907): 193.

134. Monte A. Calvert, *The Mechanical Engineer in America, 1830–1910* (Baltimore: Johns Hopkins Press, 1967).

135. William Osler, "The Hospital as a College," in *Aequanimitas,* pp. 311–25.

136. Corner, *Seven Ages of a Medical Scientist,* pp. 114–15.

137. Victor A. McKusick, "A Plan for Reorganization of the Osler Medical Service," *Johns Hopkins Med. J.* 136 (1975): 231.

138. George W. Heuer, "Dr. Halsted," *Bull. Johns Hopkins Hosp.* 90 (1952): 1. See also William S. Halsted, "The Training of the Surgeon," *Johns Hopkins Hosp. Bull.* 15 (1904): 267–75.

139. Mark Ravitch, "The Surgical Residency—Then, Now, and Future," *Pharos,* Winter 1987, pp. 13–14.

140. Ebert, "Medical Education," pp. 55–81.

141. Stewart W. Shankel and Ernest L. Mazzaferri, "Teaching the Resident in Internal Medicine: Present Practices and Suggestions for the Future," *JAMA* 256 (1986): 725–29. See also Joseph E. Hardison, "The House Officer's Changing World," *N. Engl. J. Med.* 314 (1986): 1713.

Chapter 8   Full-Time Professorships

Epigraph: Robert F. Loeb, "Acceptance of the Kober Medal Award for 1959," *Trans. Assoc. Am. Phys.* 72 (1959): 39.

1. W. Bruce Fye, *The Development of American Physiology: Scientific Medicine in the 19th Century* (Baltimore: Johns Hopkins University Press, 1987), p. 110.

2. William H. Welch, "The Advancement of Medical Education," report of remarks made at the Annual Dinner of the Harvard Medical School, June 1892, in *Papers and Addresses by William Henry Welch,* 3 vols. (Baltimore: Johns Hopkins Press, 1920), 3:43.

3. Simon Flexner and James T. Flexner, *William Henry Welch and the Heroic Age of American Medicine* (New York: Viking Press, 1941), pp. 112–13.

4. Alan M. Chesney, *The Johns Hopkins Hospital and the Johns Hopkins University School of Medicine,* 3 vols. (Baltimore: Johns Hopkins Press, 1943–63), 1:88.

5. Welch, "Advancement of Medical Education," 3:43.

6. William H. Welch, "Presidential Address, Association of American Physicians," *Trans. Assoc. Am. Phys.* 16 (1901): xvi–xvii. See also Flexner and Flexner, *William Henry Welch,* pp. 112–13.

7. Kenneth M. Ludmerer, *Learning to Heal: The Development of American Medical Education* (New York: Basic Books, 1985), chap. 11.

8. Lewellys F. Barker, "Medicine and the Universities," address delivered at the meeting of western alumni of the Johns Hopkins University in Chicago, February 28, 1902, in J. McKeen Cattell, *Medical Research and Education* (New York: Science Press, 1913), p. 223–40.

9. Ibid., p. 230.

10. Ibid., p. 239.

11. William H. Welch, "The Unity of the Medical Sciences," address delivered at the dedication of the new buildings of the Harvard Medical School, Boston, September 26, 1906, in Welch, *Papers and Addresses.* 3:309.

12. Ibid.

13. Harvey Cushing, *The Life of Sir William Osler,* 2 vols. (London: Oxford University Press, 1925), 2:271.

14. William Osler to President Remsen of the Johns Hopkins University, "Whole-Time Clinical Professors," September 1, 1911.

15. Ibid. See also Chesney, *The Johns Hopkins Hospital* 3:175–85; Cushing, *Sir William Osler,* vol. 2. See also Wilbur Davison, "Osler's opposition to 'whole time clinical professors,'" in *Humanism in Medicine,* ed. John P. McGovern and Chester R. Burns (Springfield, Ill., Charles C Thomas, 1973), pp 30–33.

16. Flexner and Flexner, *William Henry Welch,* p. 314.

17. Ibid., p. 324.

18. Ibid., pp. 309–12.

19. Ibid., pp. 309–12.

20. William S. Thayer, "The Medical Education of Jones, by Smith," first published anonymously in the *Harvard Graduates' Magazine* for March 1927 and again in *Physician and Patient, etc.,* ed. Louville E. Emerson (Cambridge: Harvard University Press, 1929); William S. Thayer, *Osler and Other Papers* (Baltimore: Johns Hopkins Press, 1931), p. 51; William S. Thayer, "Teaching and Practice," *Science* 43 (1916): 691; See also Ludmerer, *Learning to Heal,* p. 212.

21. Florence Sabin to Arnold R. Rich, December 1, 1934, Sabin Papers, American Philosophical Society, Philadelphia.

22. A. McGehee Harvey, "Rufus Cole and the Hospital of the Rockefeller Institute," in *Trends in Biomedical Research,*

1901–1976, proceedings of the 2d Rockefeller Conference, December 10, 1976 (New York: Rockefeller Archives Center, 1977).

23. William H. Howell, "The Medical School as Part of the University," *Science* 30 (1909): 29.

24. Florence R. Sabin, *Franklin P. Mall, The Story of a Mind* (Baltimore: Johns Hopkins Press, 1934), pp. 260–61.

25. Abraham Flexner, *Medical Education in the United States and Canada,* Bull. no. 4 (New York: Carnegie Foundation for the Advancement of Teaching, 1910), p. 53.

26. Flexner and Flexner, *William Henry Welch,* p. 306.

27. Ibid., p. 320.

28. Chesney, *The Johns Hopkins Hospital* 3:256.

29. Lewellys F. Barker, "Some Tendencies in Medical Education in the United States," address at convocation exercises, McGill University, June 5, 1911, in Cattell, *Medical Research and Education,* p. 241.

30. Ibid., p. 257.

31. A. McGehee Harvey, *Science at the Bedside* (Baltimore: Johns Hopkins University Press, 1981), pp. 153–59.

32. Theodore C. Janeway, "Outside Professional Engagements by Members of Professional Faculties," *JAMA* 90 (1928): 1315.

33. Ibid.

34. Ibid.

35. Ibid.

36. Ibid.

37. Dana Atchley, "The Uses of Elegance," *Ann. Intern. Med.* 52 (1960): 887.

38. Thayer, "Teaching and Practice," p. 961.

39. Ibid.

40. Harvey, *Science at the Bedside,* pp. 168–69.

41. G. Canby Robinson, *Adventures in Medical Education* (Cambridge: Harvard University Press, 1957).

42. Harvey, *Science at the Bedside,* pp. 172–74. See also A. McGehee Harvey, "The Story of Warfield T. Longcope," *Trans. Stud. Coll. Phys. Phila.* 3 (1981): 3; William S. Tillett, "Warfield Theobald Longcope—March 29, 1877–April 25, 1953," *Biographical Memoirs of the National Academy of Sciences,* no. 33 (New York: Columbia University Press, 1959), p. 205.

43. Harvey, *Science at the Bedside,* p. 161.

44. Edwards A. Park, "John Howland," *Science* 64 (1926): 80.

45. Thomas B. Turner, *Heritage of Excellence* (Baltimore: Johns Hopkins University Press, 1974), pp. 528–31.

46. Ibid., pp. 531–34.

47. Turner, *Heritage of Excellence,* p. 531; Austin Lamont to Warfield M. Firor, 1965, National Library of Medicine.

48. Turner, *Heritage of Excellence,* pp. 416–19.

49. Ibid., p. 534.

50. Ibid., p. 535.

51. Ibid., p. 536; William W. Scott, *Urology at Hopkins: A Chronicle,* vol. 1, 1889–1986 (Baltimore: Williams & Wilkins, 1987).

52. William Lloyd Fox, *Dandy of Johns Hopkins* (Baltimore: Williams & Wilkins, 1984).

53. George B. Udvarhelyi, "Tribute to Dr. A. Earl Walker," *J. Nerv. Ment. Dis.* 147 (1968): 3–13.

54. A. McGehee Harvey, "Halsted's Innovative Ventures in the Surgical Specialties: Samuel J. Crowe and the Department of Otolaryngology," *Johns Hopkins Med. J.* 140 (1977): 101.

55. A. McGehee Harvey, "Orthopedic Surgery at Johns Hopkins: A Heritage of Excellence in Clinical Practice, Teaching, and Research," *Johns Hopkins Med. J.* 150 (1982): 221.

56. Turner, *Heritage of Excellence,* p. 431.

57. Howard W. Jones, Georgeanna S. Jones, and William E. Ticknor, *Richard Wesley TeLinde* (Baltimore: Williams & Wilkins, 1986).

58. Lawrence D. Longo, "John Whitridge Williams and Academic Obstetrics in America," *Trans. Stud. Coll. Phys. Phila.* 3 (1981): 221–54.

59. Joseph C. Aub and Ruth K. Hapgood, *Pioneer in Modern Medicine: David Linn Edsall of Harvard* (Boston: Harvard Medical Alumni Association, 1970), pp. 171–72.

60. Ibid., p. 172.

61. Deryl Hart, *The First 40 Years at Duke and the P.D.C.* (Durham, N.C.: Duke University, 1971).

62. Donald Fleming, "The Full-Time Controversy," *J. Med. Educ.* 30, no. 7 (1955): 398–406.

Chapter 9   The Export of Hopkins Physicians

Epigraph: William H. Welch, "The Advancement of Medical Education," in *Papers and Addresses by William H. Welch,* 3 vols. (Baltimore: Johns Hopkins Press, 1920), 3:44.

1. Kenneth M. Ludmerer, *Learning to Heal: The Development of American Medical Education* (New York: Basic Books, 1985).

2. W. Bruce Fye, *The Development of American Physiology* (Baltimore: Johns Hopkins University Press, 1987).

3. George W. Heuer, "Dr. Halsted," *Bull. Johns Hopkins Hosp.* 90 (1952): 1; Samuel J. Crowe, *Halsted of Johns Hopkins: The Man and His Men* (Springfield, Ill.: Charles C Thomas, 1957).

4. A. McGehee Harvey, "The Influence of William Stewart Halsted's Concept of Surgical Training," *Johns Hopkins Med. J.* 148 (1981): 215.

5. William Andrus, "George W. Heuer's Contributions and

His Place in American Surgery," *Surgery* 23 (1948): 321–25.

6. B. N. Carter, "The Fruition of Halsted's Concept of Surgical Training," *Surgery* 32 (1952): 518.

7. Walter L. Bierring, *A History of the Department of Internal Medicine, State University of Iowa College of Medicine, 1870–1958* (Ames: State University of Iowa, 1958).

8. Merle Curti and Vernon Carstensen, *The University of Wisconsin: A History, 1848–1925* (Madison: University of Wisconsin Press, 1949); Paul F. Clark, *The University of Wisconsin Medical School: A Chronicle, 1848–1948* (Madison: University of Wisconsin Press, 1967); Allan G. Bogue and Robert Taylor, *The University of Wisconsin: One Hundred and Twenty-Five Years* (Madison: University of Wisconsin Press, 1975).

9. Albert R. Lamb, *The Presbyterian Hospital and the Columbia-Presbyterian Medical Center, 1868–1943* (New York: Columbia University Press, 1955).

10. G. Canby Robinson, *Adventures in Medical Education* (Cambridge: Harvard University Press, 1957).

11. John F. Fulton, *Harvey Cushing* (Springfield, Ill.: Charles C Thomas, 1946), p. 306.

12. Edwin Mims, *History of Vanderbilt University* (Nashville: Vanderbilt University Press, 1946); Rudolph H. Kampmeier, *Recollections: The Department of Medicine, Vanderbilt University School of Medicine, 1925–1959* (Nashville: Vanderbilt University Press, 1980).

13. G. Canby Robinson, "The Use of Full-Time Teachers of Clinical Medicine," address to the Southern Medical Association, *South. Med. J.* 15 (1922): 1009.

14. John Romano et al., eds., *To Each His Farthest Star* (Rochester, N.Y.: University of Rochester Medical Center, 1975).

15. Ibid., p. 45.

16. Ibid., p. 72.

17. A. McGehee Harvey, *Science at the Bedside* (Baltimore: Johns Hopkins University Press, 1981), p. 312.

18. James F. Gifford, Jr., *The Evolution of a Medical Center: A History of Medicine at Duke University to 1941* (Durham, N.C.: Duke University Press, 1972); Deryl Hart, *The First Forty Years at Duke in Surgery and the P.D.C.* (Durham, N.C.: Duke University Press, 1971); Jay M. Arena and John P. McGovern, eds., *Davison of Duke: His Reminiscences* (Durham, N.C.: Duke University Medical Center, 1980).

19. Arena and McGovern, eds., *Davison of Duke*, p. 111.

20. Hart, *First Forty Years*, p. 78.

21. Ibid., p. 109.

22. Dan McNamara, "The Original Pediatric Cardiologist: Helen B. Taussig, 1898–1986," pamphlet containing text of memorial tribute, the Johns Hopkins Medical Institutions, June 26, 1986, Alan M. Chesney Medical Ar-chives, the Johns Hopkins Medical Institutions.

23. Ibid.; Richard S. Ross, "Presentation of the George M. Kober Medal (posthumously) to Helen B. Taussig," *Trans. Assoc. Am. Phys.* 100 (1987): cxii.

24. A. McGehee Harvey, *Adventures in Medical Research* (Baltimore: Johns Hopkins University Press, 1974), pp. 217–24.

25. Thomas B. Turner, "Nobel Prize Winners Who Knew Baltimore," *Hopkins Medical News* 4, no. 1 (March 1979): 5–6.

26. Paul Talalay to Susan L. Abrams, personal communication, 1988.

27. Horace W. Davenport, *Fifty Years of Medicine at the University of Michigan, 1891–1941* (Ann Arbor: University of Michigan School of Medicine, 1986).

28. Richard Shryock, *The Unique Influence of The Johns Hopkins University in American Medicine* (Copenhagen: Ejnar Munksgaard, 1953), p. 61.

29. John Stobo to A. McGehee Harvey, personal communication, 1987.

30. Ibid.

Chapter 10 Johns Hopkins Medicine and the Community

Epigraph: Hospital Plans: Five Essays Relating to the Construction, Organization, and Management of Hospitals (New York, William Wood & Co., 1875), p. xvi.

1. Catherine DeAngelis, quoted in "Celebrating 75 Years of Children's Health Care," brochure published by the Johns Hopkins Children's Center, Office of Public Affairs, November 1987, Alan M. Chesney Medical Archives, the Johns Hopkins Medical Institutions, unpaged.

2. Thomas B. Turner, *Heritage of Excellence* (Baltimore: Johns Hopkins University Press, 1974), pp. 314–17.

3. Ibid.; also see Annual Reports of the Director of the Johns Hopkins Hospital, 1929–1952, Alan M. Chesney Medical Archives, the Johns Hopkins Medical Institutions.

4. John C. Harvey, personal communication, 1976; Turner, *Heritage of Excellence*, pp. 314–17. Also see Annual Reports of the Director of the Johns Hopkins Hospital, 1948–1967, Alan M. Chesney Medical Archives, the Johns Hopkins Medical Institutions.

5. Turner, *Heritage of Excellence*, pp. 313–14.

6. Annual Reports of the Director of the Johns Hopkins Hospital, 1948–1967, Alan M. Chesney Medical Archives.

7. John C. Harvey, personal communication, 1976.

8. Annual Reports of the Director of the Johns Hopkins

Hospital, 1948–1967, Alan M. Chesney Medical Archives.

9. Ibid.

10. Richard J. Johns, memorandum, "Columbia and the Department of Medicine," November 5, 1968, Alan M. Chesney Medical Archives, the Johns Hopkins Medical Institutions.

11. Thomas B. Turner, *Accounting of a Stewardship* (Baltimore: Johns Hopkins University School of Medicine, 1969), p. 49.

12. Robert M. Heyssel and Henry M. Seidel, "The Johns Hopkins Experience in Columbia, Maryland," *N. Engl. J. Med.* 295 (1976): 1225–31.

13. J. Richard Gaintner, memorandum, "Health Maintenance Organizations and Academic Medical Centers: The Hopkins Experience," August 8, 1980, Alan M. Chesney Medical Archives, the Johns Hopkins Medical Institutions.

14. Ibid.

15. Russell A. Nelson, "Hospital Administration Oral History, 1985," Alan M. Chesney Medical Archives, the Johns Hopkins Medical Institutions, p. 12.

16. David E. Rogers and Robert M. Heyssel, "One Medical School's Involvement in New Health Care Delivery Models: Its Problems and Its Pleasures," *Arch. Intern. Med.* 127 (1970): 57–64; David E. Rogers, "Research and Development in New Health Care Programs: An Expanded Hopkins Mission," *Johns Hopkins Med. J.* 128 (1971): 1–2; Clifton Gaus, "Who Enrolls in a Prepaid Group Practice: The Columbia Experience," *Johns Hopkins Med. J.* 128 (1971): 9–14; Malcolm L. Peterson, "The First Year in Columbia: Assessments of Low Hospitalization Rate and High Office Use," *Johns Hopkins Med. J.* 128 (1971): 15–23; Heyssel and Seidel, "Johns Hopkins Experience in Columbia," pp. 1225–31.

17. Gaintner, memorandum, "Health Maintenance Organizations and Academic Medical Centers," August 8, 1980, Alan M. Chesney Medical Archives, p. 15.

18. Clarence Burns, quoted in *Hopkins Medical News,* Fall 1986, p. 10.

19. Nelson, "Hospital Administration Oral History, 1985," Alan M. Chesney Medical Archives, pp. 11–12; Robert J. Blendon and Clifton R. Gaus, "Problems in Developing Health Services in Poverty Areas: The Johns Hopkins Experience," *J. Med. Educ.* 46 (1971): 447–84.

20. Gaintner, memorandum, "Health Maintenance Organizations and Academic Medical Centers," August 8, 1980, Alan M. Chesney Medical Archives, p. 16.

21. Robert J. Blendon, "The Age of Discontinuity: The Financing of Innovative Health Care Programs in Poverty Areas," *Johns Hopkins Med. J.* 128 (1971): 24–29.

22. Robert M. Heyssel, "The Hopkins Experience: The Hospital Perspective," address delivered at Duke University Medical Center, March 9, 1987; Blendon and Gaus, "Health Services in Poverty Areas," pp. 477–84.

23. Gaintner, memorandum, "Health Maintenance Organizations and Academic Medical Centers," August 8, 1980, Alan M. Chesney Medical Archives, p. 18.

24. Heyssel, "The Hopkins Experience," address delivered at Duke University Medical Center, March 9, 1987.

25. Ibid.

26. Ibid.

27. Gaintner, memorandum, "Health Maintenance Organizations and Academic Medical Centers," August 8, 1980, Alan M. Chesney Medical Archives; Heyssel and Seidel, "Hopkins Experience in Columbia," pp. 1225–31; Rogers and Heyssel, "New Health Care Delivery Models," pp. 57–64; Nelson, "Hospital Administration Oral History, 1985," Alan M. Chesney Medical Archives, p. 12.

28. Heyssel, "The Hopkins Experience," address delivered at Duke University Medical Center, March 9, 1987.

29. Ibid.

Chapter 11　　The Nature of Discovery

Epigraph: John Jacob Abel, cited in A. McGehee Harvey, *Adventures in Medical Research* (Baltimore: Johns Hopkins University Press, 1974), p. 58.

1. Alfred Blalock, "The Nature of Discovery," *Ann. Surg.* 144 (1956): 289.

2. Ibid.

3. Florence R. Sabin, *Franklin Paine Mall, The Story of a Mind* (Baltimore: Johns Hopkins Press, 1934), pp. 57–59, See also Franklin P. Mall, "Die Blut- und Lymphwege in Dünndarm des Hundes," *Abhandl. math.-phys. Cl. k. sächs. Gesellsch. Wissensch.* 14 (1887): 153.

4. Sabin, *Franklin P. Mall,* pp. 76–77.

5. Harvey, *Adventures in Medical Research,* chap. 10. For Mall's complete bibliography, see the *Bulletin of the Johns Hopkins Hospital* 29 (1918): 122.

6. Franklin P. Mall, "On the Circulation through the Pulp of the Dog's Spleen," *Am. J. Anat.* 2 (1903): 315; Franklin P. Mall, "A Study of the Structural Unit of the Liver," *Am. J. Anat.* 5 (1906): 227.

7. Harvey, *Adventures in Medical Research,* pp. 101–2.

8. Sabin, *Franklin Paine Mall,* p. viii.

9. Michael Heidelberger and Philip McMaster, "Florence R. Sabin," in *Biographical Memoirs of the National Academy of Sciences,* no. 34 (New York: Columbia University Press, 1960), p. 272.

10. Florence R. Sabin, "Studies of Living Human Blood Cells," *Johns Hopkins Hosp. Bull.* 34 (1923): 277.

11. Florence R. Sabin, "On the Origin of the Cells of the Blood," *Physiol. Rev.* 2 (1922): 38.

12. John B. MacCallum, "On the Histology and Histogenesis of the Heart Muscle Wall," *Anat. Anz. (Jena)* 13 (1897): 609, cited in Harvey, *Adventures in Medical Research,* pp. 107–13.

13. Archibald Malloch, *Short Years: The Life and Letters of John Bruce MacCallum, 1876–1906* (Chicago: Normandie House, 1938).

14. John B. MacCallum, "On the Muscular Architecture of the Ventricles of the Human Heart," *Am. J. Anat.* 11 (1910): 211.

15. Frederik G. Bang, "History of Tissue Culture at Johns Hopkins," *Bull. Hist. Med.* 51 (1977): 516.

16. Ross G. Harrison, "Observations of the Living Developing Nerve Fiber," *Proc. Soc. Exp. Biol. Med.* 4 (1907): 140.

17. John Spangler Nicholas, "Ross G. Harrison," in *Biographical Memoirs of the National Academy of Sciences,* no. 35 (New York: Columbia University Press, 1961), p. 132; Jane Oppenheimer, Dictionary of Scientific Biography, 16 vols. (NY: Scribner's, 1970–1980), 6:134–35.

18. George W. Corner, "Warren H. Lewis," in *Biographical Memoirs of the National Academy of Sciences,* no. 39 (New York: Columbia University Press, 1967), p. 323.

19. George W. Corner, Margaret R. Lewis, and Warren H. Lewis, "The Cultivation of Tissue from Chick Embryos in Solutions of NaCl, CaCl$_2$ and NaHCO$_3$," *Anat. Rec.* 5 (1911): 277; see also George W. Corner, Margaret R. Lewis, and Warren H. Lewis, "The Cultivation of Chick Tissue in Media of Known Chemical Constitution," *Anat. Rec.* 6 (1912): 207.

20. George W. Corner, Warren H. Lewis, and George O. Gey, "Clasmatocytes and Tumor Cells in Cultures of Mouse Sarcoma," *Johns Hopkins Hosp. Bull.* 34 (1923): 369.

21. Warren H. Lewis, "Pinocytosis," *Bull. Johns Hopkins Hosp.* 49 (1931): 17. See also Corner, "Warren H. Lewis," p. 323.

22. A complete list of George O. Gey's publications is available in Gey's biographical file in the Alan M. Chesney Medical Archives, the Johns Hopkins Medical Institutions.

23. George O. Gey, "Cellular Responses to Viruses in Relation to Cancer," in *Proceedings of the Third National Cancer Conference,* 1957, p. 453.

24. George O. Gey, "Some Aspects of the Constitution and Behavior of Normal and Malignant Cells in Continuous Culture," in *The Harvey Lectures,* ser. L, 1954–55 (New York: Academic Press, 1955).

25. Ibid.; Bang, "Tissue Culture at Johns Hopkins," p. 516.

26. Bang, "Tissue Culture at Johns Hopkins," p. 516.

27. George O. Gey, Ward D. Coffman, and Mary T. Kubicek, "Tissue Culture Studies of the Proliferative Capacity of Cervical Carcinoma and Normal Epithelium," *Cancer Res.* 12 (1952): 264.

28. George O. Gey and Frederik G. Bang, "Cell Structure—A Comparative Study of the Cytological Characteristics of Normal and Malignant Cells with Phase and Electron Microscopy," *Anat. Rec.* 33 (1952): 98. For a comprehensive review of tissue culture at Johns Hopkins, see Bang, "History of Tissue Culture at Johns Hopkins," p. 516.

29. Thomas R. Brown, "Studies of Trichinosis with Special Reference to the Increase of Eosinophilic Cells in the Blood and Muscle, the Origin of These Cells and Their Diagnostic Importance," *J. Exp. Med.* 3 (1898): 315.

30. Bailey Ashford, *A Soldier in Science* (New York: William Morrow & Co., 1934).

31. William Osler, "The Practical Value of Laveran's Discoveries," *Med. News Phila.* 67 (1895): 561.

32. William S. Thayer, *Lectures on Malarial Fever* (New York: D. Appleton & Co., 1897).

33. Eugene L. Opie, "On the Haemocytozoa of Birds," *Johns Hopkins Hosp. Bull.* 8 (1897): 52.

34. William G. MacCallum, "On the Haematozoan Infections of Birds," *Johns Hopkins Hosp. Bull.* 8 (1897): 235; William G. MacCallum, "Notes on the Pathological Changes in the Organs of Birds Infected with Haemocytozoa," *J. Exp. Med.* 3 (1898): 103; William G. MacCallum, "On the Haematozoan Infections of Birds," *J. Exp. Med.* 3 (1898): 117; William G. MacCallum, "On the Haematozoan Infections of Birds," *Johns Hopkins Hosp. Bull.* 9 (1898): 18.

35. William G. MacCallum and Carl Voegtlin, "On the Relation of the Parathyroid Gland to Calcium Metabolism and the Nature of Tetany," *Johns Hopkins Hosp. Bull.* 18 (1908): 244; William G. MacCallum and Carl Voegtlin, "On the Relation of the Parathyroid to Calcium Metabolism and the Nature of Tetany," *Johns Hopkins Hosp. Bull.* 19 (1908): 91; William G. MacCallum and Carl Voegtlin, "On the Relation of Tetany to the Parathyroid Glands and to Calcium Metabolism," *J. Exp. Med.* 11 (1909): 118; Harvey, *Adventures in Medical Research,* pp. 20–29.

36. James G. Hirsch, "Eugene L. Opie (1873–1971)," *Trans. Assoc. Am. Phys.* 84 (1971): 32.

37. Peyton Rous, "An Inquiry into Certain Aspects of Eugene L. Opie," *Arch. Pathol.* 34 (1942): 2.

38. Eugene L. Opie, "On the Relation of Chronic Interstitial Pancreatitis to the Islands of Langerhans and to Diabetes Mellitus," *J. Exp. Med.* 5 (1900): 419.

39. William G. MacCallum, "On the Relation of the Islands

of Langerhans to Glycosuria," *Johns Hopkins Hosp. Bull.* 20 (1909): 265.

40. Vernon R. Mason, "Sickle Cell Anemia," *JAMA* 79 (1922): 1318.

41. John Huck, "Sickle Cell Anemia," *Johns Hopkins Hosp. Bull.* 34 (1923): 335.

42. C. Lockard Conley, "Sickle Cell Anemia—the First Molecular Disease," in M. M. Wintrobe, *Blood Pure and Eloquent* (New York: McGraw-Hill, 1980), p. 334.

43. Irving J. Sherman, "The Sickling Phenomenon, with Special Reference to the Differentiation of Sickle Cell Anemia from the Sickle Cell Trait," *Bull. Johns Hopkins Hosp.* 67 (1940): 309.

44. Linus Pauling et al., "Sickle Cell Anemia: A Molecular Disease," *Science* 110 (1949): 543. See also Harvey, *Adventures in Medical Research,* pp. 302–5.

45. Ernest W. Smith and C. Lockard Conley, "Filter Paper Electrophoresis of Human Hemoglobin with Special Reference to the Incidence and Clinical Significance of Hemoglobin C," *Bull. Johns Hopkins Hosp.* 93 (1953): 94.

46. Ernest W. Smith and John A. Torbert, "Study of Two Abnormal Hemoglobins with Evidence for a New Genetic Locus for Hemoglobin Formation," *Bull. Johns Hopkins Hospital* 102 (1958): 38–45.

47. C. Lockard Conley, et al., "Heredity Persistence of Fetal Hemoglobin: A Study of 79 Affected Persons in 15 Negro Families in Baltimore," *Blood* 21 (1963): 261–81.

48. For additional references see Conley, "Sickle Cell Anemia," p. 319.

49. Maxwell M. Wintrobe et al., "A Familial Hemopoietic Disorder in Italian Adolescents and Adults: Resembling Mediterranean Disease (Thalassemia)," *JAMA* 114 (1940): 1530–38.

50. Vernon Ingram and A. O. W. Strefton, "Genetic Basis of the Thalassemias," *Nature* 184 (1959): 1903.

51. David Weatherall, John Clegg, and Michael Naughton, "Globin Synthesis in Thalassemia: An In Vitro Study," *Nature* 208 (1965): 1061.

52. John J. Abel and Albert C. Crawford, "On the Blood-Pressure-Raising Constituent of the Suprarenal Capsule," *Trans. Assoc. Am. Phys.* 12 (1897): 461.

53. Leonard G. Rowntree and John T. Geraghty, "An Experimental and Clinical Study of Functional Activity of the Kidney by Means of Phenolsulfonphthalein," *J. Pharmacol. Exp. Ther.* 1 (1910): 579.

54. John J. Abel, Leonard G. Rowntree, and Benjamin B. Turner, "On the Removal of Diffusible Substances from the Circulating Blood by Means of Dialysis," *Trans. Assoc. Am. Phys.* 28 (1913): 51.

55. John J. Abel, "Plasma Removal with Return of Corpus-

cles [Plasmapheresis]: First Paper," *J. Pharmacol. Exp. Ther.* 5 (1914): 627.

56. The Guillian-Barré Syndrome Study Group, "Plasmapheresis and Acute Guillain-Barré Syndrome," *Neurology* 35 (1985): 1096–1104.

57. Eli K. Marshall, Jr., "A New Method for the Determination of Urea in Urine," *J. Biol. Chem.* 15 (1913): 487.

58. Thomas H. Maren, "Eli Kennerly Marshall, Jr. (1889–1966)," *Bull. Johns Hopkins Hosp.* 119 (1966): 247.

59. Eli K. Marshall, Jr., and James L. Vickers, "The Mechanism of Elimination of Phenolsulfonphthalein by the Kidney—A Proof of Secretion by the Convoluted Tubules," *Johns Hopkins Hosp. Bull.* 34 (1923): 1.

60. Maren, "Eli Kennerly Marshall, Jr.," p. 247.

61. Ibid.

62. Ibid.

63. E. Kennerly Marshall, Jr., "Scientific Principles, Methods, and Results of Chemotherapy," *Medicine* 26 (1947): 155.

64. Sir Sheldon R. Dudley, *Our National Health Service: An Essay on the Preservation of Health* (London: Watts & Co., 1953).

65. Maren, "Eli Kennerly Marshall, Jr.," p. 247.

66. Harvey, *Adventures in Medical Research,* pp. 340–47.

67. Ibid., p. 342.

68. Joel Elkes, "Behavioral Medicine: The Early Beginnings," *Psych. Annals* 11, no. 2 (1981): 22.

69. M. Brewster Smith, presentation of D.Sc. degree to Curt Richter, University of Chicago.

70. Arnold R. Rich, "The Role of Hypersensitivity in Periarteritis Nodosa as Indicated by Seven Cases Developing during Serum Sickness and Sulfonamide Therapy," *Bull. Johns Hopkins Hosp.* 71 (1942): 123.

71. Arnold R. Rich and John E. Gregory, "The Experimental Demonstration that Periarteritis is a Manifestation of Hypersensitivity," *Bull. Johns Hopkins Hosp.* 72 (1943):65.

72. Frederick G. Germuth, Jr., and George E. McKinnon, "Studies on the Biological Properties of Antigen-Antibody Complexes: I. Anaphylactic Shock Induced by Soluble Complexes in Unsensitized Guinea Pigs," *Bull. Johns Hopkins Hosp.* 101 (1957): 13; Frank J. Dixon, "The Role of Antigen-Antibody Complexes in Disease," The *Harvey Lectures,* ser. 58P, 1962–63 (New York: Academic Press, 1964).

73. David J. Gocke et al., "Association between Polyarteritis and Australia Antigen," *Lancet* 2 (1970): 1149.

74. Arnold R. Rich, "The Formation of Bile Pigment from Hemoglobin in Tissue Cultures," *Bull. Johns Hopkins Hosp.* 35 (1924): 415.

75. Arnold R. Rich, "The Pathogenesis of the Forms of

Jaundice," *Bull. Johns Hopkins Hosp.* 37 (1930): 338.

76. Arnold R. Rich and Howard A. McCordock, "An Enquiry Concerning the Role of Allergy, Immunity and Other Factors of Importance in the Pathogenesis of Tuberculosis," *Bull. Johns Hopkins Hosp.* 44 (1929): 273.

77. Arnold R. Rich, "Significance of Hypersensitivity in Infection," *Physiol. Rev.* 21 (1941): 70.

78. A. McGehee Harvey, *The Association of American Physicians (1886–1986)* (Baltimore: Association of American Physicians, 1986), p. 298.

79. Arnold R. Rich, *The Pathogenesis of Tuberculosis* (Springfield, Ill.; Charles C Thomas, 1944); Ella H. Oppenheimer, "Arnold Rice Rich (1893–1968)," in *Biographical Memoirs of the National Academy of Sciences,* no. 50 (New York: Columbia University Press, 1979), p. 331.

80. Arnold R. Rich, "Acceptance of Kober Medal," *Trans. Assoc. Am. Phys.* 71 (1958): 48.

81. Daniel C. Gilman, report, December 2, 1878, in Alan M. Chesney, "Two Documents Relating to Medical Education at the Johns Hopkins University," *Bull. Hist. Med.* 41 (1936): 491.

82. George W. Heuer, "Dr. Halsted," *Bull. Johns Hopkins Hosp.* 90 (1952): 20.

83. Ibid.

84. William Osler, "Inner History of the Hopkins," *Johns Hopkins Med. J.* 125 (1969): 189.

85. Ibid.

86. Heuer, "Dr. Halsted," p. 1.

87. Ibid.

88. Gert H. Brieger, "A Portrait of Surgery: Surgery in America, 1875–1889," *Surg. Clin. North Am.* 67, no. 6 (1987): 1181–1216.

89. William H. Welch, "The Interdependence of Medicine and Other Sciences of Nature," address of the retiring president of the American Association for the Advancement of Science, delivered at meeting in Chicago, December 20, 1907, published in *Science,* January 10, 1908, reprinted in J. McKeen Cattell, *Science and Education,* vol. 2, *Medical Research and Education* (New York: Science Press, 1913), pp. 143–64.

90. Harvey Cushing, "On Routine Determination of Arterial Tension in Operating Room and Clinic," *Boston Med. Surg. J.* 148 (1903): 250.

91. Harvey Cushing, "Concerning the Poisonous Effect of Pure Sodium Chloride Solutions on Nerve-Muscle Preparation," *Am. J. Physiol.* 6 (1901): 77.

92. Harvey Cushing, "A Method of Extirpation of the Gasserian Ganglion for Trigeminal Neuralgia by a Route Through the Temporal Fossa and Beneath the Meningeal Artery," *JAMA* 34 (1900): 1035.

93. Harvey Cushing, "The Sensory Distribution of the Vth Nerve," *Johns Hopkins Hosp. Bull.* 15 (1904): 23.

94. Harvey Cushing, "Sexual Infantilism with Optic Atrophy in Cases in Tumor Affecting the Hypophysis Cerebri," *J. Nerv. Mental Dis.* 33 (1906): 704.

95. John F. Fulton, *Harvey Cushing: A Biography* (Springfield, Ill.: Charles C Thomas, 1946), p. 281.

96. Harvey Cushing, "Experimental Hypophysectomy," *Johns Hopkins Hosp. Bull.* 21 (1910): 127.

97. Harvey Cushing, "The Hypophysis Cerebri—Clinical Aspects of Hyperpituitarism and of Hypopituitarism," *JAMA* 53 (1909): 255.

98. Harvey Cushing, "The Basophil Adenomas of the Pituitary Body and Their Clinical Manifestations," *Bull. Johns Hopkins Hosp.* 50 (1932): 137.

99. Samuel J. Crowe, *Halsted of Johns Hopkins: The Man and His Men* (Springfield, Ill.: Charles C Thomas, 1957), p. 91.

100. Walter E. Dandy, "Ventriculography following the Injection of Air into the Cerebral Ventricles," *Ann. Surg.* 68 (1918): 5.

101. Crowe, *Halsted of Johns Hopkins,* p. 89.

102. Walter E. Dandy and Kenneth D. Blackfan, "Experimental and Clinical Study of Internal Hydrocephalus," *JAMA* 61 (1913): 2216.

103. William L. Fox, *Dandy of Johns Hopkins* (Baltimore: Williams & Wilkins, 1984).

104. Harvey, *Adventures in Medical Research,* p. 282.

105. Helen B. Taussig to A. McGehee Harvey, personal communication, 1975.

106. Alfred Blalock and Helen B. Taussig, "The Surgical Treatment of Malformations of the Heart in Which There Is Pulmonary Stenosis or Atresia," *JAMA* 128 (1945): 189.

107. Harvey, *Adventures in Medical Research,* p. 283.

108. "Citation: Albert Lasker Clinical Medical Research Awards," *JAMA* 226 (1973): 876.

109. Harvey, *Adventures in Medical Research,* pp. 285–87.

110. George J. Taylor et al., "Importance of Prolonged Compression during Cardiopulmonary Resuscitation in Man," *N. Engl. J. Med.* 296 (1977): 1515–17; George J. Taylor et al., "External Cardiac Compression: A Randomized Comparison of Mechanical and Manual Techniques," *JAMA* 240, no. 7 (1978): 644–48.

111. Michael T. Rudikoff et al., "Mechanism of Blood Flow during Cardiopulmonary Resuscitation," *Circulation* 61 (1980): 345–52; Nisha Chandra, Michael T. Rudikoff, and Myron L. Weisfeldt, "Simultaneous Chest Compression and Ventilation of High Airway Pressure during Cardiopulmonary Resuscitation," *Lancet* 1 (1980): 175–78.

112. G. L. Kissel, A. H. Blaufuss, and J. Michael Criley, "Self-administered cardiopulmonary resuscitation by

cough-induced internal compression. *Clin. Res.* 24: 139A, 1976.

113. Mieczyslaw Mirowski et al., "Termination of Malignant Ventricular Arrhythmias with an Implanted Automatic Defibrillator in Human Beings," *N. Engl. J. Med. 303* (1980): 322; Mieczyslaw Mirowski et al., "Successful Conversion of Out-of-Hospital Life-Threatening Arrhythmias with the Implanted Automatic Defibrillator," *Am. Heart J.* 103 (1982): 147; Mieczyslaw Mirowski et al., "Clinical Treatment of Life-Threatening Ventricular Tachyarrhythmias with the Automatic Implantable Defibrillator, *Am. Heart J.* 102 (1981): 265; Edward V. Platia et al., "Treatment of Malignant Ventricular Arrhythmias with Endocardial Resection and Implantation of the Automatic Cardioverter-Defibrillator," *N. Engl. J. Med.* 314 (1986): 213–16.

114. Lewis Thomas, "Notes of a Biology Watcher: The Technology of Medicine," *N. Engl. J. Med.* 285 (1971): 366.

115. John Howland and W. McKim Marriott, "Observations upon the Calcium Content of the Blood in Infantile Tetany and upon the Effect of Treatment by Calcium," *Q. J. Med.* 11 (1918): 289; John Howland and Benjamin Kramer, "Calcium and Phosphorus in the Serum in Relation to Rickets," *Am. J. Dis. Child.* 22 (1921): 105; John Howland and Benjamin Kramer, "Factors Concerned in the Calcification of Bone," *Trans. Am. Pediatr. Soc.* 34 (1922): 204; Benjamin Kramer and John Howland, "Factors Which Determine the Concentration of Calcium and of Inorganic Phosphorus in the Blood Serum of Rats," *Johns Hopkins Hosp. Bull.* 33 (1922): 313; W. McKim Marriott and John Howland, "A Micro Method for the Determination of Calcium and Magnesium in Blood Serum," *J. Biol. Chem.* 32 (1917): 233; Elmer V. McCollum et al., "Studies on Experimental Rickets: I. The Production of Rachitis and Similar Diseases in the Rat by Deficient Diets," *J. Biol. Chem.* 45 (1921): 333; Elmer V. McCollum et al., "Studies on Experimental Rickets: IV. Cod Liver Oil as Contrasted with Butter Fat in the Protection against the Effects of Insufficient Calcium in the Diet," *Proc. Soc. Exp. Biol. Med.* 18 (1921): 275; Elmer V. McCollum et al., "Studies on Experimental Rickets: VIII. The Production of Rickets by Diets Low in Phosphorus and Fat-Soluble," *Am. J. Biol. Chem.* 47 (1921): 507; Elmer V. McCollum et al., "Studies on Experimental Rickets: XII. Is There a Substance Other Than Fat-Soluble A Associated with Certain Fats Which Plays an Important Role in Bone Development?" *J. Biol. Chem.* 50 (1922): 5; Elmer V. McCollum et al., "Studies on Experimental Rickets: XVL. A Delicate Biological Test for Calcium-Depositing Substances," *J. Biol. Chem.* 51 (1922): 41; Elmer V. McCollum et al., "Studies on Experimental Rickets: XV. The Effects of Starvation on the Healing of Rickets," *Johns Hopkins Hosp. Bull.* 33 (1922): 31.

116. William H. Howell, "The Purification of Heparin and Its Chemical and Physiological Reactions," *Bull. Johns Hopkins Hosp.* 42 (1928): 119.

117. Jay McLean, "The Thromboplastic Action of Cephalin," *Am. J. Physiol.* 41 (1916): 256.

118. Harvey, *Adventures in Medical Research,* p. 94.

119. Howard A. Howe and David Bodian, *Neural Mechanism in Poliomyelitis* (New York: Commonwealth Fund, 1942).

120. Howard A. Howe, David Bodian, and Isabel M. Morgan, "Subclinical Poliomyelitis in the Chimpanzee and Its Relation to Alimentary Infection," *Am. J. Hyg.* 51 (1950): 85; Saul Benison, *Tom Rivers: Reflections on a Life in Medicine and Science* (Cambridge: MIT Press, 1967), chaps. 7, 8. See also David Bodian and Howard Howe, "Non-Paralytic Poliomyelitis in the Chimpanzee," *J. Exp. Med.* 81 (1945): 255.

121. Benison, *Tom Rivers,* chaps. 7, 8.

122. Isabel M. Morgan, "Level of Serum Antibody Associated with Intracerebral Immunity in Monkeys Vaccinated with Lansing Poliomyelitis Virus," *J. Immunol.* 62 (1949): 301. Also see Isabel M. Morgan, Howard A. Howe, and David Bodian, "The Role of Antibody in Experimental Poliomyelitis: II. Production of Intracerebral Immunity in Monkeys by Vaccination," *Am. J. Hyg.* 45 (1947): 379.

123. David Bodian, Isabel M. Morgan and Howard A. Howe, "Differentiation of Types of Poliomyelitis Viruses: III. The Grouping of 14 Strains into 3 Basic Immunologic Types," *Am. J. Hyg.* 449 (1949): 234.

124. David Bodian, "A Reconsideration of the Pathogenesis of Poliomyelitis," *Am. J. Hyg.* 55 (1952): 414; David Bodian, "Emerging Concept of Poliomyelitis Infection," *Science* 122 (1955): 105.

125. David Bodian, "Viremia in Experimental Poliomyelitis: II. Viremia and the Mechanism of the "Provoking" Effect of Injections or Trauma," *Am. J. Hyg.* 60 (1954): 358; David Bodian and R. S. Paffenbarger, Jr., "Poliomyelitis Infection in Households: Frequency of Viremia and Specific Antibody Response," *Am. J. Hyg.* 60 (1954): 83; Harvey, *Adventures in Medical Research,* pp. 408–15.

126. Howard Schatz and Arnall Patz, "Exudative Senile Maculopathy: I. Results of Argon Laser Treatment," *Arch. Ophthalmol.* 90, no. 3 (1973): 183–96; Howard Schatz and Arnall Patz, "Exudative Senile Maculopathy: II. Complications of Argon Laser Treatment," *Arch. Ophthalmol.* 90, no. 3 (1973): 197–202; Arnall Patz, "Current Concepts in Ophthalmology: Retinal Vascular Diseases," *N. Engl. J. Med.* 298 (1978): 1451–54; F. L. Ferris and Arnall Patz, "Macular Edema: A Complication of Diabetic Retinopathy," *Surv. Ophthalmol.* 28, suppl. (1984): 452–61.

127. Caroline B. Thomas, personal communication, 1975; Caroline B. Thomas, "The Prophylactic Treatment of Rheumatic Fever by Sulfanilamide," *Bull. N.Y. Acad. Sci.* 18 (1942): 508.

128. Perrin H. Long and Eleanor A. Bliss, "Para-amino-benzene-sulfonamide and Its Derivatives," *JAMA* 108 (1937): 32–36.

129. Harvey, *Adventures in Medical Research,* chap. 25; Eleanor A. Bliss, personal communication; Perrin H. Long and Eleanor A. Bliss, "Observations on the Mode of Action of Sulfanilamide," *JAMA* 109 (1937): 1524; Perrin H. Long and Eleanor A. Bliss, "Para-amino Benzene Sulfonamide and Its Derivatives: Clinical Observations on Their Use in the Treatment of Infections Due to Beta Hemolytic Streptococci," *Arch. Surg.* 34 (1937): 351; Marin, "Eli Kennerly Marshall, Jr.," p. 247; Paul Talalay, Eli Kennerly Marshall, Jr. (1889–1966)," minutes of the Advisory Board of the Medical Faculty, the Johns Hopkins University School of Medicine, January 21, 1966; William S. Tillett, "Perrin H. Long (1899–1965), *Trans. Assoc. Am. Phys.* 79 (1966): 59.

130. Edwards A. Park, "John Howland," *Science* 64 (1926): 80; Edwards A. Park, "Acceptance of the Kober Medal Award," *Trans. Assoc. Am. Phys.* 63 (1950): 26; Harvey, *Adventures in Medical Research,* chap. 17.

131. John Howland and W. McKim Marriott, "Acidosis Occurring with Diarrhea," *Am. J. Dis. Child.* 11 (1916): 309.

132. Kenneth D. Blackfan and Kenneth F. Maxcy, "Intraperitoneal Injection of Saline Solution," *Am. J. Dis. Child.* 15 (1918): 19.

133. James L. Gamble, "The Metabolism of Fixed Base during Fasting," *J. Biol. Chem.* 57 (1923): 633; James L. Gamble, "Presentation of the Kober Medal to Dr. Edwards A. Park," *Trans. Assoc. Am. Phys.* 63 (1950): 21; James L. Gamble, S. G. Ross, and F. F. Tisdall, "A Study of Acidosis Due to Ketone Acids," *Trans. Am. Pediatr. Soc.* 34 (1922): 289.

134. Robert F. Loeb, "Presentation of the Kober Medal to James L. Gamble," *Trans. Assoc. Am. Phys.* 64 (1951): 32.

135. Gamble, Ross, and Tisdall, "Acidosis Due to Ketone Acids," p. 289.

136. Loeb, "Presentation of the Kober Medal," p. 33.

137. Walter Cannon, *The Way of an Investigator* (New York: W. W. Norton & Co., 1945), p. 68.

138. John E. Howard, "Adventures in Clinical Research on Bones and Stones," *J. Clin. Endocrinol. Metab.* 21 (1961): 1254; John E. Howard, "Treatment of Thyrotoxicosis," *JAMA* 202 (1967): 706; John E. Howard et al., "Relief of Hypertension of Nephrectomy in Four Patients with Unilateral Renal Vascular Disease," *Trans. Assoc. Am. Phys.* 66 (1953): 164; John E. Howard, "The Recogni-

tion and Isolation from Urine and Serum of a Peptide Inhibitor to Calcification," *Johns Hopkins Med. J.* 120 (1967): 119; Harvey, *Adventures in Medical Research,* pp. 355–60.

139. David Marine, "On the Occurrence and Physiological Nature of Glandular Hyperplasia of the Thyroid [Dog and Sheep], Together with Remarks on Important Clinical [Human] Problems," *Johns Hopkins Hosp. Bull.* 18 (1907): 359.

140. Alan M. Chesney, Thomas A. Clawson, and Bruce Webster, "Endocrine Goiter in Rabbits: I. Incidence and Characteristics," *Bull. Johns Hopkins Hosp.* 43 (1928): 261.

141. Bruce Webster, Thomas A. Clawson, and Alan M. Chesney, "Endemic Goiter in Rabbits: II. Heat Production in Goitrous and Non-Goitrous Animals," *Bull. Johns Hopkins Hosp.* 43 (1928): 278.

142. Bruce Webster and Alan M. Chesney, "Endemic Goiter in Rabbits: III. Effect of Administration of Iodine," *Bull. Johns Hopkins Hosp.* 43 (1928): 291.

143. Bruce Webster and Alan M. Chesney, "Studies in the Etiology of Simple Goiter," *Am. J. Pathol.* 6 (1930): 275; David Marine, et al., "Effect of Drying in Air on the Goiter-Producing Substance in Cabbage," *Proc. Soc. Exp. Biol. Med.* 27 (1930): 1025; Bruce Webster, David Marine, and Anna Cipra, "The Occurrence of Variations in the Goiter of Rabbits Produced by Feeding Cabbage," *J. Exp. Med.* 53 (1931): 81.

144. Edwin B. Astwood, "Chemotherapy of Hyperthyroidism," *The Harvey Lectures,* ser. 40, 1944–45 (New York: Academic Press, 1946), p. 195; Cosmo G. Mackenzie and Julia B. Mackenzie, "Effect of Sulfonamides and Thioureas on Thyroid Gland and Basal Metabolism," *Endocrinology* 32 (1943): 185; Cosmo G. Mackenzie, Julia B. MacKenzie, and Elmer V. McCollum, "Effects of Sulfanilyl Guanidine on Thyroid of Rat," *Science* 94 (1941): 518; Julia B. Mackenzie and Cosmo G. Mackenzie, "Effect of Prolonged and Intermittent Sulfonamide Feeding on the Basal Metabolic Rate, Thyroid and Pituitary," *Bull. Johns Hopkins Hosp.* 74 (1944): 85.

145. S. Sherry, "William Smith Tillett (1892–1974)," *Trans. Assoc. Am. Phys.* 88 (1975): 32.

146. George Taplin et al., "Suspensions of Radioalbumin Aggregates for Photoscanning the Liver, Spleen, Lung, and Other Organs," *J. Nucl. Med.* 5 (1964): 259.

147. Henry N. Wagner, Jr., et al., "Regional Pulmonary Blood Flow in Man by Radioisotope Scanning," *JAMA* 187 (1964): 601.

148. Urokinase Pulmonary Embolism Trial Study Group, "Urokinase Pulmonary Embolism Trial: Phase 1 Results," *JAMA* 214 (1970): 2163; Urokinase Pulmonary Embolism Trial Study Group, "Urokinase Pulmonary

Embolism Trial: Phase 2 Results," *JAMA* 229 (1974): 1606.

149. Alan D. Guerci et al., "A Randomized Trial of Intravenous Tissue Plasminogen Activator for Acute Myocardial Infarction with Subsequent Randomization to Elective Coronary Angioplasty," *N. Engl. J. Med.* 317 (1987): 1613.

150. Harvey, *Adventures in Medical Research,* chap. 19.

151. Leslie N. Gay and Nathan B. Herman, "The Treatment of 100 Cases of Asthma with Ephedrine," *Bull. Johns Hopkins Hosp.* 443 (1928): 185.

152. Leslie N. Gay, "The Treatment of Hay Fever and Pollen Asthma in an Air Conditioned Atmosphere," *JAMA* 100 (1933): 1382.

153. Edmund L. Keeney, J. A. Pierce, and Leslie N. Gay, "Epinephrine-in-Oil: A New Slowly Absorbed Epinephrine Preparation," *Arch. Int. Med.* 63 (1939): 119.

154. Paul E. Carliner, H. Melvin Radman, and Leslie N. Gay, "Treatment of Nausea and Vomiting of Pregnancy with Dramamine—Preliminary Reports," *Science* 110 (1949): 215; Leslie N. Gay and Paul E. Carliner, "The Prevention and Treatment of Motion Sickness," *Bull. Johns Hopkins Hosp.* 84 (1949): 470.

155. Leslie N. Gay to A. McGehee Harvey, personal communication, 1976.

156. Louis Hamman, "Diagnosis of the Causes of Heart Failure," *N. Engl. J. Med.* 219 (1938): 289.

157. John C. Harvey, "The Writings of Louis Hamman," *Bull. Johns Hopkins Hosp.* 95 (1957): 178; article contains Hamman's complete bibliography.

158. Harvey, *Adventures in Medical Research,* p. 139.

159. Ibid., p. 142.

160. Ibid.

161. John E. Howard, "Serendipity in Clinical Investigation," *JAMA* 207 (1969): 736.

162. Ibid., p. 738.

163. Alan M. Chesney, "Immunity in Syphilis," *Medicine* 5 (1926): 459.

164. Harvey, *Adventures in Medical Research,* pp. 289–93.

165. Victor A. McKusick, "On the X Chromosome of Man," *Q. Rev. Biol.* 37 (1962): 69; Victor A. McKusick, *Heritable Disorders of Connective Tissue,* 4th ed. (St. Louis: C. V. Mosby, 1972); Victor A. McKusick, ed., *Medical Genetic Studies of the Amish: Selected Papers* (Baltimore: Johns Hopkins University Press, 1978); Victor A. McKusick, *Mendelian Inheritance in Man,* 5th and successive editions (Baltimore: Johns Hopkins University Press, 1978–1988); Victor A. McKusick and Frank H. Ruddle, "The Status of the Gene Map of the Human Chromosomes," *Science* 196 (1977): 390; Victor A. McKusick, "The Morbid Anatomy of the Human Genome: A Review of Gene Mapping in Clinical Med-

icine," *Medicine* 65 (1986): 1–33; 66 (1987): 1–63, 237–96; 67 (1988): 1–19.

166. John C. Whitehorn, "Adolf Meyer, 1866–1950," *Bull. Johns Hopkins Hosp.* 89, suppl. (1951): 51.

167. Ibid., pp. 53–56.

168. Jerzy E. Rose, "Adolf Meyer's Contributions to Neuroanatomy," *Bull. Johns Hopkins Hosp.* 89, suppl. (1951): 56.

169. Whitehorn, "Adolf Meyer," p. 54.

170. Rose, "Adolf Meyer's Contributions to Neuroanatomy," p. 58.

171. Wendell S. Muncie, "Adolf Meyer's Contributions to Clinical Psychiatry," *Bull. Johns Hopkins Hosp.* 89, suppl. (1951): 60–61.

172. Ibid.

173. Ibid.

174. Franklin P. Ebaugh, "Adolf Meyer's Contribution to Psychiatric Education," *Bull. Johns Hopkins Hosp.* 89, suppl. (1951): 65.

175. Ibid., p. 67.

176. Joel Elkes, "Self-Regulation and Behavioral Medicine: The Early Beginning," *Psych. Annals* 11, no. 2 (1981): 19.

177. Vernon M. Mountcastle, "Philip Bard," *Physiologist* 18 (1975): 1.

178. Clinton W. Woolsey, Wade H. Marshall, and Philip Bard, "Representations of Cutaneous Tactile Sensibility in the Cerebral Cortex of the Monkey as Indicated by Evoked Potentials," *Bull. Johns Hopkins Hosp.* 70 (1942): 399.

179. Philip Bard, "Studies on The Cortical Representation of Somatic Sensibility," in *The Harvey Lectures,* ser. 33, 1937–38 (New York: Academic Press, 1939), p. 143.

180. Mountcastle, "Philip Bard," p. 1.

181. Vernon B. Mountcastle to A. McGehee Harvey, personal communication, 1987; Alissa Swerdloff, "Mountcastle—A View from Within," Hopkins Medical News 10, no. 1 (1986): 2–5; Vernon B. Mountcastle and Elwood Henneman, "The Representation of Tactile Sensibility in the Thalamus of the Monkey," *J. Comp. Neurol.* 97 (1952): 409; Jerzy E. Rose and Vernon B. Mountcastle, "Activity of Single Neurons in the Tactile Thalamic Region of the Cat in Response to a Transient Peripheral Stimulus," *Bull. Johns Hopkins Hosp.* 94 (1954): 238; Vernon B. Mountcastle, "Modality and Topographic Properties of Single Neurons in the Cat's Somatic Sensory Cortex," *J. Neurophysiol.* 20 (1957): 408.

182. Swerdloff, "Mountcastle–A View from Within"; "Mountcastle Shares Columbia's Horwitz Prize," *Hopkins Medical News* 3, no. 5 (Nov./Dec. 1978).

183. Vernon B. Mountcastle, "An Organizing Principle for

Cerebral Function: The Unity Module and the Distributed System," in Gerald M. Edelman and Vernon B. Mountcastle, *The Mindful Brain: Cortical Organization and a Selective Theory of Brain Function* (Cambridge: MIT Press, 1978).

184. Vernon B. Mountcastle, "The Neural Mechanisms of Cognitive Functions Can Now Be Studied Directly," *Trends in Neuroscience* 10 (1986): 505–508; M. A. Steinmetz et al., "The Functional Properties of Parietal Visual Neurons: The Radial Organization of Directionalities within the Visual Field," *J. Neuroscience* 7 (1987): 177–91; Vernon B. Mountcastle et al., "Common and Differential Effects of Attentive Fixation upon the Excitability of Parietal and Prestriate (V44) Cortical Visual Neurons in the Macaque Monkey," *J. Neuroscience* 7 (1987): 2239–55.

185. A. McGehee Harvey and M. Richard Whitehill, "Prostigmine as an Aid in the Diagnosis of Myasthenia Gravis," *JAMA* 108 (1937): 1329.

186. A. McGehee Harvey, "The Actions of Quinine on Skeletal Muscle," *J. Physiol.* 95 (1939): 45; A. McGehee Harvey, "The Mechanism of Action of Quinine in Myotonia and Myasthenia," *JAMA* 112 (1939): 1562.

187. A. McGehee Harvey and Richard L. Masland, "A Method for the Study of Neuromuscular Transmission in Human Subjects," *Bull. Johns Hopkins Hosp.* 68 (1941): 81.

188. A. McGehee Harvey and Richard L. Masland, "The Electromyogram in Myasthenia Gravis," *Bull. Johns Hopkins Hosp.* 69 (1941): 1.

189. A. McGehee Harvey and Joseph L. Lilienthal, Jr., "Observations on the Nature of Myasthenia Gravis: The Intra-Arterial Injection of Acetylcholine, Prostigmine and Adrenaline," *Bull. Johns Hopkins Hosp.* 69 (1941): 566; A. McGehee Harvey, Joseph L. Lilienthal, Jr., and Samuel A. Talbot, "On the Effects of Intraarterial Injection of Acetylcholine and Prostigmine in Normal Man," *Bull. Johns Hopkins Hosp.* 69 (1941): 529; A. McGehee Harvey, Joseph L. Lilienthal, Jr., and Samuel A. Talbot, "Observations on the Nature of Myasthenia Gravis," *Bull. Johns Hopkins Hosp.* 69 (1941): 547.

190. David Grob, Joseph L. Lilienthal, Jr., and A. McGehee Harvey, "On Certain Vascular Effects of Curare in Man: The Histamine Reaction," *Bull. Johns Hopkins Hosp.* 80 (1947): 299.

191. Alfred Blalock et al., "The Treatment of Myasthenia Gravis by Removal of the Thymus Gland—Preliminary Report," *JAMA* 117 (1941): 1529.

192. A. McGehee Harvey, Joseph L. Lilienthal, Jr., and Samuel A. Talbot, "Observations on the Nature of Myasthenia Gravis: The Effect of Thymectomy on Neuromuscular Transmission," *J. Clin. Invest.* 21 (1942): 579.

193. Ibid.

194. C. C. Chang and C. Y. Lee, "The Electrophysiological Study of the Neuromuscular Blocking Action of Cobra Neurotoxin," *Br. J. Pharmac. Chemother.* 28 (1966): 172.

195. Douglas M. Fambrough, Daniel B. Drachman, and S. Satyamurti, "Neuromuscular Junction in Myasthenia Gravis: Decreased Acetylcholine Receptors," *Science* 182 (1973): 293–95.

196. S. Satyamurti, Daniel B. Drachman, and Fred Slone, "Blockade of Acetylcholine Receptors: A Model of Myasthenia Gravis," *Science* 187 (1975): 955–57.

197. Klaus V. Tokya et al., "Myasthenia Gravis: Passive Transfer from Man to Mouse," *Science* 190 (1975): 397–99.

198. Daniel B. Drachman et al., "Effect of Myasthenic Immunoglobulin on ACh Receptors of Cultured Muscle," *Trans. Am. Neurol. Assoc.* 102 (1977): 96–100.

199. Daniel B. Drachman et al., "Myasthenic Antibodies Cross-Link Acetylcholine Receptors to Accelerate Degradation," *N. Engl. J. Med* 298 (1978): 1116–22.

200. Daniel B. Drachman et al., "Mechanisms of Acetylcholine Receptor Loss in Myasthenia Gravis," in *Diseases of the Motor Unit,* ed. D. L. Schotland (New York: John Wiley & Sons, 1982) chap. 16, pp. 215–32.

201. Daniel Drachman's complete bibliography can be found in his biographical file, Alan M. Chesney Archives, the Johns Hopkins Medical Institutions.

202. William H. Howell, "Vagus Inhibition of the Heart and its Relation to Inorganic Salts of the Blood," *Am. J. Physiol.* 15 (1906): 380.

203. David Grob et al., "The Administration of Diisopropylfluorophosphate (DFP) to Man: III. Effect on the Central Nervous System with Special Reference to the Electrical Activity of the Brain," *Bull. Johns Hopkins Hosp.* 81 (1947): 257.

204. See biographical folder for Pedro Cuatrecasas in Alan M. Chesney Medical Archives, the Johns Hopkins Medical Institutions.

205. Candace B. Pert and Solomon H. Snyder, "Opiate Receptors: Demonstration in Nervous Tissue," *Science* 179 (1973): 1011.

206. Michael J. Kuhar, Candace B. Pert, and Solomon H. Snyder, "Regional Distribution of Opiate Receptor Binding in Monkey and Human Brain," *Nature* 245 (1973): 447.

207. Candace B. Pert, Gavril Pasternak, and Solomon H. Snyder, "Opiate Agonists and Antagonists Discriminated by Receptor Binding in Brain," *Science* 182 (1973): 1359.

208. Carol Lamotte, Candace B. Pert, and Solomon H. Snyder, "Opiate Receptor Binding in Primate Spinal Cord: Distribution and Changes after Dorsal Root Section," *Brain Research* 112 (1976): 407.

209. "New Department Links Brain Chemistry with Behavior, Drugs, and Disease," *Hopkins Medical News,* September 1980, pp. 2–5; Solomon H. Snyder to A. McGehee Harvey, personal communication, 1987; Solomon H. Snyder, "An Historical Overview of Neurotransmitter Receptor Binding," in *Neurotransmitter Receptor Binding,* ed. H. I. Yamamura, S. J. Enna, and M. J. Kuhar (New York: Raven Press, 1978), pp. 1–11; Solomon H. Snyder, "Opiate Receptors and Morphine-like Peptides," The *Harvey Lectures,* ser. 73, 1977–78 (New York: Academic Press, 1979), pp. 291–314; Solomon H. Snyder, "The Molecular Basis of Communication between Cells," *Scientific American* 253 (1985): 132–41.

210. Henry N. Wagner, Jr., et al., "Assessment of Dopamine Receptor Activity in the Human Brain with Carbon-11 N-methyl Spiperone," *Science* 221 (1983): 1264–66.

211. Henry M. Wagner, personal communication; also see Henry N. Wagner, "Positron Emission Tomography (PET) Imaging and the Neurobiogical Revolution," *New Developments in Medicine* 1 (1980): 3–17.

212. The account of current research in the Department of Anatomy and Cell Biology is based on a personal communication from Thomas D. Pollard, 1987.

213. A complete list of articles published by members of the Department of Anatomy and Cell Biology appears in the department's annual report to the dean of the School of Medicine, Alan M. Chesney Medical Archives, the Johns Hopkins Medical Institutions.

214. Paul Talalay, personal communication, 1987.

215. Gilbert Mudge and Irwin M. Weiner, "Renal Excretion of Weak Organic Acids and Bases," in *Proceedings of the First International Pharmacology Meeting, Stockholm 1961,* vol. 4, p. 157.

216. Irwin Weiner and Gilbert Mudge, "Renal Tubular Mechanisms for Excretion of Organic Acids and Bases," *Am. J. Med.* 36 (1964): 743.

217. Irwin M. Weiner, Robert I. Levy, and Gilbert H. Mudge, "Studies in Mercurial Diuresis: Renal Excretion, Acid Lability and Structure-Activity Relationships of Organic Mercurials," *J. Pharmacol. Exp. Ther.* 138 (1962): 96.

218. Paul Talalay to Susan L. Abrams, personal communication, 1988.

219. Barbara Hurlock and Paul Talalay, "Enzymatic Estimation of Urinary Steroids," *Proc. Soc. Exp. Biol. Med.* 93 (1956): 560–64.

220. Frank S. Kawahara and Paul Talalay, "Crystalline Δ^5-3-Ketosteroid Isomerase," *J. Biol. Chem.* 235 (1960), PC1.

221. A complete list of articles published by members of the Department of Pharmacology and Molecular Sciences appears in the department's annual report to the dean of the School of Medicine, Alan M. Chesney Medical Archives, the Johns Hopkins Medical Institutions.

222. For references to Lehninger's publications, see A. McGehee Harvey, "The Department of Physiological Chemistry: Its Historical Evolution," *Johns Hopkins Med. J.* 139 (1976): 237.

223. A complete list of articles published by members of the Department of Biological Chemistry appears in the department's annual report to the dean of the School of Medicine, Alan M. Chesney Medical Archives, the Johns Hopkins Medical Institutions.

224. Untitled article, *Hopkins Medical News* 3, no. 5, (November/December 1978). Complete bibliographies for Daniel Nathans and Hamilton O. Smith can be found in their biographical files in the Alan M. Chesney Medical Archives, the Johns Hopkins Medical Institutions.

225. Hamilton O. Smith and K. W. Wilcox, "A Restriction Enzyme from *Hemophilus influenzae:* I. Purification and general properties," *J. Mol. Biol.* 51 (1970): 379; Thomas J. Kelly and Hamilton O. Smith, "A Restriction Enzyme from *Hemophilus influenzae:* II. Base Sequence of the Recognition Site," *J. Mol. Biol.* 51 (1970): 393.

226. Kathleen Danna and Daniel Nathans, "Specific Cleavage of Simian Virus 40 DNA by Restriction Endonucleases," *Proc. Natl. Acad. Sci. USA* 68 (1971): 2913.

227. Louis Pasteur, "Pourquoi la France n'a pas trouvé des hommes supérieurs au moment du péril," *Revue Scientifique,* 2d ser., I, July 22, 1871, pp. 73–76; reprinted in *Oeuvres de Pasteur,* ed., Pasteur Vallery-Radot, 7 vols. (Paris: Masson et Cie, 1939) 7:211–13.

Epilogue

Epigraph: Alan M. Chesney, *The Johns Hopkins Hospital and the Johns Hopkins University School of Medicine,* 3 vols. (Baltimore: Johns Hopkins Press, 1943–63), 2:320.

1. Richard Shryock, *The Unique Influence of the Johns Hopkins University on American Medicine* (Copenhagen: Ejnar Munksgaard, 1953), p. 9.

2. George Rosen, "Critical Levels in Historical Process—A Theoretical Exploration Dedicated to Henry Ernest Sigerist," *J. Hist. Med.* 13 (1958): 179.

3. Arnold R. Rich, "Reflections on the Relation of the Curriculum to Certain Problems in Medical Education," *Bull. Johns Hopkins Hosp.* 49 (1931): 121.

4. Alan Gregg, "Dr. Welch's Influence on Medical Education," *Bull. Johns Hopkins Hosp.* 87, suppl. (1950): 35–36.

5. Daniel C. Gilman, *The Launching of a University* (New York: Dodd, Mead & Co., 1906), pp. 134–35.

6. William H. Welch, "Address at the Twenty-Fifth Anniversary of the Johns Hopkins Hospital, 1889–1914," *Johns Hopkins Hosp. Bull.* 25 (1914): 364.

7. William H. Welch, in Lewellys F. Barker, manuscript account of talk with Welch in Johns Hopkins Hospital, July 14, 1933, Barker Papers, Alan M. Chesney Medical Archives, the Johns Hopkins Medical Institutions.

8. John Shaw Billings, "The National Board of Health," *Plumber and Sanitary Engineer* 3 (1880): 47, cited in Kenneth M. Ludmerer, *Learning to Heal: The Development of American Medical Education* (New York: Basic Books, 1985), p. 64.

9. William Osler, "The Natural Method of Teaching the Subject of Medicine," *JAMA* 36 (1901): 1673.

10. Ludmerer, *Learning to Heal,* chap. 1, pp. 16–19, 69–70.

11. William Osler, "Looking Back: Communication from Osler at the Twenty-fifth anniversary of the Johns Hopkins Hospital, 1889–1914," *Johns Hopkins Hosp. Bull.* 25 (1914): 354.

12. Chesney, *The Johns Hopkins Hospital* 3:280.

13. Shryock, *Influence of The Johns Hopkins University,* p. 69.

INDEX